WP 815 HAR

DATE DUE

13/11/13	
25/3/16	
21/4/16	
20/5/16	

GAYLORD   PRINTED IN U.S.A.

MAKING THE DIAGNOSIS
A Practical Guide to Breast Imaging

MAKING THE DIAGNOSIS
A Practical Guide to Breast Imaging

Jennifer A. Harvey, MD, FACR
Director, Division of Breast Imaging
Co-Director, University of Virginia Breast Care Program
Professor of Radiology
University of Virginia
Charlottesville, Virginia

David E. March, MD
Director of Breast Imaging
Radiology & Imaging Inc. and Baystate Medical Center
Springfield, Massachusetts
Assistant Professor of Radiology
Tufts University School of Medicine
Boston, Massachusetts

ELSEVIER
SAUNDERS

1600 John F. Kennedy Blvd.
Ste 1800
Philadelphia, PA 19103-2899

Notices

Knowledge and best practice in this field are constantly changing. As new research and experience
broaden our understanding, changes in research methods, professional practices, or medical
treatment may become necessary.

Practitioners and researchers must always rely on their own experience and knowledge in
evaluating and using any information, methods, compounds, or experiments described herein. In
using such information or methods they should be mindful of their own safety and the safety of
others, including parties for whom they have a professional responsibility.

With respect to any drug or pharmaceutical products identified, readers are advised to check the
most current information provided (i) on procedures featured or (ii) by the manufacturer of each
product to be administered, to verify the recommended dose or formula, the method and duration
of administration, and contraindications. It is the responsibility of practitioners, relying on their
own experience and knowledge of their patients, to make diagnoses, to determine dosages and the
best treatment for each individual patient, and to take all appropriate safety precautions.

To the fullest extent of the law, neither the Publisher nor the authors, contributors, or editors,
assume any liability for any injury and/or damage to persons or property as a matter of products
liability, negligence or otherwise, or from any use or operation of any methods, products,
instructions, or ideas contained in the material herein.

Library of Congress Cataloging-in-Publication Data
Harvey, Jennifer A.
  Making the diagnosis : a practical guide to breast imaging / Jennifer A. Harvey, David E. March.
     p. ; cm.
  Includes bibliographical references and index.
  ISBN 978-1-4557-2284-6 (hardcover : alk. paper)
  I. March, David E.   II. Title.
  [DNLM: 1. Breast Diseases—diagnosis.   2. Breast Neoplasms—diagnosis.   3. Mammography—
methods. WP 815]
  RG493.5.D52
  618.1′90754—dc23
                                                                                    2013005683

Content Strategist: Donald Scholz
Content Development Specialist: Roxanne Halpine Ward, Lisa Barnes
Publishing Services Manager: Pat Joiner
Senior Project Manager: Joy Moore
Design Manager: Steven Stave

Printed in China

Last digit is the print number: 9   8   7   6   5   4   3   2   1

We dedicate this book to the courageous women and men who face a diagnosis of breast cancer.

Preface

This book is intended to provide practical information on breast imaging, with the goal of improving breast cancer detection. This is not meant as a reference book or as a guide to prepare for board examinations. There are other books better suited for those purposes. The material in our book will be most useful to radiology residents and fellows, to generalists, and to those radiologists who subspecialize in another area and who also interpret breast imaging examinations.

This book provides information in an accessible format that will enable the reader to expand his or her fund of knowledge in breast imaging. The style is somewhat informal, which hopefully will make for enjoyable reading. The twenty chapters, divided into six sections, span a wide range of topics that are commonly encountered in breast imaging. Each chapter includes many practical scenarios intended to help radiologists decide how findings should be described, what to include in the differential diagnosis, and how the finding should be managed. Key points are summarized at the end of each chapter.

Each chapter is followed by cases carefully chosen to reinforce key points. The case material is the backbone of this book, and hundreds of images are included, highlighting the use of different modalities in many cases. This approach—rather than strict organization by modality—reflects the multimodality approach that is essential to breast imaging today. In reviewing the cases, the reader will benefit most by carefully analyzing the images and arriving at a conclusion before reviewing the answers. This will more closely simulate a true prospective clinical experience and encourage the reader to reach a conclusion on his or her own. However, if the finding is not clear, don't be discouraged! Some of the findings are quite subtle. Take what you can from these cases and understand that the finding would have been much more obvious to you on a high-resolution monitor.

Those who have experience in breast imaging will recognize that the most meaningful findings are often quite difficult to detect. Most texts, however, are limited to figures that show obvious findings. In working with the Elsevier team, one of our greatest challenges was to include more subtle cases in order to realistically portray findings commonly seen in practice. You may need to look really hard to see and understand these findings, and we advise that you review this text in excellent lighting (or, with electronic format, in high-resolution display)!

This book can be used in a number of ways. For the most industrious radiologist, it can be read in its entirety. If you are in training or new to breast imaging, this will give you a solid foundation for the practice of breast imaging. However, we understand that your time is precious, and this book can also be used to quickly review a specific topic. Review of the figure and case images is a good visual exercise when the findings are correlated with the ultimate diagnosis.

Although the material in this book is based on our combined experience of 40+ years in breast imaging, it should not be viewed in any sense as a standard of care for the practice of breast imaging. There is often more than one approach to a situation. For example, our good friend, Val Jackson, loves rolled views, whereas we would rather have spot compression views and an ultrasound. Either approach will work just fine. Our individual skills in breast imaging develop over time through different experiences and the use of different tools. This book is intended to give you many practical options in your approach. With experience, you will learn what techniques work best for you and your patients.

In breast imaging, we have the opportunity to detect and diagnose many malignancies at a time when the chance for cure is very high or to reassure patients when the findings are benign. We hope the material in this book will help you make the most of these opportunities. Our patients are counting on us. We can save lives.

Jennifer A. Harvey
David E. March

Acknowledgments

I am honored to have written this book with my good friend, David March. When I told an acquaintance that we were working on a book together, they replied, "And you're still friends?!" Presumably the demands of writing a book can undo a previously solid friendship. I am delighted to report that David remains a very good friend and colleague whom I very much respect. David is a very sharp, organized man. His passion for improving patient care is evident throughout this book. At times in the process, I believe my role was only to put in a few jokes.

My sons, Brendon, Taylor, Alexander, and Benjamin, were exceedingly tolerant of Mom working on the laptop at all hours. I am grateful for their humor and love. You will often see them in various slides during my lectures, such as my 12-year-old being well behaved and benign like a fibroadenoma. They have kindly indulged us with the opening picture to the Physics chapter (excluding Taylor) by doing their best geek imitation. They are my joy.

I would like to thank the many people that have given me a chance: Paul Capp, Bruce Hillman, Val Jackson, Larry Bassett, Etta Pisano, Tony Proto, the entire ABR and RSNA offices, and so many others. I would like to thank my many colleagues who let me question them so that we could learn together: Carl D'Orsi, Ed Sickles, Martin Yaffe, and Dan Kopans. I would like to thank my very, very good friends: Val Jackson, Mary Mahoney, Larry Bassett, and Michael Linver—you make me believe in myself. I would like to thank my fellow UVa breast imaging radiologists: Brandi Nicholson, Heather Peppard, Carrie Rochman, and Michael Cohen (who is a Virginian by heart)—you are not only my colleagues but also my friends. I would like to thank my technologists and staff—you treat every patient as though they were family. You are the best!

I would like to thank all of my residents and fellows for putting up with my merciless requests for recitation of differential diagnoses and facts and also for not asking too much of me in the mornings before I've had a really strong cup of tea. I love teaching you. Your questions make me think.

Finally, I am grateful to my patients and their families. You inspire me to be better.

Jennifer A. Harvey

There are numerous individuals who contributed either directly or indirectly to the preparation of this book. To those deserving of acknowledgment whose names I did not include, please accept my sincere apology for the oversight.

First, I would like to thank my wife, Carolyn, for her unwavering support and encouragement throughout this project, as well as for her expert editorial insights. I also appreciate the understanding of our sons, Kevin and Daniel March, and the encouragement of my mother, Susan March, my sister, Jocelyn Dreier, my brother, Christopher March, and their families.

My interest in breast imaging was sparked by the brilliant teaching of Dr. Stephen Feig during my residency at the Thomas Jefferson University Hospital. This book would surely never have been written without his dedication to teaching. I am also grateful to Dr. W. Max Cloud, who served as a role model at Radiology & Imaging through his leadership in establishing mammography in the region and by setting high standards for its interpretation.

One of the greatest privileges of my career has been to volunteer for the American Board of Radiology and to work with the phenomenal volunteers and staff associated with the Board. The Board's commitment to quality has attracted some of the most highly accomplished and dedicated breast imaging radiologists in the field. Exposure to the professional qualities embodied by these individuals has inspired my own efforts.

Through the Board, I was fortunate to meet my coauthor and friend, Dr. Jennifer Harvey. Working with Jennifer has been a remarkable educational experience on many levels. After working with Jennifer, "dedicated" and "driven" have taken on new meanings. Often, as I began early morning work on a chapter before the start of my clinical day, I would discover that Jennifer had been hard at work on the chapter the night before, signing off just a few hours before I woke up. I am grateful to Jennifer for sharing her remarkable experience and fund of knowledge in this text.

I would like to thank all of the technologists I have had the honor to work with while at Radiology & Imaging, Baystate Radiology & Imaging, the Baystate Comprehensive Breast Center, InMed Diagnostic Services, and the Baystate Breast & Wellness Center. These individuals currently include Jennie Benford, Susan Boucher, Grace Bryda, Lisa Cody, Elizabeth Daniel, Carol Day, Kimberly Duclos, Cathy Dusseault, Megan Fuss, Linda Garvey, Ann Marie Gentile, Gail Gladu, Catherine Grosh, Jean Hagner, Francine Johnson, Tina Juliano, Donna King, Ashley LaFortune, Diane Lane, Janice Miller, Roberta O'Neill, Edmarie Parrilla, Susan Pearson, Maureen Peczka, Sherry Piantoni, Joanne Picard, Amy Rivera, Carrie Rooney, Lauren Rosa, Nicole Sarrette, Carrie Silvia, Oksana Slivka, April Tabb, Danielle Thibault, and Danielle Toledo. The excellent work these individuals do every day has enabled the diagnosis of thousands of women with breast cancer, and I appreciate their dedication to patient care. A special acknowledgment goes to Janet Harp, our operations manager, Connie Desjardins, our Systems Analyst and Administrator, and Richard French, our IT Director, for their support and excellent work keeping things running smoothly at the Center.

I would like to thank the administration of Baystate Medical Center for their administrative expertise in planning and seeing to completion the beautiful, elegant, and patient-centered Baystate Breast & Wellness Center. I wish Baystate continued success in the pursuit of its mission to improve the health of the people in our communities with quality and compassion.

Special acknowledgment goes to my friends, Dr. Howard and Judy Raymond, for their support during this project, and to Dr. Holly Mason, my co-director at the Baystate Breast & Wellness Center. I also thank my breast imaging colleagues at Radiology & Imaging, especially Dr. Jennifer Hadro and Dr. Vivian Miller, for their assistance with challenging cases and their contributions to the breast imaging program at Baystate.

Finally, I thank our talented team at Elsevier, including Lisa Barnes, Joy Moore, Roxanne Halpine Ward, Kathryn DeFrancesco, and Steven Stave, whose expertise and patience helped bring this project to completion.

David E. March

Contents

APPROACH AND TECHNIQUE

CHAPTER 1

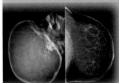

The First Question

The first question that a radiologist should consider when interpreting any study is, "Is this an adequate study?" That topic encompasses many points in breast imaging:

- *Is this the correct patient?*
- *Is this the correct study for this patient?*
- *Is the positioning adequate?*
- *Are any images blurry?*
- *Do the images have any correctable artifacts?*

Correct Patient/Correct Study

A quick check of patient name and an additional identifier such as date of birth or medical record number ensures that the correct patient is being reviewed. Checking the study date also confirms that the current study is being read (and not last year's study!). Another good check is to glance at the charge code and the study performed to ensure that they match. Finally, checking the number of images in the study will help make sure none are skipped during your review.

Knowing the indication for the study and the patient history are also important. Occasionally women may have completed a screening mammogram before informing the technologist about a palpable lump or other newly discovered clinical finding. These findings should be described in your report and diagnostic imaging should be recommended. If the patient referred for screening shares clinical complaints prior to the examination, she should optimally be rescheduled for diagnostic imaging.

- *Screening mammography* typically consists of two views of each breast: the craniocaudal (CC) and mediolateral oblique (MLO) views. Screening is performed for women with no symptoms of breast cancer, so they should not have any new breast lumps, palpable thickening, or worrisome nipple discharge. Screening mammography can be performed for women with a prior lumpectomy for breast cancer if their mammograms have shown benign findings for a number of years

(typically 2 to 5 years after diagnosis in our practices). Screening performed at multiple sites in the community provides easy access for women. Direct supervision by a radiologist is not required (i.e., a radiologist does not have to be present).

- *Diagnostic mammography* is performed to evaluate a breast symptom that may be due to breast cancer (e.g., palpable lump or breast thickening) or to evaluate an abnormal screening mammogram. Women with recent breast cancer typically undergo diagnostic mammography. Ultrasound is often performed in conjunction with diagnostic mammography. Diagnostic mammography is nearly always performed under the direct supervision and interpretation of a radiologist on site.

Positioning

A poorly performed mammogram is a significant disservice to the patient. Radiologists may fear that a report stating that the examination is technically inadequate will hurt a technologist's feelings or that referring physicians will think poorly of the facility. However, everyone has a bad day now and then. No technologist is perfect. Every technologist occasionally will have patients who are just not positioned well. If feedback is given in a kind and supportive manner, it is often appreciated. If there is a trend of individual technologists having a high technical recall rate, focused feedback and training are helpful. Likewise, a facility often gains respect from referring health care providers if they understand that the radiologists expect the highest quality care for all patients. In our experience, consistent recall to repeat technically inadequate mammograms with feedback to the technologist is vital in creating and maintaining excellence.

An important point in understanding positioning for mammograms is that the upper inner quadrants of each breast (the cleavage area) are relatively fixed in position, whereas the inferior and lateral aspects of the breast are very mobile. This is why the technologist raises the image or film receptor when performing the CC view. There are cartoons jesting at why women have to stand on their toes for a mammogram. Now you know why! If you have never had a mammogram or seen one performed, ask a technologist if you can observe a screening mammogram. A good technologist is highly skilled at positioning even the most difficult patient. Ask her how she deals with women with very small breasts or who have a large abdomen. Watch how she works with the patient to obtain optimal compression. Your understanding (and respect for technologists) will be considerably elevated.

The Mediolateral Oblique View

The MLO view is positioned with the image receptor parallel to the pectoralis major muscle (typically between

a 60- and 45-degree angle) and extends into the axilla. The pectoralis major muscle should be seen to at least the level of the *posterior nipple line* (Fig. 1-1).

Ideally, the inframammary fold should be visualized (Fig. 1-2). The last maneuver of the technologist in positioning the MLO view is to move the breast "up and out" (see Fig. 1-2). This means that the breast is pulled up and away from the pectoralis muscle, which allows for optimal compression of the breast. If the breast is not pulled up and out, the breast may droop with a "camel nose" appearance.

When the pectoralis muscle is thick, it may be difficult to obtain good compression of the front of the breast, particularly in large-breasted women. Some manufacturers address this issue by offering compression paddles that angle to allow compression of the anterior and posterior portions of the breast. Another approach is to obtain separate MLO views of the front of the breast, without the pectoralis muscle (front compression MLO views), to improve compression of the anterior breast (Fig. 1-3). It is helpful to get patients to relax their shoulders to get the pectoralis muscle (and breast tissue) into the MLO view (Box 1-1; Fig. 1-4).

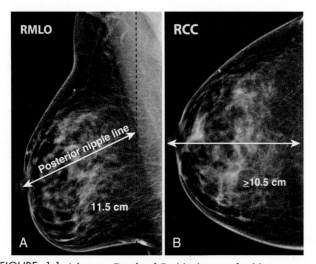

FIGURE 1-1 **Adequate Depth of Positioning on the Mammogram.** **A,** The depth on the mediolateral oblique (MLO) view is judged by the intersection of the pectoralis muscle with the posterior nipple line (*double arrow*). Therefore, the dashed line represents the minimal depth to be considered an adequate mammogram. **B,** If the posterior line measures 11.5 cm on the MLO view, then the posterior nipple line on the craniocaudal view must measure at least 10.5 cm to be adequately positioned for depth.

BOX 1-1   How to Get Great Muscle on Mediolateral Oblique Views

If you do this simple exercise, you will forever understand how your best technologists get great muscle and why others do not. Hang your arm relaxed down by your side. Now, grab your pectoralis muscle at the top of your axilla. See how the muscle is nice and soft and fat? Next, raise your shoulder. Feel how the muscle becomes concave? The best technologists get patients to relax their shoulders down, pushing the pectoralis muscle (and breast tissue) into the mediolateral oblique (MLO) view. Technologists who are nervous or don't get the patient to relax will struggle with MLO positioning (Fig. 1-4).

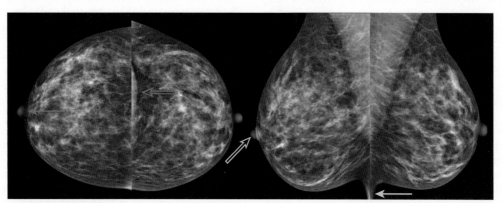

FIGURE 1-2 **Nicely Positioned Mammogram.** On the craniocaudal views (*left*), the nipples are well centered (*blue arrow*) and the pectoral muscle is seen on the left side (*blue open arrow*). On the mediolateral oblique views (*right*), the pectoralis muscles are convex and visualized well below the posterior nipple line. The breasts have been pulled "up and out" nicely in this mammogram so that the nipples are high on the image (*yellow open arrow*). This also results in opening up the inframammary fold without overlying skinfolds (*yellow arrow*).

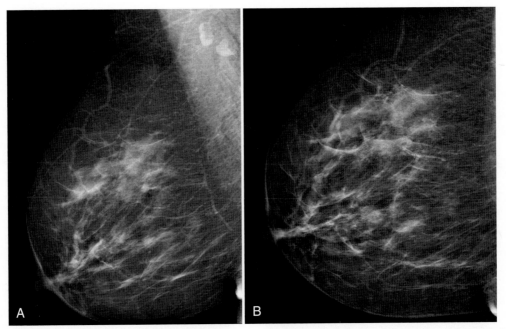

FIGURE 1-3 **Front Mediolateral Oblique (MLO) Views.** Sometimes it is difficult to obtain adequate compression of the front of the breast on the MLO views (**A**) if the pectoralis muscle is thick. Compression of just the front of the breast (**B**) in the MLO projection can improve sharpness.

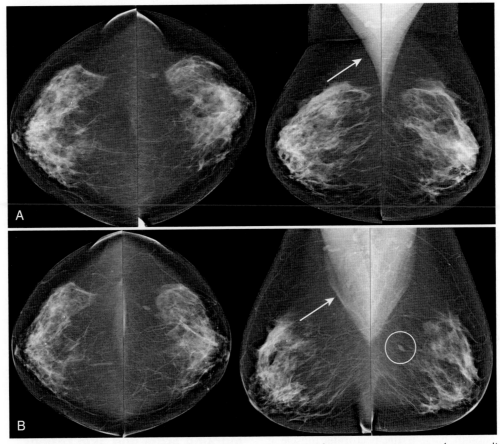

FIGURE 1-4 **Tense Versus Relaxed Pectoralis Muscles. A,** Bilateral mammogram with concave appearance to the pectoralis muscles (*arrow*). **B,** Bilateral mammogram the next year with a different technologist with a convex appearance to the pectoralis muscles (*arrow*). This is due to the muscle being relaxed. Note that a small oval mass in the lateral left breast is not visualized on the mediolateral oblique view on the first mammogram, but is readily apparent on the second (*circle*).

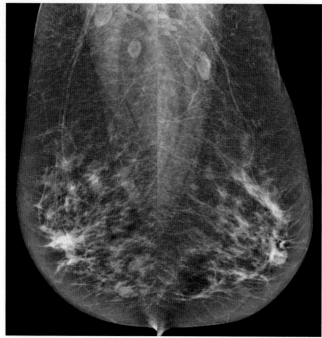

FIGURE 1-5 **Using the Lateral Medial Oblique (LMO) View.** A 67-year-old woman presents for screening. She has moderate pectus excavatum. LMO views were obtained instead of mediolateral oblique (MLO) views, allowing better visualization of the posterior breast. The appearance is similar to that obtained with MLO views.

When to Use a Lateral Medial Oblique View

The LMO (lateral medial oblique) view is obtained in the same projection as the MLO except that the machine is flipped over so that the image receptor is in the cleavage and the tube head is nearer the floor. In certain situations the LMO view may be preferable to the MLO view. The smaller size of the image receptor near the patient's head makes the LMO view useful for women with kyphosis or pectus excavatum (Fig. 1-5). An LMO view may also require less manipulation of hardware when internal devices such as a pacemaker or port are present in the cleavage area.

The Craniocaudal View

The CC view is typically performed horizontal to the floor, though the receptor may be rotated about 5 degrees toward the axilla if needed. Again, the receptor should be elevated in order to mobilize the inferior breast and image the superior breast. The nipple should be centered in the image and not pointing toward the lateral corner of the image. The cleavage of the contralateral breast should remain on the receptor; if it is pushed back, then medial tissue from the breast of interest will also be pushed off the receptor.

The pectoralis muscle should be visualized on at least 30% of CC views (see Fig. 1-2). Obviously the image is positioned far enough back if the pectoralis muscle is seen. So how can one tell if a CC view is positioned well if the pectoralis muscle is not present? Let's go back to the MLO view. The measured posterior nipple line should

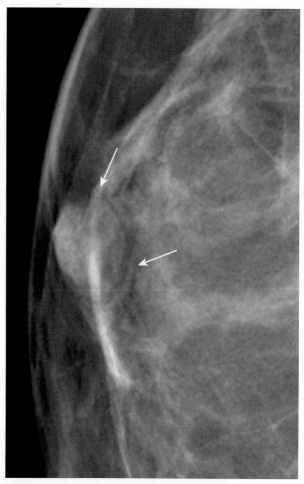

FIGURE 1-6 **Nipple Simulating a Mass.** The nipple may mimic a mass if not in profile. A halo of air (*arrows*) entrapped around the nipple helps to verify that the "mass" is the nipple.

equal or be within at least 1 cm of the same line on the CC view (see Fig. 1-1). If it is not, then the CC view should be repeated.

For women who are very kyphotic, the CC from below (CCFB) view may improve visualization of the posterior breast tissue. This view is obtained by flipping the entire gantry upside down. The receptor (which is much smaller) is then in the area of the patient's face, rather than the tube head.

Nipple in Profile

The nipple should be in profile in one of the two views if possible. Sometimes the nipple can be mistaken for a mass and converging ducts as architectural distortion if it is not in profile (Fig. 1-6). In addition, subareolar cancers can be difficult to visualize when the nipple is not in profile.

Marking Scars and Skin Lesions

Wires may be taped to the skin to mark scars. This can be helpful to ensure that architectural distortion due to prior surgical biopsy does not undergo an unnecessary workup. Marking scars from reduction mammoplasty is not typically necessary if the surgical history is provided. An alternative to marking all scars directly is for the technologist to draw them on a diagram so they can be correlated with the mammographic findings.

Marking skin lesions can also reduce screening recall to evaluate a possible breast mass. We use BBs to mark skin lesions, but other markers are also available.

Blur

Blur can be due to generalized patient motion or breathing motion. Breathing motion often results in blur that predominates along the back of the image. Blur can also be due to inadequate compression, usually along the anterior portion of the breast or the inferior breast on the MLO view. In film-screen mammography, focal blur can occur when debris elevates the film away from the screen, causing poor film-screen contact.

Blur can be difficult to perceive on mammography. The easiest way to assess for blur is to look at the Cooper ligaments, which appear as white lines in the fat. They should be thin and crisp. If they are thick or fuzzy, then there is either breast edema or blur (Fig. 1-7). If there is edema, then there should also be skin thickening. If not, it is likely due to blur. Looking at the sharpness of calcifications and comparing their appearance with prior mammograms can also help determine whether blur is present.

With digital mammography, blur that is obvious on a five-megapixel monitor may be hard to see on the small lower resolution monitors in the acquisition room.

Technologists may have a difficult time perceiving blur if only using the lower resolution monitors to review the images. We encourage the technologists to use the digital zoom to quickly check their images for blur before letting a screening patient go.

Correctable Artifacts

Artifacts have been considerably reduced with the elimination of film processors. If you are performing film-screen mammography, there are numerous artifacts that one must know about and understand well (pickoff from dirty rollers, temperature changes, dirty screens, fixer retention, static). We will be focusing on digital mammography in this section.

Grid Lines

All mammograms, except for magnification views, are performed with a reciprocating (moving) grid. This improves image contrast. Grid lines should normally blur out of the image because the grid is moving. Grid lines may uncommonly be visible with a properly functioning grid if there is a very short or a very long exposure; in these cases the grid lines have not had enough exposure time to blur or become superimposed during a lengthy exposure.

Grid lines are probably the most common correctable mammography artifact, particularly on film-screen, and may be difficult to recognize by an untrained eye. On most film-screen mammography and some digital units (General Electric), grid lines are visualized as fine, dark,

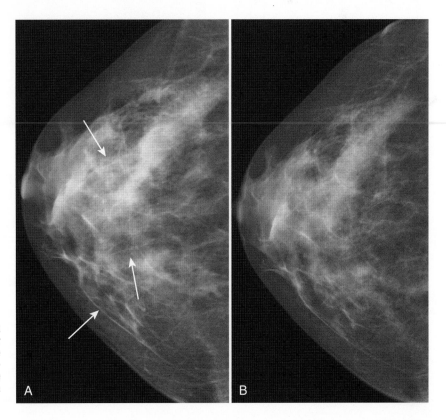

FIGURE 1-7 **Blur.** Craniocaudal (CC) views from the same patient. **A,** The Cooper ligaments appear thickened and fuzzy (*arrows*) due to blur, similar to Kerley B lines on a chest radiograph with pulmonary edema. **B,** Repeat CC view shows that the Cooper ligaments are very thin and normal in appearance.

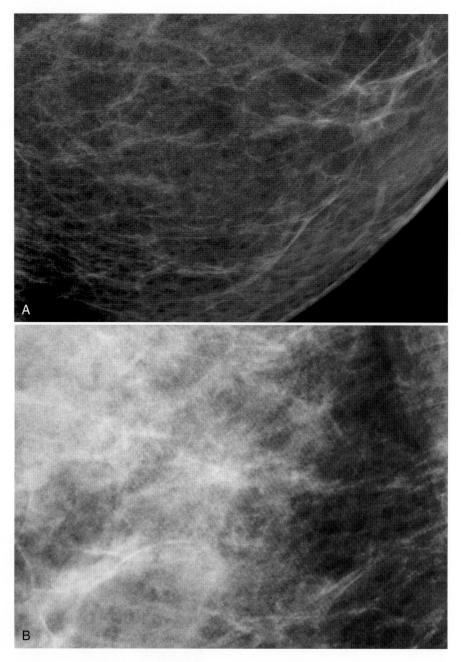

FIGURE 1-8 **Grid Lines. A,** Most mammography machines use grids that consist of thin parallel metal bars. When this type of grid is not functioning properly, fine, dark, horizontal lines are visible on the image. **B,** Some manufacturers use a different type of grid structure. When these grids malfunction, fine dark lines appear that are oriented at 45 degrees from the horizontal, creating sloping lines in an X-shaped pattern.

horizontal lines (Fig. 1-8). Some film-screen (Hologic) and many digital (Hologic, Siemens) units use mesh metallic grids that are oriented like an "X" on the image (see Fig. 1-8). The grid lines will be visualized as very fine, dark lines oriented obliquely across the image. If the grid is not functioning, a service call is needed to repair the unit before it can be used.

External Artifacts

Hair, patient gown, deodorant, talc, and tattoos can create artifacts on mammography. Ideally, the technologist will recognize and correct most of these problems at the time of the study. Deodorant has a typical appearance (Fig. 1-9) and is usually not confused with calcifications

in the axilla. If there is an artifact on the mammogram, the technologist will ask the patient to remove or move the item and will repeat the image(s) in question. Talc and ointments are more problematic than deodorant because they often overlie the breast tissue.

Internal Artifacts

Internal artifacts include pacemakers, catheters, bullet fragments, retained hookwires, shunt tubing, and Dacron cuffs from Hickman catheters. They obviously cannot be removed but should be recognized for what they represent. For women with pacemakers or port catheters, an LMO view may be safer and easier to perform than an MLO view. With an LMO view, the pacemaker or

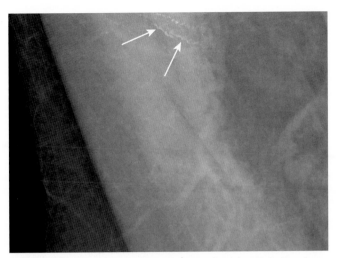

FIGURE 1-9 **Deodorant Artifact.** Close-up of a right MLO view shows high-density artifact (*arrows*) overlying the high axilla, characteristic of the appearance of deodorant. It is often clumpy and linear, as in this case.

catheter is placed next to the receptor and the compression plate is moved toward it, reducing motion.

Optimizing the Diagnostic Mammogram

Palpable abnormalities should be identified with a radiopaque marker over the area. This could be a triangle or metallic BB pellet. If a BB is used, then skin lesions such as moles should be marked with a different type of radiopaque identifier.

Spot compression views are typically obtained in CC and MLO projections with or without magnification. Spot compression views with magnification may have a small reduction in contrast. On the other hand, magnification allows better delineation of margins. Whether to magnify or not on spot compression views is a personal preference. Leaving the collimator open for spot compression views allows a larger view of the region to help ensure that the correct area was included and that the

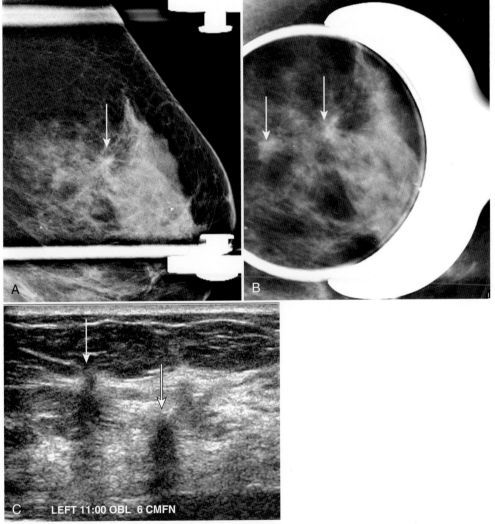

FIGURE 1-10 **Spot Compression Views with Large and Small Paddle.** This 49-year-old woman was recalled from screening for evaluation of a focal asymmetry in the left breast. **A,** On the MLO spot compression view using a large paddle, there is a subtle area of architectural distortion present (*arrow*). **B,** On the MLO spot compression view obtained using the small compression paddle, two areas of architectural distortion are clearly identified (*arrows*). **C,** Ultrasonography confirmed two adjacent, highly suspicious masses (*arrows*). Biopsy showed multifocal invasive ductal carcinoma.

lesion did not slip out from under the compression paddle. The use of a smaller paddle will result in better focal compression of the potentially abnormal area than that obtained with a large compression paddle (Fig. 1-10). A larger paddle allows good visualization of landmarks.

For women presenting with a palpable finding, spot compression views performed in CC and MLO projections, or tangentially to the palpable finding, often help visualize and characterize lesions more effectively than the routine views alone. These views should be taken with a radiopaque marker overlying the lump.

Magnification views are obtained in the CC and mediolateral (ML) projections. A true lateral view is used rather than MLO magnification so as not to miss milk of calcium. Collimating the beam to the area of concern and using spot compression reduces blur and improves contrast. Magnification views are optimal when scattered radiation is minimized (see discussion of physics in Chapter 2).

True lateral view: ML or LM? For screening recalls a true lateral view is often helpful for localizing a lesion. This is especially useful for one-view findings and when stereotactic biopsy will be performed. To make the lesion sharper, it should be as close as possible to the image receptor. Therefore, if the lesion is in the lateral breast, then an ML view is preferred. If the lesion is medial, then a lateral medial (LM) view will optimize lesion sharpness. If the lesion is not well seen on the CC view, then an ML view is obtained because most breast cancers (about 70%) occur in the lateral breast.

Final Comments

Imaging should be optimized for every patient. This approach is important if we are to provide the best patient care. The first question of those reviewing

KEY POINTS

- The first question: Can you read this study? Is it the right patient? Is it the right examination? Is the study technically adequate for interpretation?
- Use the posterior nipple line to assess for adequate positioning on both the MLO and CC views.
- Check for blur and other correctable artifacts.
- Leave the collimator open for spot compression views when they are obtained for a mass or focal asymmetry.

medicolegal cases is typically, "Is the study adequate?" If a cancer is missed due to poor positioning, blur, or a correctable artifact, the radiologist may have little ground to stand on.

Optimal imaging may not be possible for every patient. If suboptimal images are obtained, the reason for the limitation may be included in the report. For example, the MLO views may be suboptimal in women with a torn rotator cuff or stroke. Including this disclaimer in the report may reduce liability if the patient is later diagnosed with cancer in the posterior breast.

Reference

Bassett LW, Hirbawi IA, DeBruhl N, Hayes MK. Mammographic positioning: Evaluation from the view box. Radiology 1993; 188(3):803-806.

CASE 1-1. A 72-year-old woman with prior right mastectomy presents for screening of the left breast. Is this mammogram acceptable for interpretation?

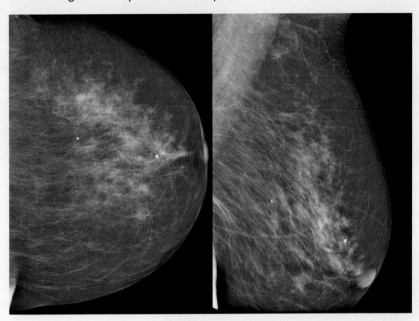

CASE 1-2. How can this screening mammogram be improved?

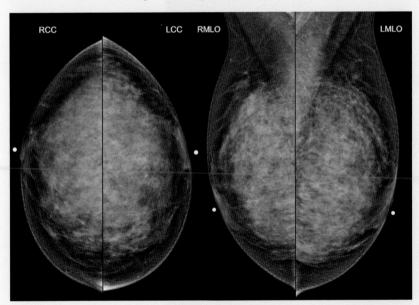

CASE 1-3. A 53-year-old woman presents for screening. Are there any preventable artifacts?

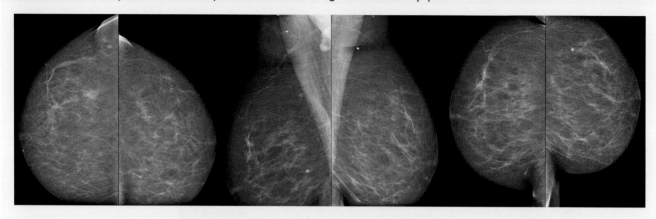

CASE 1-4. A 43-year-old woman presents for baseline screening. What is your BI-RADS assessment category given this image?

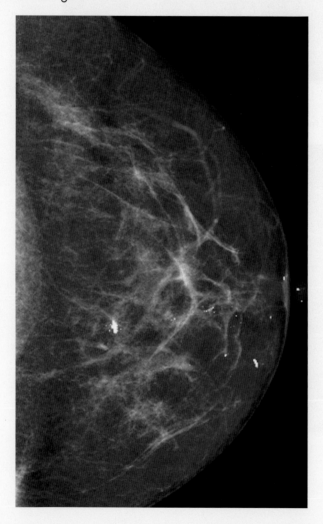

CASE 1-5. A 49-year-old woman with lumpectomy 4 years ago presents for follow-up. Is this study adequate for interpretation?

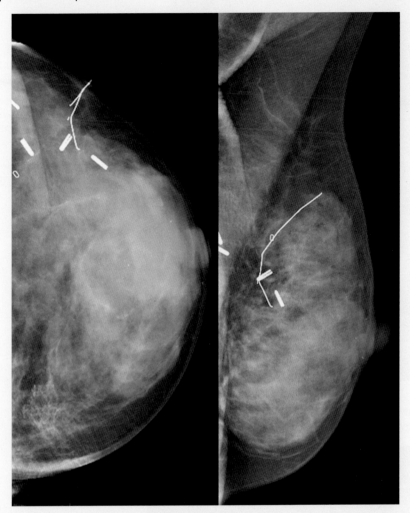

CASE 1-6. Close-up of a right MLO view. What is the artifact (*arrows*)?

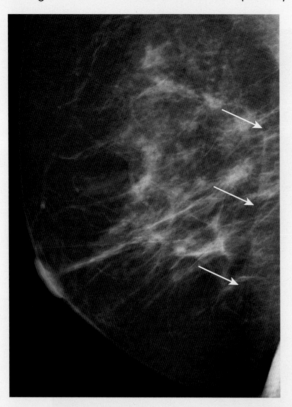

CASE 1-7. What is the most likely cause of the finding in the medial right breast (*arrow*)? How might recall of this patient have been avoided?

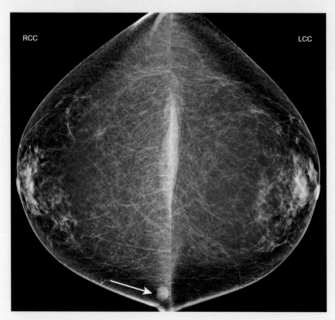

CASE 1-8. A 61-year-old woman had a palpable mass questioned in her right breast. How could the technologist include more tissue on the CC view?

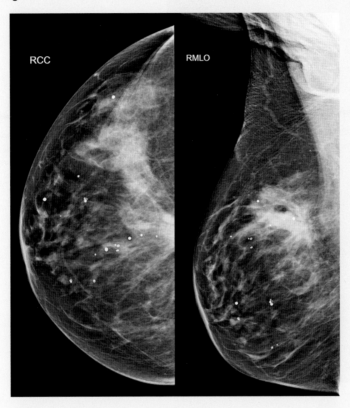

CASE 1-9. An experienced technologist performed a screening mammogram on a 50-year-old woman. She felt that she had excluded tissue on her initial views and, therefore, performed a second CC view to include more medial tissue. What is the result of her efforts?

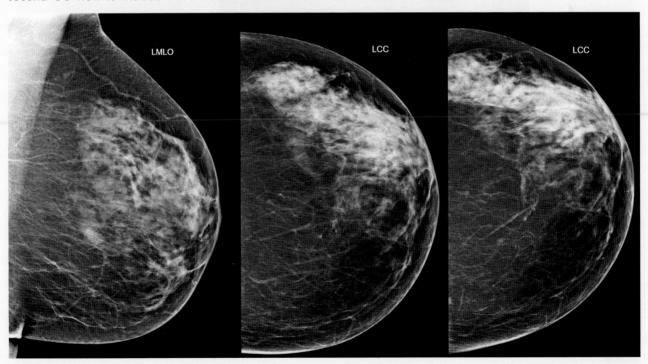

CASE 1-10. How could this left CC view be improved?

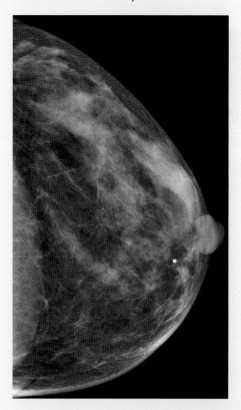

CASE 1-11. What is the artifact? Does the study need to be repeated?

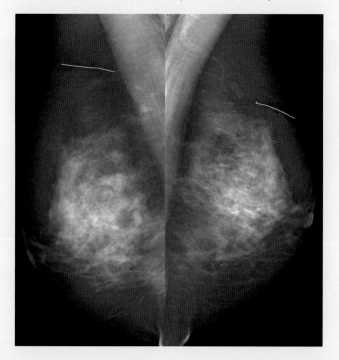

CASE 1-12. A 60-year-old woman presents for a screening mammogram. Is this study adequate?

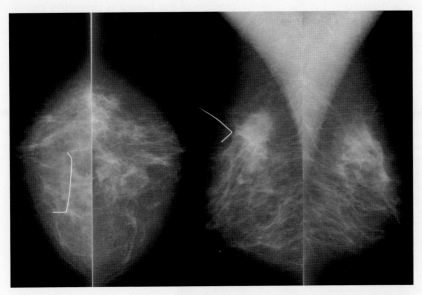

CASE 1-1. No! The CC view is adequate, but the anterior portion of the breast is drooping on the MLO view ("camel nose"). In addition, the inferior portion of the breast has been cut off on the MLO view. The repeat image has much improved positioning with the breast pulled "up and out." Notice the position of the nipple compared with that seen in the original mammogram.

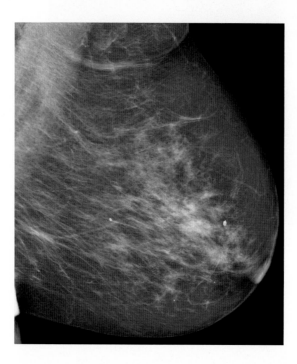

CASE 1-2. First, the nipples are pointing toward the top of the image on the CC views (*arrows*), so much of the lateral breast is not being seen on this study. Second, the pectoralis muscle is not visualized down to the posterior nipple line on either MLO view (*double arrows*).

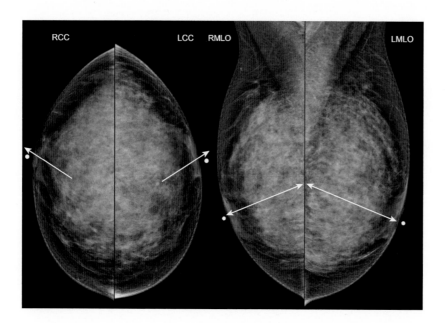

CASE 1-3. Do you see the high-density artifact? This is due to deodorant. If you look closely, you'll notice that the artifact is in the same location on three of the views. There is a clump of deodorant that stuck to the image receptor that overlies the left MLO, the left front compression MLO, and the right MLO views. Note that the artifact is in the same place (*arrows*) because it is on the receptor, not the patient's skin. Cleaning the image receptor (which should be done routinely after every patient anyway) will get rid of the problem. These views were repeated and the artifact was no longer present.

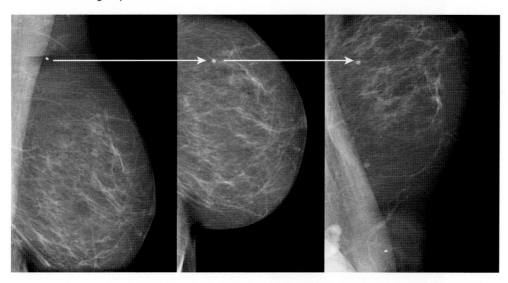

CASE 1-4. BI-RADS 2 (or 1). Metallic densities are present in a linear distribution in the medial left breast. The patient had a gunshot wound to her chest many years earlier. The metallic densities represent bullet debris.

CASE 1-5. No! There is hair overlying the medial breast on the CC view. Here are close-up and repeat CC views.

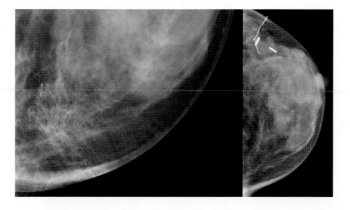

CASE 1-6. The patient's gown has fallen over the breast. The image should be repeated.

CASE 1-7. Screening CC views show a circumscribed mass medially on the right. This is a common location for sebaceous cysts and at recall, it was discovered that she had a known sebaceous cyst in this region. Recall for skin lesions can be avoided if a radiopaque marker is placed over them prior to the mammogram.

CASE 1-8. The inferior aspect of the breast is very mobile. By raising the image receptor and elevating the breast, the technologist was able to include much more posterior tissue on a repeat CC view (*below*). This revealed a spiculated mass that represented invasive ductal carcinoma.

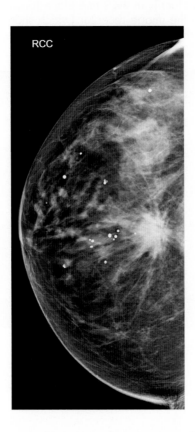

CASE 1-9. The repeated view reveals an irregular asymmetry (*arrow*) at the edge of the image for which the patient was recalled for diagnostic evaluation. The finding persisted in the CC projection only (*closed arrow*) and was not seen by ultrasonography. Do you see that the medial aspect of the contralateral breast is present on the CC view (*open arrow*)? Keeping the contralateral breast on the image receptor allows more medial tissue to be visualized on the image. Magnetic resonance imaging showed an enhancing mass with plateau kinetics (*arrow*). Diagnosis: invasive lobular carcinoma.

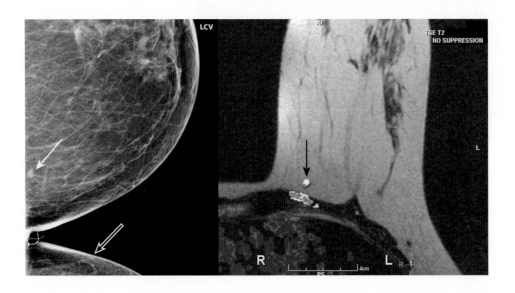

CASE 1-10. There is a skinfold in the central breast (*arrows*). Folds can mimic a dilated duct. Here is the original together with the repeat view.

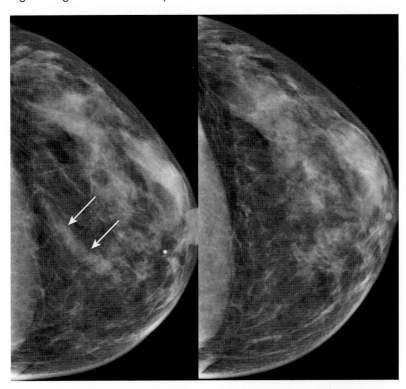

CASE 1-11. There is a radiopaque artifact overlying the left MLO view (*arrow*). This patient previously had a Hickman catheter, which has been removed. The density is a cuff that anchored the catheter into place that persisted when the catheter was removed. The image does not need to be repeated.

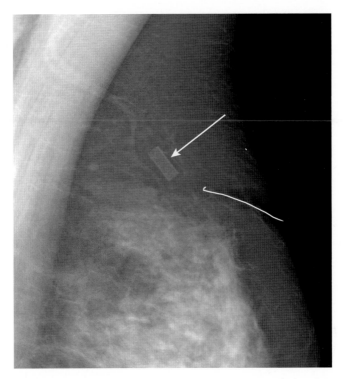

CASE 1-12. No! The most important problem is the lack of depth on the right CC view. A repeat CC view shows a large mass in the upper outer quadrant (*arrow*). Biopsy showed invasive ductal carcinoma. Did you get this one? Congratulations! You may have just saved a life.

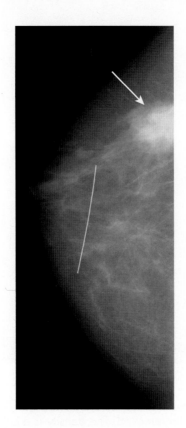

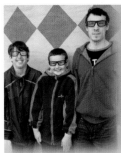

CHAPTER 2

Physics Facts That WILL Improve Your Images

Many readers will skip this chapter. Don't be one of them. Most of us learned physics in order to pass boards, but we never really made the leap to understanding how physics knowledge really can improve our images.

Optimizing Mammography

Because the breast is a soft tissue organ, there is little internal contrast. High contrast is necessary to distinguish cancers from the surrounding breast tissue. Most of the improvements with mammography over the last 30 years have been related to contrast. These include the use of single emulsion film, extended processing, and the use of molybdenum targets and grids. More recently, digital mammography has improved contrast compared with film-screen mammography. This section will focus on digital mammography because the majority of facilities use this equipment.

Contrast

The lower the kilovolt peak (kVp), the higher the contrast. Digital machines operate with an automatic exposure device (AED) that selects an appropriate target, filter, kVp, and milliampere second (mAs). This works very well ... most of the time.

Molybdenum anode targets were used almost exclusively in film-screen mammography because of the resulting lower energy spectrum due to molybdenum's characteristic radiation at approximately 18 and 20 keV. Occasionally the rhodium target would be used for women with dense breasts to have a slightly higher energy spectrum (characteristic radiation at about 20 and 23 keV) in order to adequately penetrate the breast tissue.

In digital mammography, the image contrast can be adjusted via the window and level settings of the display, so the target material and goal of obtaining the lowest possible beam energy are less important. Most digital exposures use either a tungsten or a rhodium target, and occasionally fall back to a molybdenum target. One advantage of using a higher energy x-ray spectrum is better breast penetration, so x-rays are more likely to pass through the breast and contribute to forming the image and the exposure is faster, reducing the chance of motion artifacts. Another advantage is lower radiation dose because fewer x-rays are absorbed in the breast. Digital mammography is about 30% lower in radiation dose than film-screen mammography.

Mammography filters are also made from molybdenum or rhodium and are used to remove x-rays that are lower or higher in energy than the desired spectrum. On digital mammography machines, the filter selection is also automated.

So if all of this is automated, why know any of this? There are times when the AED will not provide an appropriate technique. The most common situations where this occurs are when a patient has breast implants or hardware (Fig. 2-1). A high-density implant or hardware that overlies the AED will cause an exposure setting that is too high for the breast parenchyma, resulting in overexposure of the tissue and low contrast. A manual technique is required for women with implants and may also optimize contrast in women with hardware.

With film-screen mammography, poor technique is usually obvious because the film is too light or dark, or low in contrast. However, poor technique can be hard to recognize with digital mammography. The image will appear uncharacteristically noisy (Fig. 2-2). Windowing of the image may result in some improvement, though repeating the exposure is often preferred (Box 2-1).

For some women, their breasts become very thin (less than 2 cm) when compressed—"pancake breasts." The internal contrast is extremely low because these women tend to have very little body fat (Fig. 2-3). The breast may appear to be very dense, when there is actually very little breast tissue present. A manual technique using the molybdenum target/filter at the lowest kVp possible can improve the image contrast.

Specimen radiographs, whether core or surgical, likewise, are usually quite thin, and a manual technique using a molybdenum target/filter combination and the lowest possible kVp will result in the best image contrast.

Reducing Scatter

The reduction of scattered x-ray photons is a key part of optimizing contrast. There are several ways to reduce scatter:
• Beam collimation
• Breast compression
• Grid
• Air-gap

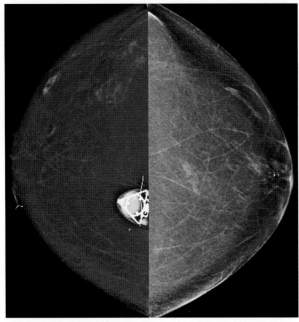

FIGURE 2-1 **Overexposure Due to Port Catheter.** The right craniocaudal (CC) view is overexposed (kVp 32, mAs 237) but the left CC view technique is good (kVp 31, mAs 53). The port catheter overlies the region of the automatic exposure device, resulting in overexposure.

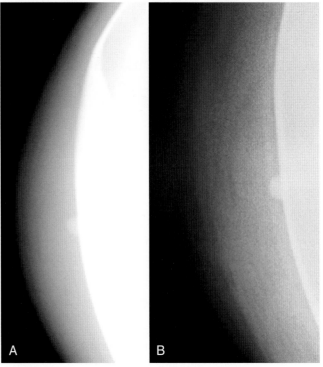

FIGURE 2-3 **Low Contrast Due to Low Body Fat. A,** In this patient who weighs 85 lb with large saline implants, the contrast is very low. The breast tissue is uniformly gray. The technique used was 30 kVp and 261 mAs. **B,** The kVp was decreased to 25 (mAs 125) with improvement in contrast.

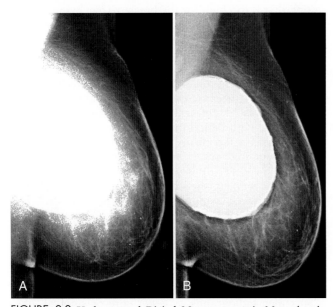

FIGURE 2-2 **Underexposed Digital Mammogram. A,** Manual technique (28 kVp, 100 mAs) was used due to the implant. The breast adjacent to the implant is underexposed. **B,** The repeat view was performed with a higher exposure (140 mAs) and the image is now adequate for interpretation.

> **BOX 2-1 Situations in Which the Technique May Need Adjusting**
>
> - Implants
> - Very thin breasts
> - Specimen radiographs
> - Overlying hardware

landmarks helps assure that the area of interest is included on the image.

Compression reduces the thickness of the breast, thereby reducing the exposure and scattered radiation. Using spot compression during magnification views focally compresses the tissue even more than the compression used during routine mammographic views. This further reduces scatter, and improves image contrast.

Grids improve image contrast on mammography by reducing scatter. However, magnification views are not obtained using a grid because the exposure time, which is already increased due to the lower output of the small focal spot used for magnification views, would be too long.

Even without a grid, most scatter in magnification views is eliminated using the air-gap technique. Because of the large gap between the breast and the receptor, most scattered photons diverge from the primary beam and will not strike the image receptor.

So how can you use this information in your practice? By performing spot compression magnification views

Beam collimation ("coning") is helpful for reducing scatter when obtaining magnification views to assess calcifications. For this purpose, a wider field of view is not needed because visualization of the calcifications on the magnified images confirms that the correct area was included. However, when using spot compression views to evaluate masses or focal asymmetries, the image is not collimated. In this case, visualization of the surrounding

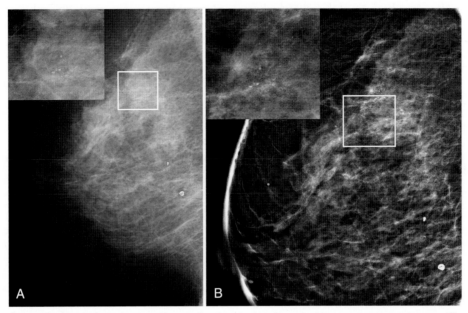

FIGURE 2-4 **Different Magnification Techniques. A,** Full magnification view performed without spot compression or collimation down to the size of the area of interest. Inset shows enlarged area of calcifications. **B,** Magnification view of the same patient performed with spot compression and coning of the x-ray beam to the region of interest. The contrast is improved due to decreased scatter. Inset shows that the calcifications are much sharper and more calcifications are visualized using this technique.

BOX 2-2 How to Get Beautiful Magnification Views

- Use spot compression and coning for calcifications (see Fig. 2-4). Spot compression reduces the breast thickness and thus exposure time. Coning of the image reduces scattered radiation.
- Obtain true geometric magnification views, which are better than zoomed views of digital mammograms (see Fig. 2-5).
- Get magnification views in the craniocaudal and mediolateral (not mediolateral oblique) projections as your routine practice so as not to miss milk of calcium.

with collimation and taking advantage of the air-gap technique, you can obtain incredible detail on your magnification views (Box 2-2; Figs. 2-4 and 2-5).

Resolution

Digital mammography units vary in detector element size from 40 to 100 μm, corresponding to limiting spatial frequency of 12.5 to 5.0 line pairs (lp) per millimeter, respectively. Note that the actual spatial resolution in digital mammography is determined by the focal spot size and blurring elements in the detector, primarily in the scintillator or phosphor screen in indirect conversion detectors. Thus the detector element size only sets an upper limit on resolution that may or may not actually be obtained. Digital mammography is not actually higher in resolution than film-screen mammography, which has a resolution of

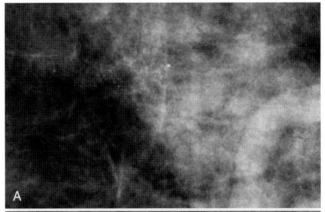

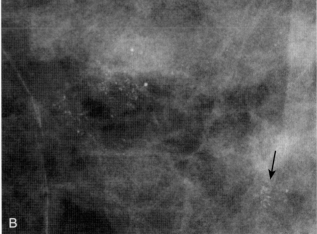

FIGURE 2-5 **Zoom Versus Magnification View.** Zoomed digital image (**A**) does not depict calcifications with the same clarity as a true geometric magnification view (**B**). The morphologic appearance and extent are much better evaluated on the true magnification view. Did you notice the second group of calcifications (*arrow*)? Both areas were ductal carcinoma in situ, intermediate grade.

about 14 lp per mm. However, because of the much higher noise introduced by the film and film processing, the signal-to-noise ratio of film-screen mammography in practice is lower. The primary improvements gained through digital mammography are elimination of film granularity noise and a large increase in the dynamic range of x-ray intensities that can be measured. The minor differences in resolution between digital units have not been shown to impact cancer detection.

Optimizing Ultrasonography

Whether the radiologist, trainee, or technologist performs the ultrasonography (US) examination, careful attention to technical parameters can optimize the study (Box 2-3).

Resolution

Higher frequency transducers are higher in resolution but have lower tissue penetration. Because the breast is a superficial organ, a very high frequency transducer can be used. The most common transducer used for breast imaging is a 7 to 15 MHz gradient linear array transducer, though a higher frequency (10-17 MHz) transducer yields beautiful images in smaller breasts.

Adjust the Depth

Fill your screen with the area of interest! The field of view should include only the breast tissue and the anterior

---

> ### BOX 2-3   Optimizing Breast Ultrasonography
>
> - *Depth*—include only breast and pectoral muscle in the field of view
> - *Focal Zones*—adjust to breast tissue for survey scanning or specifically to a lesion once identified
> - *Gain*—adjust to be uniform in the image; a straight time-gain curve works well in breast ultrasonography.

---

pectoral muscle (Fig. 2-6). The ribs and lung should not be seen on breast US unless the breast is thin. With a large breast, the default depth may actually need to be increased to include the posterior tissues. Otherwise, a deep lesion could be missed. The depth may also need to be increased to demonstrate the posterior acoustic enhancement of a cyst or shadowing of a mass.

Focal Zone Positioning

When surveying the breast, the focal zone should include the area of the breast tissue from just under the skin to the pectoral muscle (Fig. 2-7).

Once a lesion is identified, improvement in image quality can be gained by narrowing the focal zone to the area of the lesion (see Fig. 2-7). Classic teaching is that the focal zone should be positioned deep to a lesion. However, that only holds true when using a single focal zone. Most US machines now use multiple focal zones to create a focal area. The focal zone should be centered *at* the lesion rather than behind it.

Setting the Gain

Setting the overall gain and the time-gain curve (TGC) to the optimal levels is essential for accurately characterizing cystic or solid masses. The overall gain should be set so that fat lobules are midlevel gray and the TGC adjusted so that the fat lobules at all depths of the breast have the same echogenicity (Fig. 2-8). The TGC should be relatively straight in breast imaging.

Adenosis, lymph nodes involved by tumor, or lymphomatous masses may appear markedly hypoechoic and can be mistaken for cysts. When questioning a cyst within the axilla, keep in mind that cysts in this location are very uncommon, and a pathologic lymph node should be suspected. Color Doppler usually demonstrates the solid nature of the mass in these cases (Fig. 2-9).

Tissue Harmonic Imaging

Harmonic imaging is a feature that improves contrast resolution and is widely available on current US

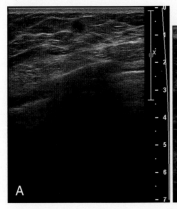
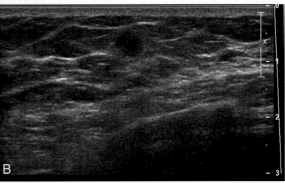

FIGURE 2-6 **Adjusting the Field of View (Depth). A,** Field of view is too deep. We don't need to see the lung and chest wall! **B,** Depth is decreased to optimize the field of view for this patient. The screen is filled with only the area of interest. This is a beautiful ultrasound image.

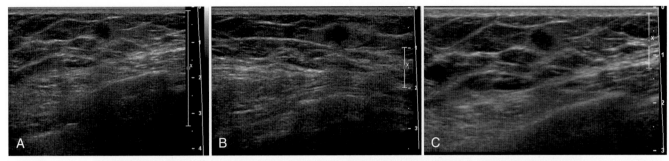

FIGURE 2-7 **Focal Zone Positioning. A,** The focal zone is too broad; it does not need to include the chest wall! **B,** The focal zone is too low. **C,** The focal zone is just right! It includes the breast tissue, but excludes the pectoral muscle and chest wall.

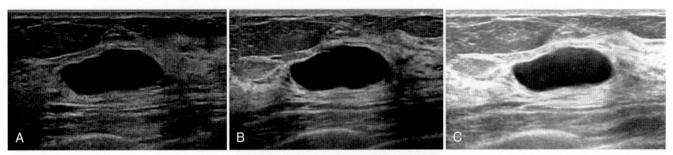

FIGURE 2-8 **Simple Cyst with Different Gain Settings.** With the gain too low (**A**) the fat lobules are too hypoechoic. With this setting, a solid or complex mass can appear anechoic. With an optimal gain setting (**B**), the fat lobules are midlevel gray. With the gain too high (**C**), the cyst is filled with artifactual echoes.

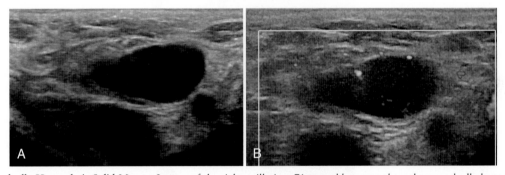

FIGURE 2-9 **Markedly Hypoechoic Solid Masses.** Images of the right axilla in a 71-year-old woman show three markedly hypoechoic masses (**A**) that could be mistaken for cysts. However, color Doppler examination (**B**) confirms internal flow within the largest mass, indicating a solid lesion. The findings represented axillary adenopathy due to metastatic breast carcinoma.

equipment. An ultrasound beam transmitted at one center frequency creates higher harmonic frequencies as it passes through tissue. In tissue harmonic imaging (THI), the returning harmonic frequencies are used to form the image, and the lower frequency component of the beam is removed by a processing technique. This step removes artifact that is present in the lower frequency beam component, resulting in improved contrast.

By reducing reverberation and speckle artifacts, THI is useful for characterizing cysts and distinguishing them from solid lesions. The reduction in reverberation artifact can also be helpful in the evaluation of implants. Solid masses generally appear more hypoechoic with THI, which can make them more conspicuous.

THI is particularly useful in identifying and guiding biopsy of lesions that, on conventional imaging, are nearly isoechoic with the surrounding tissue (Fig. 2-10).

It can also make subtle abnormalities of tissue echo-texture, such as lesions appearing mammographically as architectural distortion, much more conspicuous (Fig. 2-11).

Compound Imaging

Compound imaging is another feature available on many US units that can be used to improve contrast and spatial resolution. In conventional US, the beam is transmitted at a 90-degree angle to the transducer, and the resulting image creates a single frame. With compound imaging, additional sweeps are generated at different angles, and the returning echoes are compounded to produce the image. The resulting image has reduced artifact compared with conventional imaging.

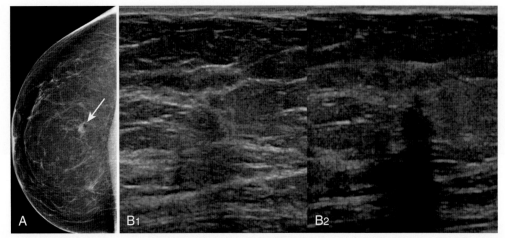

FIGURE 2-10 **Harmonic Imaging of an Isoechoic Mass. A,** Mammogram of a 42-year-old woman with a history of reduction mammoplasty shows an irregular mass in the right breast (*arrow*). **B,** The lesion is much more conspicuous with tissue harmonic imaging (right image, **B2**), and its shadowing is accentuated. Harmonic imaging was used to guide core biopsy, which revealed fat necrosis.

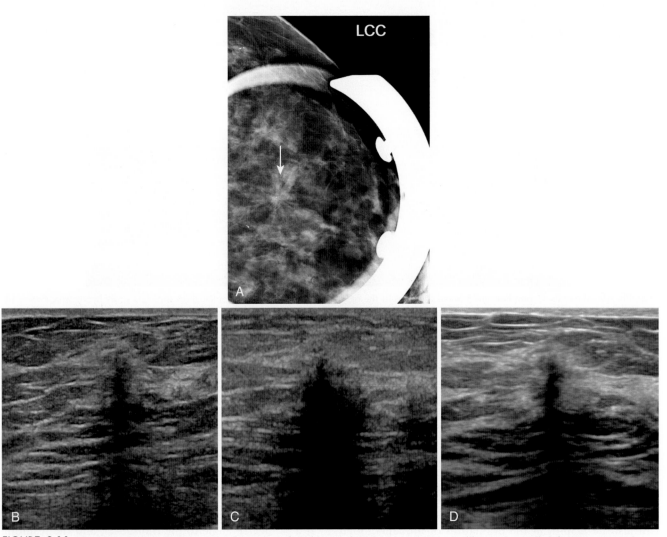

FIGURE 2-11 **Harmonic Imaging and Compound Imaging of Architectural Distortion.** A 61-year-old woman recalled from screening due to suspected architectural distortion. **A,** Distortion is confirmed in the lateral left breast (*arrow*). **B,** Ultrasonography with routine processing shows a corresponding shadowing hypoechoic lesion. **C,** With harmonic imaging there is marked accentuation of shadowing, making the lesion more conspicuous. **D,** With compound imaging, the shadowing is reduced and there is improved evaluation of margin detail. Biopsy revealed invasive ductal carcinoma and ductal carcinoma in situ.

The added information obtained with compound imaging can improve evaluation of the margins and internal architecture of masses (Figs. 2-12 and 2-13). Evaluation of the deep margins of masses may be particularly improved, for example, if the posterior margin is not well assessed because of shadowing.

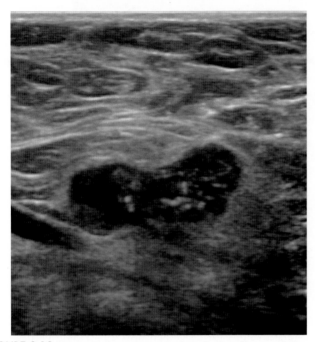

FIGURE 2-12 **Compound Imaging to Evaluate Lesion Characteristics.** The use of compound imaging permits detailed evaluation of this axillary lymph node. The image has high contrast, and the shape, margins, and internal characteristics of the lesion are well assessed. The echogenic foci represent calcifications due to metastatic tumor involvement.

It is important for the sonographer and radiologist to realize that the posterior acoustic features of a lesion may be greatly reduced or eliminated by compound imaging (see Fig. 2-13). The shadowing of a subtle lesion, which may be the only feature that permits its detection, may be removed by this technique. Compound imaging is therefore most useful for characterizing a lesion that has already been detected, rather than in survey scanning or screening of a large region.

Elastography

When you examine a palpable lump in the breast, you are evaluating the relative stiffness of the breast tissue. Cancers tend to be firmer on clinical examination, and likewise stiffer on elastography. Elastography maps the relative stiffness of the breast tissue, typically using a color map.

There are currently two methods of breast elastography. The first method uses external manual compression force. Strain is measured perpendicular to the skin surface. This method uses both size and stiffness criteria; cancers appear larger on the elastogram. Manual techniques are limited by operator variability. Vibration elastography (shear wave) uses a variant of Doppler imaging to generate tissue motion (Fig. 2-14). Shear wave technology may be more reproducible because it is obtained without manual compression.

Elastography is a newer technique, and the literature is evolving. Elastography may improve specificity in the evaluation of breast masses. For example, a small mass with low level echoes and a benign elastogram may improve confidence that the lesion represents a cyst. On the other hand, moderate stiffness may increase the level of suspicion. The results of elastography must be

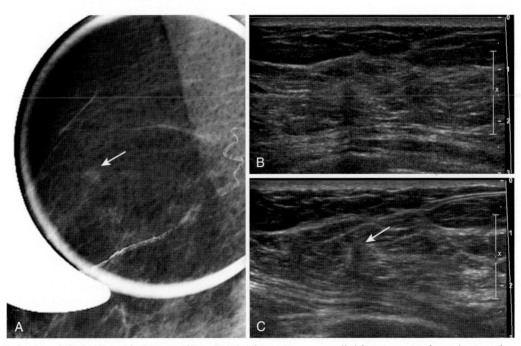

FIGURE 2-13 **Reduction of Shadowing with Compound Imaging. A,** This patient was recalled from screening for evaluation of a subtle developing asymmetry (*arrow*). Images of this malignant mass obtained with conventional (**B**) and compound imaging (**C**). Shadowing is less apparent with this technique. During survey scanning a subtle area of shadowing may be overlooked when using compound imaging.

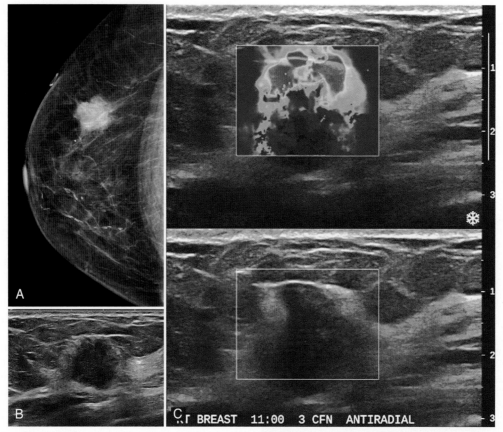

FIGURE 2-14 Shear Wave Elastography. A, Diagnostic mammogram demonstrates an irregular, high-density mass with spiculated margins that corresponds to a palpable lump. **B,** Ultrasonography demonstrates a round hypoechoic mass with microlobulated margins and an echogenic rim. **C,** Shear wave elastogram demonstrates very stiff tissue at the anterior border of the mass (*red*). Biopsy showed invasive ductal carcinoma NOS (not otherwise specified).

considered in the context of other US findings, prior mammograms, and other imaging.

Optimizing Breast Magnetic Resonance Imaging

High-quality breast magnetic resonance imaging (MRI) mandates the use of a 1.5 T (tesla) or higher field strength magnet, a dedicated breast coil, uniform fat saturation (FS), and intravenous contrast. Timing of dynamic sequences must balance spatial and temporal resolution.

Magnet and Coils

A 1.5 or 3 T field strength yields the best results. The closer the coils are to the breast, the higher signal strength will be. The geometry of the coil is more important than the number of channels. A 7-channel or higher coil is typically preferred.

Sequences

Scanning in either the axial or sagittal planes is acceptable. Ductal abnormalities are beautifully seen in the

> **BOX 2-4 Typical Breast Magnetic Resonance Imaging Protocol for Cancer Evaluation**
>
> - Scout
> - T2 with fat saturation (FS) or STIR
> - T1 no FS
> - Dynamic axial T1 with FS
>   - Intravenous gadolinium
>   - 3 to 5 repetitions
>   - Less than 2 minutes per acquisition
> - Sagittal high resolution T1 with FS

sagittal plane, but side-by-side comparison is more manageable in the axial plane. Using isotropic voxels (a cube) allows viewing of the sequence in any plane without distortion, so the scan plane becomes less important. There is variability in the noncontrast scan sequences that are obtained. A T2 or STIR (short T1 inversion recovery) sequence with FS provides information about water content of lesions. A T1 sequence without FS prior to contrast injection is very helpful for evaluating fat-containing masses and scars (Box 2-4).

FS may be difficult in some women, especially those with very little body fat, very large fatty breasts, or implants (Fig. 2-15). The fat peak is usually selected by automated software; when this method is not successful, the peak can be hand selected by the technologist. Inhomogeneous FS is usually due to field inhomogeneity, which can be improved by reshimming the magnet. Signal flare can resemble inhomogeneous FS but is simply due to contact of the breast with the coil (Fig. 2-16).

The dynamic sequence should commence about 30 seconds after injection of contrast agent. Gadobenate

dimeglumine (MultiHance, Braco) has a higher relaxivity resulting in improved lesion detection over gadopentetate dimeglumine (Magnevist, Bayer Healthcare) (Fig. 2-17). In a multicenter study including 162 women who underwent MRI with each of the agents, sensitivity improved from 81% with gadopentetate dimeglumine to 92% with gadobenate dimeglumine. Three to five dynamic sequences are obtained; each dynamic sequence should be less than 2 minutes.

Curve-ology (Color Display)

The dynamics of lesion contrast enhancement are predictive of the likelihood of cancer. Contrast enhancement is considered in two phases: initial (rapid, medium, or slow) and delayed (washout, plateau, persistent). Computer-aided display (CAD) provides review of this dynamic information using color coding.

Why do some lesions show color but other lesions that are clearly enhancing do not? Lesions that enhance more than a specified percentage (usually 60%) over precontrast background signal are considered to have rapid initial enhancement and show color (Fig. 2-18). Lesions with slow or medium initial phase enhancement will not show color. Suspicious lesions are less likely to demonstrate rapid initial enhancement in a woman with low cardiac output (e.g., congestive heart failure) because of the slow circulation of contrast. Lowering the color threshold to below 60% of background may help in the evaluation of these women.

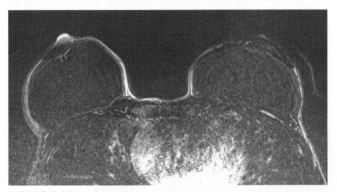

FIGURE 2-15 **Poor Fat Saturation Due to Implants and Small Volume of Breast Tissue.** Despite multiple attempts to obtain good fat saturation, fat signal is still bright on the T1 sequence (after contrast). When fat saturation is poor, subtraction images can be used to identify enhancing masses if there is no patient motion.

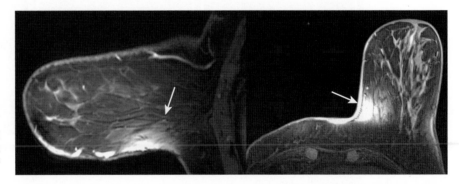

FIGURE 2-16 **Signal Flare.** There is increased signal (*arrows*) where the breast is touching the coil, mimicking inhomogeneous fat saturation.

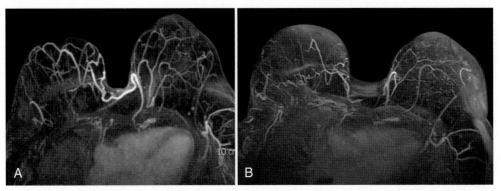

FIGURE 2-17 **Different Contrast Agents.** Maximum intensity projection images from screening MRI using gadobenate dimeglumine (MultiHance) (**A**) shows greater conspicuity of the vessels and lymph nodes compared with the prior MRI using gadopentetate dimeglumine (Magnevist) (**B**) in the same patient.

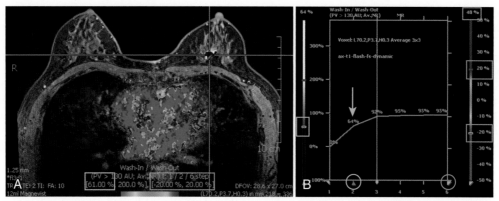

FIGURE 2-18 **MRI Computer-Aided Display (CAD).** Notice that parameters can be found on the image (**A**) as well as the curve (**B**). Areas that display in color on MRI CAD enhance over a specified minimum. This value is typically set at 60% (*yellow boxes*) on the first time point after contrast (*yellow circle*). The lesion at the intersection of the reference lines (a small focus of ductal carcinoma in situ) enhances to 64% over background (*yellow arrow*). The specific color that is assigned is based on the percentage change in enhancement between the first (*yellow circle*) and last (*green circle*) time points. For a persistent curve (*blue*), there is an increase of more than 20%, and a washout curve (*red*) is a decrease of over 20%. These thresholds are indicated by bars on the color spectrum on the right side of the image (*pink boxes*). Anything in between is a plateau curve (*yellow/green*). Enhancement of the lesion shown increases by 48% (*green box*) between the first and last sequences, which is persistent and therefore blue on the axial image.

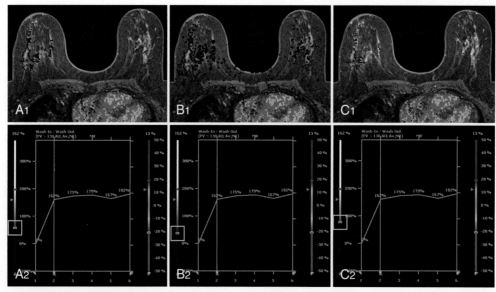

FIGURE 2-19 **Changing CAD Color Threshold.** As we change the color threshold (*yellow boxes*), only the amount of color on the images changes; the curves and numbers do not change, nor does the color (*red, yellow/green, blue*) assigned. **A,** The color threshold is typically set at 60%. **B,** The color threshold has been decreased to 40%. There is more color in the image. **C,** The threshold for color has been increased to 80% over background and there is less overall color.

Sometimes, everything seems to be enhancing. Raising the threshold for color assignment to above 60% may decrease background coloring in the images of women with diffuse parenchymal enhancement or multiple enhancing foci (Fig. 2-19).

The specific color of a lesion is determined by delayed enhancement. Basically, a change in the later sequences of greater than 20%, less than 20%, or in between correlates with persistent (blue), washout (red), or plateau (yellow/green) curves. This can go wrong if the scanning is started too early after contrast; a lesion that should show washout will display as plateau. The threshold criteria for assigning different colors can be changed (Fig. 2-20), although this is less useful.

A patient with very slow flow due to low cardiac output may peak at the second time point after contrast agent is given. In this case, the time point used to determine color assignment can be changed from the first to the second postcontrast sequence (Fig. 2-21).

Positioning and Motion

Just as in mammography, positioning counts! MRI technologists may be in the habit of having patients position themselves by simply laying down on the breast coil. Because of coil design, most women will position themselves too high on the coil so as to reduce shoulder

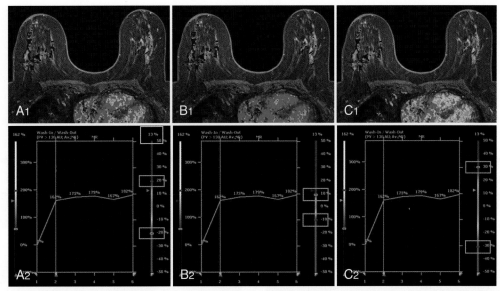

FIGURE 2-20 **Changing CAD Color Coding Range.** As we change the enhancement range assigned to plateau (*pink boxes*), the color coding changes. The threshold is held steady at 60%, so the total amount of color on the images remains the same. **A,** Typical setting with the color coding range set at ±20%. This lesion is green (plateau) because it increases in enhancement by 13% (*yellow box*) over the first postcontrast image, falling within this ±20% range. **B,** The color coding has now been set to ±10%. The lesion is therefore blue (persistent) because 13% is outside the ±10% coding range. **C,** The color coding range is now set at ±30%. The lesion is now green again because 13% is less than the 30% threshold to be blue.

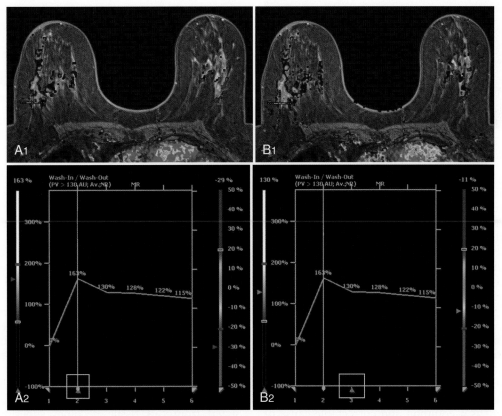

FIGURE 2-21 **Changing CAD Time Points. A,** Typically the first postcontrast sequence is subtracted from the final sequence to determine color assignment. **B,** In this view, we've subtracted the second postcontrast study, which is indicated by the yellow box. As a result, there is overall more color in the image and there is a higher percentage of red and yellow. This can be useful for women with low cardiac output when the peak contrast bolus occurs on the second sequence after contrast injection.

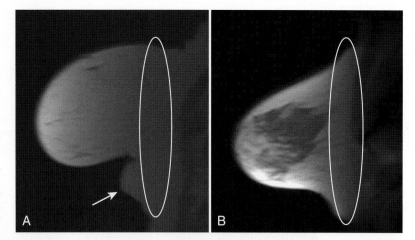

FIGURE 2-22 **Positioning of the Breast in the Coil Aperture. A,** The breast is not centered in the aperture (*circle*). Abdominal fat has dropped into the aperture (*arrow*). The patient needs to move toward her feet. The breasts need to be pulled into the aperture. **B,** The breast is well centered in the aperture (*circle*) on this study.

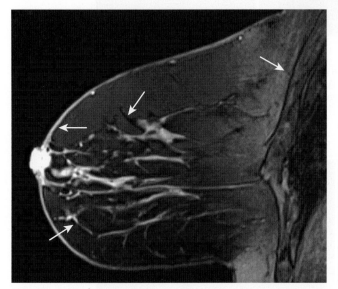

FIGURE 2-23 **Chemical Shift Artifact.** There are dark lines at the skin-fat, fat-tissue, and fat-muscle interfaces (*arrows*).

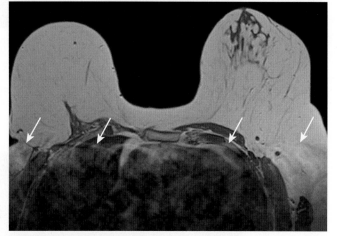

FIGURE 2-24 **Phase Encoding Artifact.** Cardiac motion is propagated in the phase encoding direction. In the axial plane, the phase encoding direction must be left to right or the smear artifact will overlie the breast tissue.

discomfort (Fig. 2-22). However, the breast needs to be centered within the aperture and most women will need to be coached to scoot toward their feet. The breast should be pulled down into the coil. Motion degrades the subtraction images, maximum intensity projections (MIPs), color maps, and enhancement curves. Soft cushioning with towels or light compression, coaching, and communication are all effective ways of reducing motion.

Common Magnetic Resonance Imaging Artifacts

The same artifacts that affect scanning techniques elsewhere also affect breast MRI.

Chemical shift is a common and correctable cause of image degradation. It looks like a child took a permanent marker and drew black lines at every tissue interface (Fig. 2-23). At 1.5 T, water and fat are in-phase at echo times of 0, 4.4, 8.8 ms, and so on. They are out of phase at echo times of 2.2, 6.6, 11.0 ms, and so on. Where fat and water overlap, their out-of-phase signals cancel each

other out, producing a dark band at tissue interfaces. Chemical shift artifact can be corrected by increasing the bandwidth or the echo time so that the fat and water are in-phase.

Phase encoding artifact is due to normal respiratory, vascular, and cardiac motion, which is always propagated in the phase encoding direction (Fig. 2-24). This normal motion degrades the image. We can't stop cardiac and respiratory motion, but we can minimize its effect by putting the phase encoding direction where the artifact will not overlap the breast. The phase encoding direction should therefore be left-to-right in the axial plane and top-to-bottom in the sagittal plane.

Wrap around or *phase wrap* occurs when not all of the signal-producing tissue is within the field of view. The signal from this tissue becomes superimposed on the tissue in the field of view (Fig. 2-25). Can you guess that phase wrap occurs in the phase encoding direction? And who is buried in Grant's Tomb?

Zebra artifact occurs when excited tissue outside the field of view wraps into the area of interest and there are tissues that are both in and out of phase. This is

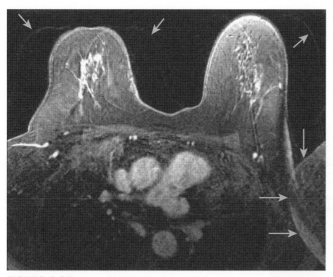

FIGURE 2-25 **Phase Wrap (Aliasing).** This patient was unable to put her right arm over her head for the study. Tissue from her right arm, which was down along her side, was included in the field of view, resulting in phase wrap or aliasing of the arm over the left side of the image (*yellow arrows*). More subtle phase wrap of the breasts is also present (*blue arrows*).

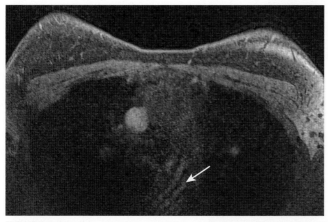

FIGURE 2-26 **Zebra Artifact.** This is the sixth slice in from the top of the breasts. Zebra artifact is commonly seen overlying the spine and thorax on these early slices (*arrow*). The study does not need to be repeated if confined to these areas.

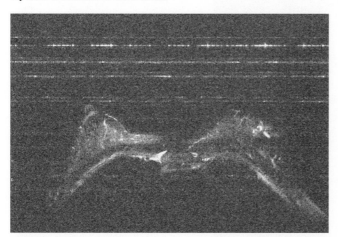

FIGURE 2-27 **Radiofrequency (RF) Interference Artifact.** The parallel white lines are due to RF signal noise. When there is this much present, it typically means that the door to the scanner was not shut tightly.

KEY POINTS

- Underexposed digital mammograms appear very noisy and should be repeated.
- Use a manual technique with a molybdenum target/filter combination and the lowest possible kVp to improve contrast for women with very thin breasts and for specimen radiographs.
- Reduce scatter in magnification views by collimating the beam (coning) and using spot compression.
- Optimize US resolution by using the highest frequency transducer possible and by decreasing depth to include only the breast tissue.
- Optimize US lesion evaluation by narrowing and centering the focal zone to the breast tissue during survey scanning and then to the level of the lesion once it is identified.
- Breast positioning is important in breast MRI. Learn to recognize and correct artifacts such as chemical shift that can degrade image quality.

commonly seen on the first and last image or two of the sequence (Fig. 2-26). If this is seen in the center of the sequence, that is bad news—there is something terrible going on. It may be that the images were obtained using the body coil when the breast coil was not selected or the field of view is much too small. Get help!

Radiofrequency interference is a very uncommon artifact that may be difficult to recognize. Essentially, extraneous radio signal is leaking into the room or being generated within the room. It presents as variable white lines in the phase encoding direction (Fig. 2-27). This may considerably degrade image quality by increasing noise. It may be due to a problem with the door seal or equipment in the room.

References

Harvey JA, Hendrick RE, Coll JM, et al. Breast MR imaging artifacts: How to recognize and fix them. Radiographics 2007;27(Suppl 1):S131-S145.

Martincich L, Faivre-Pierret M, Zechmann CM, et al. Multicenter, double-blind, randomized, intraindividual crossover comparison of gadobenate dimeglumine and gadopentetate dimeglumine for breast MR imaging (DETECT Trial). Radiology 2011;258(2):396-408.

Ojeda-Fournier H, Choe KA, Mahoney MC. Recognizing and interpreting artifacts and pitfalls in MR imaging of the breast. Radiographics 2007;27:S147-S164.

Pediconi F, Catalano C, Occhiato R, et al. Breast lesion detection and characterization at contrast-enhanced MR mammography: Gadobenate dimeglumine versus gadopentetate dimeglumine. Radiology 2005;237(1):45-56.

Rausch DR, Hendrick RE. How to optimize clinical breast MR imaging practices and techniques on your 1.5-T system. Radiographics 2006;26(5):1469-1484.

Stavros AT. Breast Ultrasound. Philadelphia, Lippincott Williams & Wilkins, 2004, pp 25-33, 66-67, 948-950.

Weinstein SP, Conant EF, Sehgal C. Technical advances in breast ultrasound imaging. Semin Ultrasound CT MRI 2006;27:273-283.

CASE QUESTIONS

CASE 2-1. One of your technologists brings you these images to check. Here is a close-up of a mediolateral oblique view.

What is the problem? Can it be corrected?

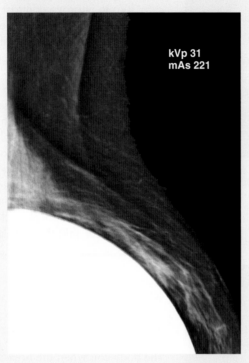

kVp 31
mAs 221

CASE 2-2. Close-up of a right craniocaudal view (26 kVp, 22 mAs, 12 mm compression, GE unit).

What is the artifact? Is it correctable?

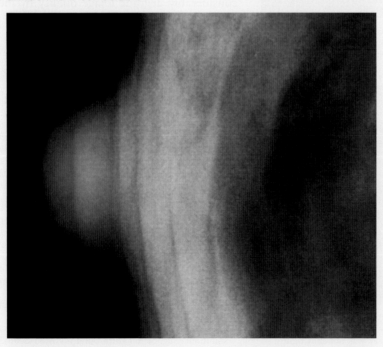

CASE 2-3. Close-up of a left craniocaudal view (kVp 27, mAs 104, compression 41 mm, Hologic unit).

What is the artifact? Is it correctable?

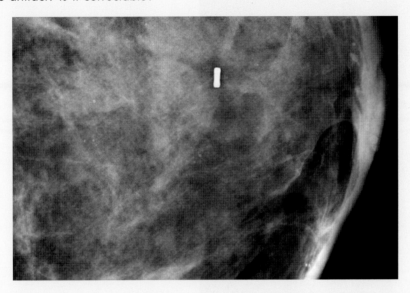

CASE 2-4. One of your technologists brings you this image and asks how to fix it.

What would you recommend?

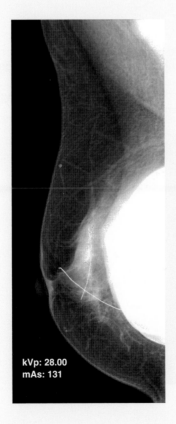

CASE 2-5. What is this artifact? Is it correctable?

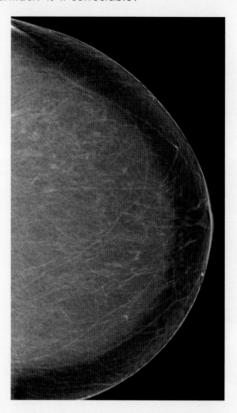

CASE 2-6. A 28-year-old woman presents with a palpable lump. Her health care professional thought it was probably a fibroadenoma. The technologist returns with this image.

Can we let her go? P.S.: The technologist loves scanning with compound imaging because the images are really pretty. What are your assessment and recommendation?

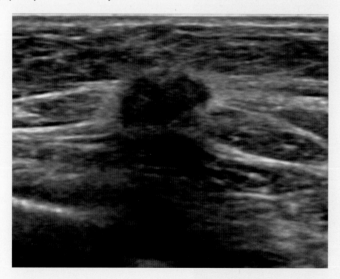

CASE 2-7. A 42-year-old woman with a palpable lump in the left breast.

What is your recommendation?

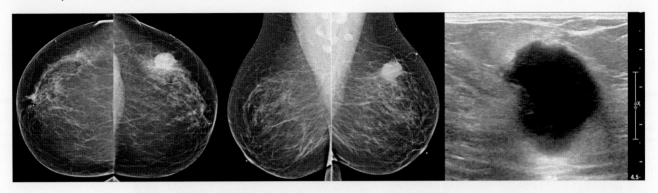

CASE 2-8. A patient is referred for aspiration and possible biopsy of the mass shown here.

What are the technical limitations of this image? How can they be corrected?

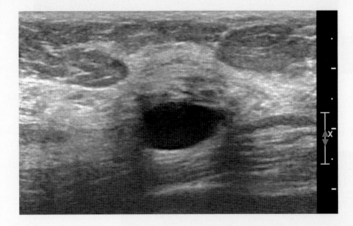

CASE 2-9. A 69-year-old woman is recalled from screening because of a mass in the lateral left breast (*arrow*). Your sonographer brings you the following ultrasound image and states that the finding is a cyst.

Do you agree? What do you recommend?

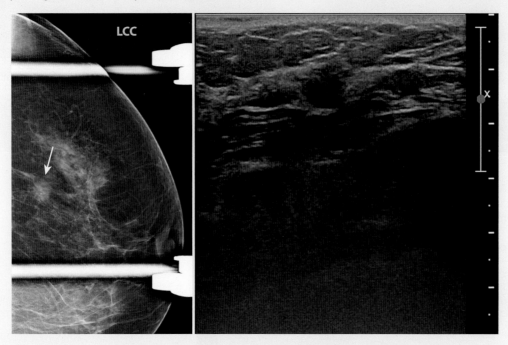

CASE 2-10. What is the artifact? Is it correctable?

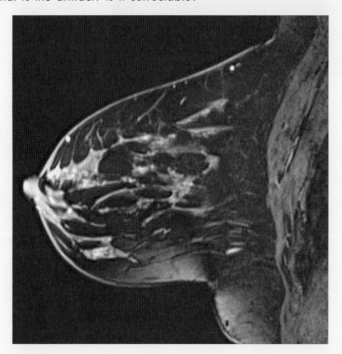

CASE 2-11. You have noticed that your breast MRI studies seem to be getting noisy. This is a close-up from one of your screening MRI patients.

What could the noise be due to?

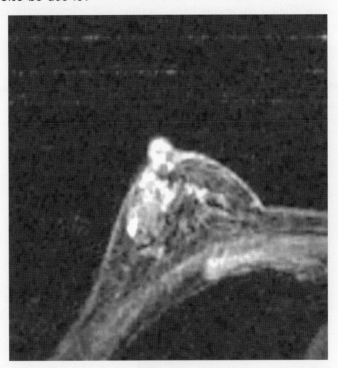

CASE 2-12. This is a screening MRI on a young woman at high risk for breast cancer. She has marked background parenchymal enhancement.

How can we adjust the parameters to reduce the coloring of the background parenchyma without changing the curve of the tissue at the indicator lines?

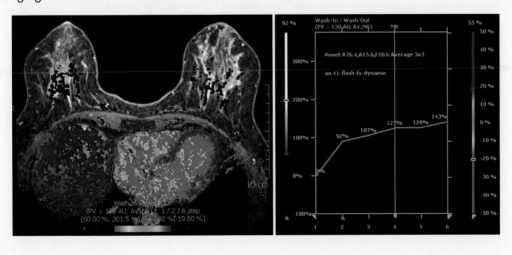

CASE 2-1. Did you notice the irregular edge at the skin line? The image is overexposed. A manual technique should be used for women with implants. It looks like the technologist may have accidentally used an automatic exposure. The repeat image here obtained with a lower exposure shows improved visualization of the subcutaneous tissues.

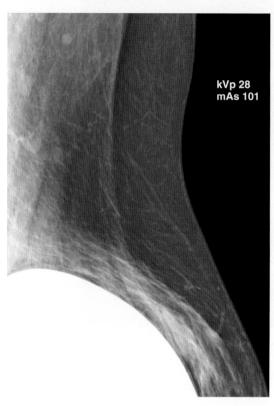

CASE 2-2. Faint gridlines are seen as fine horizontal dark lines extending across the image. The exposure is very low, not allowing the gridlines to blur. This artifact is probably not correctable for this patient.

CASE 2-3. Gridlines in the oblique plane are seen as dark lines going from the lower left corner to the upper right corner. Different manufacturers use different grids. This type of grid has a different appearance than gridlines on film-screen and GE digital units. In this case, the gridlines are due to a malfunctioning grid rather than low exposure, which is correctable. Here is the repeat image obtained after the machine was serviced.

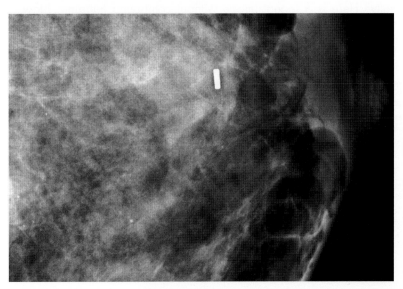

CASE 2-4. A manual technique was used because of the implant. The chosen technique is too low—the image is underexposed. The repeat image here was performed with a higher kVp, and the technique is now adequate.

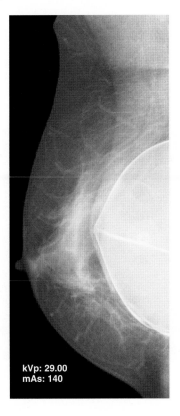

CASE 2-5. The outer edge of the breast is darker than the rest of the image. This "breast-within-a-breast" artifact is due to image processing and is not a correctable artifact.

CASE 2-6. Fibroadenoma? Really? Here is a repeat image without compound imaging. Now what do you think? What are your BI-RADS assessment and recommendation? Although fibroadenomas can occasionally demonstrate some posterior acoustic shadowing, this is quite a lot of shadowing, particularly for a fibroadenoma in a young woman. Did you notice the echogenic halo best seen with compound imaging? This is invasive ductal carcinoma.

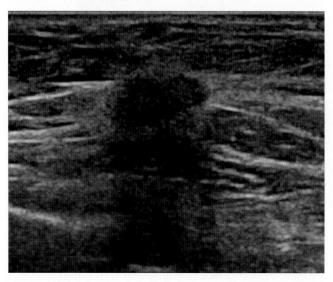

CASE 2-7. The round mass with ill-defined margins in the left breast corresponds to the palpable finding. On the ultrasound image, this appears to represent a cyst (and this is what the patient was told). However, the focal zone is a bit low, and the image was obtained with harmonic imaging. Here is a repeat ultrasound image obtained without compound or harmonic imaging, which shows a solid mass with duct extension. Biopsy showed invasive ductal carcinoma, grade III.

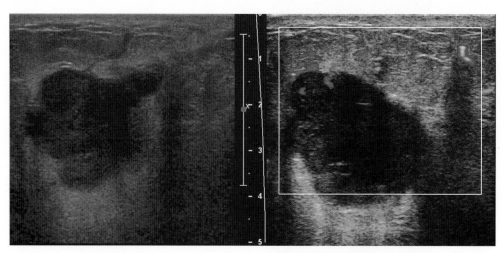

CASE 2-8. The gain setting is too high, and the focal zone is positioned a little too deep. There are artifactual echoes within the mass. The gain was adjusted and the focal zone centered on the finding. The resulting image shows the finding to be a simple cyst.

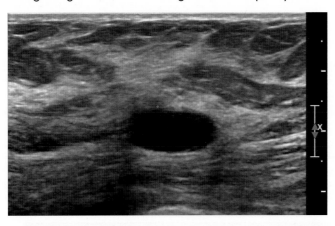

CASE 2-9. The technical limitations of the image do not permit adequate assessment of the lesion. The patient should be rescanned. The following adjustments should be made: depth, focal zone, and gain.

First, the depth should be decreased. There is no need to include the chest wall and lung. The focal zone should also be narrowed and centered on the lesion. Last, the time-gain curve should be adjusted so the fat lobules at all depths are the same shade of gray. Note how the superficial fat is more echogenic than the deep fat on the initial image. These adjustments are shown on the image here. Compound imaging was also used to increase contrast and enhance evaluation of the margins. The mass is shown to be solid and irregular in shape with spiculated margins. Biopsy revealed invasive ductal carcinoma and ductal carcinoma in situ.

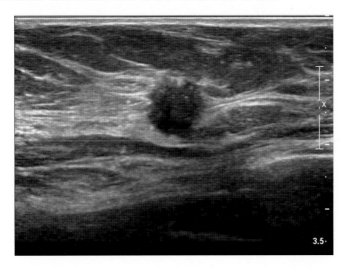

CASE 2-10. Do you notice the dark lines at the skin-fat and fat-tissue interfaces? This is chemical shift artifact. This looks like a marker was used to draw along the lines. This artifact is not uncommon and is relatively easy to correct by adjusting the bandwidth and ensuring that fat and water are both in-phase.

CASE 2-11. Did you notice the horizontal white lines? They are due to radiofrequency interference. This case is more subtle than when someone neglects to shut the door tightly. The artifact may be due to a leak in the door seal or electrical equipment nearby.

CASE 2-12. Let's increase the minimum threshold for color from 60% to 80% over baseline (*solid yellow arrow, yellow box*). Here are the results: Only the overall amount of color in the image has decreased. The shape and type of curve of the tissue at the indicator lines have not changed. The indicated area increased in enhancement by 55% over baseline (*open arrow*) on both images.

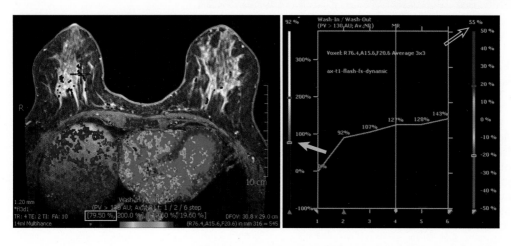

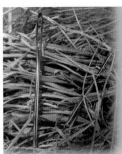

CHAPTER 3

Screening Mammography 101 and Beyond

You get on the elevator. The woman in the elevator smiles at you. The door closes. She clears her throat and says, "I know you don't remember me, but you saved my life." She's right—you don't recognize her. "You read my screening mammogram five years ago—and I'm doing great. I had a small cancer, and my lymph nodes were clear. Thank you for all that you do." You are blushing, but that just made your day!

Screening mammography is the most widely used modality for detecting breast cancer and the only one proven to reduce the mortality rate from the disease. Reading these studies, we have the chance to intervene in the natural history of a potentially fatal disease on behalf of the patient. It is a time when we can really make a difference in the life of an asymptomatic woman who feels fine. None of our other activities in breast imaging is more important.

You may recognize the names and faces of some of the women entering your mammography suite for screening. These are our colleagues, neighbors, teachers, and others who live in or near our community. They are willing to undergo the discomfort of mammography because they believe that our interpretation may provide them with the chance to have a malignancy diagnosed at a stage when cure is more likely. They are relying on us to be well trained, up to date, and free of distractions so that our attention and skills will be fully devoted to reading their mammograms.

If we are to make an impact on the breast cancer mortality rate in our local population of women, we need to be really good at interpreting screening mammograms. This assignment is unlike any other in radiology and requires different skills. We are trying to find those 3 to 8 cancers out of 1000 mammograms. Detection of those cancers can depend on perception of subtle mammographic changes that occur gradually over years. Lack of recall for a suspicious finding may be due to an error of perception (didn't see it) or judgment (saw it and dismissed it as benign). In about 15% of cases, cancers produce no detectable signs on screening.

There are several ways to improve screening performance. Small modifications in your group practice can help optimize screening. Developing a consistent approach to reading screening mammograms reduces the chance of cancers being overlooked. Greater familiarity with the more subtle presenting signs of breast cancer will increase the cancer detection rate. Learning about common errors in judgment can push up the cancer detection rate even more. Finally, monitoring the screening performance of the overall practice and of each individual radiologist provides feedback for continual improvement.

The Prerequisites: Optimizing Your Group Practice

Stratify Screening and Diagnostic Patients

From the patient's perspective, screening should require little time and effort. It should be convenient, quick, and performed in a pleasant environment. Providing screening facilities in the community rather than deep within the hospital increases the likelihood that women will be screened. Compliance with screening drops precipitously when the facility is more than 20 miles away, even if the test is free. Having dedicated screening facilities also allows for batch interpretation of studies. Once an abnormal finding is detected at screening, women will drive a hundred miles and even negotiate their way through your parking garage to get an answer.

Obtaining the Best Possible Images for Each Patient

A cancer can't be detected if it is excluded from the image or cannot be seen because of blur. Thankfully, the vast majority of technologists are dedicated and passionate about our patients. They want to provide excellent care and will work hard to obtain high-quality images. Review of Chapter 1, The First Question, will provide some tools for reviewing and optimizing mammographic techniques.

When patients are recalled because of a quality issue, the technologist should review the case to make it a learning experience. A detailed audit of image quality over a period of time can provide additional specific feedback for improvement. Review quality recalls by technologist, reason (blur, positioning, other), and view. One technologist may have difficulty getting enough depth on the right craniocaudal (CC) view. Another technologist may have difficulty identifying blur (time for new glasses...). Bringing in an expert in mammographic positioning to work with your technologists every few years is a good investment.

Finally, happy technologists and staff equal happy patients. Happy patients are relaxed so they are easier to position and will also be more likely to return for annual mammography. Put staff satisfaction on the agenda for discussion at group meetings. Your staff should know that they are highly valued and that their job satisfaction is important to the radiologists and management.

Having the Right Equipment

Investing in digital mammography has had a positive impact on the quality of our practices. It has higher sensitivity and specificity than film-screen mammography for women who have dense tissue, are premenopausal, or are under age 50. Digital mammography also improves workflow and makes it easier to compare with previous mammograms.

We also recommend using computer-aided detection (CAD), which is easily integrated into the workflow using digital systems. If you take the approach of using any available information to help find cancers, the decision to use CAD is easy. Why not make use of technology that reportedly marks over 80% of screening cancers and may increase screening cancer detection by over 19%? Although the results of studies for CAD are mixed, we all have days when we are tired or distracted. CAD is especially great for marking malignant calcifications.

Digital breast tomosynthesis (DBT) is an application of digital mammography with the first commercial unit receiving Food and Drug Administration (FDA) approval in 2011. With DBT, the x-ray tube moves through an arc and multiple low-dose exposures are obtained at different angles. The data are then reconstructed into multiple tomographic images that are reviewed by scrolling through the images on a workstation. The tomosynthesis images are frequently obtained with a conventional digital mammogram (dual acquisition). This technology is intended to overcome the two major limitations of mammography: false-positive findings caused by overlapping normal and benign structures, and false-negative studies caused by obscuration of cancers by normal tissues. Tomosynthesis appears to be of greatest value in detecting and evaluating soft tissue density findings (masses, asymmetries, focal asymmetries, and architectural distortion), particularly for women with dense tissue.

The clinical use of DBT is evolving. DBT is associated with a significant reduction in recall rate of 40% to 60%. In one study, the recall rate for DBT and mammography was 4.9% compared with a rate of 11.9% for mammography alone. Between the two groups, this study found similar recall rates for masses and calcifications but a significantly lower (1.8% vs. 8.2%) recall rate for asymmetries within the DBT group. A recent prospective study of a screened population compared the performance of digital mammography alone with digital mammography and DBT. This study showed that the addition of DBT resulted in a significantly higher cancer detection rate—especially of invasive cancers—together with a decrease in the rate of false-positive findings. It therefore seems that DBT is particularly suited for use in the screening setting.

Who Reads the Screens?

High-volume readers generally have higher sensitivity and specificity for screening mammography. Ideally, each radiologist should read at least 1000 screening mammograms

per year. In medium-size to large group practices, a subset of radiologists can be identified to batch-read screening studies. This approach is preferred over one that has more radiologists reading fewer studies. Radiologists who read screening mammograms should also see diagnostic patients and perform breast biopsy. The feedback from seeing which recalled patients are subsequently dismissed, which are recommended for biopsy, and correlating the imaging findings with pathologic findings provides the basis for continuing improvement.

Batch Versus Online Interpretation

The practice of interpreting screening mammograms in batches and recalling patients as needed for diagnostic evaluation is much more efficient than interpreting studies "online" and performing diagnostic studies during the same appointment. Batch interpretation also benefits your patients by reducing the recall rate and increasing the cancer detection rate, including the percentage of minimal and early-stage cancers. On the other hand, if your patient has limited mobility, drove hours to have her mammogram, has difficulty with transportation, or may not reliably return for recall, then an immediate reading may improve patient compliance.

Optimizing the Reading Environment

"Time to read the screens" means different things to different radiologists. For some it means it's time for a caffeine boost. For others it's time to put on the headphones. Whatever your personal routine, keep in mind that the mammographic signs of malignancy can be difficult to detect in even the best of conditions, and that surrounding influences in the workspace can affect the quality and efficiency of interpretation.

The optimal setting is a darkened quiet room where screening studies are reviewed in batches and reported with few interruptions. Let those emails on your smartphone wait until later. Minimize disruptive background noise. Your eyes will be at their best when background lights and computer screens are directed away from the workstation monitors and your line of sight. Computer monitors or view boxes placed away from or at a 90-degree angle to the workstation monitors minimize the effects of extraneous light.

Focus Equals Efficiency

Is your practice concerned about the efficiency of the radiologists? Whose isn't these days! Getting into the screening mindset by batch reading and minimizing distractions focuses the radiologist on finding cancers. Getting through a worklist of screens can be very efficient with this mindset.

Learn to manage your interruptions. Interpretation of screening mammograms involves holding a visual image of a tissue pattern or questioned abnormality in mind and relating it to findings on other images as you go through the study. Let's say that you have opened a screening study and notice a small asymmetry in the medial left breast. You keep that image in your mind while you are reviewing the rest of the study to see if it's also on the mediolateral oblique (MLO) view and on prior mammograms. Now let's say your technologist interrupts you in the middle and asks you to check a specimen radiograph. Do you finish the case first? Do you check the specimen and go back to where you left off? Or do you start over after you check the specimen radiograph? When you are interrupted (and you will be!), it is difficult if not impossible to remember the appearance of that asymmetry in the medial left breast. For this reason, when you are interrupted, either complete the current case first or start the whole case over after you address the issue.

Managing paperwork, preparing cases for interpretation, requesting outside studies and other patient information, and hanging and taking down analog images are functions best left to other personnel. Use of templates in voice recognition programs increases efficiency and reduces reporting errors. Standardized reporting using specific breast imaging reporting software further increases efficiency and retains data in a computerized tracking system for the medical audit.

Screening 101: Approach to Screening

Reviewing the History

Before interpreting the images, review the information provided by the technologist for history that may affect your interpretation or your callback threshold. Note any risk factors, such as a personal or family history of breast cancer. If the patient has a history of lumpectomy or benign surgery, review the location of any scars.

Occasionally, during an appointment for screening mammography, the patient will inform the technologist that she has noticed a recent change, such as a palpable finding, bloody nipple discharge, or nipple changes. The referring provider may not yet be aware of the new concern. The technologist should record this information, and it should also be described in your report. When we become aware of potentially significant new history, we schedule the patient for diagnostic evaluation.

Image Interpretation and Comparison

Establishing a systematic approach for reviewing mammograms and comparing with prior studies improves consistency and efficiency of interpretation. Current workstations for digital mammography permit great flexibility in image "hanging" protocols and sequencing of images for review. The specifics of the protocol details are a matter of personal preference; however, they should include review of all images in their entirety on high-resolution monitors, at full-pixel resolution, with enlargement or magnification.

An example of a review protocol for digital mammography is shown in Figure 3-1. Whether you use our

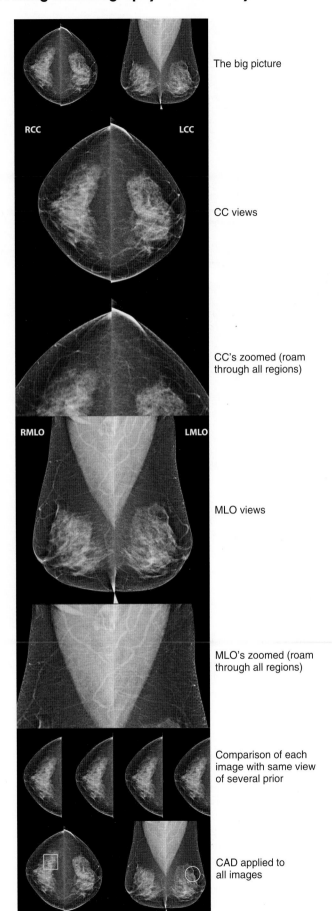

FIGURE 3-1 **A Review Protocol for Digital Mammography.** Example of a sequence reviewing and comparing digital screening mammograms on a two-monitor workstation.

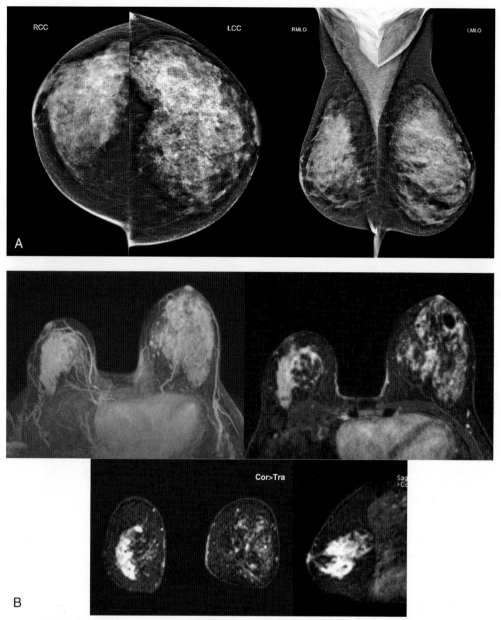

FIGURE 3-2 **Asymmetry in Breast Size at Overview. A,** Screening mammogram of a 45-year-old woman shows asymmetry in breast size, with the right breast considerably smaller than the left. The asymmetry was new since her previous mammograms. **B,** Postcontrast magnetic resonance imaging (maximum intensity projection, axial, coronal, and sagittal images) shows the asymmetry in size and also reveals extensive nonmass enhancement in the lateral right breast. Diagnosis: invasive lobular carcinoma (ILC) in the right breast.

protocol or a different one, it should be used consistently for every case. Our approach can be adapted for the interpretation of film-screen mammograms, using a hand-held magnifying glass rather than digital magnification.

Interpretation begins with an overview of the current images in mirror-image display. In this step, look for findings that may be more obvious from a distance than close up, such as asymmetry of breast size and density, masses, suspicious tissue contours, axillary lesions, and skin or nipple abnormalities (Figs. 3-2 and 3-3). More subtle findings may also be detected on the big-picture overview.

Next, carefully review zoomed images, covering all regions of the breasts on all views, searching for, yes, calcifications, but also for subtle masses, asymmetries, and architectural distortion. Closely examine any findings detected on the big-picture overview. Assess the borders of the fibroglandular tissue and examine the adjacent fat. Adjust contrast and brightness as needed to optimize evaluation of different regions.

Comparison with prior studies is often needed to determine whether a finding on the current study is significant. Some findings, such as developing asymmetries or changes in the tissue contour, may resemble normal fibroglandular

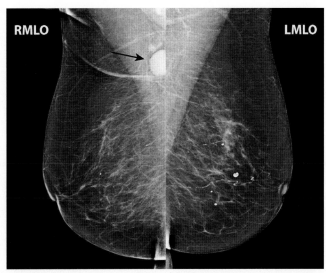

FIGURE 3-3 Screening-Detected Adenopathy. Screening mammogram on a 78-year-old woman reveals an enlarged, dense lymph node in the right axilla (*arrow*). This finding can be easily appreciated on the case overview. Biopsy revealed previously unsuspected non-Hodgkin lymphoma.

tissue on the current study and only be recognized as abnormal by the changes that have occurred. Stability on comparison also allows us to disregard many questioned findings.

Compare with mammograms from at least 2 years prior; even longer-term comparison may be helpful in many cases. Sometimes an apparent change from the most recent mammograms is simply due to differences in positioning that will be replicated on an earlier mammogram. In other cases, it may become more obvious that a finding is developing when comparison is made with several older mammograms. Availability of prior digital studies makes it easier to compare the current image with the corresponding previous ones in the same orientation, which can be helpful in detecting subtle changes.

Comparing images is an active process. Identify and compare specific findings, such as masses, calcifications, asymmetries, and lymph nodes with concerning features. Also compare the tissue pattern and contours in different regions (Fig. 3-4). If nipple retraction is present, see whether it is stable mammographically. Malignant findings may appear stable over years. Just because your colleague called it normal last year doesn't mean that the finding is benign!

Finding Cancers Where They Live and Hide

Masses and asymmetries in any region of the breast may represent malignancy. However, there are certain regions where these findings deserve your particular attention for a number of reasons. Cancers in these regions are more likely to be visible on only a single view or to be obscured by normal tissues. They may occur in areas where soft tissue density findings do not commonly develop, and should therefore be viewed with higher

suspicion (Fig. 3-5). These regions include the axilla (see Fig. 3-3), retroglandular fat (Fig. 3-6), medial breast (Fig. 3-7), inferior breast (Fig. 3-8), apex of the fibroglandular tissue (Fig. 3-9), and subareolar region (Fig. 3-10).

Screening 201: Pushing Up the Cancer Detection Rate

Expand Your Breast Cancer Encyclopedia

Early in training, residents learn the classic mammographic signs of breast cancer. However, only 39% of screening-detected cancers present with classically malignant findings. As the resident sits with the attending, he or she realizes that finding early cancers requires recognition of more subtle and less specific signs, such as asymmetries and architectural distortion. (For more information on these topics, please refer to Chapters 9 and 10.) Suddenly, the resident starts marking every little dot on the mammogram for recall. The attending smiles and says, "Cancer doesn't look like that. That's normal tissue." How does the attending know what to recall and what to leave alone? Through years of experience, attendings have acquired a really big encyclopedia of the imaging appearances of breast cancer.

Familiarity with the varied appearances of malignancy is essential to increasing cancer detection on mammography. Finding breast cancer is like looking for a familiar face in a crowd. Our eyes quickly scan over the crowd with an image of the person in mind. When our eyes cast over the familiar face, recognition is usually instantaneous. We don't search consciously for individual features, such as facial bone structure or hair color; we recognize the person who embodies a composite of these features. The more people we know in the crowd, the more faces we will recognize.

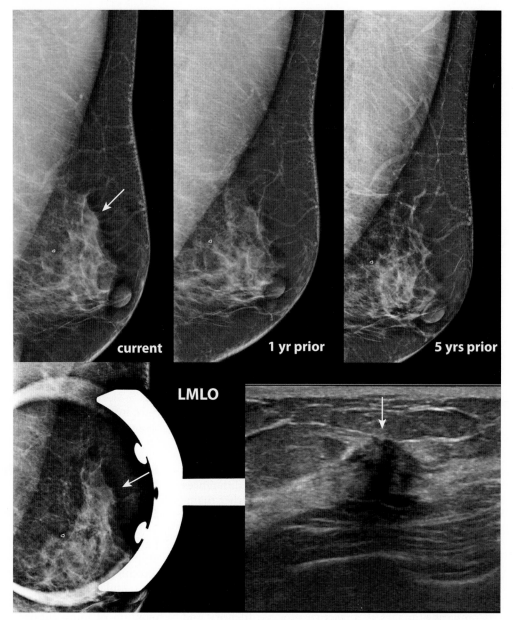

FIGURE 3-4 **Screening-Detected Change in Tissue Contour due to ILC.** Screening mammogram on a 57-year-old woman. The clip is from previous benign biopsy. There is new convex protrusion ("*speed bump*") at the border of the fibroglandular tissue (*arrow*). This finding persists on a spot compression view, and US shows an irregular hypoechoic mass mostly within the echogenic fibroglandular tissue, with its margin extending into the adjacent fat (*arrows*).

There is evidence that the same is true in detecting the many faces of cancer on screening mammograms. Kundel and colleagues evaluated search time and gaze tracking during analysis of a series of mammograms, half with subtle malignant findings. They found evidence for a very rapid holistic process for detecting and analyzing subtle signs of malignancy that was most highly developed among the more proficient observers. Less experienced observers relied more heavily on a search-to-find approach, which was slower and associated with more errors. These observers were less likely to detect malignant findings on rapid holistic review and also less likely to recognize the significance of the malignant findings that were detected. As we become more familiar with the subtle presentations of malignancy, our eyes will be increasingly drawn to them.

How do we gain experience recognizing these subtle findings? Look at every breast cancer that you can! Every

time that you read a mammogram on a patient who has had breast cancer, pull up the mammograms from the time of her diagnosis. And then, if you *really* want to see what early breast cancer looks like, pull up the mammograms from a year or 2 before that. It is common to see some evidence of the cancer on preceding mammograms. It doesn't mean that your colleagues made a mistake, but it will help you burn those faces of cancer into your brain. Use of educational materials that demonstrate numerous case images of malignancies will also accelerate the learning process. Adding these images to your repertoire of the signs of malignant lesions will make it easier to recognize similar findings as they are encountered prospectively.

It is also important to become very familiar with the mammographic appearance of findings that do not represent cancer. Performing diagnostic mammography in addition to screening builds experience with the varied

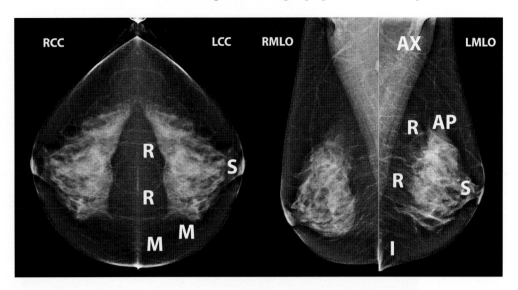

M	Medial breast	Normal asymmetric tissue uncommon; may be excluded from MLO view.
AX	Axillary region	Axillary mass may be mistaken for normal lymph node; density of pectoralis muscle may make lesions less conspicuous.
I	Inferior posterior breast	May be excluded from CC view.
AP	Apex of fibroglandular tissue	Overlapping dense tissue can obscure lesion.
R	Retroglandular fat	Normal asymmetric tissue uncommon; common location for missed cancer.
S	Subareolar	Complex anatomy with overlapping ducts; nipple not in profile may cause confusion; compression may be less than other regions; mammography less sensitive in this region.

FIGURE 3-5 **Living in the Wrong Neighborhood.** Masses and asymmetries in certain regions of the breast deserve special scrutiny.

appearance of normal tissue patterns and will also aid in the recognition of findings where those patterns are altered. Practices where radiologists read only screens are at a disadvantage because they do not get the benefit of working up findings and learning which are normal and which require biopsy.

Balancing the Decision to Recall

Reading screening mammograms is all about the odds. How likely is a finding to represent cancer? Radiologists understand that over 99% of screening mammograms will *not* reveal cancer. How do we know if we're calling back too few or too many patients?

In the past, the recommended callback rate was a number specifying an upper limit of acceptability, usually 10%. In 2010, Carney and associates defined an acceptable callback *range* of 5% to 12%. Establishing a lower limit acknowledges that recalling fewer than 5% of patients makes it very difficult to detect and diagnose many of the more subtle malignancies that present with less specific findings. The emphasis is usually placed on how to lower the recall rate, and that is important.

However, a low recall rate is unimportant if the cancer detection rate is low. Both recall rate and cancer detection rate should be looked at together to assess performance.

The highest priority in screening is to establish a high cancer detection rate. Recently trained radiologists often need support early in practice to gain experience and develop effective practice habits. Early on, these radiologists tend take longer to interpret cases and recall a higher percentage of patients than radiologists with more experience. This is to be expected, and usually, as experience is gained, efficiency increases and the callback rate decreases. Findings to consider for recall are summarized in Box 3-1.

"Is that anything? Should I call her back for THAT?" How many times have you had that conversation with yourself? So here you are reading the screening mammograms in a nice, dark, quiet room. You may have already called back several women in a session and want to avoid recalling too many. You may be looking at a vague one-view asymmetry or possible area of distortion. It may be late in the day, and you may be tired. And most of us have a natural tendency to hope that a patient will not have cancer. Although it is understandable to consider all

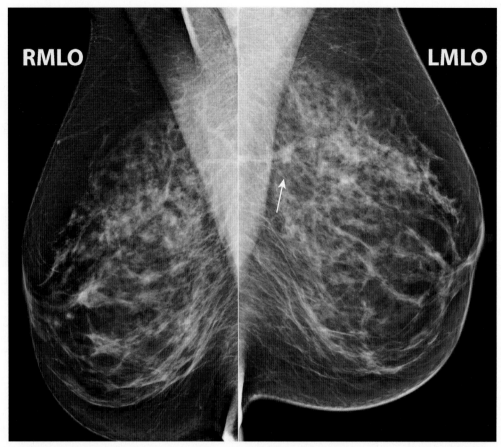

FIGURE 3-6 **Cancer in the Retroglandular Fat.** Screening mammogram on a 54-year-old woman reveals a one-view asymmetry in the retroglandular fat of the left breast. Diagnostic evaluation confirmed a mass in this region. Diagnosis: invasive ductal carcinoma (IDC) and ductal carcinoma in situ (DCIS).

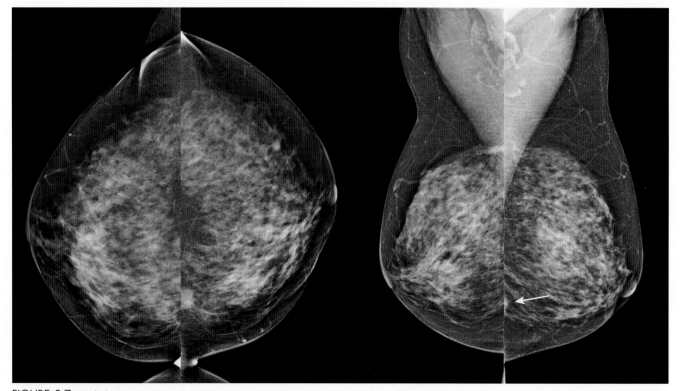

FIGURE 3-7 **Medial Mass Representing IDC.** Screening mammogram on a 55-year-old woman with a history of right breast carcinoma shows a mass in the posterior medial left breast. This is only partially included on the MLO view (*arrow*).

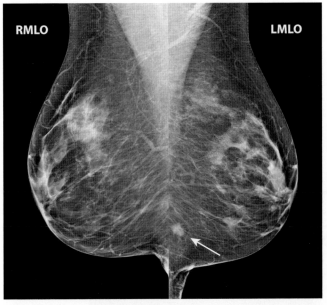

FIGURE 3-8 **Cancer in the Inferior Breast.** Initial screening mammogram of a 49-year-old woman shows a dense irregular mass in the posterior inferior left breast. Diagnosis: IDC.

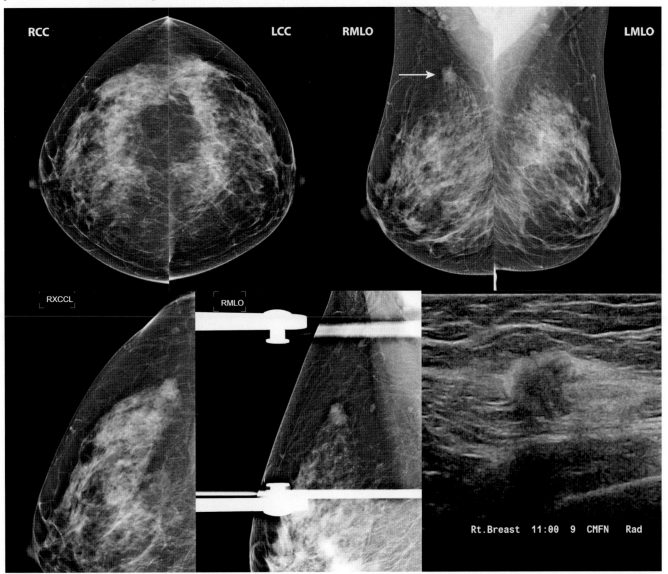

FIGURE 3-9 **Cancer at the Apex of the Fibroglandular Tissue.** Screening mammogram on a 48-year-old woman shows a suspected mass in the superior right breast visible on the MLO view only (*arrow*). An irregular mass with spiculated margins is confirmed on exaggerated CC and spot compression MLO views and ultrasonography. Diagnosis: IDC.

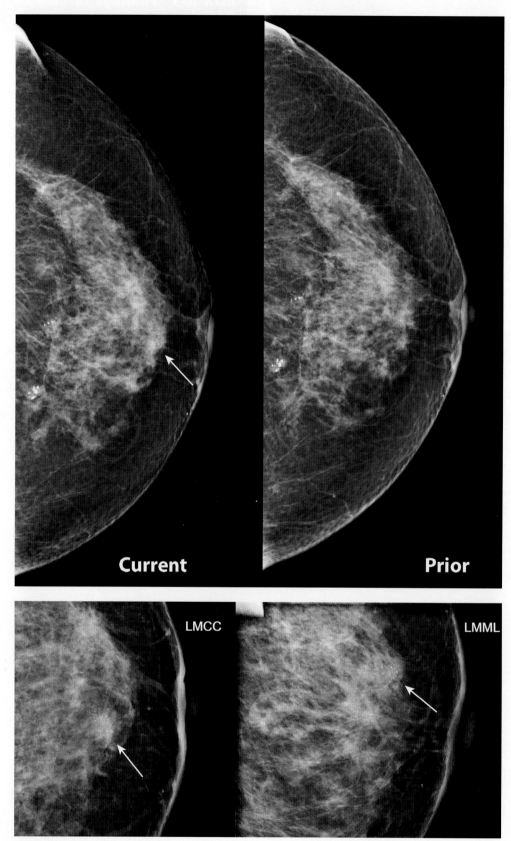

FIGURE 3-10 **Subareolar Cancer.** Screening CC view of a 64-year-old woman shows a developing asymmetry with calcifications in the retroareolar region of the left breast (*arrow*). There are two additional clusters of coarse heterogeneous calcifications in the posterior third of the breast that were stable. Magnification views show clustered fine pleomorphic calcifications with an associated focal asymmetry in the subareolar region (*arrows*). Diagnosis: IDC and DCIS.

of these factors, they should not influence your decision about whether to recall an individual patient! Remember that the inconvenience of recalling a patient cannot be compared with a missed chance to diagnose a potentially curable cancer.

So what can we do in these situations? Compare with as many previous mammograms as needed. Ask your colleague's opinion. See if it's marked by CAD. Forget about the last three callbacks. And make a decision. What if you still can't decide? Or if you decide to let it go but then have second thoughts? Deciding not to recall a patient should not be a difficult decision. If you find yourself wrestling with the pros and cons of recalling a patient or being influenced by factors unrelated to the specific case, do yourself and the patient a favor. Call her back!

Screening 301: Understanding How We Miss Cancers

At some point, every driver has accidentally run a red light and driven straight through an intersection without stopping. It may be that the light was hard to see because of sun in your eyes or perhaps there was only a flashing yellow light there before. Maybe you misjudged the timing of the traffic signal. There are patterns to our errors that also apply to breast cancer detection. (Just *please* don't say that you were texting!)

Overlooked Cancer

We have all overlooked cancer. And we do mean "we." Breast cancer is sly. It hides among multiple masses. It's in the opposite breast from where you just found a cancer. It's in the typical location for a lymph node. Cancers are also more difficult to detect when the tissue is dense or when there are multiple or distracting findings.

Dense Tissue
The sensitivity of mammography is reduced in women with dense tissue and cancers are more likely to be missed. Many cancers can still be detected in these women, although the findings are often quite subtle. For a review of the mammographic findings of malignancy in women with dense tissue and an approach to interpreting these studies, please refer to Chapter 12.

Distracting Lesions
Did you notice the second needle in the hay in the image at the beginning of this chapter? Distracting lesions are a leading cause for missing cancers that present as either masses or calcifications. When reading a case with an obvious finding, we need to be careful to avoid the pitfall of satisfaction of search. This is a phenomenon in which the detection of one finding reduces our chance of detecting or recognizing the significance of one or more additional findings. When one abnormality is identified, disregard it for the moment and continue to complete your search routine. Once all of the images of both

breasts have been completely reviewed, return to the initial finding and analyze it in detail.

When one lesion has been detected, we may be reluctant to recommend diagnostic evaluation of a second or third potentially suspicious finding. None of us wants to appear to be going overboard by recommending a "mega-workup," but sometimes it is necessary to fully evaluate the patient.

Multiple Findings
When interpreting cases with multiple masses or extensive calcifications, not only can the multiple findings be distracting, but it can also be tempting to jump to the conclusion that all of the findings are benign based on the rule of multiplicity—even before they have been thoroughly examined (Fig. 3-11). In these cases, we need to search for the lesion that appears different from the others. Please see Chapter 8, Multiple Masses, for more information on this topic.

Misjudged Cancer

In this case, we see the cancer but then dismiss it. These are errors of judgment rather than lack of perception of the finding. Breast cancer may be located right where the patient had a benign surgical biopsy 5 years ago. Or maybe it doesn't look that different from last year. When a finding catches your eye, look closely and don't jump to conclusions.

One-View Findings
It can be tempting to disregard a finding because it is seen on only a single view. However, asymmetries and other one-view findings can represent early signs of breast cancer. When a potentially suspicious finding is seen on only one view, diagnostic evaluation is often warranted if the finding could have been excluded from the second view or obscured by tissue (Fig. 3-12).

Change Is Due to Positioning or Technique
Maybe it is, but you need to be sure. In this case, pull back older studies to see if the area had a similar appearance on a prior mammogram. If not, recall may be needed.

Looks Like a Scar
Architectural distortion from postsurgical scarring decreases over time. Comparison with older studies is very helpful. Most benign scars have little or no distortion after 5 to 10 years. See Chapters 9 and 18 to find tips on evaluating architectural distortion and the postsurgical breast.

History of Trauma
Although trauma can result in bruising and fat necrosis, the findings of distortion or a mass that is not an oil cyst is very uncommon. If the finding is not clearly due to trauma, very short-term follow-up (2 to 3 months) will often show partial or complete resolution. If not, biopsy may be indicated.

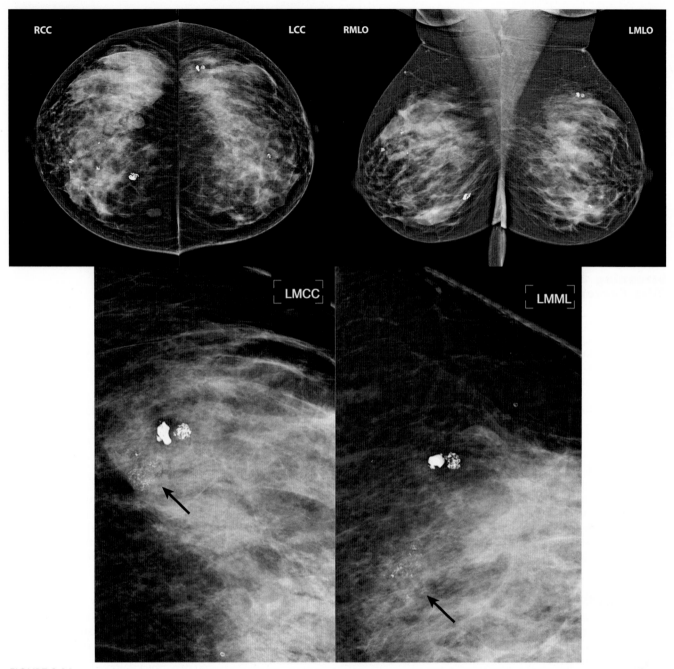

FIGURE 3-11 **Not Another Degenerating Fibroadenoma.** This 41-year-old woman was recalled from screening because of new coarse heterogeneous calcifications (*arrows*). It would be easy to assume that these represent yet another degenerating fibroadenoma like her other benign calcifications. Diagnosis: DCIS, high-grade.

It's Stable

Some cancers grow slowly over time. Comparison with studies that are at least 2 years old is standard, but sometimes even older studies are needed. Comparing with older studies may make a suspicious change more obvious or increase your confidence that a lesion is truly stable or decreasing in size (Fig. 3-13).

Prior Benign Core Biopsy

Core biopsy is a great test; the sensitivity is about 98%. Unfortunately, this means that a few women now and then will have a cancer that is missed at core biopsy. A

cancer unrelated to the previously biopsied lesion may also develop in the same region. If there is an interval change, such as enlargement of a mass or increase in calcifications, repeat core biopsy or excisional biopsy may be indicated (Fig. 3-14). Even if the lesion is unchanged but the finding is suspicious and was not explained by the prior biopsy, further evaluation may be needed.

Prior Negative Workup

Your colleague saw that same spot last year. The workup was negative, but it still catches your eye. Look closely

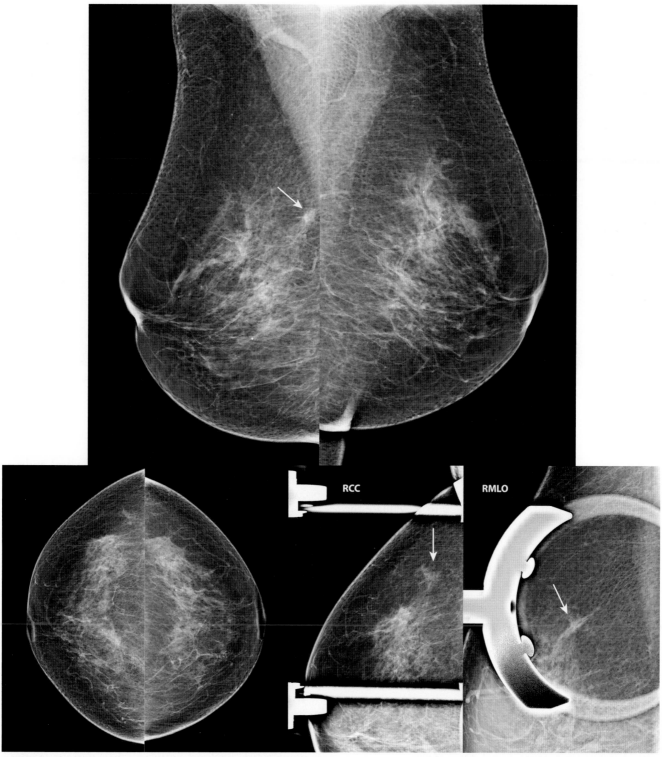

FIGURE 3-12 **Carcinoma Presenting as One-View Asymmetry.** Screening mammogram on a 69-year-old woman shows asymmetry in the retro-glandular fat on the MLO view (*arrow*). A corresponding finding is not clearly seen on the CC view. On spot compression views the lesion persisted as a focal asymmetry in the lateral breast. Biopsy revealed ILC.

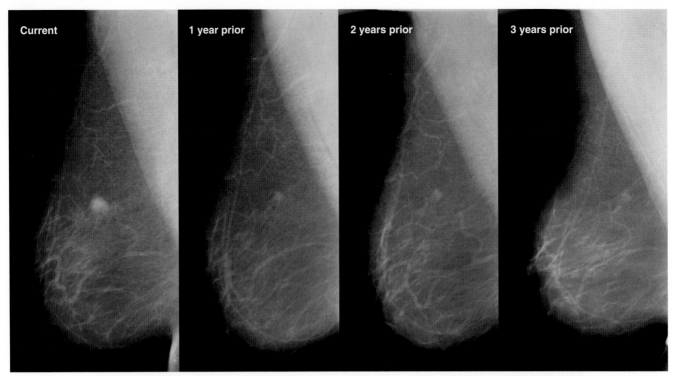

| Current | 1 year prior | 2 years prior | 3 years prior |

FIGURE 3-13 **It's Not Actually Stable.** On the prior mammograms taken over 3 years, the mass in the superior breast showed little change. The cancer was not diagnosed until it had clearly enlarged. This is not uncommon for IDC, grade I. The good news: she was still node negative.

at the current images and the previous diagnostic images and ultrasound study, if one was performed. Compare with multiple previous mammograms. If there is still any question in your mind, bring her back to reevaluate the finding (Fig. 3-15).

Is It Really a Lymph Node?

Small masses overlying the pectoralis muscle on the MLO view or in the upper outer quadrant may look like a normal lymph node at first glance. However, if it is dense or round, if there is no fatty hilum, or if the margins are ill-defined, it may not represent a lymph node and recall may be indicated, especially if it is new or larger than on previous studies (Fig. 3-16). When a lymph node that previously appeared normal enlarges or becomes more round and dense, it may represent adenopathy from occult breast cancer or be associated with extramammary disease (Fig. 3-17).

Final Examination: Find Out How You're Doing and Adjust As Needed

The Medical Audit

So how are we doing? Gulp. Feedback can be hard, but in reality we're fortunate to have it. If we use the information to see where we stand individually and as a practice, the data can suggest specific adjustments that can significantly improve our individual and practice

performance. So instead of viewing the medical audit as an onerous event, think of it as your personal guide to becoming a better screener—or as objective confirmation that your performance is already where you want it to be.

To fulfill the requirements of the U.S. Food and Drug Administration Mammography Quality Standards Act (MQSA), a limited medical audit and outcome analysis is performed at least every 12 months. Each facility must identify and follow-up patients with positive mammograms, have a system for attempting to obtain pathology results for all biopsies, have a method for correlating pathology results with the final assessment category, and review the medical outcome audit data for the aggregate of interpreting physicians as well as for each individual physician.

To obtain the most useful information on the performance of a screening mammography program, we need to go beyond the minimum requirements. Analysis of screening data is simplified and enhanced by the use of computerized tracking software that permits analysis of data for screening mammography separately from diagnostic data. The cancer detection rate will be overestimated if screening and diagnostic mammography data are combined. We suggest investing in tracking software and designating personnel to obtain pathology reports and other information needed to keep the tracking database current. High-quality tracking data provide a powerful tool for evaluating a practice and guiding changes needed to improve performance. It permits detailed

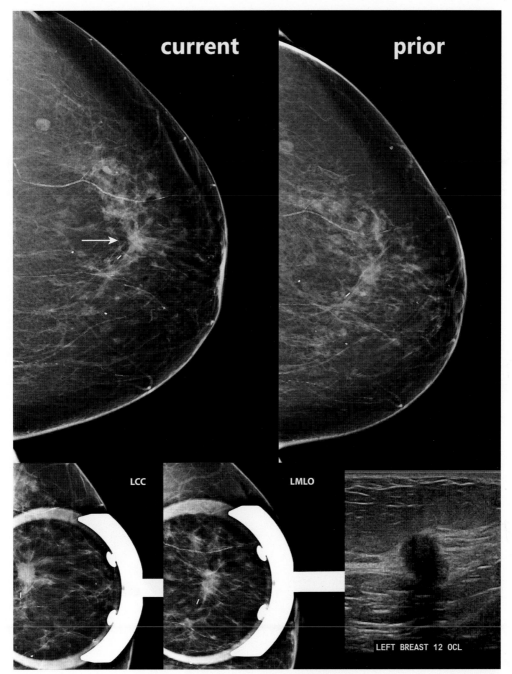

FIGURE 3-14 **Change After Core Biopsy.** Screening CC view of a 69-year-old woman. She has a history of successful stereotactic biopsy of left breast calcifications 4 years prior with benign pathologic findings. Mammography now shows new spiculation near the clip. Spot compression views and ultrasonography confirm a spiculated mass. Diagnosis: IDC with DCIS.

comparison of individual and practice performance with published benchmarks. If mammography volume is low, cumulative data and combined data from multiple sites can increase the statistical power of the analysis.

So how do I know where I stand and if I need to improve? Carney and associates (2010) published an important paper outlining minimally acceptable performance criteria for screening mammography (Table 3-1). The authors decided on cut points for these criteria

with the understanding that radiologists whose performance data did not meet the performance thresholds would be recommended to consider additional training. Incorporating performance thresholds such as these into the audit is useful in identifying radiologists for whom additional education and training should be considered.

Even if you've been reading mammograms for a while, directed feedback can be really helpful. Look at the big

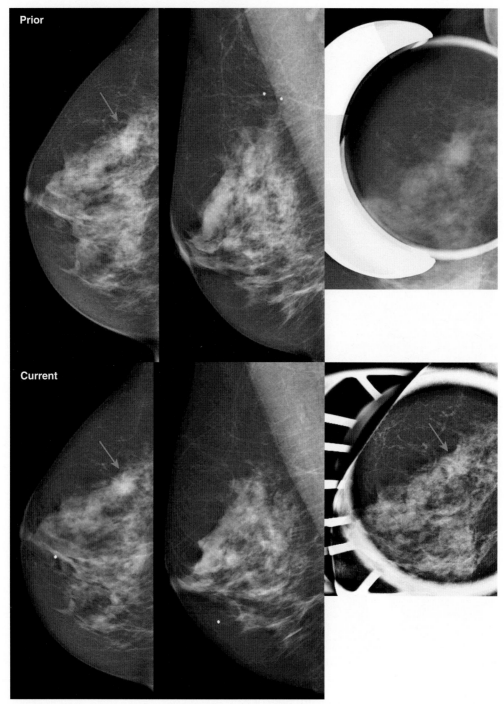

FIGURE 3-15 **Workup Was Negative/Benign Last Year.** This patient was recalled the prior year because of a one-view asymmetry (*arrow*). The finding was thought not to persist and US was negative. On the current study, the finding remains concerning. Architectural distortion is now apparent on the spot compression view. US confirmed a suspicious mass at 9 o'clock. Biopsy showed ILC.

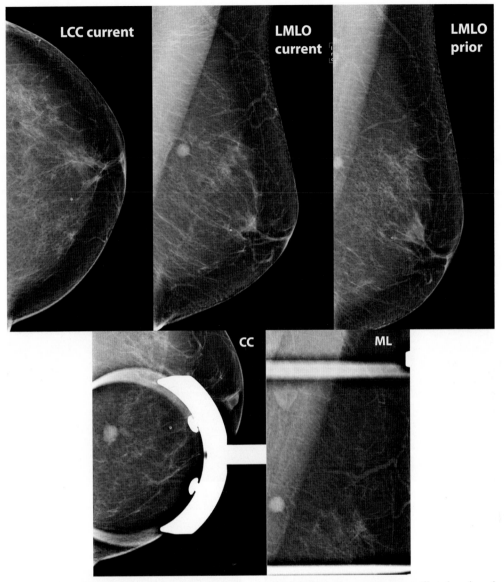

FIGURE 3-16 **It's Not a Lymph Node.** Although the location and shape on the screening views suggest an axillary lymph node, closer inspection shows that the mass is round, does not have a fatty hilum, and has an ill-defined margin. On diagnostic imaging, the mass is not located in the axilla, but actually is in the upper inner quadrant. Diagnosis: IDC.

picture: your cancer detection rate, positive predictive value (PPV), and recall rate. Then dig in to the finer details. Look at the percentage of cancers that are minimal (<1 cm), ductal carcinoma in situ (DCIS), and cancers that were masses versus calcifications, and compare yourself to your partners.

Not finding as many cancers as you would like? Build that encyclopedia of the faces of cancer. Have your breast imaging colleagues second-read your screens for a while and give you feedback. It doesn't have to be every day or every case. Do you find a lot of those small invasive cancers but not very many calcifications that are DCIS? You may need to lower your threshold for recalling calcifications. Read a couple of book chapters on calcifications. Do you have a high cancer detection rate but also a really high recall rate? Get someone in your practice to overread your recalls to help you become more confident in deciding which findings can be let go.

It's well known that there are significant differences in interpretive performance among practices and that much of this variability is due to differences among individual radiologists. Routine analysis of practice data will identify those radiologists who are less successful in detecting screening cancers than their colleagues. If additional education and training of these individuals were to result in the detection of one or two more screening cancers per thousand, the positive impact on women's health would be substantial (Box 3-2).

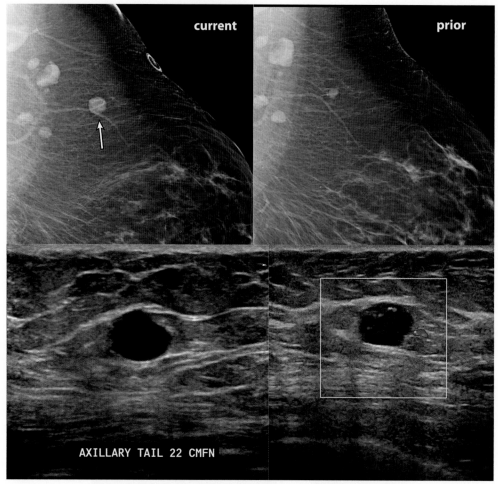

FIGURE 3-17 **Enlarging Lymph Node.** Screening MLO view of the left breast shows enlargement of one lymph node (*arrow*) that previously appeared normal. This node was markedly hypoechoic on US with flow demonstrated on color Doppler. Core biopsy revealed previously unsuspected non-Hodgkin lymphoma.

TABLE 3-1   Minimally Acceptable Performance Criteria for Screening Mammography

MEASURE	LOW PERFORMANCE THRESHOLD
Sensitivity (%)	<75
Specificity (%)	<88 or >95
Recall rate (%)	<5 or >12
PPV1 (%)*	<3 or >8
PPV2 (%)†	<20 or >40
Cancer detection rate (per 1000)	<2.5

*Proportion of all women with positive screening mammograms (BI-RADS Category 0, 4, or 5) who are diagnosed with breast cancer.
†Proportion of all women with positive screening mammograms (BI-RADS Category 0, 4, or 5) and a recommendation for biopsy at the end of imaging workup (BI-RADS Category 4 or 5) who are diagnosed with breast cancer.
From Carney PA, Sickles EA, Monsees BS, et al. Identifying minimally acceptable interpretive performance criteria for screening mammography. Radiology 2010;255:354-361.
BI-RADS, Breast Imaging Reporting and Data System; PPV1, PPV2, positive predictive values 1 and 2.

BOX 3-2   Be a Better Screener

- Optimize your group practice for screening
- Read both screening and diagnostic mammograms
- Read at least 1000 screening mammograms per year
- Ask other radiologists for their opinions
- Build your encyclopedia of the faces of cancer
- Look at the mammogram from the year *before* the cancer was diagnosed
- Understand common reasons for overlooked or misjudged cancer
- Review pathology reports for your recalls and recommended biopsies and correlate with the imaging
- Review your audit results and make a plan of what you would like to do better

KEY POINTS

- Optimize the work environment for focused and efficient interpretation of screening mammograms. Perform batch interpretation in a dark room with few interruptions and distractions.
- Use a systematic approach for reviewing and comparing the images to aid consistency and efficiency of interpretation. Compare with previous mammograms that are at least 2 years old. CAD is recommended.
- The "wrong neighborhood" regions on mammograms deserve your close attention during case review.
- Be aware that some cases—such as those with dense tissue, multiple findings, or potentially distracting lesions—are more difficult and may require more time and closer scrutiny than other cases.
- Understand common pitfalls of missed cancer such as dismissing a finding because it is only seen on one view or assuming that a finding is due to postsurgical scar or a benign lymph node.
- When in doubt, recall the patient.
- Generate and review audit data for the group and for each radiologist at least annually to identify areas of potential improvement.

References

American College of Radiology. ACR BI-RADS: Mammography. In ACR Breast Imaging Reporting and Data System, Breast Imaging Atlas, 4th ed. Reston, VA, American College of Radiology, 2003.

Bird RE, Wallace TW, Yankaskas BC. Analysis of cancers missed at screening mammography. Radiology 1992;184:613-617.

Birdwell RL, Ikeda DM, O'Shaughnessy KF, Sickles EA. Mammographic characteristics of 115 missed cancers later detected with screening mammography and the potential utility of computer-aided detection. Radiology 2001;219:192-202.

Burnside ES, Park JM, Fine JP, Sisney GA. The use of batch reading to improve performance of screening mammography. AJR 2005;185:790-796.

Carney PA, Sickles EA, Monsees BS, et al. Identifying minimally acceptable interpretive performance criteria for screening mammography. Radiology 2010;255:354-361.

Catherine S, Giess CS, Keating DM, et al. Retroareolar breast carcinoma: Clinical, imaging, and histopathologic features. Radiology 1998;207:669-673.

Freer TW, Ulissey MJ. Screening mammography with computer-aided detection: Prospective study of 12,860 patients in a community breast center. Radiology 2001;220:781-786.

Ghate SV, Soo MS, Baker JA, et al. Comparison of recall and cancer detection rates for immediate versus batch interpretation of screening mammograms. Radiology 2005;235:31-35.

Kundel HL, Nodine CF, Conant EF, Weinstein SP. Holistic component of image perception in mammogram interpretation: Gaze-tracking study. Radiology 2007;242:396-402.

Linver MN, Osuch JR, Brenner RJ, Smith RA. The mammography audit: A primer for the Mammography Quality Standards Act (MQSA). AJR 1995;165:19-25.

Majid AS, de Paredes ES, Joherty RD, et al. Missed breast carcinomas: pitfalls and pearls. RadioGraphics 2003;23:881-895.

Philpotts L, Raghu M, Durand M, et al. Initial experience with digital breast tomosynthesis in screening mammography. AJR 2012;198(5 Suppl):180 (abstract).

Poplack SP, Tosteson TD, Logel CA, Nagy HM. Digital breast tomosynthesis: Initial experience in 98 women with abnormal digital screening mammography. AJR 2007;189:616-623.

Sickles EA. Mammographic features of "early" breast cancer. AJR 1984:143:461-464.

Sickles EA. Mammographic features of 300 consecutive nonpalpable breast cancers. AJR 1986;146:661-663.

Sickles EA. Periodic mammographic follow-up of probably benign lesions: Results in 3,184 consecutive cases. Radiology 1991;179:463-468.

Skaane P, Bandos AI, Gullien R, et al. Comparison of digital mammography alone and digital mammography plus tomosynthesis in a population-based screening program. (Online) January 7, 2013, doi:10.1148/radiol.12121373.

U.S. Food and Drug Administration Mammography Quality Standards Act and Program, 2009; www.fda.gov.

Wallace TW, Yankaskas BC. Analysis of cancers missed at screening mammography. Radiology 1992;184:613-617.

CASE QUESTIONS

CASE 3-1. Screening mammogram of a 62-year-old woman. What are the findings? What are your BI-RADS assessment and recommendation?

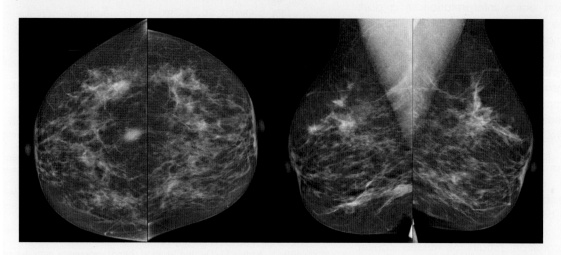

CASE 3-2. Screening mammogram of a 49-year-old woman with a family history of breast cancer. What are the findings? Your BI-RADS assessment?

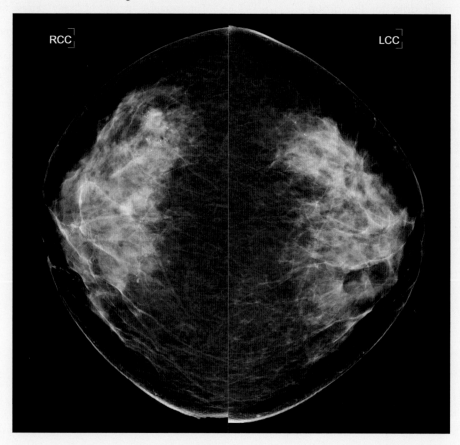

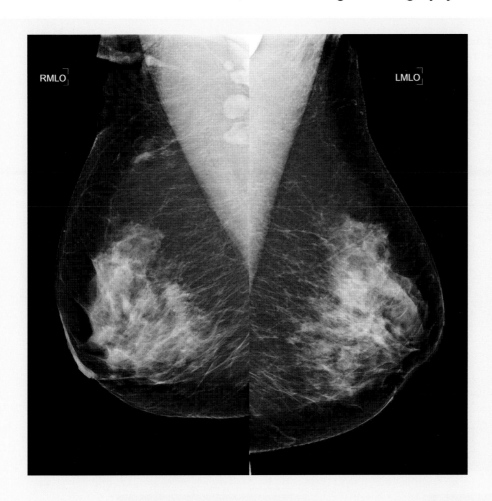

CASE 3-3. Screening mammogram of a 63-year-old woman. What are the findings? What are your BI-RADS assessment and recommendation?

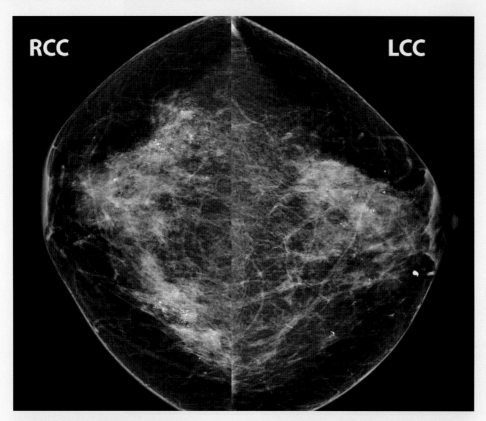

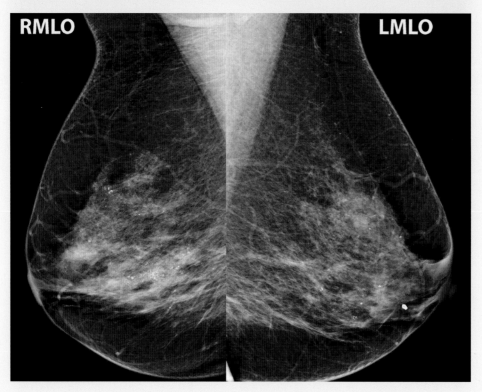

CASE 3-4. Screening mammogram of a 66-year-old woman. What do you see? What would you do?

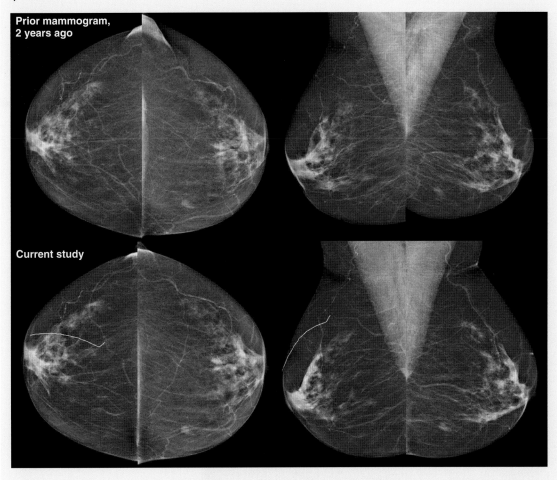

CASE 3-5. Screening mammogram of a 58-year-old woman. What are the findings? What are your BI-RADS assessment and recommendation?

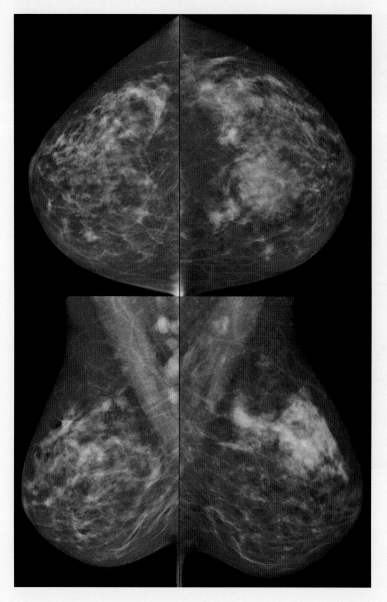

CASE 3-6. Screening mammogram of an 81-year-old woman with a history of melanoma excised from her abdomen 25 years prior. What are the findings? What do you recommend?

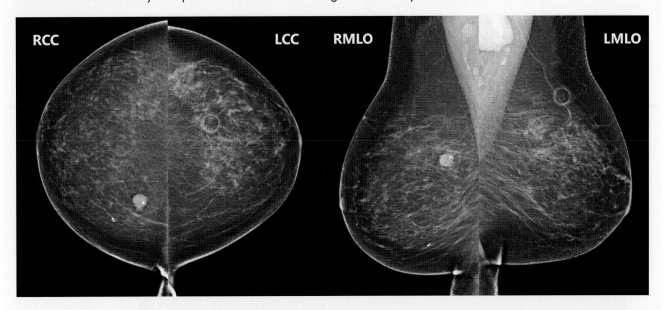

CASE 3-7. Screening MLO view of the left breast on a 61-year-old woman. What change has occurred since the prior study?

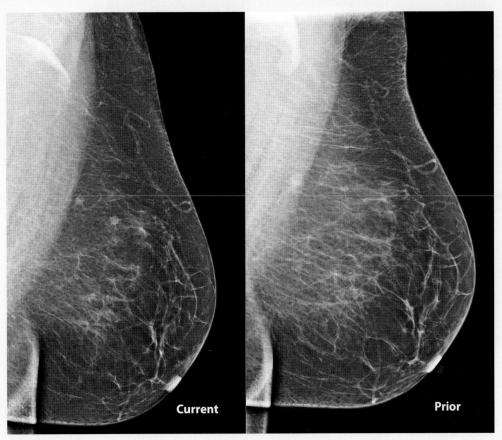

CASE 3-8. Screening mammogram on a 76-year-old woman. What is the most significant finding? What do you recommend?

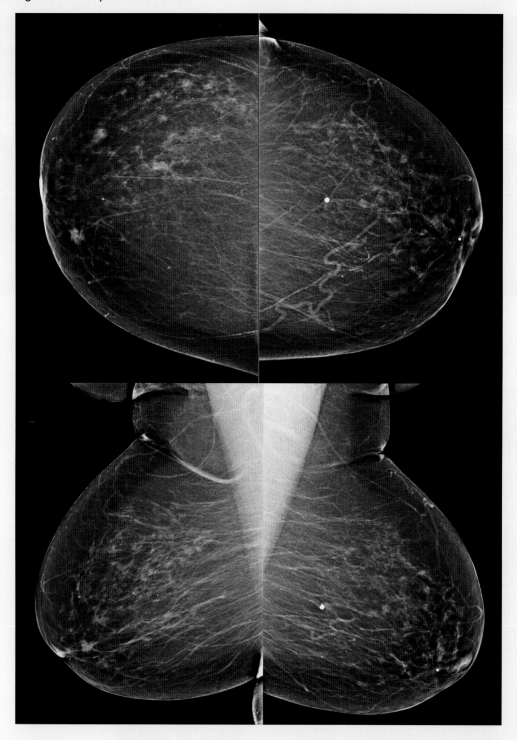

CASE 3-9. This 58-year-old woman had an US-guided core biopsy 1 year ago for a mass that showed stromal fibrosis. A flag marker clip was placed (*arrows*). She missed her 6-month follow-up, but is having no problems. What are your BI-RADS assessment and recommendation?

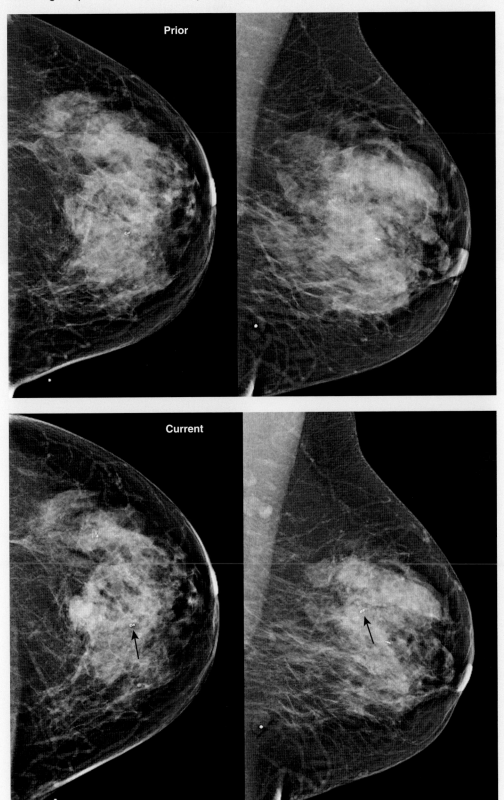

CASE 3-10. A 63-year-old woman presents for screening mammography. What is the finding? What is your BI-RADS category?

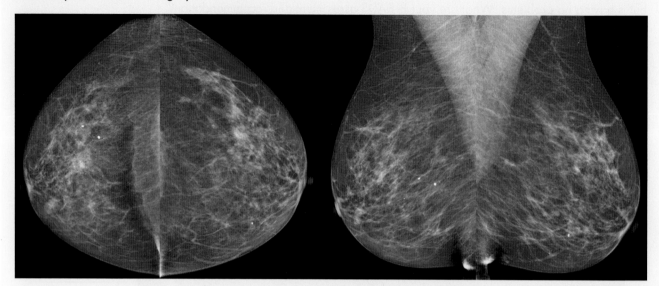

MEDICAL AUDIT QUESTIONS

MEDICAL AUDIT QUESTION 3-1. A medical audit was performed in your practice that includes 4 years of screening data for the entire practice. You are shown the results for Radiologist A, who interprets between 2000 and 4000 screening mammograms per year. How would you interpret this radiologist's performance? What do you recommend?

CANCER DETECTION RATE

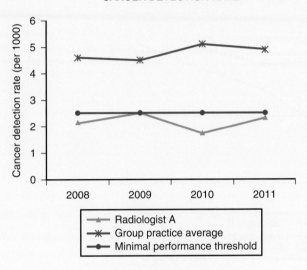

RECALL RATE

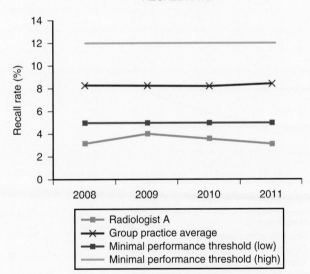

MEDICAL AUDIT QUESTION 3-2. You are reviewing data from your practice medical audit that covers 4 years of screening data. Let's look at the performance of Radiologist B, who interprets between 2800 and 3200 screening mammograms per year. In 2008, because of a concerning audit profile, additional individual training was recommended, focusing on recognizing the more subtle presenting signs of malignancy. Recall of a higher percentage of patients with more subtle, less specific findings was recommended. How would you interpret this individual's response to these recommendations?

CANCER DETECTION RATE

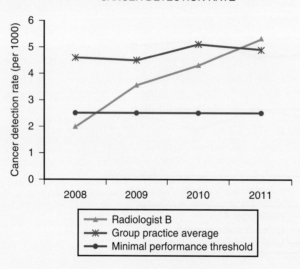

RECALL RATE

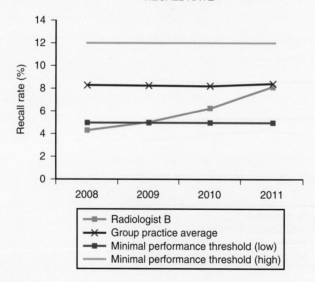

CASE ANSWERS

CASE 3-1. BI-RADS 0: Needs additional imaging. There is an oval mass in the retroglandular fat of the right breast at 6 oclock, posterior third. This mass is living in the wrong neighborhood, which makes it more suspect. Recommend recall for diagnostic imaging. Spot compression views and ultrasonography confirm the suspicious nature of this mass. BI-RADS 5: Malignant findings. Diagnosis: invasive ductal carcinoma.

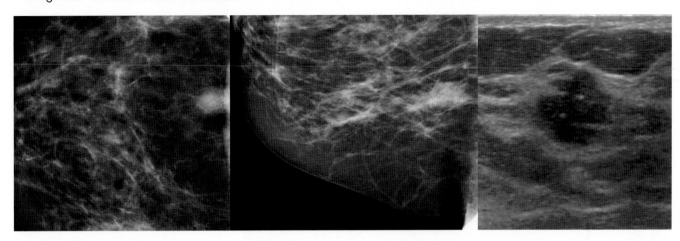

CASE 3-2. There is an obscured mass with coarse heterogeneous calcifications in the lateral right breast. A much more subtle area of architectural distortion is seen in the lateral left breast, anterior third. BI-RADS 0. Recommend spot compression views and US of both breasts.

Spot compression views show an irregular mass with obscured margins and associated calcifications on the right. Architectural distortion is confirmed on the left. Bilateral US shows corresponding irregular hypoechoic masses. Diagnosis: IDC and DCIS both breasts.

When an obvious finding is present, complete your review protocol and look carefully at all areas before returning to examine the obvious finding more closely.

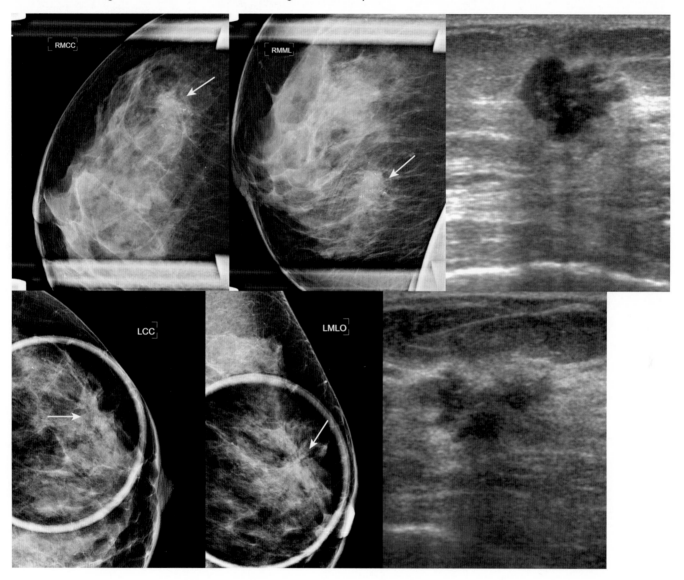

CASE 3-3. There are multiple clustered and scattered predominantly coarse calcifications bilaterally. Calcifications in the medial right breast appear different from the others because there are more calcifications in this area and they are associated with a focal asymmetry. BI-RADS 0, recommend magnification views.

Magnified views are shown here. There are coarse heterogeneous calcifications with segmental distribution in the posterior medial right breast. BI-RADS 5, recommend biopsy. Diagnosis: High-grade DCIS with microinvasion.

In cases with multiple findings, a common pitfall is to assume that all of the findings are benign. Evaluate all of the findings closely to identify any that are more suspicious than the predominant ones.

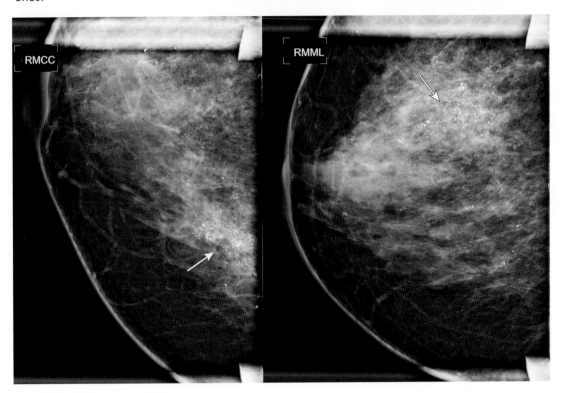

CASE 3-4. There is a focal asymmetry in the left breast at 8 o'clock. It may be increasing in size. Let's look at some older studies for this patient. Below is her left mammogram from 4 years ago. Notice how the asymmetry is actually smaller than 4 years ago. In fact, she was recalled that year and the area was found to be a cyst. This case highlights the utility of pulling older studies to make decisions about recall if stability or change is unclear when compared to the images from 2 years ago.

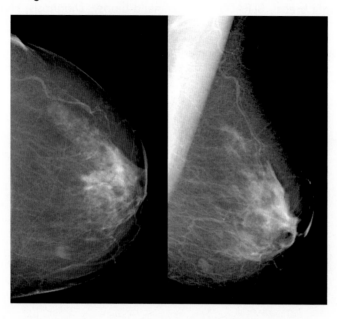

CASE 3-5. Did you notice the right axillary adenopathy? This should make you look even harder at the right breast. BI-RADS 0: Needs additional evaluation. There is subtle architectural distortion at 10 o'clock, posterior third, that persists on spot compression views. US confirms a suspicious mass. Diagnosis: IDC with metastasis to axillary lymph nodes.

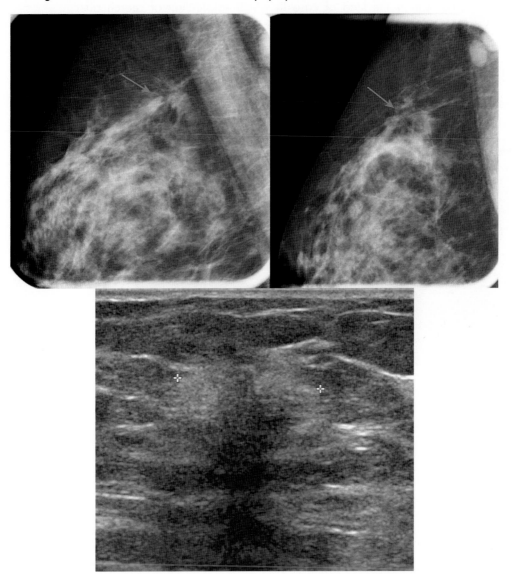

CASE 3-6. There is a circumscribed mass with coarse peripheral calcification in the medial right breast. This finding was stable and consistent with a hyalinized fibroadenoma. There is also a left axillary mass consistent with an enlarged lymph node. The patient was recalled and axillary ultrasonography showed a hypoechoic vascular mass. Core biopsy revealed previously unsuspected non-Hodgkin lymphoma. This is the kind of case in which satisfaction of search after detecting the right breast mass could cause the radiologist's review to be curtailed and the adenopathy overlooked.

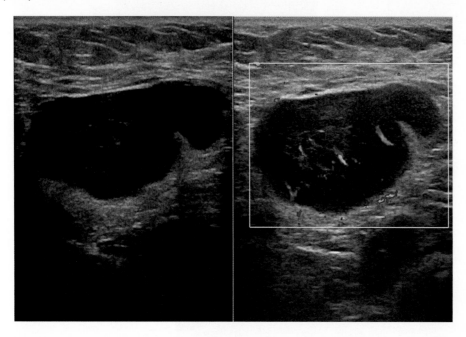

CASE 3-7. There is a mass in the upper outer quadrant of the left breast (*arrow*) that is larger than on the previous study. This lies anterior to an intramammary lymph node (*circle*). On spot magnification views, the mass (*arrow*) is more dense than the node and has spiculated margins. US shows a hypoechoic shadowing mass as well as the adjacent lymph node. Diagnosis: IDC.

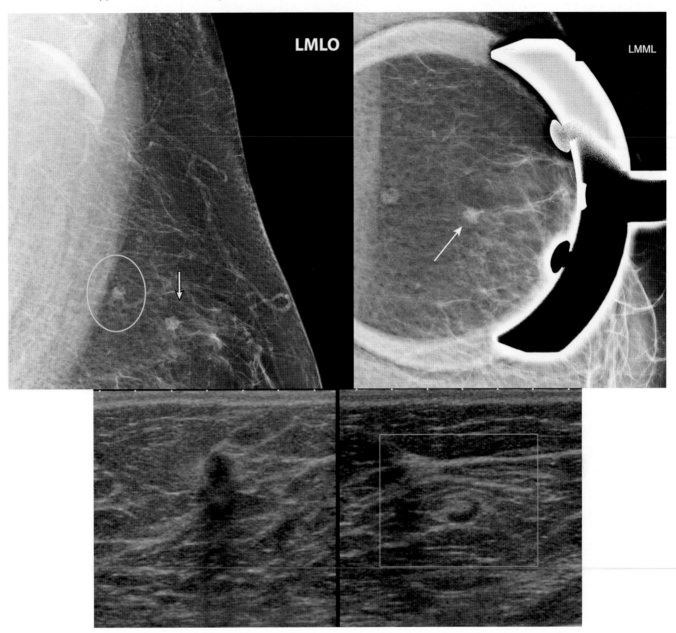

CASE 3-8. There are multiple bilateral masses, most with benign features. When multiple findings are seen, they should be examined individually to see if one is more suspicious than the others. This is the case for the dense irregular mass in the anterior medial right breast (*arrows*). A spot compression view confirms an irregular mass and shows the margins to be spiculated. US shows the lesion to have an echogenic halo. Diagnosis: Infiltrating carcinoma with ductal and lobular features.

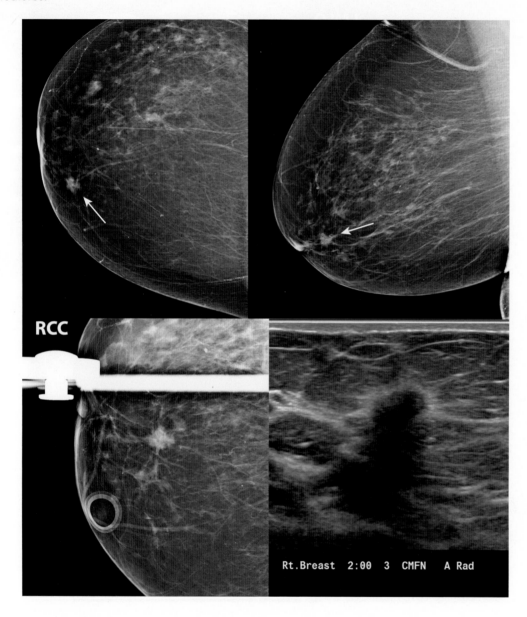

CASE 3-9. There is a new biopsy clip in the left breast at 1 o'clock from the benign biopsy last year. Did you get distracted? There is a new mass in the left breast at 12 o'clock (*arrow*). The US is below. So she needed another biopsy this year. It showed IDC.

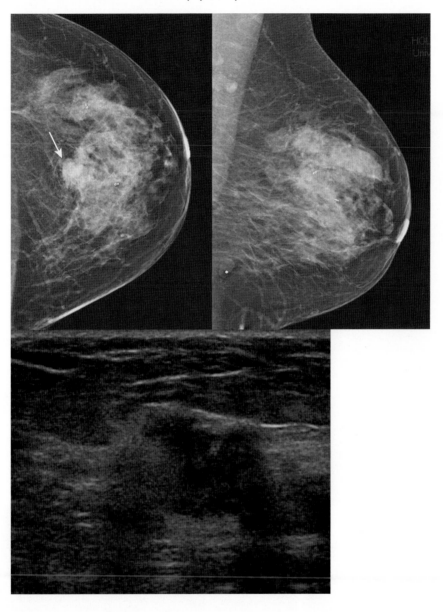

CASE 3-10. There is a focal asymmetry in the retroglandular fat of the left breast at 2 o'clock, posterior third (*arrows below*). At first glance, this asymmetry appears to represent a lymph node on the MLO view. However, on the CC view, the location and appearance are not typical. This should be BI-RADS 0.

On spot compression views, the finding is clearly a mass. US features are highly suspicious. US-guided biopsy showed IDC.

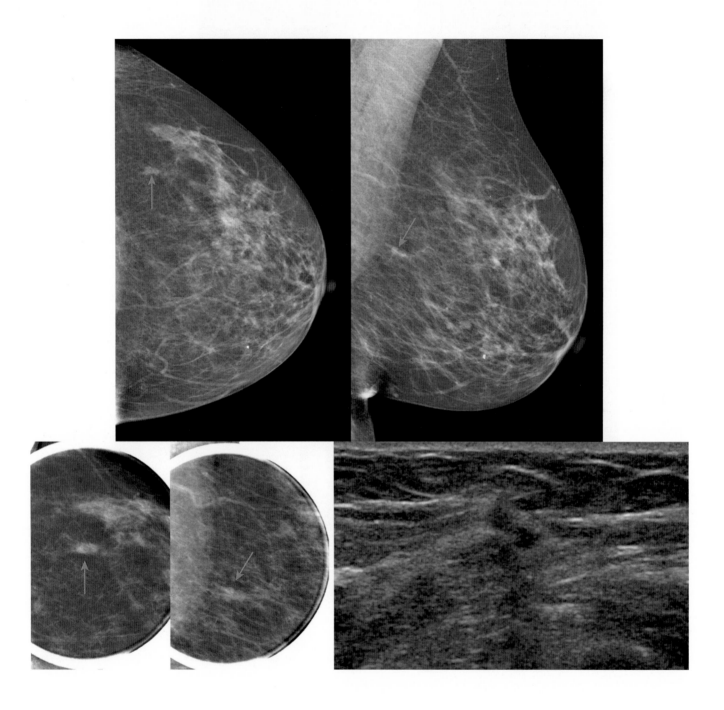

MEDICAL AUDIT ANSWER 3-1. The results of the medical audit regarding Radiologist A are very concerning. A low cancer detection rate outweighs all other considerations. This radiologist's cancer detection rate has only reached the minimally acceptable cutoff point for performance 1 out of 4 years. Cancer detection is also much lower than the average for the practice, indicating an individual performance problem rather than a finding related to the makeup of the screened population. In addition, Radiologist A's recall rate was below the minimally acceptable range during all 4 years and averaged less than half of the recall rate for the practice.

Radiologist A needs to be a little more worried about missing breast cancer! Additional education and training, focusing on the presenting signs of breast cancer on screening mammography, may be beneficial and could include conference attendance and educational materials for self-study. Second reading of screens by subspecialized breast imagers within the group may provide helpful feedback. The goal is to improve recognition of the signs of malignancy and more aggressive recall of patients with subtle findings. The audit profile should be closely monitored to ensure that these measures result in significantly improved performance.

MEDICAL AUDIT ANSWER 3-2. These charts show the results of successful retraining! In 2008 this radiologist's cancer detection rate and recall rate were below the threshold for minimal performance. Cancer detection has since ascended to a level above the practice average. Way to rock!

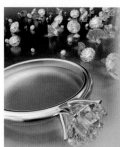

CHAPTER 4

The Recalled Patient: Now What?

Let's see. A screening recall. Is it a real finding? It looks kind of ugly on the screening views. The mediolateral oblique (MLO) spot looks fine, but the craniocaudal (CC) spot may still have something there. What next? Rolled CC views? Ultrasonography (US)? Magnetic resonance imaging (MRI)? Should I just let her go? It's not always easy to decide if a screening finding is significant.

Is it real, or is it cubic zirconium? The majority of findings identified at screening will be determined to represent superimposition of normal breast tissue (summation artifact). The role of diagnostic evaluation is to separate benign findings from those that are potentially malignant. The important questions include whether the finding is new or developing, persists on spot compression, and is suspicious based on its imaging features. If the finding is suspicious, then location becomes important. A one-view finding must be localized if possible prior to biopsy.

In this chapter, we will focus on the diagnostic evaluation of the patient recalled from screening for a mass or asymmetry. We will give you tools to localize lesions in two orthogonal projections. Then we'll need to decide on our level of suspicion for the lesion and whether biopsy is warranted. Evaluation of breast calcifications is discussed further in Chapter 6: Calcifications Made Easy.

The Screening Recall

Our routine imaging for an abnormal screening mammogram includes a true lateral view (mediolateral [ML] or lateromedial [LM]) and spot compression views of the finding (Fig. 4-1). Additional imaging often follows and may include additional mammographic views and US.

The goals of the workup are to decide whether the finding represents a true lesion and, if so, to localize it in two orthogonal projections, and determine its level of suspicion. These goals are often achieved simultaneously. For example, an ML view obtained to evaluate a finding seen in the MLO view may show that the finding represents superimposed breast tissue. Alternatively, if the finding represents a true mass, the ML view may help localize it to the medial or lateral breast.

True Lateral View

The true lateral view is helpful in determining the location of the finding because this can be misjudged on the MLO view. Obtaining a true lateral view is also very helpful for planning if stereotactic or wire-localized biopsy is performed.

The true lateral view may be ML or LM. So, which to choose? Remember that the view is named for the direction of the x-ray beam. We want the lesion to be as close to the image receptor as possible to maximize sharpness. If the lesion is in the lateral breast, then an ML view will put the lesion closest to the receptor. If the lesion is medial, then the LM view is preferred. If we are not sure whether the finding is medial or lateral, then an ML is performed because statistically, most cancers are located in the lateral breast.

Spot Compression Views

Spot compression views are often helpful in deciding whether a finding represents summation artifact or a true lesion. They are also used to confirm the location of a finding and to help determine the level of suspicion. Although it may seem more efficient to go straight to US when a mammographic finding is seen in two projections, spot compression views result in an increase in cancer detection of about 18%.

When a cancer undergoes focal (spot) compression, the abnormal tissue will typically appear more dense than the surrounding tissues, and mass borders are more clearly seen. These views may show a one-view asymmetry to represent a focal asymmetry or a mass. A mass with obscured margins may be shown to have spiculated margins on spot compression views. Associated findings such as architectural distortion are often better seen than on the screening views. When normal tissue undergoes spot compression, it will spread out and become less dense; the normal, respectful breast architecture becomes more apparent.

Spot compression views ("spots") should be obtained in both CC and MLO projections if the finding is seen on both views. Spot compression views may be performed with or without magnification ("spot mags"). The advantage of using magnification with spot compression is the ability to see fine architecture and calcifications well, although the disadvantage is lower contrast. Whether or not to use magnification with spot compression is really one of personal preference. As you can see from our many case studies, we typically perform spot compression without magnification.

Go ahead and skip the spot compression views when the mass for which the patient is being recalled is very likely to represent a cyst (Fig. 4-2). Spot compression

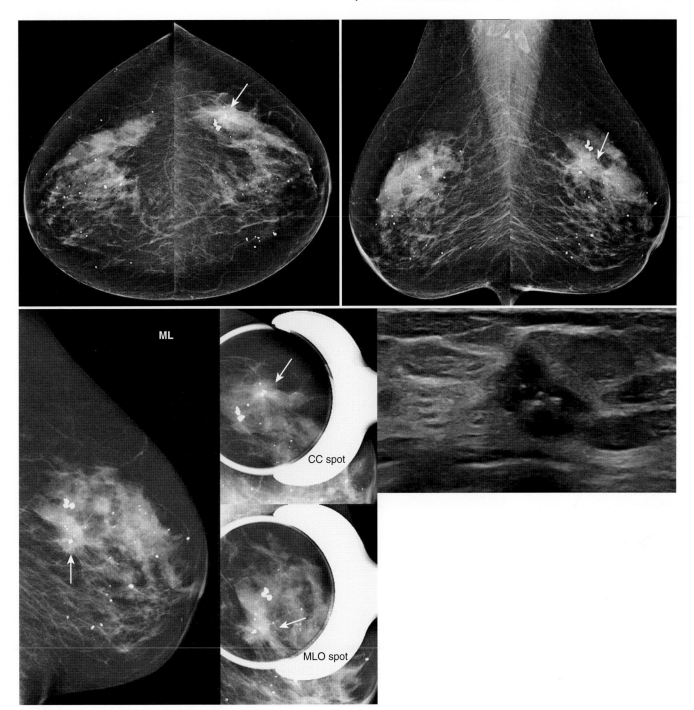

FIGURE 4-1 **Typical Screening Recall Workup.** This 78-year-old woman was recalled for a possible mass in the left breast at 2 o'clock (*arrows*). The diagnostic evaluation included an ML view, spot compression in the CC and MLO projections, and US. These additional images confirm that there is an irregular mass with spiculated margins. BI-RADS 5. Ultrasound-guided biopsy showed invasive ductal carcinoma (IDC).

views are often uncomfortable, but when there is a large cyst present they can be downright painful. So spare your patient the discomfort and start with US if the mass is likely to be a cyst.

Tomosynthesis and Other Imaging

Digital breast tomosynthesis (DBT) gives us a not-quite three-dimensional evaluation of the breast. The use of DBT in diagnostic breast imaging is evolving. Many other

mammographic views (rolled CCs, off-angle, tangential views, etc.) can be very helpful in both localizing the lesion and assessing the level of suspicion. Be creative!

Ultrasonography can be invaluable in identifying breast cancer, but we must first know when and where to look. As in spot compression views, an additional 20% of cancers will be detected when US is used appropriately as a part of the diagnostic evaluation. More on this later.

Breast MRI is rarely needed in the diagnostic evaluation of a mammographic finding. Here's the problem: a negative MRI does not mean that the mammographic

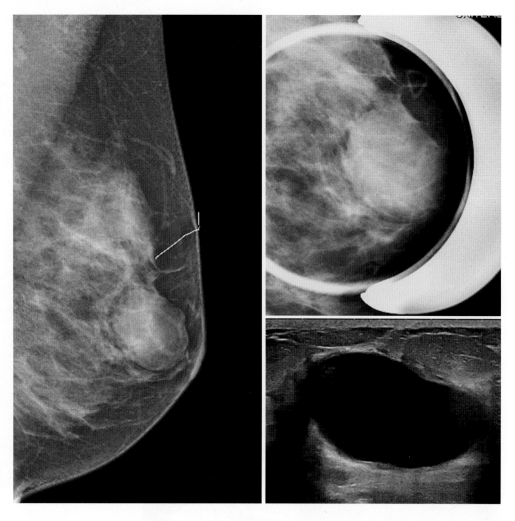

FIGURE 4-2 **Skip the Spots!** A large mass in the subareolar region of the left breast on the screening mammogram is almost surely a cyst. The spot compression view adds no useful information. The US confirms a simple cyst and could have been performed first. If the US did not show a simple cyst, spot compression views can still be performed after the US if needed.

finding is not cancer. Additional mammographic views and US should be used to evaluate the finding and establish the level of suspicion. Occasionally, MRI is useful to localize a suspicious mammographic finding seen in one view that is not amenable to US or stereotactic biopsy.

Determining the Location of a Two-View Finding

When we see a finding that we think is concerning, we will want to localize it in two orthogonal views. Sometimes this is easy, but it may be especially challenging on a complex or dense mammogram. Even when the location on the CC and MLO views is obvious, we'll need to remember that the MLO cannot be treated like a true lateral view when determining the location of a lesion. Localization is important because we will need to know where to focus our attention before we do an US.

There are a few things to keep in mind when localizing a finding. The lesion should have similar size, shape, and imaging characteristics in both CC and MLO views. The depth of the lesion should be similar on all mammographic views so long as the nipple is in profile.

Lesion Depth

A finding should have similar depth (distance from the nipple) on all mammographic views as long as the nipple is in profile (Fig. 4-3). A mass that is in the anterior breast on the CC view will not correspond to a finding in the posterior breast on the MLO view as long as the nipple is relatively in profile. If the nipple rolls under the breast on the CC view or to the side on the MLO view, the depth of the lesion could appear much different on the CC and MLO views (Fig. 4-4).

Account for Obliquity on the MLO View

For a finding seen in both CC and MLO views, we need to remember that an MLO view is typically obtained at a 30- to 60-degree angle, although a true lateral view is obtained at 90 degrees. We have to mentally account for the differences in obliquity between the MLO and a true lateral view (Fig. 4-5). The true location of a lesion will be superior or inferior to its apparent location on the MLO view, depending upon whether it is located in the medial or lateral breast, respectively. The location of a far lateral or far medial finding will be more affected by

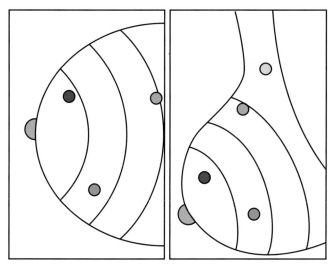

FIGURE 4-3 **Determine Lesion Depth.** The distance from the nipple should be similar between the CC and MLO views so long as the nipple is in profile. Each of the colored dots on the CC view can only represent the same color dots on the MLO view and vice versa. For example, the green dot on the CC view cannot represent the red or orange dots on the MLO view. However, if the nipple is not in profile on one of the views, then the depth can be different on the other view. Note that the yellow dot may not be viewed on the CC view because of the far posterior location.

the obliquity on the MLO view than a more centrally located finding.

Correlating between Mammography and Ultrasonography

Understanding the location of a lesion on mammography prior to US or biopsy is important. Using the information available from the mammogram, it is often possible to have a good idea of the location and US appearance of a finding before you scan. If US is performed in the incorrect location, a mammographic finding may incorrectly be assumed benign (Fig. 4-6).

The size, shape, and other characteristics of the lesion on the mammogram should be similar to the appearance on US (Fig. 4-7). Other landmarks can also sometimes be used to increase your confidence that you are examining the correct finding. For example, a calcified oil cyst, fibroadenoma, or intramammary lymph node adjacent to the suspicious finding may be identified by US.

In addition to the "o'clock position" and depth of a lesion, it can be helpful to consider the location of a lesion relative to the central core of fibroglandular tissue. Ask yourself whether the lesion is at the border of the fibroglandular tissue, more centrally within this tissue, or in the retroglandular fat. Finding a lesion by US with the same position with respect to the fibroglandular tissue

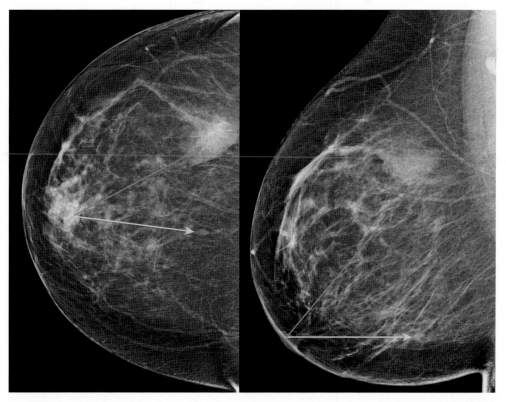

FIGURE 4-4 **Inaccurate Depth.** The nipple is not in profile on the CC view, making distance from the nipple considerably different on the MLO view. A focal asymmetry in the upper outer quadrant is farther from the nipple on the MLO than predicted on CC (*blue arrows*), although a small oval mass is the same distance from the nipple on both views (*yellow arrows*).

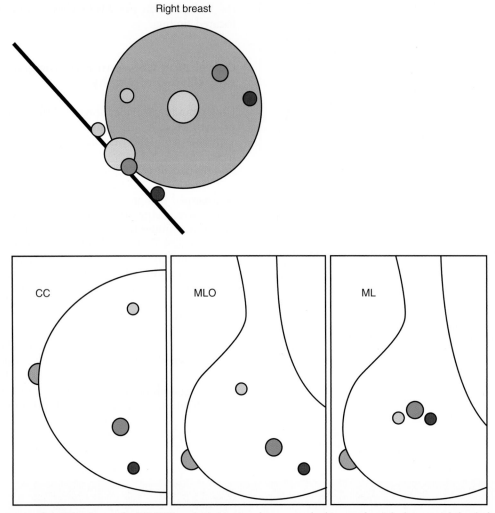

FIGURE 4-5 **Accounting for Obliquity on the MLO View.** Let's imagine that we are looking at the right breast and the dark line represents the image receptor for an MLO view. A mass seen in the lateral breast (*yellow*) will project higher on the MLO view than its true location as seen on the ML view. The opposite is true for a mass in the medial breast (*red*), which will project lower on an MLO view than its true location. A more central medial mass (*green*) will not shift so much in location between the MLO and ML views compared with a far medial lesion (*red*).

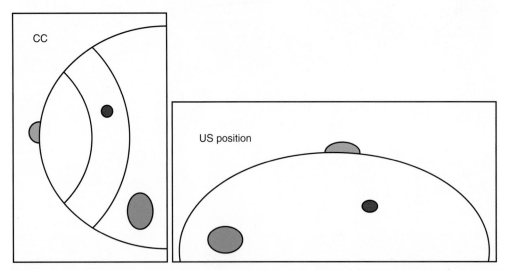

FIGURE 4-6 **Correlation of Mammographic and US Location.** Try to visualize the location of the mammographic finding on US before scanning. The breast will flatten in the supine position used for US. The red lesion on the mammogram will be about 1 cm lateral to the nipple and about halfway between the skin and the pectoral muscle. The green lesion will be 6 to 8 cm medial to the nipple in an average-sized breast and relatively close to the skin.

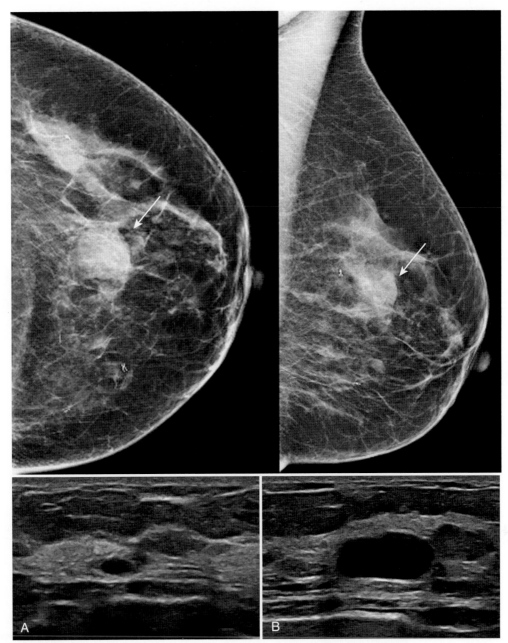

FIGURE 4-7 **Size Discrepancy.** The mass in the left breast at 12 o'clock (*arrows*) cannot correlate with the first cyst identified (**A**), which is too small and was located at 2 o'clock. The second cyst (**B**) identified at 12 o'clock is a much more appropriate correlate both by size and location.

increases confidence that it corresponds to the mammographic finding.

Keep in mind that with mammography, the technologist pulls the breast tissue away from the chest wall. For US, the patient is recumbent and the breast tissue flattens toward the chest wall. As a result, lesions may appear closer to the pectoral muscle than one might expect based on the mammographic location. For example, a mass in the middle third of the breast on mammography may appear to abut the pectoralis muscle on US.

If you are uncertain whether the US and mammographic findings are the same lesion, but the US and mammographic findings individually are both suspicious enough to warrant biopsy, there is no real need to prove that they correspond before performing a biopsy. Place a

clip after ultrasound-guided core biopsy and perform postprocedure mammography, which will show whether they correspond. Be ready, however, to also perform a stereotactic biopsy if the clip is not located in the suspicious mammographic finding. Hey, it happens.

Determining the Location of a One-View Finding

Let's say that your colleague identified a suspicious one-view asymmetry on screening and now you are seeing her for diagnostic evaluation. We need to find it in an orthogonal projection before we do US so we can look in the correct location.

Our first step is to determine lesion depth (see Fig. 4-3). If the depth is such that the finding should be included on the other projection (see Fig. 4-3, red, green, and most orange dots), then it is either due to superimposition of breast tissue or obscured on the other projection. If obscured, there are several techniques that we can use to determine the location in the orthogonal projection. If the lesion depth is far posterior (see Fig. 4-3, yellow and some orange dots), then a different approach will be needed.

Obscured in the Other Projection

We have several views to help us. The "best guess" spot compression, true lateral, or stepped oblique views can help whether the finding is best seen in the CC or MLO view. If a lesion is seen well only in the CC projection, rolled CC views can be very helpful. For an MLO finding, a true lateral view is typically the most helpful.

"Best Guess" Spot Compression View

This is a good place to start for a one-view finding that may be obscured in the other projection. Go ahead and get your spot compression view in the projection that you are most worried about. Then make your best guess about where the finding may be located in the other projection. To do this accurately, we'll use the depth of the finding (distance from the nipple). Then look at that depth on the other projection, which should be similar between views as long as the nipple is in profile (Fig. 4-8).

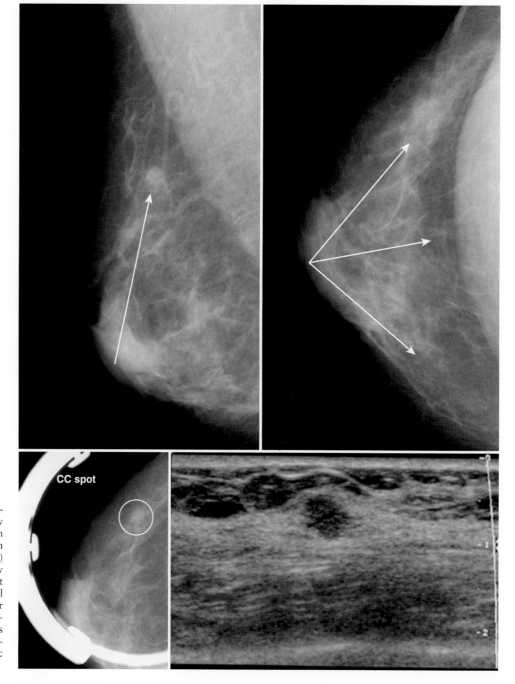

FIGURE 4-8 **Best Guess Spot Compression View.** There is a one-view asymmetry in the superior breast on the MLO view. The distance from the nipple in the MLO view (*arrow*) must be similar in the CC view (*arrows*). Because there is only fat at this depth in the central and medial breast, the most likely location for this finding is lateral. CC spot compression view of this area confirms the finding. US shows a corresponding suspicious solid mass. Histologic diagnosis: IDC.

Sometimes there is more than one suspect and both may need to undergo spot compression.

Shallow or Stepped Oblique Views

In these techniques, full mammogram views are obtained at slightly different angles from the original CC or MLO view in which the finding is seen. Shallow oblique (or off-angle) views are obtained at plus and minus 10 to 15 degrees from the original angle. Stepped oblique views are similar in concept; full images are obtained at 10- to 15-degree intervals between the CC and MLO views. The finding can be tracked over the views to determine the location. We do not use these often because other techniques can usually determine the location with fewer

exposures. In some cases, though, either shallow or stepped oblique views can localize a finding when our other tricks haven't helped.

Rolled CC Views for a CC Finding

If a lesion is seen only on the CC view, the location in the superior or inferior breast must be determined. For rolled CC views, the breast is placed on the image receptor and the superior breast is rolled lateral (CCRL) or medial (CCRM). The inferior breast may also be rolled in the opposite direction during positioning. If a lesion moves laterally on the CCRL, then it is located in the superior breast (Fig. 4-9). If it moves medially or does not shift in position, then it is in the inferior or central breast. These

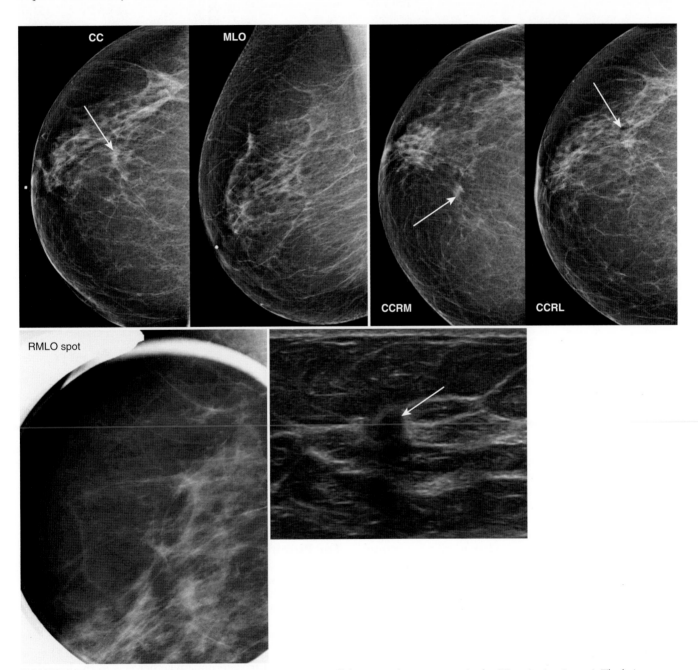

FIGURE 4-9 **Rolled CC views to Determine Location.** Screening recall for a one-view asymmetry in the CC projection (*arrow*). The lesion moves lateral on the CCRL and medial on the CCRM (*arrows*), indicating that the lesion is located in the superior breast. The MLO spot compression view is not helpful, but US does show a small hypoechoic solid mass at 11 o'clock. BI-RADS 4. Ultrasound-guided core needle biopsy showed IDC.

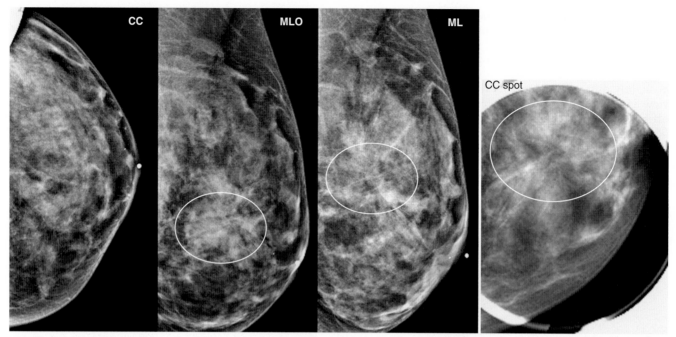

FIGURE 4-10 ML View to Localize an MLO Finding. Architectural distortion is present in the superior left breast on the MLO view (*circle*), but not seen on the CC view. Because the area of distortion moves up on the ML view (*circle*), the lesion must be located in the medial breast. This is confirmed on a CC spot compression view (*circle*). Excisional biopsy showed radial sclerosing lesion.

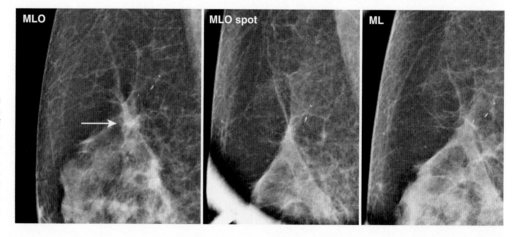

FIGURE 4-11 **ML to Resolve Lesions at the Breast Apex.** There is a focal asymmetry at the apex of the breast (*arrow*) that appears more concerning on the MLO spot compression view. The area is shown to be normal on the ML view. Overlap of breast tissue at the apex of the breast can result in summation, forming a pseudolesion.

are similar in concept to shallow oblique views. Rolled CC views may also "unsuperimpose" normal structures and may be quite helpful in proving that a finding represents summation artifact rather than a true lesion.

ML View for an MLO Finding
We reviewed earlier how a lateral lesion shifts lower from the MLO to the ML view and a medial lesion shifts up (see Fig. 4-5). We can use this to our advantage for lesions seen only in the MLO view (Fig. 4-10). An ML or LM view may also reveal a finding that was initially seen only on the CC view.

ML View for the Apex of the Breast
An ML view is also helpful in evaluating lesions at the apex of the breast. Most of the fibroglandular tissue is located in the upper outer quadrant. The breast tissue

often bunches up in the apex of the breast. An ML view can often help us discern if a one-view finding in the apex is due to summation artifact or a concerning lesion (Fig. 4-11).

Far Posterior Lesions

If a lesion is in the posterior third of the breast tissue or overlying the pectoral muscle, it may not overlie the image receptor on the other projection.

On the MLO View
When a lesion is located far posterior on the MLO view only, we need to determine whether it is in the lateral or medial breast. These lesions are often not seen on an ML view, so we need a different approach. About 70% of

breast cancers are located in the lateral breast, and the CC view often does not include all of the tail of the breast. Therefore, we'll start our search with an exaggerated craniocaudal lateral (XCCL) view to look at the lateral tissue (Fig. 4-12).

The XCCL view will identify the lesion most of the time. If not, then we need to look in the medial breast. We typically see most of the medial breast on the CC view. So where could the lesion be hiding? Let's go back to our anatomy for a moment. The skin of the upper

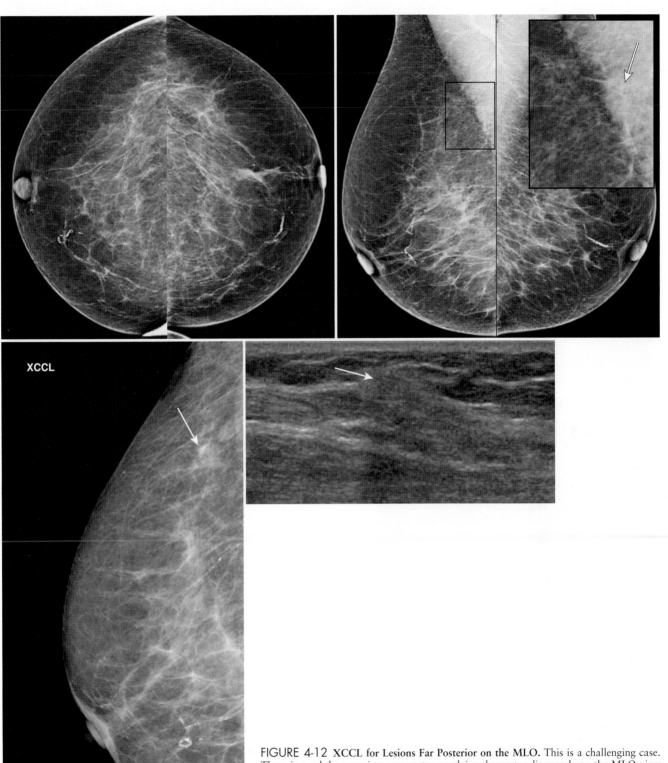

FIGURE 4-12 XCCL for Lesions Far Posterior on the MLO. This is a challenging case. There is a subtle, one-view asymmetry overlying the pectoralis muscle on the MLO view (*arrow*). Statistically, this is more likely to be located in the lateral breast than the medial, so let's start with an XCCL. And there it is (*arrow*)! The finding is confirmed to be located at 10 o'clock, 10 cm from the nipple on US (*arrow*). Ultrasound-guided biopsy showed IDC.

inner breast is not very mobile. When positioning the patient for the CC view, the technologist raises the image receptor and lifts up the inferior breast onto the receptor. However, if the lesion is very high and medial, the CC positioning may still not be adequate. In order to see some high medial lesions, the image receptor must be raised very high (Fig. 4-13). We want to see everything below the clavicle. It can be difficult to include this tissue on the mammogram, so beware of the high upper inner quadrant lesion!

On the CC View

Far posterior lesions seen only on the CC view are very uncommon. When present, they are usually located in the central or medial breast. Doing an ML or LM view in which the technologist knows you really want to see the

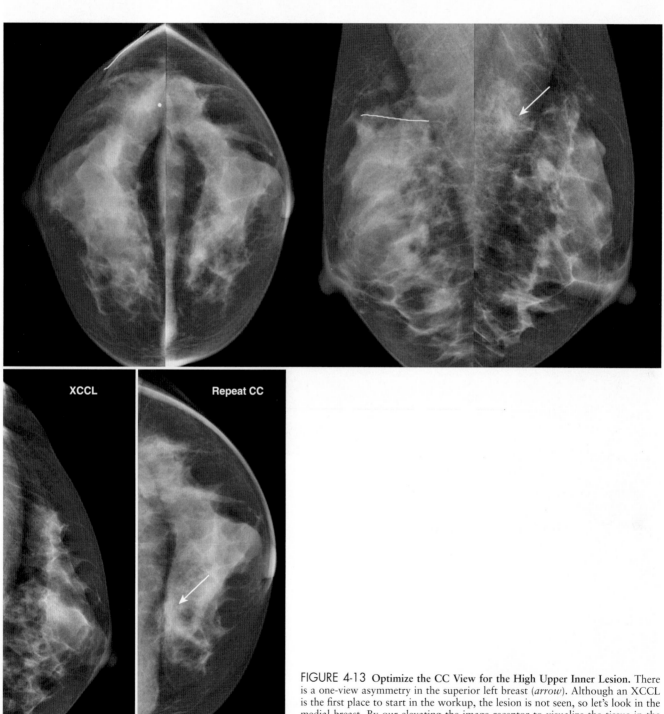

FIGURE 4-13 **Optimize the CC View for the High Upper Inner Lesion.** There is a one-view asymmetry in the superior left breast (*arrow*). Although an XCCL is the first place to start in the workup, the lesion is not seen, so let's look in the medial breast. By our elevating the image receptor to visualize the tissue in the superior breast, the lesion is now well seen (*arrow*). Ultrasound-guided core biopsy and excisional biopsy showed radial scar with atypical ductal hyperplasia.

medial and central breast will often do the trick (Fig. 4-14).

Still Can't Find It

Sometimes it is difficult to localize a lesion in two orthogonal views because the lesion is small and low density. If the one-view asymmetry is considered suspicious (often because it is a new or enlarging), there are several other alternatives.

Ultrasonography with BB Shot

US can be helpful, particularly for larger lesions seen in only one view. For smaller lesions, it becomes more difficult to know if an US finding correlates with the mammographic finding. Place a BB over the candidate lesion seen on US followed by mammographic views for confirmation (Fig. 4-15).

Stereotactic Biopsy

A suspicious one-view asymmetry can often undergo biopsy using stereotactic guidance, even if you are unsure

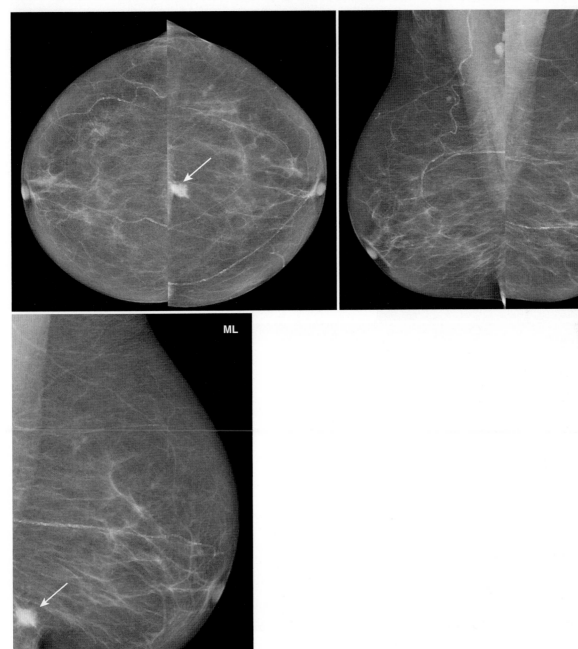

FIGURE 4-14 **An ML View for the Far Posterior CC Finding.** There is a very suspicious asymmetry in the posterior central left breast on the CC view (*arrow*). In this case, there is nothing seen in the superior breast, so the lesion must be located in the inferior breast. This location is confirmed on the ML view (*arrow*). Histologic diagnosis: IDC.

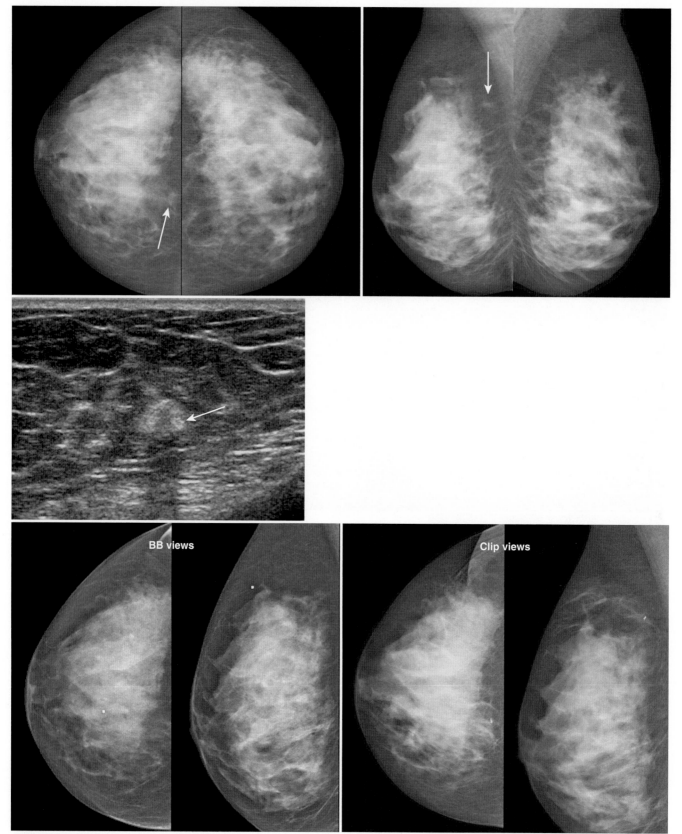

FIGURE 4-15 **BB Views to Confirm Correlation of an US finding.** There is a small focal asymmetry in the right breast at 1 o'clock, posterior third (*arrows*). The lesion persisted on spot compression views (not shown). A possible correlate is identified on US (*arrow*). To increase confidence that the US finding represents the mammographic finding, a BB was placed over the US finding and CC and ML views performed. The BB is near the finding. Ultrasound-guided core biopsy was performed. Postbiopsy CC and ML views document that the metallic marker (clip) is within the lesion and confirms that the US finding was the correlate. Histologic examination showed stromal fibrosis, which was considered concordant.

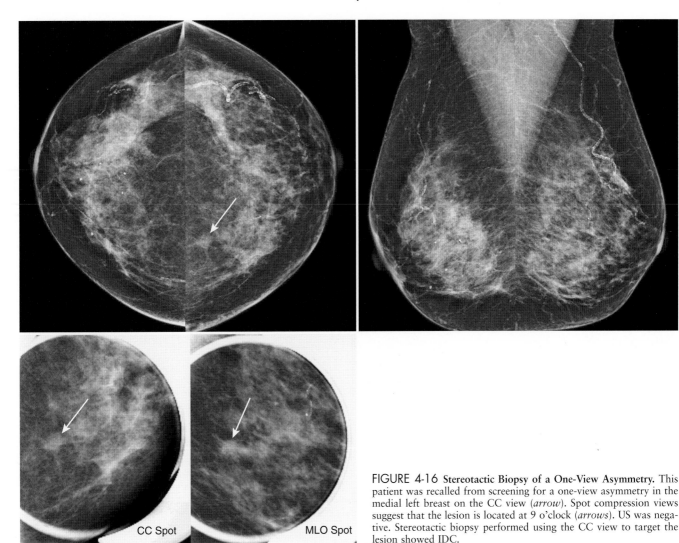

FIGURE 4-16 **Stereotactic Biopsy of a One-View Asymmetry.** This patient was recalled from screening for a one-view asymmetry in the medial left breast on the CC view (*arrow*). Spot compression views suggest that the lesion is located at 9 o'clock (*arrows*). US was negative. Stereotactic biopsy performed using the CC view to target the lesion showed IDC.

CC Spot

MLO Spot

of the location of the finding in the other projection (Fig. 4-16). If the finding overlies the pectoral muscle or the compressed breast thickness is less than about 30 mm, you'll need to find another method to sample the finding.

Digital Breast Tomosynthesis

Multiple low-dose radiation images are obtained in an arc over the breast. These angled or projection images can be viewed directly. More commonly, they are viewed by scrolling through reformatted 1-mm slices of the breast. Although tomosynthesis is probably used to best advantage to reduce recalls from screening, it can also be useful in the diagnostic setting to localize an asymmetry that is only well seen in one view (Fig. 4-17). Note that suspicious lesions are typically not high in density on tomosynthesis images even when they are dense on the non-DBT images. The architecture of the tissue is more important for cancer detection than the density of a lesion on tomosynthesis images.

MRI for Localization

Sometimes a very suspicious one-view asymmetry cannot be localized despite the best attempts. The next step

would typically be stereotactic biopsy. If the lesion is not amenable to stereotactic biopsy, MRI can be helpful to localize the finding (Fig. 4-18). Note that the goal of the MRI is localizing the lesion, not determining the level of suspicion. Your level of suspicion should be established based on the mammographic findings.

How Suspicious Is It?

Each image must be evaluated to determine the level of suspicion of a lesion. Is it a concerning finding that needs biopsy? Is there no persistent finding? There are several ways to determine the level of suspicions (Box 4-1).

Pretest Probability

Did you look at the screening views and think, "This is almost surely going to be a cancer?" If the spot compression views do not confirm a suspicious finding, you may want more reassurance that it is really okay. Diagnostic views for small findings in women with dense tissue can be particularly misleading because a true lesion can be

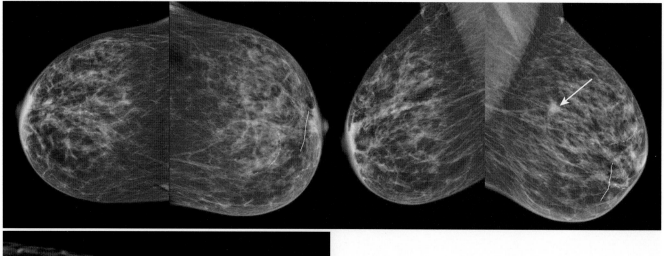

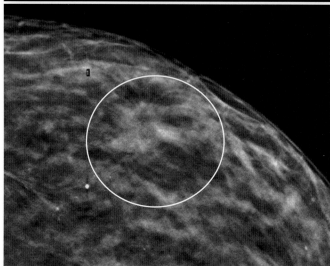

FIGURE 4-17 **Digital Breast Tomosynthesis for Lesion Localization.** An 82-year-old woman recalled for one-view asymmetry on the MLO (*arrow*). CC tomosynthesis slice shows a corresponding irregular spiculated mass in the lateral breast (*circle*). Note that the mass is not high in density on the tomosynthesis slice. Biopsy showed IDC.

BOX 4-1 Techniques for Assessing Level of Suspicion

- Pretest probability. Is it ugly on the screening views? Is it new or larger than on prior studies? Consider US or stereotactic biopsy.
- Spot compression views. Does it R-E-S-P-E-C-T the breast architecture or does it become denser with straight Cooper ligaments?
- True lateral (ML or LM). A possible mass or distortion on the MLO view may clearly represent only breast tissue on the true lateral.
- Repeat view. Does it appear the same when you take the same view on the day of her diagnostic?
- Tomosynthesis may help distinguish summation from a true lesion.
- US may add information if the diagnostic views are equivocal.

obscured on these views. In cases like these, you may still want to perform an US (Fig. 4-19).

R-E-S-P-E-C-T

Yes, you are dating yourself if you know that great song by Aretha Franklin, but we are with you! Does the finding represent breast tissue or persist as a suspicious finding on the spot compression views? If the finding is due to summation of normal tissue, the structures should respect the normal architecture of the breast (Fig. 4-20). The Cooper ligaments should be soft and round, without straight or radiating lines. The area should become less dense on spot compression views. Findings that become more dense, have outwardly convex margins, or are associated with straight lines are more concerning (Fig. 4-21).

Repeat the View

Repeating the same view as the original finding may also immediately answer the question (Fig. 4-22).

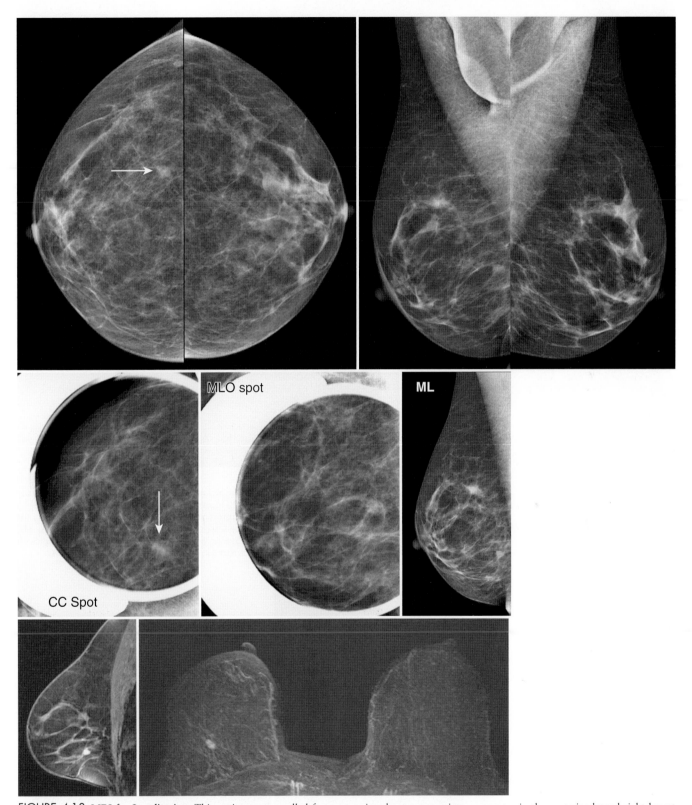

FIGURE 4-18 **MRI for Localization.** This patient was recalled from screening due to a one-view asymmetry in the posterior lateral right breast on the CC view (*arrow*). The finding persists on the CC spot compression view. It may be in the inferior breast on the MLO spot, but on the ML view it may actually be located in the superior breast. US was negative. Stereotactic biopsy was attempted, but this low-density lesion could not be targeted. Contrast-enhanced MRI shows an enhancing mass at 7 o'clock. MRI-guided biopsy showed IDC.

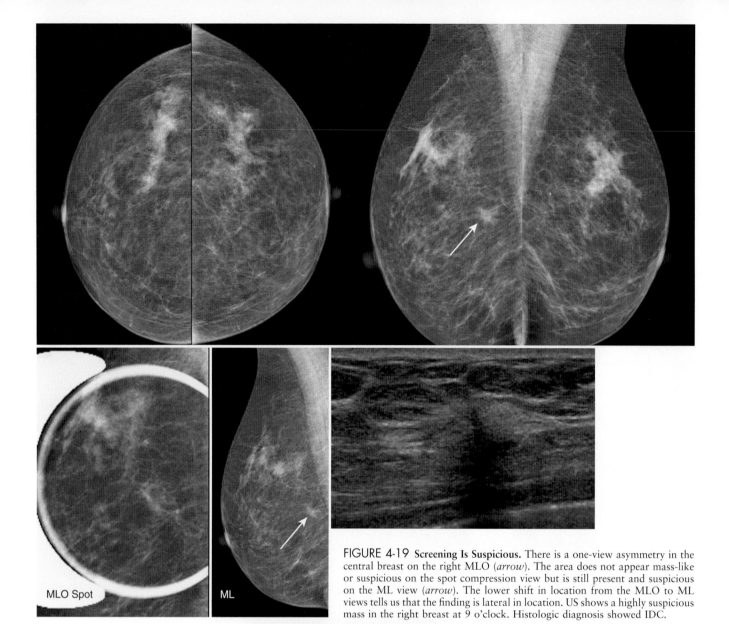

FIGURE 4-19 Screening Is Suspicious. There is a one-view asymmetry in the central breast on the right MLO (*arrow*). The area does not appear mass-like or suspicious on the spot compression view but is still present and suspicious on the ML view (*arrow*). The lower shift in location from the MLO to ML views tells us that the finding is lateral in location. US shows a highly suspicious mass in the right breast at 9 o'clock. Histologic diagnosis showed IDC.

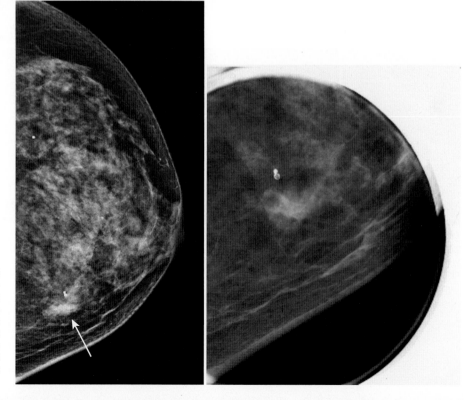

FIGURE 4-20 **Does Not Persist.** Patient was recalled for workup of a one-view asymmetry (*arrow*). On the spot compression view, the tissue becomes less dense, has no outward convex margin, and respects the normal breast architecture; curvilinear Cooper ligaments and vessels run through the area rather than to a central point within it. BI-RADS 1. Recommend routine screening.

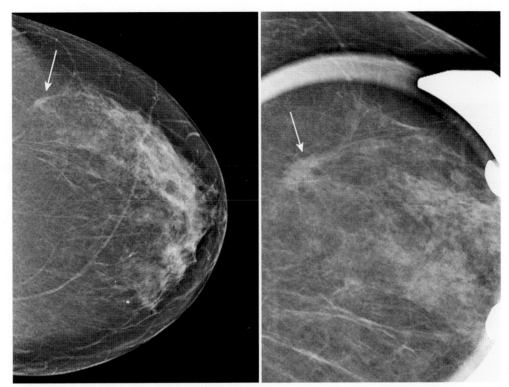

FIGURE 4-21 **Persistent Finding.** This focal asymmetry on screening (*arrow*) becomes more dense and has an outward convex margin on the spot compression view (*arrow*). Subtle straight lines radiate from the lesion; these differ from overlapping lines that appear to extend through it. Biopsy showed IDC.

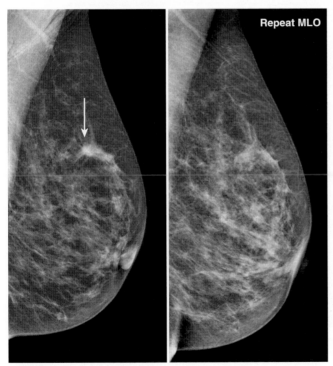

FIGURE 4-22 **Repeat the Screening View.** There is a one-view asymmetry in the superior left breast (*arrow*). The MLO view was repeated and has an appearance similar to that on the prior mammogram. The asymmetry is due to summation artifact.

Digital Breast Tomosynthesis

DBT can be useful in the diagnostic setting to distinguish summation artifact from a true lesion (Fig. 4-23).

Ultrasonography

US can be useful to identify suspicious findings when the additional mammographic views are not convincingly negative or if a lesion could be obscured by dense tissue (Fig. 4-24). Don't get us wrong. US is not needed for every recall. The large majority of screening recalls can be dismissed as summation artifact without US. However, if something about the mammographic appearance is causing you lingering concern, US can often be of great value in the decision-making process.

Putting It All Together

During the diagnostic evaluation of a screening-detected finding, the mammographic views obtained will be used to determine or confirm location as well as the level of suspicion. For example, you may obtain rolled CC views with the purpose of determining location but then deduce that the finding is due to summation when you review the images.

As you progress through a diagnostic case, the location, size, and imaging characteristics should correlate between views and modalities. The depth of the lesion on

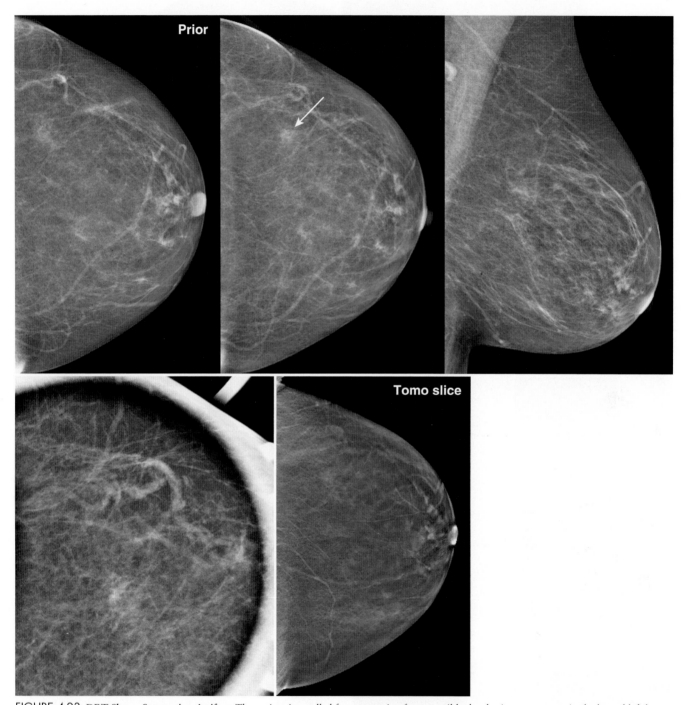

FIGURE 4-23 **DBT Shows Summation Artifact.** The patient is recalled from screening for a possible developing asymmetry in the lateral left breast (*arrow*). The spot compression view is not that helpful; there may still be a lesion. However, the tomosynthesis images only show normal, respectful tissue in this area.

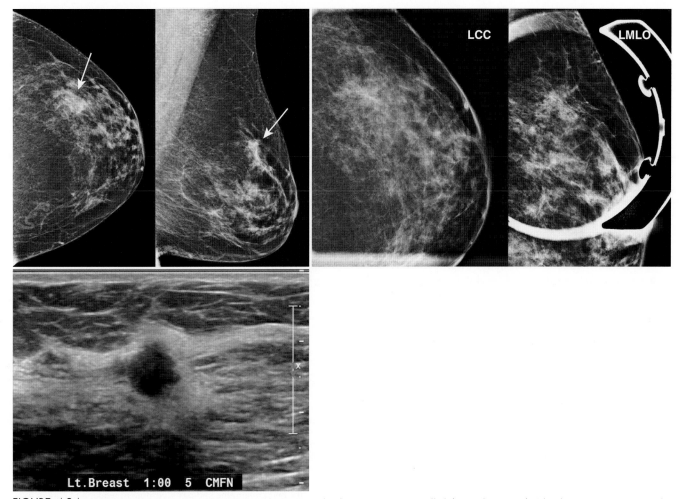

FIGURE 4-24 US **When the Diagnostic Mammogram Is Equivocal.** This patient was recalled for evaluation of a developing asymmetry in the upper-outer quadrant of her left breast (*arrows*). Spot compression views are equivocal—the finding does not efface but appears similar to the adjacent dense tissue. US shows a suspicious mass within the echogenic fibroglandular tissue. Biopsy revealed IDC grade 1 and ductal carcinoma in situ (DCIS).

mammography is not the same as the distance from the nipple on US (see Fig. 4-7). Differences between the compressed breast, supine positioning, and prone positioning must all be taken into account. The relationship to other breast landmarks such as a cyst or island of breast tissue can be helpful for locating an adjacent lesion on another modality. A mass on mammography should have a similar size and shape on US or MRI (see Fig. 4-7). An irregular mass or architectural distortion on the mammogram cannot be explained by a circumscribed mass such as a simple cyst on US.

Ready for More?

The evaluation and management of masses and asymmetries are reviewed in more depth in Chapters 7 and 10.

KEY POINTS

- The diagnostic evaluation should determine whether a finding is real and potentially significant and, if so, establish its location and level of suspicion. These goals are usually accomplished simultaneously using additional mammographic views and often US.
- Localizing a lesion involves determining its depth, accounting for the effects of obliquity on the MLO view, and using additional mammographic views as needed.
- Summation artifacts respect the normal breast architecture on spot compression views and can usually be shown to "unsuperimpose" on views taken at different angles or on rolled views.
- Level of suspicion should be determined using information from all views. Consider the appearance on screening, spot compression, and the true lateral views. Repeating the same view and tomosynthesis can also be helpful. Think about adding US if these views remain concerning or are equivocal.
- Close correlation of the location, size, and features of an US finding with the mammographic finding helps ensure that the same lesion is being examined.
- Occasionally a finding is suspicious on the screening views but less so on the diagnostic views (e.g., a developing asymmetry that persists but resembles normal tissue on the spot views and is not seen by US). In this situation, biopsy should still be considered, especially if the finding is new or larger than on previous mammograms.

References

Faulk RM, Sickles EA. Efficacy of spot compression-magnification and tangential views in mammographic evaluation of palpable breast masses. Radiology 1992;185:87-90.

Harvey JA, Nicholson BT, Cohen MA. Finding early invasive breast cancers: A practical approach. Radiology 2008;248:61-76.

Leung JWT, Sickles EA. Developing asymmetry identified on mammography: Correlation with imaging outcome and pathologic findings. Am J Roentgenol 2007;188:667-675.

Majid AS, de Paredes ES, Joherty RD, et al. Missed breast carcinomas: Pitfalls and pearls. RadioGraphics 2003;23:881-895.

Pearson KL, Sickles EA, Frankel SD, Leung JWT. Efficacy of step-oblique mammography for confirmation and localization of densities seen on only one standard mammographic view. Am J Roentgenol 2000;174(3):745-752.

Shetty MK, Watson AB. Sonographic evaluation of focal asymmetric density of the breast. Ultrasound Q 2002;18:115-121.

Sickles EA. Findings at mammographic screening on only one standard projection: Outcomes analysis. Radiology 1998;208:471-475.

Sickles EA. The spectrum of breast asymmetries: Imaging features, work-up, management. Radiol Clin North Am 2007;45:765-771.

Venkatesan A, Chu P, Kerlikowske K, et al. Positive predictive value of specific mammographic findings according to reader and patient variables. Radiology 2009;250:648-657.

CASE QUESTIONS

CASE 4-1. What potential abnormality is shown on this screening mammogram below? How would you work it up?

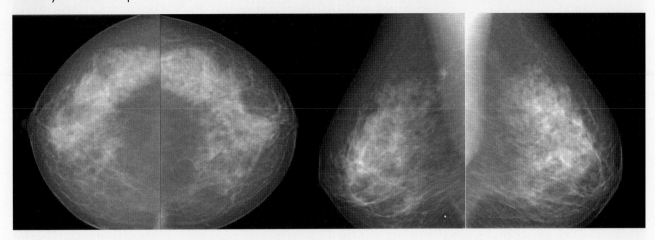

CASE 4-2. This patient has been recalled from screening for a one-view asymmetry in the medial left breast on the CC view (*arrow*). What views would you ask the technologist to obtain and why?

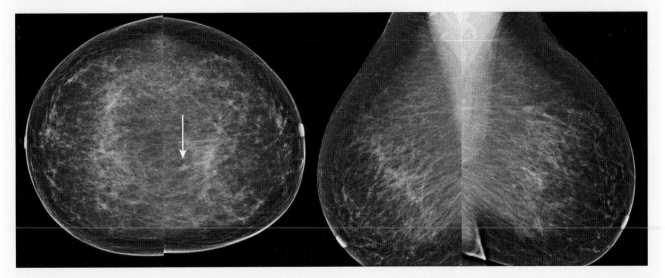

CASE 4-3. This 66-year-old woman is recalled from screening for a focal asymmetry in the right breast (*arrows*). The spot compression views are provided. US was negative. What are your BI-RADS assessment and recommendation?

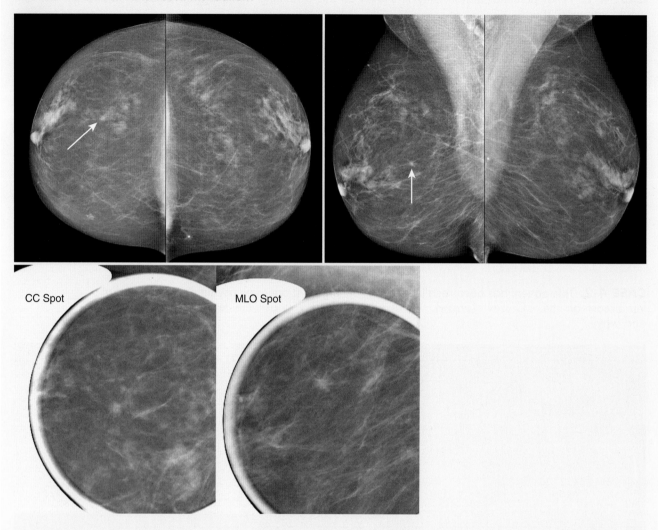

CC Spot

MLO Spot

CASE 4-4. This is a 45-year-old woman for screening recall of a one-view asymmetry on the MLO view only (*arrow*). Where will you spot on the CC view? Yellow or blue arrow?

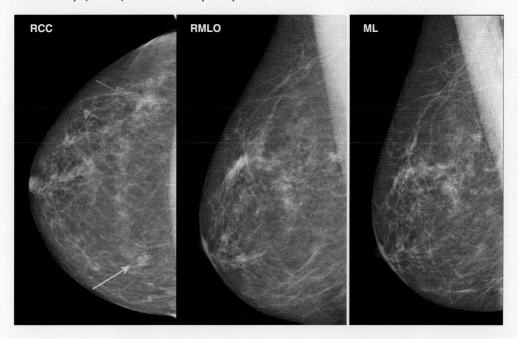

CASE 4-5. A 70-year-old woman is recalled from screening to work up a one-view asymmetry (*circle*). Here are her diagnostic views. A "best guess" spot compression view was performed of the lateral breast because there is so little tissue in the medial breast at the same distance from the nipple. US identified a mass at 11 o'clock, 3 cm from the nipple. What do you think?

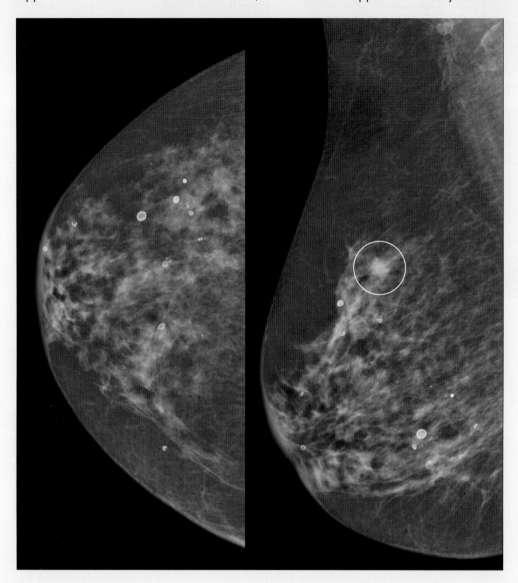

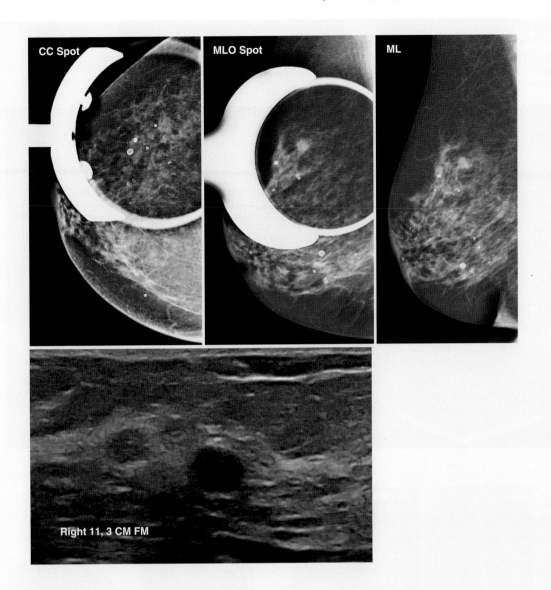

CASE 4-6. This 64-year-old woman is recalled for a new one-view asymmetry on the right MLO view (*arrow*). Here are her MLO spot compression and ML views. To localize the lesion in the CC projection, spot compression views in the lateral, central, and medial breast were obtained. Where is the lesion? What would you do next?

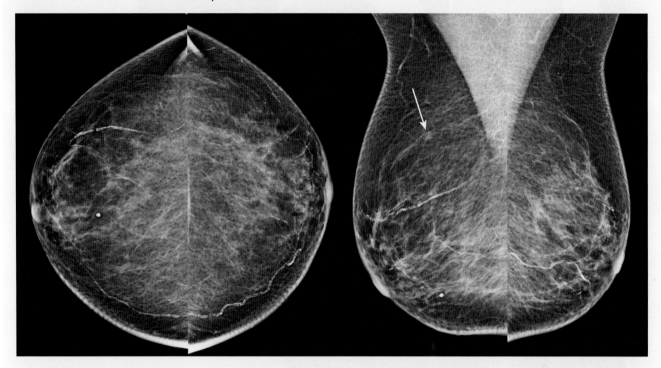

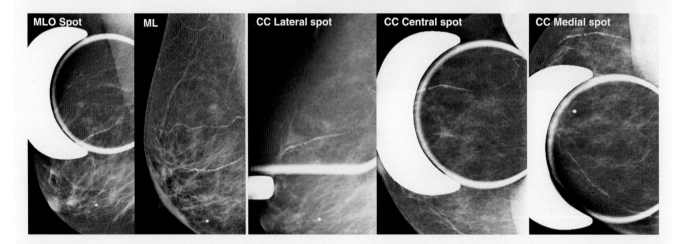

CASE 4-7. A 63-year-old-woman recalled from screening for a focal asymmetry in the left breast at 8 o'clock (*arrows*) that may be increasing in density compared with the findings of the prior study. Her diagnostic mammogram and US are shown here. What are your BI-RADS category and recommendation?

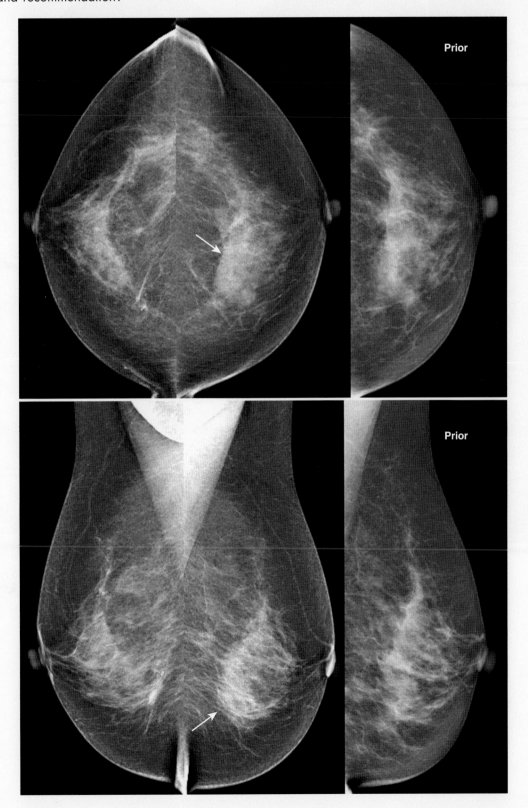

Figure continued on the next page.

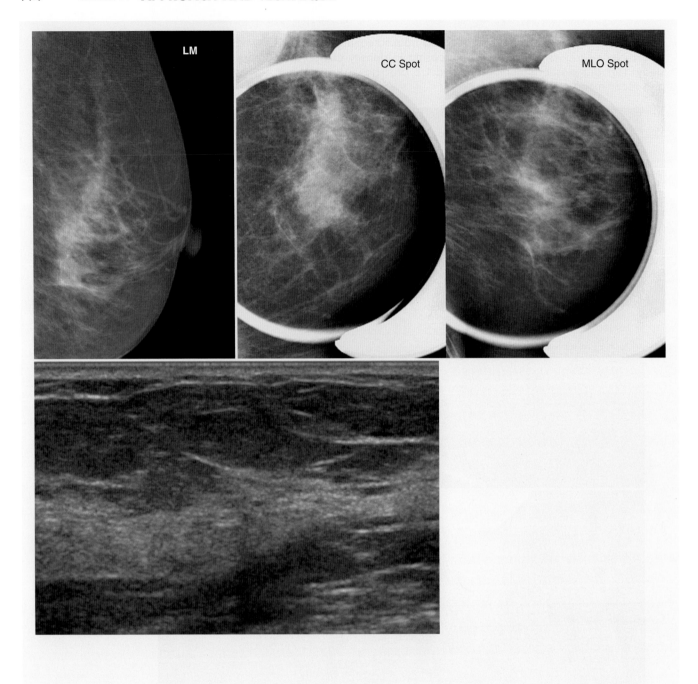

CASE 4-8. This 44-year-old woman was recalled from screening to evaluate a small mass protruding into the superficial fat (*arrow*). Which cyst corresponds to the mammographic finding? *A* or *B*?

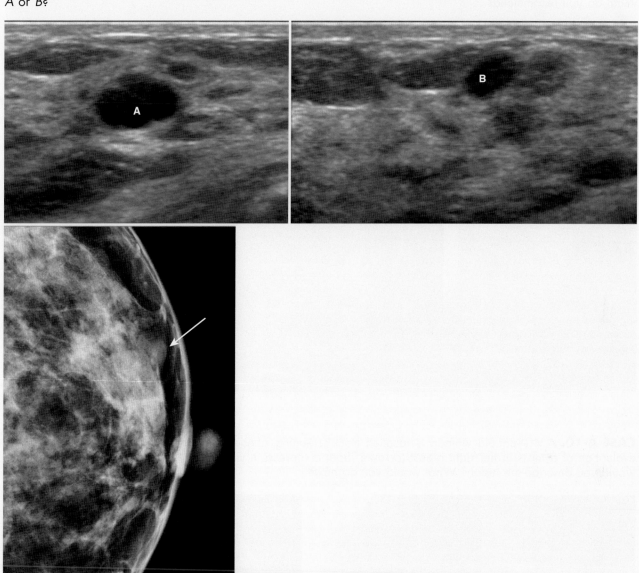

CASE 4-9. A 48-year-old woman is recalled from her first mammogram for an asymmetry seen on the right MLO view (*arrow*). A spot compression view is performed. Does the finding persist? What do you recommend?

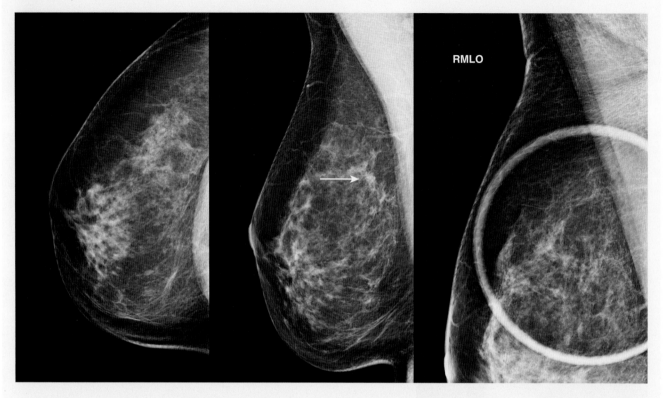

CASE 4-10. A 40-year-old woman is recalled from screening after her first mammogram for evaluation of a mass in her right breast (*arrows*). Spot compression views are performed. How would you describe the lesion? What would you do next?

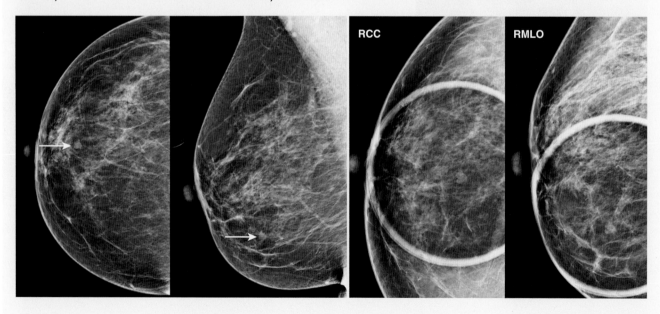

CASE 4-11. A 60-year-old woman is recalled from screening due to an asymmetry in the central breast on the CC view (*arrow*). The location on the MLO view is not obvious. Given the tomo-synthesis slice here, where is the mass located? What are your BI-RADS assessment and recommendation?

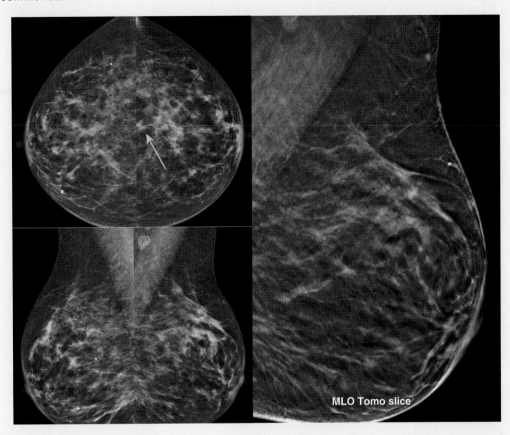

MLO Tomo slice

CASE 4-12. A 64-year-old woman recalled from screening for a focal asymmetry in the left breast (*arrows*). BB is on a skin lesion. What do you think of her diagnostic mammogram? What is your recommendation?

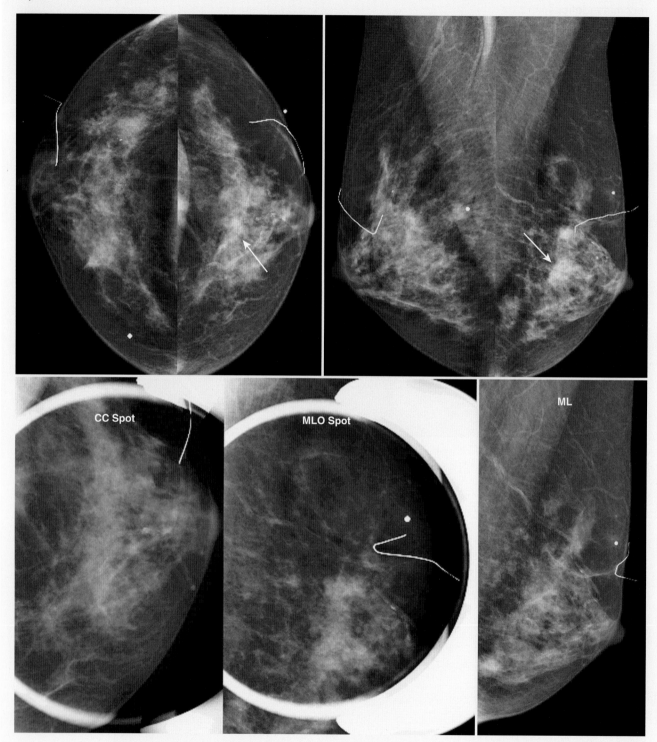

CASE 4-1. Did you remember to look over the pectoralis muscle? First, we need to confirm that the one-view asymmetry on the right MLO view is a concerning finding by doing a spot compression view. Then we need to localize the lesion in the CC projection. We can compare the position of the lesion on the MLO and ML; it shifts lower so it is lateral. An XCCL spot followed by an US confirms that it is located in the 10 o'clock position. Diagnosis: IDC.

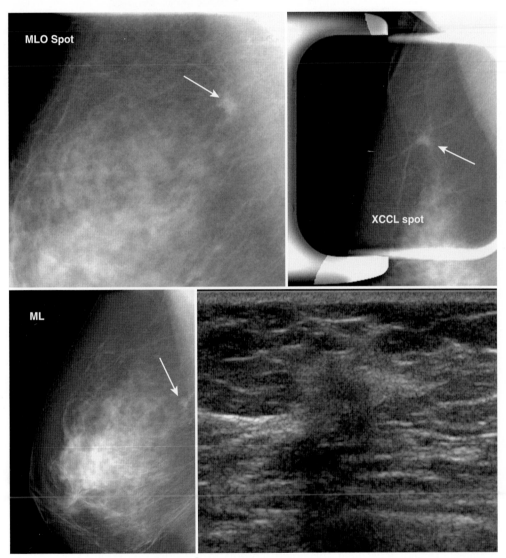

CASE 4-2. First, we want a CC spot compression view to evaluate the level of suspicion. We will also want a true lateral view. Because the asymmetry is in the medial breast, we will get an LM view rather than an ML. Let's also get a best-guess spot compression view in the MLO view— it's probably in the superior breast. The lesion is much better seen on the LM than on the MLO view. A medial lesion is closer to the image receptor and thus sharper on an LM view than on an ML or MLO view. US confirms the 11 o'clock location. Ultrasound-guided core biopsy showed IDC.

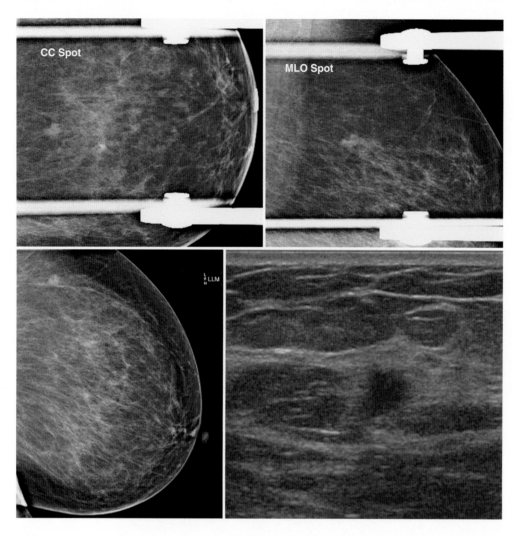

CASE 4-3. There is a small, irregular mass with spiculated margins in the right breast at 11 o'clock, middle third. This is BI-RADS 4; recommend stereotactic biopsy. A negative US does not change the assessment or need for biopsy. Histologic diagnosis: IDC.

CASE 4-4. Because the lesion moves superior on the ML view, it is located in the medial breast. The yellow arrow is the best choice for a CC spot compression view. Biopsy showed IDC.

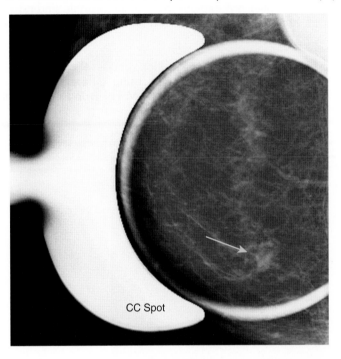

CC Spot

CASE 4-5. The lateral location is confirmed on the ML view because the lesion moves lower compared with the original MLO view. The US shows what may be a cyst, although there is no posterior acoustic enhancement, but a cyst would not explain the mammographic finding of a mass with ill-defined margins, and 3 cm from the nipple seems too close. Let's go take a look. Here is her repeat US.

This mass with suspicious features is a better correlate in size, position, and level of suspicion for the mammographic finding. Biopsy of both masses was performed, using different markers for each. Ultrasound-guided biopsies showed sclerosing adenosis at 3 CM FN (wing marker, *blue arrow*), and IDC at 6 CM FN (coil marker, *yellow arrow*).

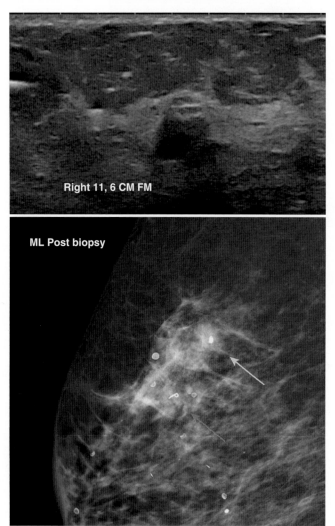

CASE 4-6. The asymmetry shifts down only slightly on the ML view compared with the MLO. Therefore, the lesion should be located at 11 o'clock. Unfortunately, the CC spot compression views do not help us confidently locate the lesion in that projection. Let's use US to see if we can confirm our thought that the lesion is at 11 o'clock. We were right on! There are two ways we can confirm that the US finding represents our mammographic finding—BB shot or mammogram views after the ultrasound-guided core biopsy showing the marker in the same location. Biopsy showed invasive lobular carcinoma (ILC).

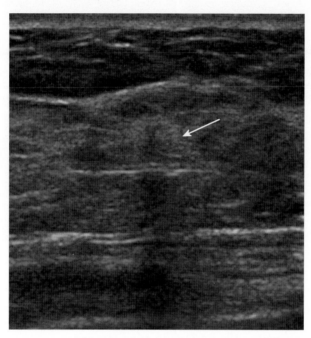

CASE 4-7. Although the area looked like there may have been a change, the tissue looks very respectful on the spot compression views. In addition, the US shows only normal breast tissue. This case is here to keep you honest! BI-RADS 1. Routine screening recommended.

CASE 4-8. The mass for which the patient was recalled is superficial. Cyst *A* is *within* the hyperechoic breast tissue and represents a cyst that is deeper and larger than the mass on the mammogram. Cyst *B* is at the superficial border of the echogenic fibroglandular tissue and corresponds better in size and location to the mammographic finding.

CASE 4-9. A lesion is not confirmed on the MLO spot view. However, we cannot be satisfied that the finding represents summation artifact based on this single view alone. A lesion this small could easily be obscured by fibroglandular tissue. ML and XCCL views were performed, and a mass is confirmed in the upper outer quadrant (*arrows*). US identified the lesion in the 10 o'clock position, and biopsy revealed IDC and DCIS.

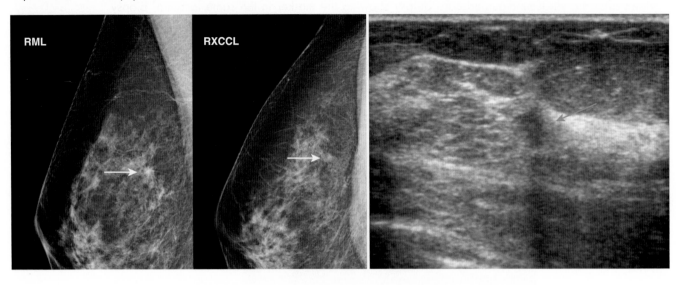

CASE 4-10. The spot views suggest a fatty hilum (*arrow*)! US confirms an intramammary lymph node in the 7 o'clock position. Although most nodes are found in the mid-upper and outer breast and along the pectoral muscle, they can occasionally be seen in other locations.

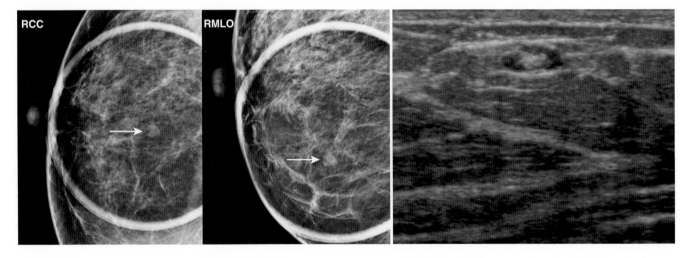

CASE 4-11. The MLO tomosynthesis slice shows architectural distortion in the superior breast (*arrow*). US confirms a highly suspicious mass in this area. Ultrasound-guided biopsy showed IDC.

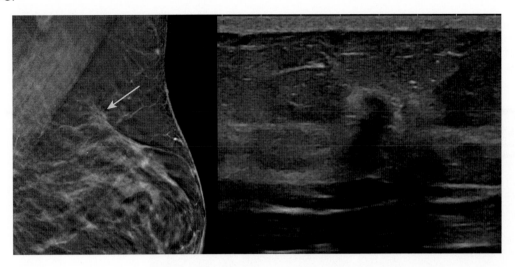

CASE 4-12. The area recalled from screening looks somewhat mass-like on the MLO spot, but improved on the CC spot. Suggest US. This did confirm a mass in the central breast, and biopsy showed IDC.

But wait, there is a second finding. Did you notice the abnormal finding at 6 o'clock on the ML and CC spot (*arrows*)? If so, GOOD JOB!
Here are her second set of spots centered at 6 o'clock. Her sagittal MRI nicely shows the two lesions. Biopsy of the second mass also showed IDC, and the patient underwent mastectomy.

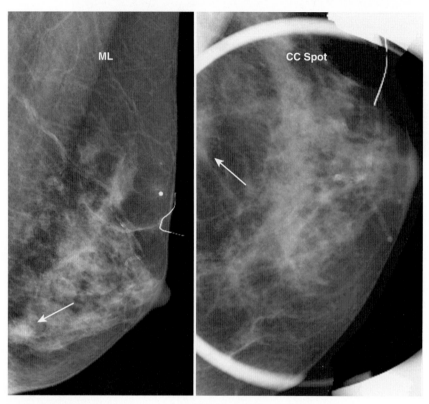

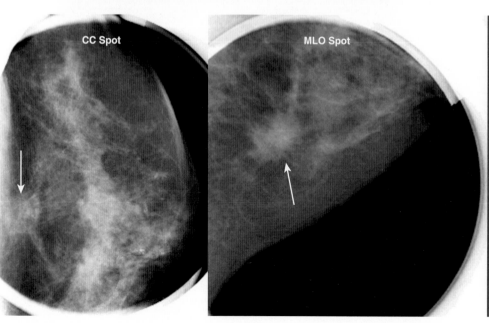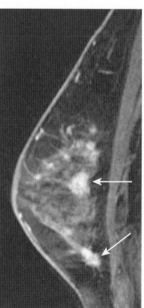

FINDINGS ON MAMMOGRAPHY

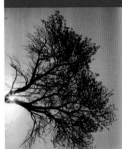

CHAPTER 5

Breast Anatomy and Physiology: Recognizing Normal Changes

A young woman presented with a palpable lump in her right axilla. She was 3 months pregnant and terrified. Her sister had been diagnosed with stage III breast cancer at age 30. This was her first child. She was thinking the worst. Before starting an ultrasound examination, the patient told us about the lump, she stated that it was enlarging and tender. The ultrasonography (US) showed axillary breast tissue, a normal variant. It was tender and enlarging because of her pregnancy. She left relieved and assured.

Breast anatomy seems pretty straightforward, so why bother to read on? Normal anatomic structures and normal physiologic changes can mimic pathology; recognition of these findings as normal can avoid unnecessary follow-up studies or interventions and reduce patient anxiety. It is also important to be familiar with the normal anatomy as visualized on mammography, US, and magnetic resonance imaging (MRI) so that findings can be correlated among the modalities. Understanding normal breast anatomy and its lymphatic drainage can also help us evaluate the extent of cancers more accurately.

Breast Anatomy

The Fibroglandular Tissue

The breast is a mound of fibrous stroma with adipose, ductal, and glandular tissue overlying the anterior chest wall (Fig. 5-1). It often extends to the axillary tail (tail of Spence).

The fibroglandular tissue is surrounded by mostly fatty tissue in the subcutaneous and retromammary (retroglandular) regions (Fig. 5-2). The upper outer quadrant typically contains more fibroglandular tissue than the other quadrants and is where cancers are most likely to develop. The superficial fascia splits into deep and superficial fascial layers that envelop the fibroglandular tissue. The

superficial fascial layer lies between the fibroglandular tissue and the subcutaneous fat, while the deep fascial layer is located between the fibroglandular tissue and the retromammary fat. The fascial layers are often difficult to identify on mammography, but may be seen on US (Fig. 5-3). The deep pectoral fascia separates the pectoralis major muscle from the retromammary fat (see Fig. 5-3).

Cooper ligaments are thin sheets of fascia that support the breast. They extend like a mesh through the breast parenchyma, attaching to the dermis and the superficial and deep fascial layers. The Cooper ligaments appear mammographically as fine, white, curvilinear lines throughout the breasts (Fig. 5-4). They are seen on US as thin, curvilinear, echogenic lines (see Fig. 5-4). Straightening and tethering of the Cooper ligaments appear as architectural distortion and spiculation, and are often due to invasive carcinoma, radial scar/complex sclerosing lesion, or scarring due to surgery. Retraction of these ligaments by cancers can cause deformity of the border of the fibroglandular tissue, skin dimpling, or nipple retraction. Familiarity with the normal patterns created by Cooper ligaments allows recognition of cases in which these patterns are distorted.

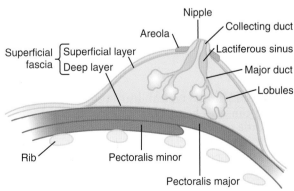

FIGURE 5-1 Cross-Sectional Anatomy of the Breast.

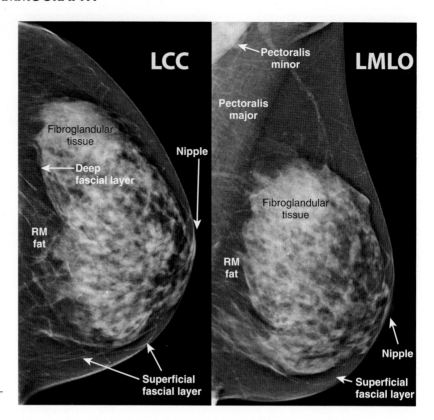

FIGURE 5-2 Anatomy Seen on Routine Mammographic Views. RM fat, retromammary fat.

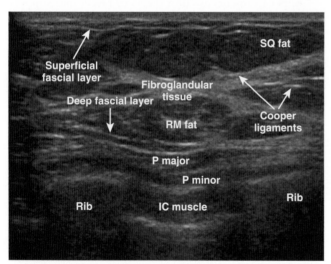

FIGURE 5-3 Breast Ultrasound Anatomy. IC muscle, intercostal muscle; P major, pectoralis major muscle; P minor, pectoralis minor muscle; RM fat, retromammary fat; SQ fat, subcutaneous fat.

Understanding the typical distribution of fibroglandular tissue can also help detect cancers. In most women, there is little or no dense tissue in the medial and inferior breast or in the retroglandular region (Fig. 5-5). Therefore, developing or focal asymmetry in these areas should be viewed with suspicion.

The border of the fibroglandular tissue has a variable appearance (Fig. 5-6). Abrupt changes in the contour of this border are uncommon in the normal patient. Cancers can produce retraction, protrusion, or spiculation at this border, disrupting the normal tissue contours.

Breast Asymmetry

Asymmetry in breast density or size is usually just a normal variation but may be due to malignancy. There may be considerably more breast tissue in one breast than the other (global asymmetry) (Fig. 5-7). This is a nearly always a normal finding provided there are no breast symptoms such as a palpable lump, breast thickening, or skin erythema, and no associated findings such as architectural distortion. Likewise, asymmetry in the size of the breasts can be quite striking, but is nearly always normal as long as there are no associated clinical or mammographic findings. Beware, however, of the finding known as the "shrinking breast," which is a sign of invasive lobular carcinoma. This diagnosis should be considered when one breast appears smaller than the other, especially when the parenchyma is dense and the size discrepancy is new or increasing (see Chapter 11, Expanding the Differential Diagnosis).

Lobules and the Terminal Duct Lobular Unit

The lobules are the milk-producing glands in the breast. They have somewhat of a flower shape (Fig. 5-8). Therefore, lobular calcifications often manifest as a group or cluster of calcifications or multiple clusters (see Fig. 5-8). The end branch of the duct and the lobule that it serves is the terminal duct lobular unit (TDLU). Most breast cancers originate in the TDLU.

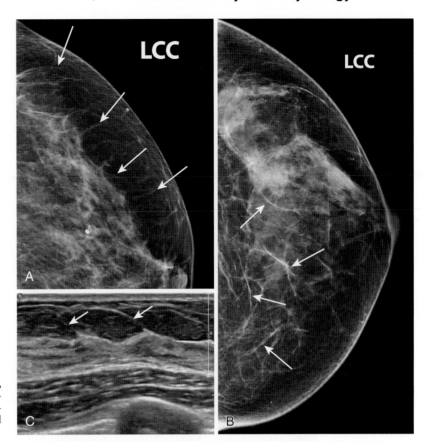

FIGURE 5-4 **Normal Cooper Ligaments. A** and **B,** The thin, white lines throughout the breast on mammography are Cooper ligaments (*arrows*). **C,** On ultrasonography, Cooper ligaments are also thin, white, and curvilinear (*arrows*).

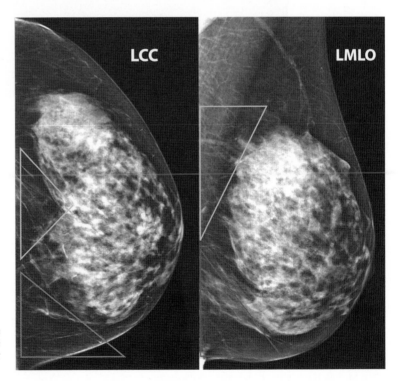

FIGURE 5-5 **Normal Distribution of Fibroglandular Tissue on Mammography.** There is usually little or no tissue in the medial breast (*blue triangle*), inferior breast (*red triangle*), or retromammary fat (*pink triangles*).

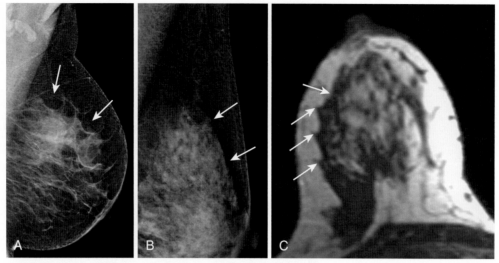

FIGURE 5-6 **Normal Fibroglandular Border. A,** Scalloped appearance of the fibroglandular tissue border. **B,** This interface may also be smooth and convex, especially when the tissue is dense. **C,** T1-weighted MRI shows peaks at the edge of the fibroglandular tissue where Cooper ligaments attach.

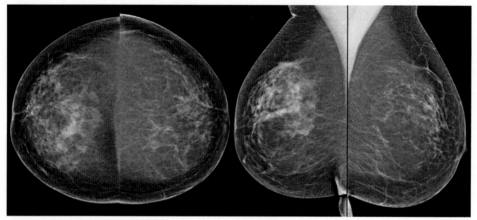

FIGURE 5-7 **Global Asymmetry.** Asymmetric distribution of breast tissue is not uncommon and is nearly always a normal finding in the asymptomatic patient.

FIGURE 5-8 **Terminal Duct Lobular Unit (TDLU). A,** Schematic of a normal TDLU showing the terminal ducts and lobules. Calcifications (blue circles) often form in the lobules. **B,** Lobular calcifications are usually round, punctate, or amorphous and develop in one or more clusters. Most are benign.

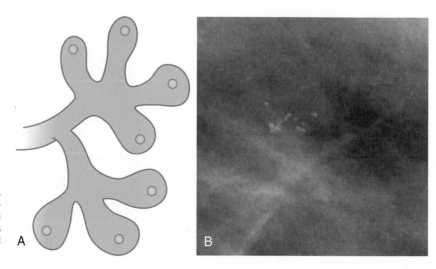

Ductal Anatomy

A good way to think of ductal anatomy is like a shrub with the base at the nipple. Look at the picture of the tree at the beginning of this chapter. Can you visualize the tree as ductal anatomy? Large branches or major ducts begin to arborize a short distance behind the nipple (Fig. 5-9). These major ducts continue to arborize into smaller and smaller ducts. The branches intertwine, just as branches

of a shrub or tree. Ductal systems of the breast are not like segments of an orange or the lobes of the lung that have well-defined anatomic boundaries. A single ductal system can extend over a wide area of the breast (see Fig. 5-9). Segmental calcifications involving most of a single ductal system may therefore appear to be regional in distribution.

Ductal carcinoma in situ (DCIS) most often manifests as calcifications within the milk duct. Calcifications that are in a linear or segmental distribution have a higher predictive value for cancer than those with grouped or regional distribution. When a suspicious lesion is identified, the regions between the finding and the nipple and the finding and the chest wall should be scrutinized because they are the most likely locations for additional disease (Fig. 5-10).

Milk produced in the lobules travels to the nipple via minor ducts that join to form major ducts (see Fig. 5-9). The major duct dilates beneath the areola to form the lactiferous sinus. This normal structure is sometimes mistaken for a breast mass on breast self-examination (Fig. 5-11). Milk collects in the lactiferous sinus during

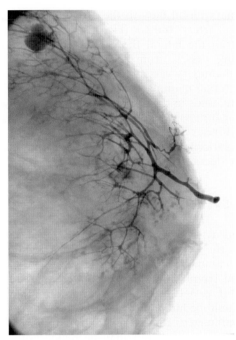

FIGURE 5-9 **Extent of One Ductal System.** This craniocaudal (CC) view from a normal galactogram (image inverted) demonstrates the large area over which a single ductal system can extend. If this entire ductal system contained calcifications, the distribution may appear regional rather than segmental. The mass in the lateral breast is a cyst.

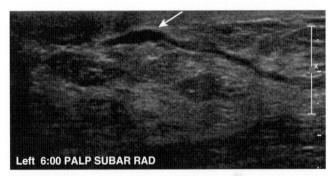

Left 6:00 PALP SUBAR RAD

FIGURE 5-11 **Lactiferous Sinus.** A normal lactiferous sinus (*arrow*) can sometimes be mistaken for a breast mass on clinical examination.

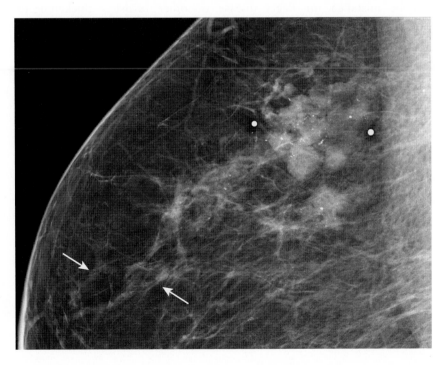

FIGURE 5-10 **An Abnormal Ductal System.** Breast cancer commonly extends throughout one duct system. In this case, segmental fine linear branching calcifications fill an entire ductal system with ductal carcinoma in situ. If you look closely, calcifications (*arrows*) can be seen between the primary finding (*marked with BBs*) and the nipple.

lactation. The duct then tapers within the nipple, where it is called the collecting duct (a misnomer, because nothing really collects here).

Nipple and Areola

The nipple has five to ten ductal openings. This is important if you are going to perform a galactogram because you will need to identify which duct is producing the abnormal discharge. If the discharging orifice cannot be identified, galactography cannot be performed.

Nipple in Profile
It is helpful to have the nipple in profile on at least one mammographic projection (CC or mediolateral oblique [MLO]). When not in profile, the nipple can be mistaken for a mass. The subareolar anatomy produces a complex mammographic appearance due to the overlapping lines of the converging milk ducts and surrounding blood vessels. The superimposition of these structures can simulate masses or obscure true lesions.

Retraction Versus Inversion
The nipple may be retracted (pulled back slightly) or inverted (invaginated into the breast) (Fig. 5-12). These variations are normal for many women. In postmenopausal women, the ducts can become enlarged or ectatic, which can result in mild nipple retraction or heme-negative nipple discharge.

If nipple retraction or inversion is of recent onset, it is concerning for breast cancer. In these cases, we routinely perform spot compression views and US of the subareolar region.

Nipple Enhancement
The nipples often enhance on contrast MRI of the breast (Fig. 5-13). This is a normal finding and should not be mistaken for Paget disease or other breast pathology.

The areola has little to do with breast imaging, except that occasionally women with a swollen Montgomery gland may present for diagnostic evaluation. The Montgomery glands are those little bumps on the areola. They can produce discharge, become infected, or produce milk during lactation.

Blood Supply

The primary blood flow to the breast is via the internal mammary artery (60%) (Fig. 5-14). Additional flow comes from the lateral thoracic artery (Fig. 5-15) and perforating vessels from the intercostal arteries. The internal mammary vessels are a good landmark for identifying internal mammary lymphadenopathy on MRI.

Of note, veins in the breast can be quite tortuous, even simulating a mass. Thrombosis of superficial veins in the breast (Mondor disease) is treated conservatively with no need for anticoagulation. Arterial calcifications can simulate early ductal calcifications.

Lymph System

The majority of lymph generated in the breast (97%) drains to the axilla, with the remainder draining to the internal mammary lymph nodes.

Normal lymph nodes can be quite large in long-axis diameter (Fig. 5-16). The cortex should be thin and the hilum should be fatty. On US, the cortex will typically be a few millimeters thick. The hilum of normal lymph nodes is hyperechoic, but may be hypoechoic centrally (see Fig. 5-16).

Blood flows into the lymph node and exits through the hilum, and the lymph channels enter the node on the capsule and exit through the hilum. Metastatic deposits therefore frequently appear as a focal bulge or thickening of the cortex (Fig. 5-17). With more significant involvement, the lymph node cortex can become

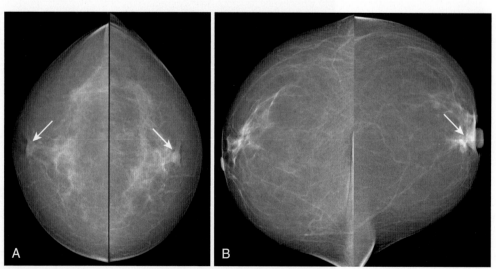

FIGURE 5-12 **Nipple Inversion and Retraction. A,** Bilateral longstanding normal nipple inversion (*arrows*). **B,** Retraction of the left nipple (*arrow*) due to a subareolar cancer.

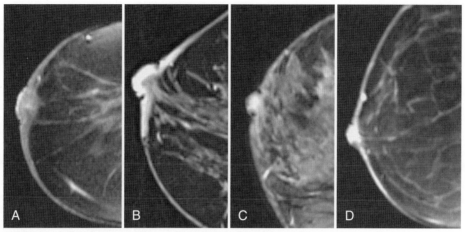

FIGURE 5-13 **Range of Normal Appearance of Nipples on MRI.** Nipples may have thin (**A**) or thick (**B**) surface enhancement, or may enhance centrally (**C**) or diffusely (**D**).

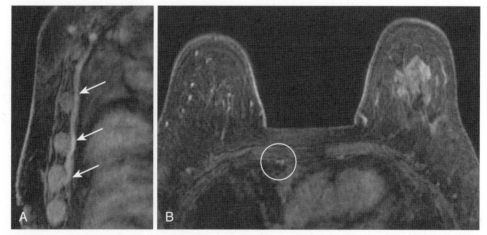

FIGURE 5-14 **Internal Mammary Artery and Vein on MRI. A,** Sagittal T1-weighted postcontrast image of the parasternal area showing the internal mammary artery (*arrows*). **B,** Axial T1-weighted image of the breast showing the location of the internal mammary artery and vein (*circle*).

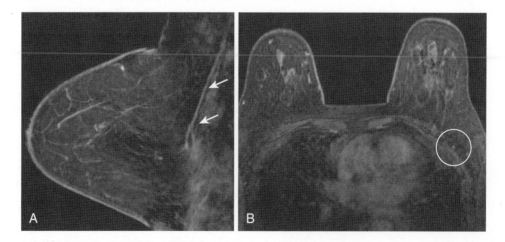

FIGURE 5-15 **Lateral Thoracic Artery on MRI. A,** Sagittal T1-weighted postcontrast image of the breast showing the lateral thoracic artery (*arrows*) adjacent to the chest wall. **B,** Axial T1-weighted postcontrast image of the breasts showing the location of the lateral thoracic artery (*circle*).

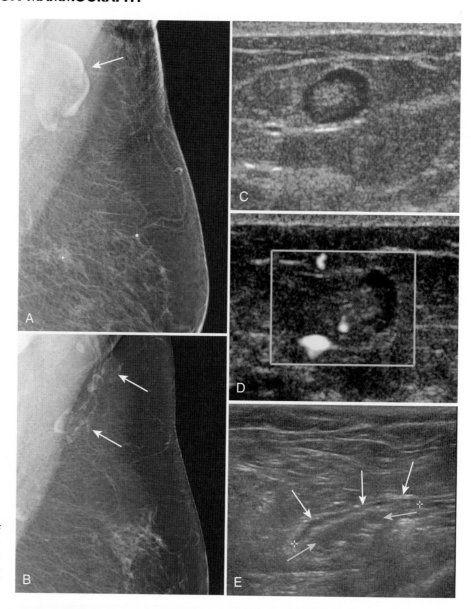

FIGURE 5-16 **Normal Appearance of Lymph Nodes on Mammography (A and B) and US (C to E).** The cortex of normal lymph nodes (*arrows*) is thin (2 to 3 mm). The hilum of lymph nodes is hyperechoic on US, but may be hypoechoic centrally (*yellow arrows*).

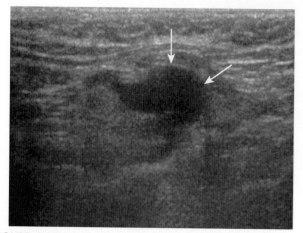

FIGURE 5-17 **Focal Metastatic Deposit.** In this patient with invasive breast cancer, the focal cortical bulge (*arrows*) represents metastasis.

diffusely thickened and there may be loss of the fatty hilum.

Intramammary lymph nodes are normal and present on most mammograms. They are typically located in the subcutaneous tissue and along the pectoral muscle and usually lie in close proximity to blood vessels (Fig. 5-18). They are not typically seen within the fibroglandular tissue.

Axillary lymph nodes are divided into levels based on their location relative to the pectoralis minor muscle (Fig. 5-19).

Anatomy of the axilla is important in considering a biopsy approach for abnormal axillary lymph nodes. The axillary lymph nodes lie in a basin formed by the latissimus dorsi muscle at the lateral wall, the pectoralis muscles at the medial wall, and the breast at the inferior wall. The axillary artery and vein are at the bottom or posterior aspect of the basin. Use of a long-throw core biopsy needle may then be hazardous because the steep angle needed to avoid the muscles may result in injury to

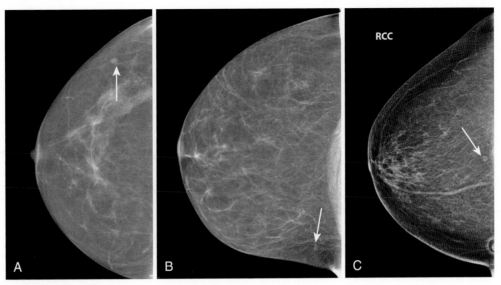

FIGURE 5-18 **Normal Location of Intramammary Lymph Nodes.** Intramammary lymph nodes in the subcutaneous tissue and near a vessel in the lateral (**A**, *arrow*) or medial (**B**, *arrow*) breast. They can also be located just anterior to the pectoralis major muscle (**C**, *arrow*).

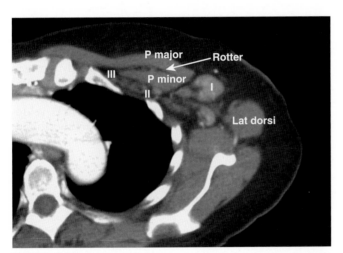

FIGURE 5-19 **Levels of Axillary Lymph Nodes.** Level I lymph nodes are lateral to the pectoralis minor muscle (P minor). Level II lymph nodes are beneath the pectoralis minor muscle. Level III lymph nodes are medial to the insertion of the pectoralis minor muscle. Rotter lymph nodes are located between the pectoralis major (P major) and minor muscles.

the vessels. Instead, a manually thrown needle (Temno, Achieve) or fine-needle aspiration (FNA) biopsy may be safer.

Internal mammary lymph nodes are located just posterior to the intercostal muscle in the second and third interspace near the sternum. When abnormal, they can be identified on US. The chance of internal mammary metastases is highest in the setting of invasive breast cancer located in the medial breast. Isolated metastasis to the internal mammary lymph nodes without concurrent metastases to the axillary lymph nodes is very uncommon, occurring in about 3% of women with invasive breast cancer. If identified, the internal mammary area may be included in the radiation field following surgery to lower the risk of recurrence.

Muscles Visualized on Mammography

The breast lies anterior to the pectoral and serratus anterior muscles. The pectoralis major muscle should be seen on all MLO mammograms and about 30% of CC mammograms unless there are factors that limit positioning. The appearance of the pectoralis major muscle can be variable on the CC view (Fig. 5-20). The pectoralis minor muscle is seen on the MLO view in some patients (see Fig. 5-2).

Poland Syndrome
This rare disorder manifests as unilateral hypoplasia of the breast and ipsilateral chest wall. The affected breast is small. The ipsilateral pectoral muscles are absent. Patients may also have ipsilateral brachysyndactyly (short, fused fingers), skin webbing, and renal agenesis.

Other Pectoralis Muscle Findings
The pectoral muscles may also be atrophic as a result of stroke or poliomyelitis. The muscles may contain calcifications that are due to trichinosis or other parasitic infection, or autoimmune disorders such as CREST syndrome (calcinosis, Raynaud's phenomenon, esophageal dysfunction, sclerodactyly, and telangiectasis).

Sternalis Muscle
This nonfunctional sliver of muscle parallels the sternum (hence the name "sternalis"). It can appear as a rounded mass just medial to the pectoralis muscle (Fig. 5-21). On mammography, it is visualized on the CC view only! About 8% of the population has this muscle. The muscle is unilateral in two thirds of cases and bilateral in the remaining third. This little muscle can prompt a long, arduous workup. On the other hand, a medial cancer can be mistaken for a sternalis muscle. If not seen on older mammograms, a diagnostic workup is usually indicated to exclude a breast cancer. Spot compression views and US can help evaluate for the presence of a mass. If needed,

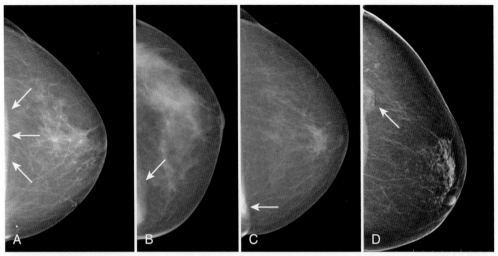

FIGURE 5-20 **Various Appearance of the Normal Pectoralis Major Muscle on the Craniocaudal (CC) View. A,** The most common appearance is a symmetric bulge located in the center of the CC view (*arrows*). **B,** The medial insertion of the pectoralis major muscle may bulge into the image (*arrows*). **C,** The medial insertion of the pectoralis major muscle can also have a triangular shape (*arrow*). **D,** The lateral aspect of the pectoralis major muscle can appear as a focal bulge (*arrow*).

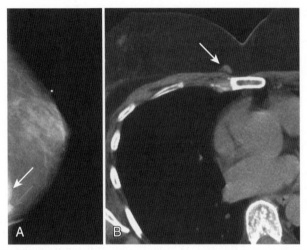

FIGURE 5-21 **Sternalis Muscle. A,** This small muscle (*blue arrow*) that parallels the sternum can appear as a round mass medial to the pectoralis muscle (*white arrow*) on the craniocaudal view. **B,** Computed tomography of another patient showing the typical appearance of this muscle.

a computed tomography (CT) scan of the chest (contrast is not needed) can show whether or not a sternalis muscle is present (see Fig. 5-21).

Other Musculoskeletal Findings

Pectus excavatum deformity, deformity from prior thoracic trauma or surgery, and severe kyphoscoliosis may limit positioning for mammography.

Essentials of Breast Development

All breast development that occurs up to the time of birth is the same for males and females and is not hormone dependent. Neonates (both male and female) can have breast enlargement or colostral milk ("witch's milk") due

to maternal hormones. In females, the hypothalamus stimulates the pituitary gland to secrete follicle-stimulating hormone (FSH) and luteinizing hormone (LH). FSH stimulates the ovaries, which produce predominantly estrogen in early puberty. This results in ductal elongation and branching. Later, when ovulation commences, progesterone levels rise, resulting in lobular proliferation. Development of the breasts is monitored clinically by the Tanner classification. Breast development can continue into the early 20s.

Milk Streak and Accessory Tissue

The milk streak (Fig. 5-22) forms in the fifth week of embryonic development. All but the part of the streak that ultimately develops into the breast normally involutes. If involution does not occur, supernumerary (accessory) nipples, accessory breasts, and axillary breast tissue can result.

Accessory nipples are most commonly located in the inframammary fold or axilla, but can be present anywhere along the milk streak (Fig. 5-23). They are often mistaken for moles. They may produce a scant amount of milk during lactation.

Accessory breast tissue is most commonly located in the axilla (Fig. 5-24), with the second most common location being the inframammary fold. This wayward breast tissue may enlarge during pregnancy and lactation, causing anxiety in expectant mothers. An overlying accessory nipple is very uncommon.

Tuberous Breasts

This disorder manifests as a small breast mound with the areola projecting as a separate mound (Fig. 5-25). This finding is likely due to incomplete breast development.

Amazia

Amazia is lack of breast development. Sadly, this is usually due to trauma or surgery that damages or removes the breast bud. For this reason, surgery is often delayed if possible for many benign disorders seen in prepubescent girls until development is more complete.

Essentials of Breast Physiology

During the follicular phase of the menstrual cycle (days 7 to 14), estrogen predominates, resulting in epithelial proliferation. Progesterone predominates during the luteal phase of the menstrual cycle (days 15 to 30), resulting in increased secretions and blood flow. Breast

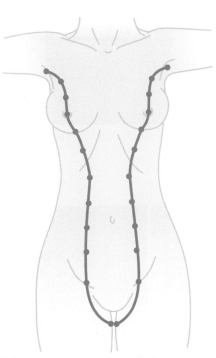

FIGURE 5-22 **Location of the Milk Streak.** Accessory nipples and breast tissue can be located anywhere along the path of the milk streak.

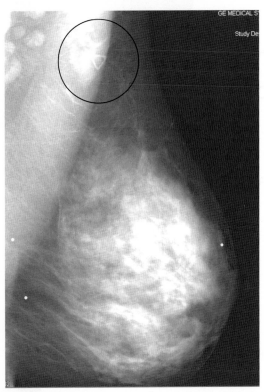

FIGURE 5-24 **Axillary Breast Tissue.** This patient palpated normal-appearing axillary breast tissue (*circle*) (the *triangle* marks the palpable lump).

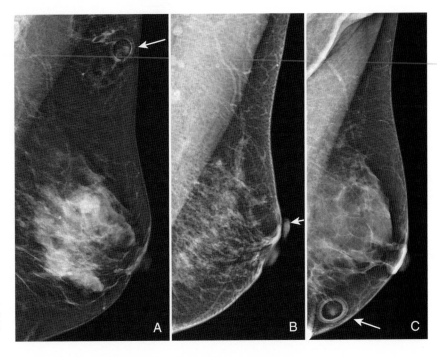

FIGURE 5-23 **Supernumerary Nipples.** Supernumerary nipples arising from the milk streak in three women. **A,** Axillary region; **B,** areolar region; and **C,** inferior breast (*arrows*).

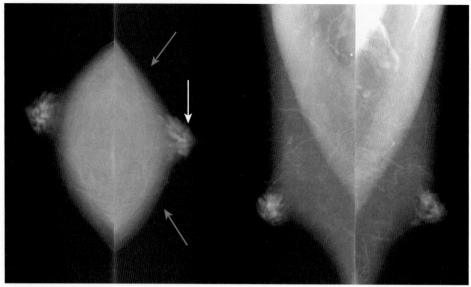

FIGURE 5-25 **Tuberous Breasts.** The breast has two distinct mounds. The primary mound (*blue arrows*) has only fat. The volume of breast tissue is low and is located in the secondary breast mound (*white arrow*).

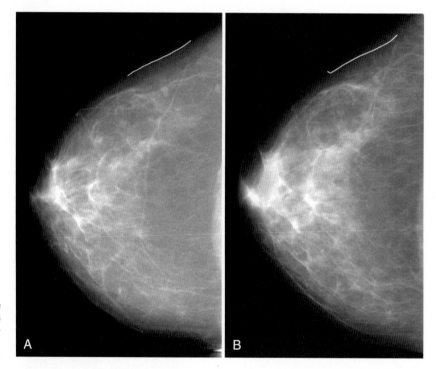

FIGURE 5-26 **Small Changes in Breast Density Due to Hormonal Fluctuations. A** and **B,** Mammograms obtained 1 year apart in a 47-year-old perimenopausal woman show a small increase in density (**B**). This is common and normal for women in their 40s.

tenderness is maximal at days 26 to 30. With the onset of menses (days 1 to 7), secretory activity regresses and edema subsides; breast volume is minimized on days 5 to 7 of the cycle. The most comfortable time for most women to undergo mammography therefore is days 5 to 10 of the menstrual cycle. Likewise, MRI of the breasts will demonstrate less physiologic enhancement if performed during the follicular phase of the cycle. Mild changes in breast density can be seen over the course of the cycle, with slightly greater density in the luteal phase than in the follicular phase. Mild fluctuations in breast density are common for premenopausal and perimenopausal women (Fig. 5-26 and Box 5-1).

Pregnancy and Lactation

Marked ductal and lobular proliferation occurs during pregnancy. Ductal proliferation begins as early as the first few weeks of pregnancy. Enlargement of the breasts

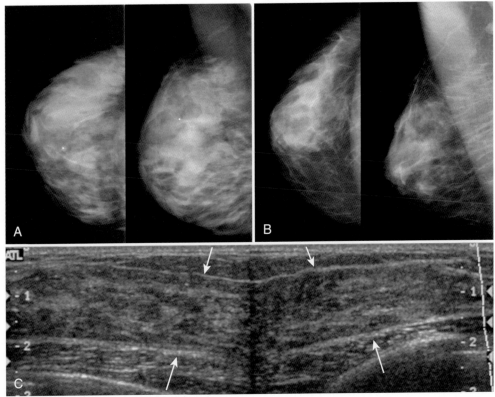

FIGURE 5-27 **Appearance of Lactating Breasts on Mammography and US. A,** The mammogram shows very dense tissue with expansion of the lobules. **B,** Mammogram of the same patient 3 years later after cessation of lactation shows marked regression of the breast tissue. **C,** Lactating breast tissue (*arrows*) is hypoechoic on US, becoming isoechoic to fat.

BOX 5-1 Causes of Bilateral Increase in Breast Density

- Hormone therapy—estrogen with progesterone more likely than estrogen alone
- Perimenopausal
- Follicular versus luteal phase in premenopausal women
- Pregnancy/lactation
- Elevated serum prolactin

---

occurs at 5 to 8 weeks, so breast pain and enlargement may be the first symptoms of pregnancy. A woman presenting to the Emergency Department with new onset of bilateral breast pain needs a pregnancy test! During the second trimester, lobular proliferation predominates and the alveoli contain colostrum. Lactation may be possible as early as 16 weeks of gestation.

Immediate withdrawal of placental hormones results in a rise in prolactin that converts mammary cells to a secretory state. The initial milk is colostrum, which is thin and watery, but high in protein. Mature milk is much higher in fat. Tactile stimulation of the nipple causes release of oxytocin, which causes contraction of the myoepithelial cells in the breast, resulting in the milk let-down release for nursing.

Changes During Pregnancy and Lactation

The breast tissue becomes markedly dense on mammography (Fig. 5-27). On US, the tissue becomes more hypoechoic (see Fig. 5-27C). Women with high serum prolactin levels due to pituitary prolactinoma or due to some medications, such as antipsychotics, may have extremely dense tissue similar to that seen during pregnancy.

Cancers *do* occur during pregnancy and lactation. US may be used as the initial imaging technique in these women, but mammography can be performed safely with shielding of the pelvis with a lead apron, if clinically indicated. Core needle biopsy or even surgical biopsy performed during the third trimester of pregnancy or during lactation may result in a milk fistula, a complication in which milk from the high-pressure ductal system extends along the biopsy track to the skin. Women must often stop lactating to eliminate the fistula. Infection of the fistula is uncommon. This potential complication should be discussed with these women prior to biopsy.

Galactocele

This word means "milk cyst." Galactoceles typically present as palpable masses in lactating women. Because human milk is very high in fat, a fat-fluid level can form.

In our experience, this layering never forms a clean, straight line.

Lactating Adenomas

These masses have imaging and histologic features that resemble fibroadenomas. There is some discussion in the pathology literature that these masses may actually be fibroadenomas "revved up" on the hormones of pregnancy. They are often multiple. Provided there are no suspicious sonographic features, we typically perform follow-up US after delivery after cessation of lactation, or at 4 to 6 months post partum. These lesions often regress rapidly after lactation ceases.

Perimenopause

With apologies to Dylan Thomas, the ovaries "do not go gentle into that good night." Hormonal fluctuation is rampant in the 5 or so years preceding menopause. The menstrual cycle typically shortens—specifically the follicular phase—so the breasts are exposed to longer periods of progesterone. This can result in increased breast density, breast pain, fibrocystic change, and development of breast cysts. The patient can be reassured that her breast symptoms will improve after menopause, unless she begins use of menopausal hormone therapy (MHT) (in which case you may become good friends during her frequent appointments for US of her cysts).

Menopause

Declining ovarian function results in regression of the breast epithelium through apoptosis. This occurs in an order that is the reverse of breast development. The lobules first undergo involution, with ducts remaining stable or even becoming ectatic until much later in menopause. Fibroadenomas undergo degeneration, decreasing in size, often with formation of popcorn-like calcifications. Large rod-like (secretory) calcifications form as the ducts degenerate, often 10 to 20 years after menopause.

Menopausal Hormone Therapy

MHT increases breast density in 17% to 75% of women, depending upon the regimen used (Fig. 5-28). Density changes are greater for combined estrogen-progesterone regimens than for an estrogen-only regimen. Most of the change occurs in the first year and is associated with mastalgia. Fibroadenomas may increase in size (see Fig. 5-28).

KEY POINTS

- Potential masses visualized on breast imaging may represent normal structures. Examples are the nipple or a sternalis muscle on mammography, a lactiferous sinus on US, or enhancing nipples on MRI.
- The sternalis muscle is never seen on the MLO view. Spot compression views, US, or CT may be needed to differentiate this muscle from a breast mass.
- Biopsy of the breast bud in prepubescent girls may disrupt normal breast development.
- Fluctuations in breast density can occur between the luteal and follicular phase of the menstrual cycle, accounting for some differences in density between screening examinations and differences in parenchymal enhancement between MRI examinations.
- Cysts and fibrocystic change predominate in the fifth decade and can continue after menopause if women use MHT.

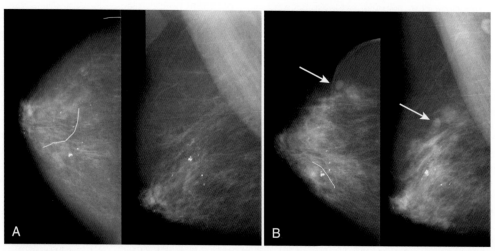

FIGURE 5-28 **Increase in Breast Density Due to MHT. A,** Mammogram prior to MHT in a postmenopausal woman. **B,** Moderate increase in breast density after beginning MHT. A new mass (*arrow*) has developed in the upper outer quadrant. Biopsy showed a fibroadenoma.

Final Comments

Normal structures and physiologic changes in the breast can be mistaken for pathologic findings. Conversely, a cancer may be mischaracterized as a normal anatomic structure or thought to represent normal physiologic changes. When such uncertainty exists, a thorough diagnostic workup should be performed to differentiate between normal and potentially abnormal findings. Although most new clinical findings during pregnancy are benign, cancers do occur. These findings should undergo appropriate diagnostic evaluation if clinically suspicious.

References

Assadi FK, Salem M. Poland syndrome associated with renal agenesis. Pediatr Nephrol 2002;17(4):269-271.

Ellis RL. Optimal timing of breast MRI examinations for premenopausal women who do not have a normal menstrual cycle. Am J Roentgenol 2009;193(6):1738-1740.

Jeung MY, Gangi A, Gasser B, et al. Imaging of chest wall disorders. Radiographics 1999;19(3):617-637.

Osborne MP. Breast development and anatomy. In JR Harris (ed). Breast Diseases, 2nd ed. Philadelphia, JB Lippincott, 1991.

CASE QUESTIONS

CASE 5-1. Screening mammogram shows a mass in the central right breast (*arrows*). What view may be helpful as part of the workup?

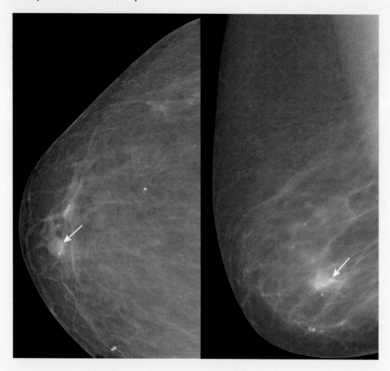

CASE 5-2. A 52-year-old woman with a palpable lump in the areolar area. **A,** Left MLO spot compression view (*BB marks the palpable lump*). **B,** US of the palpable finding. What is the cause of the finding? What is your BI-RADS assessment category?

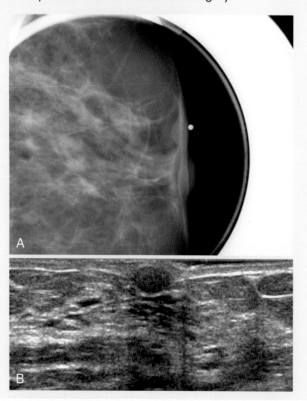

CASE 5-3. Screening magnetic resonance imaging (MRI) in a high-risk patient. Sagittal and axial T1-weighted MRI at 2 minutes after administration of contrast agent. What are your BI-RADS category and recommendation?

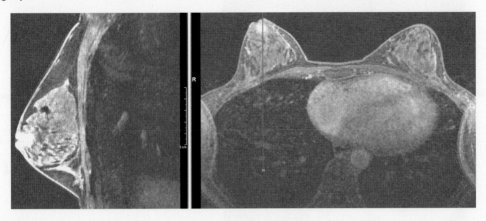

CASE 5-4. Bilateral screening mammogram showing a possible mass in the medial right breast (*arrow*). What is the most likely cause?

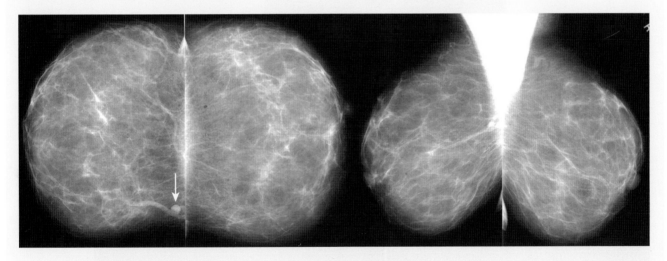

CASE 5-5. A 72-year-old woman with newly diagnosed invasive carcinoma in the left breast at 9 o'clock. US of the parasternal region oriented in the sagittal plane. What is the finding (*arrow*)?

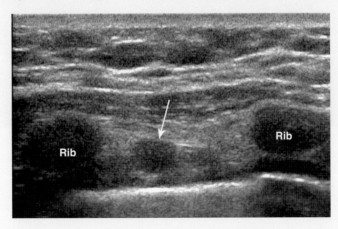

CASE 5-6. A 40-year-old woman with screening MRI T1-weighted, postcontrast images. What is the finding?

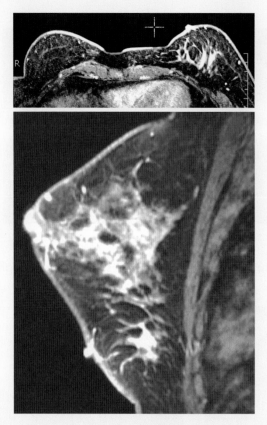

CASE 5-7. A 58-year-old woman for screening mammogram. Only the MLO views are shown. What are your BI-RADS assessment and recommendation?

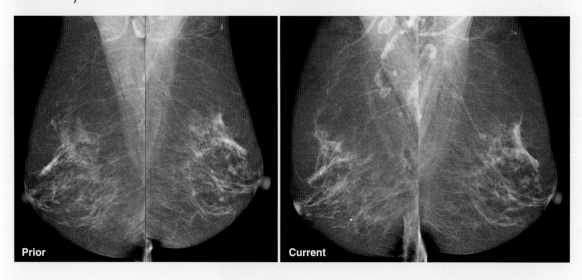

CASE 5-8. A 55-year-old woman presents for screening mammogram. What is the finding? What is your BI-RADS assessment category? What other clinical findings might you expect?

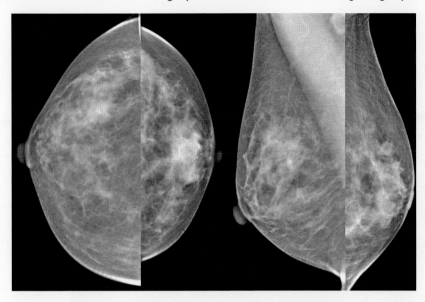

CASE 5-9. A 20-year-old woman presents with multiple bilateral palpable findings. She is 8 months pregnant. Ultrasound examination was performed. Two of the masses are shown. What do the masses likely represent? What are your BI-RADS assessment and recommendation?

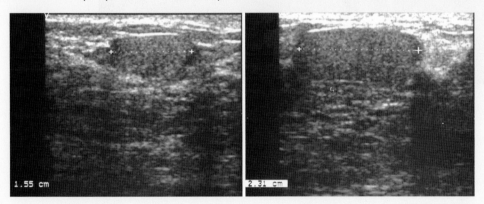

CASE 5-10. A 56-year-old woman presents for screening. What might explain the large increase in breast density? She is postmenopausal and not using menopausal hormone therapy.

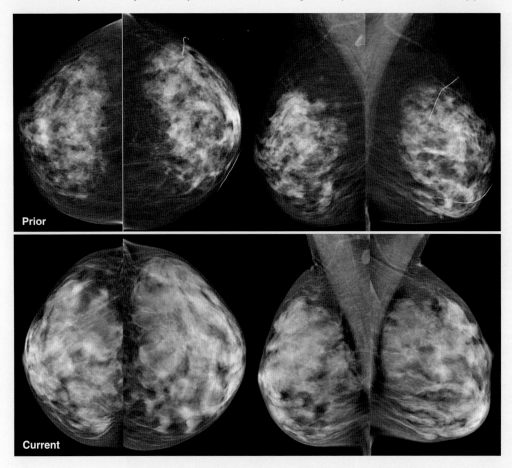

CASE 5-11. A 48-year-old woman presents for screening. What is the finding? What is your BI-RADS assessment?

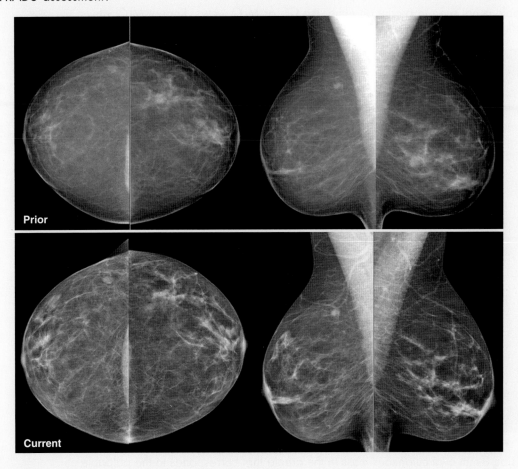

Prior

Current

CASE 5-12. This is a screening MRI in a 39-year-old woman who had left breast cancer treated with lumpectomy and radiation therapy 3 years ago. What are the findings? What are your assessment and recommendation?

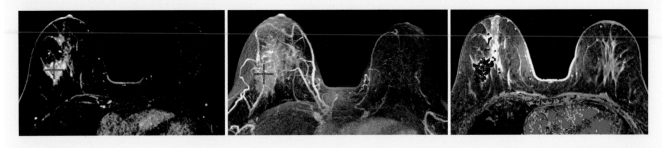

CASE 5-1. The nipple is not seen in profile on either the CC or MLO views. Repeat MLO views with the nipple (*marked with a BB, arrow*) in profile document that the "mass" was the nipple.

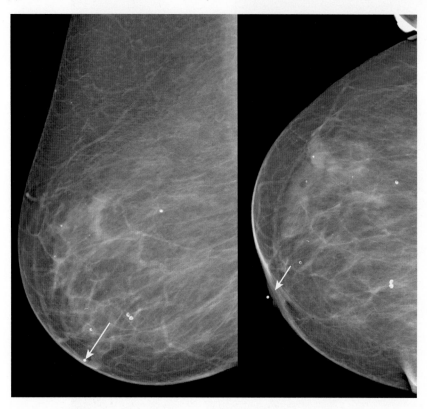

CASE 5-2. There is an 8-mm oval cutaneous mass in the areola that corresponds to the palpable finding. This is an enlarged Montgomery gland (BI-RADS 2). The patient was instructed to apply warm compresses, resulting in drainage a few days later. The lesion resolved without additional treatment.

CASE 5-3. There is an oval enhancing "mass" in the right breast, which represents an inverted nipple (BI-RADS 1 or 2 would be appropriate). Below are sagittal and axial images from the same patient through the left nipple, which was retracted. This patient had chronic nipple changes. A note from the technologist or quick phone call to the patient can confirm the chronic nature of the finding.

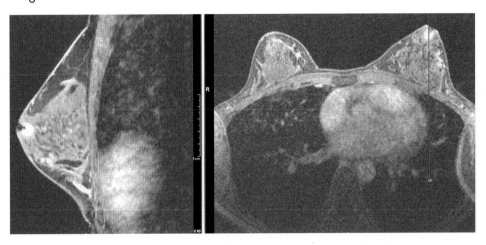

CASE 5-4. Diagnostic mammogram was not performed, which was a mistake. Excisional biopsy was recommended from the screening mammogram. An image from failed needle localization shows that the "mass" represents a tortuous vein (*arrows*).

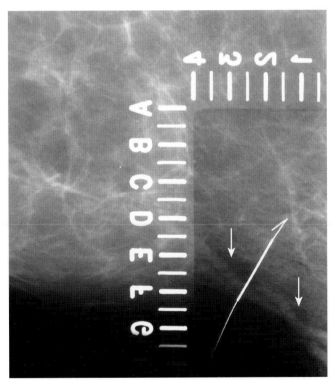

CASE 5-5. Abnormal internal mammary lymph node. These are visualized as one or more small hypoechoic masses (*arrow*) posterior to the intercostal muscles in the first or second intercostal space near the sternum. If lymph nodes are visible on ultrasonography in this region, they are abnormal. Tortuous vessels can also be seen in this area, so Doppler should be used to ensure that the lesion is not vascular.

On MRI, abnormal internal mammary lymph nodes are best seen in the sagittal plane. This T1-weighted postcontrast MRI with fat suppression shows an abnormal internal mammary lymph node (*arrow*) in a different patient.

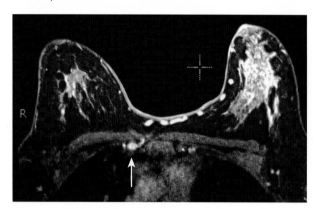

CASE 5-6. There is an enhancing dermal mass in the left breast at 6 o'clock. On the sagittal image, the mass is seen to extend into the breast. On clinical examination, the mass corresponds to an accessory nipple.

CASE 5-7. This is BI-RADS 1: Negative. The apparent increase in the number of lymph nodes on the current study is due to differences in positioning—essentially how much of the fatty tissue in the axilla the technologist was able to include on the image. The morphology of the lymph nodes is normal, so this is not concerning for lymphoma.

CASE 5-8. The left pectoralis muscle is absent. This patient has Poland syndrome. She has shortening of the middle fingers on her left hand with webbing (brachysyndactyly). She does not have renal agenesis, which can also occur with Poland syndrome.

CASE 5-9. These have an appearance suggestive of fibroadenomas. In a pregnant woman, these are most likely lactating adenomas. We gave this a BI-RADS 3 and had the patient return 3 months post partum. The follow-up images show marked interval decrease in size.

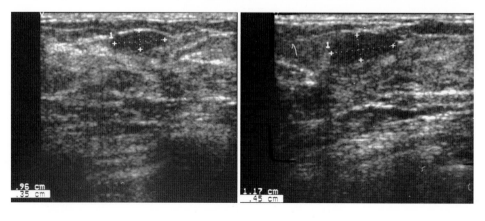

CASE 5-10. This patient began using an antipsychotic medication. Many of the antidepressants and antipsychotic medications are dopamine antagonists, resulting in an increase in serum prolactin. These patients may also present with breast pain or galactorrhea.

CASE 5-11. There is a possible developing asymmetry in the right breast at 10 o'clock (*circle*). BI-RADS 0. If you look closely at the prior and current mammograms, there is actually a subtle increase in overall breast density. The asymmetry did not persist on additional views, and ultrasonography was negative. The asymmetry represents cyclic hormonal fluctuations in normal breast tissue in this perimenopausal woman.

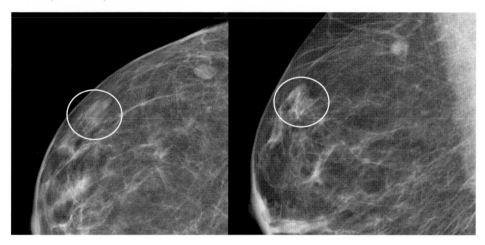

CASE 5-12. There is nonmass enhancement in the lateral right breast. In most women, comparison with the contralateral breast would help discern whether this was due to normal parenchymal enhancement or suspicious enhancement that would require biopsy. The patient has had a prior hysterectomy, so this study was not timed with regard to her cycle. Because the enhancement may have been hormonal, she was asked to have a repeat study when her serum progesterone level was less than 1.5 ng/mL. She was positioned in the biopsy coil so that biopsy could be performed if the enhancement persisted. The enhancement had resolved on the repeat study (not shown) and was consistent with physiologic parenchymal enhancement.

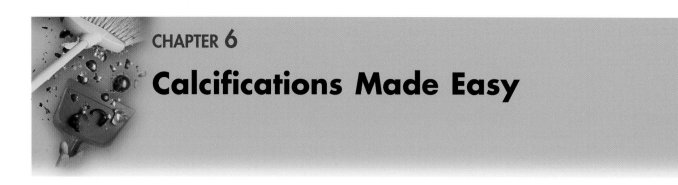

CHAPTER 6

Calcifications Made Easy

Your children have finally learned to get their own cereal in the morning. But yikes, what is that stuff on the kitchen floor? You start to reach for a paper towel. Actually, that stuff looks kind of sharp. You're going to need a broom and dustpan. Analyzing calcifications can be like deciding how to deal with a dirty kitchen floor. Do you use a paper towel because the debris is just stuff, or do you go to the closet to get the dustpan because the detritus is sharp like pieces of glass? A good way to approach calcifications is to think about the sharpness of the edges. The sharper the calcifications, the more worried you should be. So ... when you look at calcifications, would you go for the paper towel or the dustpan?

As radiologists, we have an opportunity to detect and diagnose curable breast cancer. This is especially true for ductal carcinoma in situ (DCIS); the 10-year survival rate is 98%. Once invasion occurs, the prognosis is less sure. Calcifications are the earliest sign of breast cancer, and their accurate assessment is potentially lifesaving.

Calcifications Versus Artifact

The first step in evaluating suspected calcifications is to make sure that they represent true calcifications rather than artifact. Deodorant is radiopaque because it contains aluminum compounds. It has a characteristic appearance and is typically present in the axilla. Zinc oxide in ointments and talc can mimic calcifications, especially when collected in moles and other skin lesions (Fig. 6-1). Sand on the skin, tattoo pigment, and metallic artifacts from gunshot wounds or prior surgical procedures (Fig. 6-2) can also resemble calcifications, as can pick-off artifact or dust on screens in film-screen mammography.

Describing Calcifications

Calcifications are described by distribution, morphology, laterality, and location. The key to evaluating calcifications is to accurately define their distribution and morphology. Careful analysis of these features and comparison with prior studies allows us to estimate the level of suspicion of calcifications and determine how they should be managed. Remember that assessment of calcifications is only as good as the quality of the magnification views.

Distribution

The BI-RADS lexicon defines distribution modifiers (Fig. 6-3) that range from the least suspicious (diffuse/scattered) to the most suspicious (segmental).

A ductal system in the breast resembles the branches of the tree. Ductal systems vary greatly in size and can extend over quite a large region.

The large majority of breast cancers develop within a single ductal system. Therefore, calcifications of *almost any morphologic type* that are judged to be in one ductal system are suspicious for DCIS, especially if their distribution is segmental or linear (Fig. 6-4). If widely separated calcifications of suspicious morphologic appearance are visualized, particularly within dense tissue, they may still be malignant. Because they are sparse, the initial impression may be that they are scattered; however, calcifications that appear scattered *within a segment* may still be suspicious. If you connect the dots and the resulting distribution is linear or segmental, biopsy should be considered (Fig. 6-5).

On the other end of the spectrum, the lowest suspicion distribution is bilateral scattered calcifications. Benign processes producing calcifications in the breast frequently involve more than one duct system, often in both breasts. This most commonly occurs with round & punctate calcifications that develop within lobules; when scattered and bilateral, these calcifications are typically benign (Fig. 6-6).

Morphology

The BI-RADS lexicon divides calcifications by morphology into two categories based on their risk of malignancy: (1) typically benign and (2) suspicious (Table 6-1).

Typically Benign Calcifications

Typically benign calcifications are classified by their etiology (e.g., suture, dermal) except for round & punctate. These are nearly always recognized as benign on screening mammography, although occasionally, recall for magnification or tangential views may be needed to confirm their benign status.

152

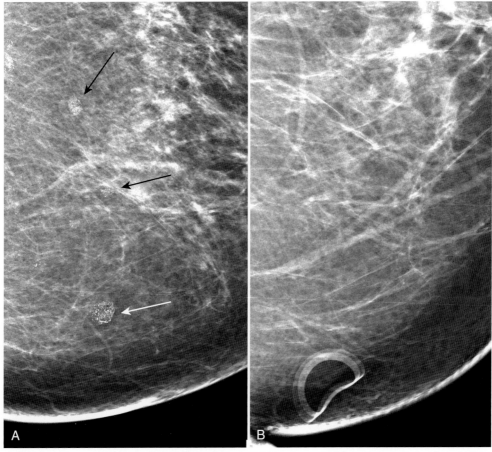

FIGURE 6-1 **Talc Artifact. A,** Talc artifact resembling calcifications (*arrows*). **B,** These features were no longer seen on a follow-up study obtained after talc use was discontinued.

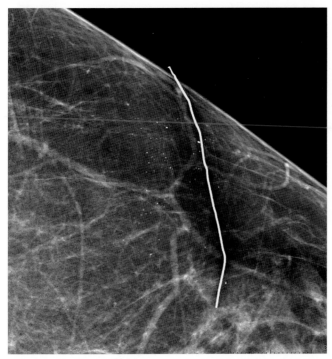

FIGURE 6-2 **Metallic Artifact Due to Surgery.** This patient had a benign excisional biopsy. There are several small metallic densities in the bed that are too white to be calcifications. They are due to metallic deposits from the electrocautery device.

TABLE 6-1	Morphology Descriptors for Calcifications	
LIKELIHOOD OF MALIGNANCY	**MORPHOLOGY**
Typically benign	Dermal
	Vascular
	Coarse, popcorn-like
	Large rod-like
	Lucent-centered or rim
	Milk of calcium
	Suture
	Dystrophic
	Round & punctate
Suspicious	Amorphous, indistinct
	Coarse heterogeneous
	Fine pleomorphic
	Fine linear or fine linear branching

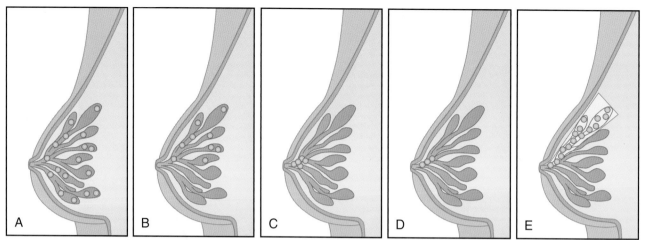

FIGURE 6-3 **Distribution of Calcifications (from Lowest to Highest Suspicion). A,** Scattered calcifications are distributed throughout most of or the entire breast. **B,** Regional calcifications are present in much of the breast, but not all. **C,** Grouped or clustered calcifications are present in a focal area. Sometimes multiple clusters may be present. **D,** Linear calcifications are distributed more or less in a line. **E,** Segmental calcifications extend from the nipple toward the chest wall.

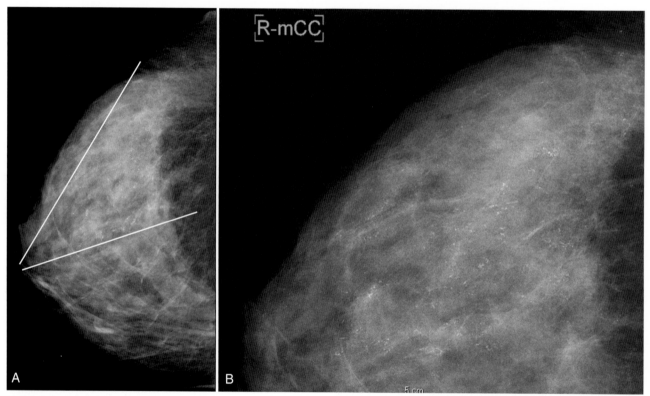

FIGURE 6-4 **Segmental Calcifications. A,** Right craniocaudal (CC) view showing segmental distribution of calcification. **B,** On the CC magnification view, fine pleomorphic calcifications extend from the nipple toward the chest wall. This is BI-RADS 5. Biopsy showed high-grade DCIS.

Dermal Calcifications

Benign dermal calcifications occur in folds where women sweat—in the inframammary fold, cleavage, and axilla (Fig. 6-7). Because dermal calcifications are fixed in the skin, they retain the same relationship to each other in each view; this is called the "tattoo sign" (Fig. 6-8). Dermal calcifications are also common in scar tissue. A

tangential view may be needed to confirm that calcifications have a dermal location.

Vascular Calcifications

Arterial calcifications usually produce parallel tracks of linear calcifications that follow the course of a vessel and can almost always be dismissed as benign. Occasionally,

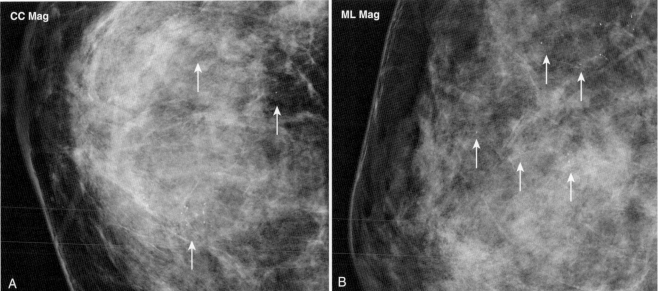

FIGURE 6-5 **Widely Separated Calcifications in a Segmental Distribution. A** and **B,** Magnified views show extremely dense tissue with fine pleomorphic calcifications in the superior and central right breast (*arrows*) in a segmental distribution. **C,** Ultrasonography (US) shows an irregular hypoechoic mass with associated calcifications in the upper breast. Core biopsy revealed invasive ductal carcinoma (IDC) and DCIS.

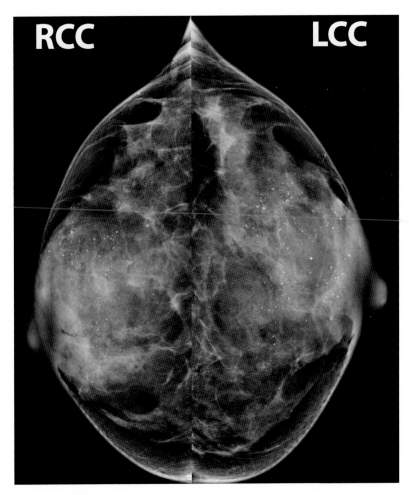

FIGURE 6-6 **Scattered Bilateral Round & Punctate Calcifications.** These calcifications are typically benign (BI-RADS 2) and require no additional evaluation.

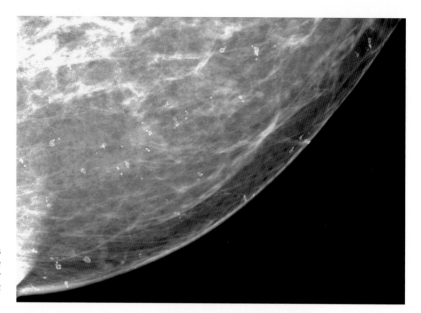

FIGURE 6-7 **Dermal Calcifications.** These calcifications have lucent centers but are smaller and finer than those due to fat necrosis. They are also often polygonal or geometric in shape rather than very round or oval like fat necrosis calcifications.

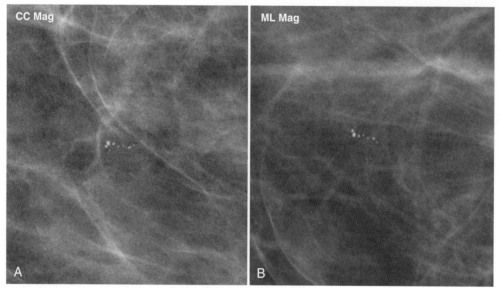

FIGURE 6-8 **Tattoo Sign.** This cluster of calcifications has the same appearance on the CC magnification view (**A**) and mediolateral (ML) magnification view (**B**) if flipped horizontally. This finding suggests a dermal location. Calcifications within the breast tissue will appear to move relative to one another on different projections.

when early, they may mimic fine pleomorphic calcifications that are in a linear distribution (Fig. 6-9).

Coarse Popcorn-like Calcifications

Coarse, popcorn-like calcifications are due to degenerating fibroadenomas. Although this late stage is usually obviously benign, the earlier appearance of coarse heterogeneous calcifications is less specific. Calcifications often develop first at the periphery of a fibroadenoma and become increasingly coarse and coalescent over time (Fig. 6-10; see Fig. 6-20).

Large Rod-like (Secretory) Calcifications

Large rod-like calcifications are ductal in origin. They are typically large (≥1 mm in diameter), well-defined linear calcifications oriented toward the nipple (Fig. 6-11). They

are often bilateral and symmetric but may be few in number and affect a single ductal system early in their development. They are usually intraluminal with a rod shape but may also be periductal, in which case they are cigar-shaped with a lucent center. Think of secretory calcifications as dashes with no dots. They are due to involution of the duct, so they are usually seen 10 to 20 years after menopause. If you identify what you think are secretory calcifications in a young woman who has not undergone early menopause, think twice!

Eggshell or Rim Calcifications

These calcifications are easy to recognize and are nearly always due to fat necrosis. Injury to a fat lobule results in healing by liquefaction necrosis, which causes an inflammatory response at the margin. Calcifications form

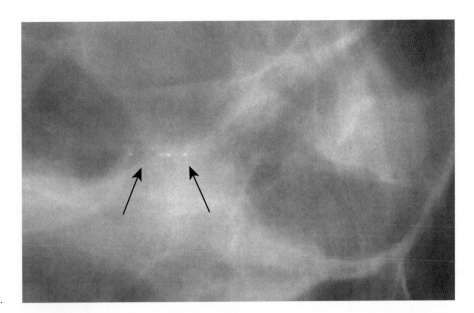

FIGURE 6-9 Early Vascular Calcifications.
These can occasionally mimic DCIS (*arrows*).

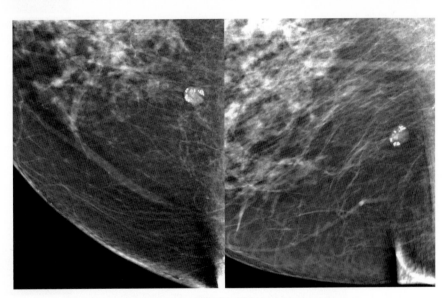

FIGURE 6-10 Coarse Popcorn-like Calcifications. There are coarse calcifications at the periphery of a circumscribed mass are consistent with fibroadenoma.

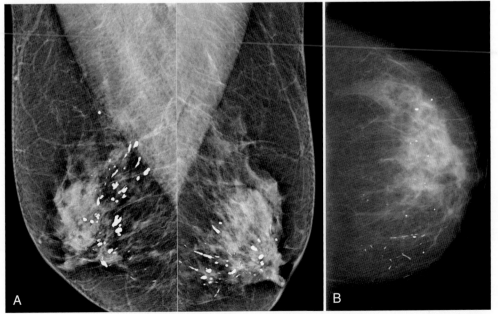

FIGURE 6-11 Large Rod-like Calcifications. Calcifications are often bilateral and symmetric (**A**), but they may be unilateral and grouped or segmental when early (**B**).

at this inflamed margin, and can disappear after a number of years.

Injury can affect a single fat lobule, resulting in small fat necrosis calcifications (Fig. 6-12). For those of you who learned Latin prior to medical school, this is also called liponecrosis microcystica. These calcifications are typically due to incidental trauma, such as an encounter with a soccer ball when playing with your kids. Larger areas of fat necrosis can also occur (liponecrosis macrocystica) (see Fig. 6-12). This type is often due to recallable trauma, like a motor vehicle collision or an encounter with a surgeon.

Recognition of the central lucency within calcifications is important in establishing them as benign. Although other types of calcifications may also have lucent centers, they are most accurately described by their specific type (e.g., dermal or large rod-like), rather than as lucent centered.

Dystrophic Calcifications

These benign calcifications are typically seen after surgery, trauma, or radiation. They are often irregular in shape but too large to be considered suspicious for malignancy (Fig. 6-13). They frequently have lucent centers (Box 6-1).

Milk of Calcium

Milk of calcium is one type of benign calcification due to fibrocystic change (FCC). When the fluid-filled lobule is enlarged and calcium forms within it, the calcium can form layer in the dependent part of the lobule (Fig. 6-14). On the CC view, this is like looking down on sugar that has settled to the bottom of a glass of iced tea. The calcifications are powdery and spread out. They may even be difficult to identify. No linear particles should be present on the CC view. On the ML view, this is like looking at the sugar from the side of the iced tea glass. The calcifications layer and form a line that may have a curved bottom ("tea-cupped" appearance). The mediolateral oblique (MLO) view is in between the CC and ML views, so the calcifications may also layer on this view. When patients are recalled from screening, magnification views should be obtained in the CC and ML projections. Although change in morphologic appearance between the CC and ML magnification views is the first clue, layering of most if not all of the calcifications on the ML view is the key to diagnosis.

Suture Calcifications

These calcifications are due to foreign body reaction to suture material after a surgical procedure. They are most

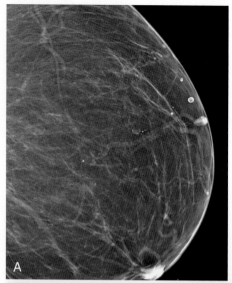
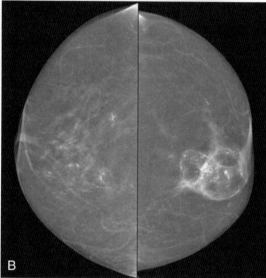
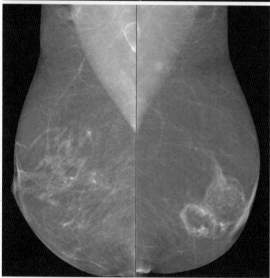

FIGURE 6-12 **Rim or Eggshell Calcifications. A,** Calcifications due to fat necrosis have thick rims and tend to be round or oval. They look like tiny eggs. **B,** Oil cysts are formed by the same process as the smaller, more common fat necrosis calcifications but are typically due to more significant trauma, such as surgery.

BOX 6-1   Differential Diagnosis of Lucent-Centered Calcifications

- Dermal
- Large rod-like (secretory)
- Rim or eggshell
- Dystrophic

common in the radiated breast. The typical appearance is regular lines or circles of calcifications; calcified knots are frequently seen as well. Suture calcifications are most often seen with catgut suture material. With the increased use of silk sutures, they are less frequently encountered than in the past.

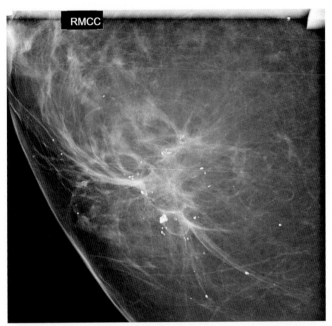

FIGURE 6-13 **Dystrophic Calcifications.** Architectural distortion with dystrophic calcifications in a patient with a history of benign surgical biopsy of this region.

Round & Punctate Calcifications

Round calcifications are typically uniform in size (≥0.5 mm) and very round—like peas in a pod (Fig. 6-15). Punctate calcifications are similar but smaller (<0.5 mm). Round & punctate calcifications usually develop within lobules (see Fig. 6-15). The differential diagnosis of lobular calcifications is broad; they are most commonly due to FCC. FCC results in an increase in fluid and sometimes debris within the lobules. Debris can then calcify.

Distribution and changes over time are the most helpful ways to assess round & punctate calcifications. This approach is comparable to that used for round and oval circumscribed masses. Multiple bilateral circumscribed masses are benign, but a single circumscribed mass or new mass is more concerning. Similarly, scattered round & punctate calcifications are considered benign but a focal or new cluster may be suspicious.

Round & punctate calcifications are considered typically benign when they are scattered throughout both breasts (see Fig. 6-6). Loose groups of identical calcifications can occur among those that are diffusely scattered and need not be considered suspicious. Think about when a bag of marbles is spilled on the floor. There will almost always be some groups just by random chance.

Round & punctate calcifications are also often unilateral or regional in distribution. Regional distribution usually implies that there is more than one ductal system involved. However, if the calcifications are unilateral and new or increasing, biopsy may be indicated.

Occasionally, round & punctate calcifications that are clustered or have a linear or segmental distribution can be due to DCIS. The positive predictive value of these

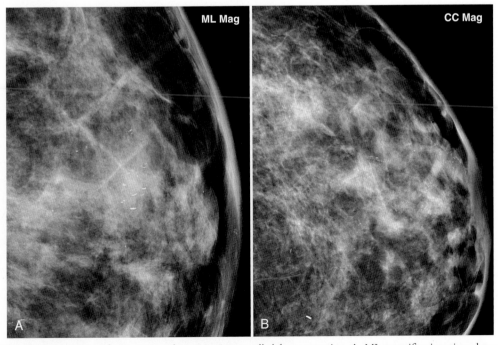

FIGURE 6-14 **Milk of Calcium.** Magnification views from a patient recalled from screening. **A,** ML magnification view shows multiple layering calcifications in the subareolar region. **B,** On the CC magnification view, the calcifications are difficult to identify as they are now less dense and smudgy in appearance. The calcifications change shape in the two views, further documenting the benign finding of milk of calcium.

calcifications is low—in the 10% to 15% range—and the DCIS is typically low or intermediate grade.

If clustered round & punctate calcifications are discovered on the patient's first mammogram, short-term follow-up can be performed, after performing a diagnostic mammogram with magnification views (BI-RADS 3).

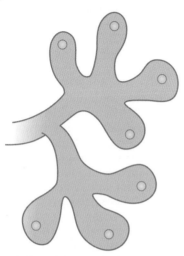

FIGURE 6-15 **Lobular Calcifications.** A line drawing of typical lobular calcifications.

If they are new or increasing, biopsy may be needed (Fig. 6-16). Round & punctate calcifications with segmental or linear distributions are suspicious and often require biopsy regardless of stability (Box 6-2; Figs. 6-17 and 6-18).

Suspicious Calcifications

Okay, you've excluded artifacts and the easy calcifications that are typically benign. Now the real work begins. How can we decide which amorphous, coarse heterogeneous, and fine pleomorphic calcifications need to undergo biopsy? Knowing four things will guide your decision making: the differential diagnosis of each morphologic type, the distribution of the calcifications, change from previous mammograms, and findings associated with the calcifications. Using this approach can improve both sensitivity and specificity in evaluating calcifications and will usually guide you to the correct management decision. We are going to give you good strategies for management. This really is easier than you think!

Amorphous Calcifications
Amorphous calcifications are tiny and somewhat smudgy in appearance (Fig. 6-19). This helps differentiate them

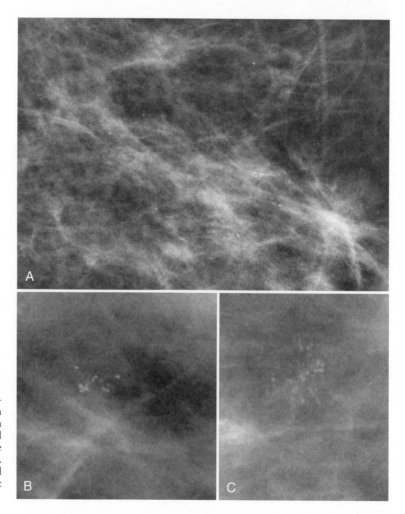

FIGURE 6-16 **Round & Punctate Calcifications. A,** Scattered, round calcifications. Both morphology and distribution are benign. **B,** Round grouped calcifications. They have been stable for over 2 years and are considered benign. **C,** Grouped punctate calcifications on a magnification view. They were new and underwent biopsy showing fibrocystic change. Although small, these calcifications can be distinguished individually (they are "countable") and therefore are not amorphous.

BOX 6-2 *Pathology of Ductal Carcinoma in Situ*

DCIS is graded as low, intermediate, or high grade. The most common histologic types are papillary, cribriform, solid, and comedocarcinoma with papillary typically being lower grade and comedo typically being higher in grade.

Low-grade DCIS is characterized by a monomorphic population of cells expanding a duct (Fig. 6-17). Low-grade DCIS is most commonly papillary or cribriform type. Calcifications form in punched-out spaces in the duct. Low-grade DCIS most commonly manifests as relatively benign-appearing calcifications—frequently either round & punctate or amorphous. The distribution of calcifications due to low-grade DCIS is often grouped or clustered. Segmental and linear distributions are less common. Unlike high-grade DCIS, the extent of low-grade DCIS is usually much greater than the extent of calcifications.

High-grade DCIS is associated with rapid growth that can result in necrosis of the central duct (Fig. 6-18). The resulting necrotic material can calcify, most commonly forming fine pleomorphic, fine linear branching, or coarse heterogeneous calcifications. The extent of

calcifications typically correlates well with the extent of calcifications. Comedocarcinoma is nearly always high-grade DCIS. Solid-type DCIS is often high grade as well.

What about intermediate-grade DCIS? Any of the histologic subtypes can be intermediate-grade DCIS.

Do we overdiagnose DCIS? Probably. However, we are not at a point where we can distinguish cases that can be followed from those that must be treated. The value of diagnosis of low-grade DCIS is underestimated in the public perspective. A retrospective study of 29 women with incompletely excised low-grade DCIS found that 11 were subsequently diagnosed with IDC in the same quadrant of the same breast; 7 were diagnosed within the first 10 years. Five of these 11 women were subsequently diagnosed with distant metastasis with death occurring 1 to 7 years after diagnosis. Genomics of breast cancer as expressed by hormone and other receptor expression is revealing more knowledge that may lead to our ability to understand which types of cancers may undergo watchful waiting and those that must be treated more aggressively.

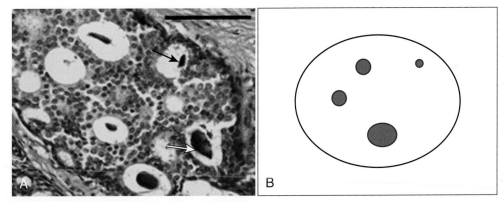

FIGURE 6-17 **Low-Grade Cribriform DCIS. A,** Note punched-out spaces containing calcifications (*arrows*). **B,** Some calcifications are round and some are more irregular. Calcifications seen on mammography can develop within these small tumor spaces or in adjacent tissues.

from round & punctate and fine pleomorphic calcifications in which the particles are easier to individually define. Think of amorphous calcifications as powdered sugar, whereas round & punctate and fine pleomorphic calcifications are more like table sugar. Amorphous calcifications are not "countable" whereas the others can be distinguished and "counted."

Distribution is the key to evaluating amorphous calcifications. Segmental, linear, or clustered distributions are concerning. If they are scattered (especially if bilateral),

biopsy is not typically indicated. Regional distribution can be tricky—if they appear to involve more than one ductal system, then biopsy may not be needed. If unilateral and possibly just in one ductal system, biopsy may be warranted.

Amorphous calcifications are considered intermediate risk for malignancy with a positive predictive value of about 20%. They are most frequently due to FCC, sclerosing adenosis, columnar cell change, or DCIS. When malignant, the DCIS is usually low or intermediate grade.

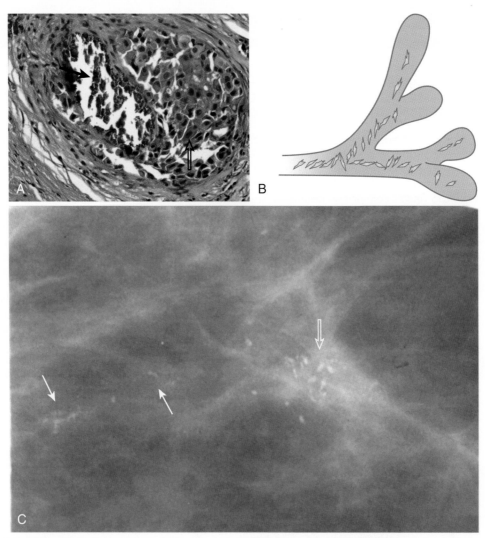

FIGURE 6-18 **High-Grade DCIS. A,** Photomicrograph showing high-grade DCIS with central comedonecrosis (*open arrow*) resulting in sharp-appearing calcifications (*arrow*). **B,** Schematic diagram showing intraductal necrotic material that results in linear/branching calcifications. **C,** High-grade DCIS commonly manifests as coarse heterogeneous (*open arrow*) or fine pleomorphic (linear/branching) calcifications (*arrows*). Both types are seen in this case.

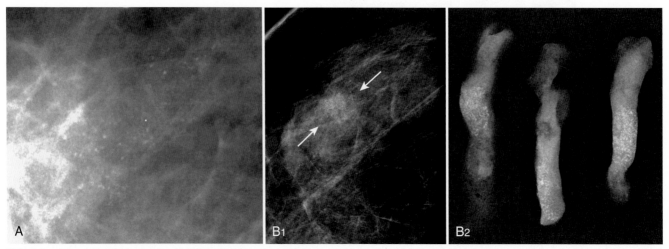

FIGURE 6-19 **Amorphous Calcifications. A,** Magnification view from a patient recalled from screening shows a tight group of amorphous calcifications. Can you count them? No. Biopsy showed low-grade DCIS. **B,** Magnification view of another patient shows amorphous calcifications (*arrows;* B1), better seen on specimen radiograph from stereotactic biopsy (B2). These were due to IDC with low- and intermediate-grade DCIS.

Because the differential diagnosis includes low-grade DCIS, mammographic stability does not prove benignity (Box 6-3).

Coarse Heterogeneous Calcifications

Coarse heterogeneous calcifications are the second type that is of intermediate concern for malignancy. They are often due to degenerating fibroadenoma, papilloma, FCC, or DCIS, which is often high grade. The first three items on this list produce findings that change slowly over time (Fig. 6-20), as opposed to high-grade DCIS, which often progresses rapidly (Fig. 6-21). Thus, comparison with prior studies is very helpful in evaluating these calcifications.

Distribution of coarse heterogeneous calcifications is also important. The benign causes of these calcifications often result in multiple similar findings (Fig. 6-22). These calcifications often occur within soft tissue density masses (fibroadenomas or papillomas). In cases of multiple bilateral calcifications, evaluate the clusters of calcifications individually to identify any that are different from the others and may be of higher suspicion (Fig. 6-23).

Segmental or linear distribution of coarse heterogeneous calcifications is highly suspicious (Fig. 6-24). Grouped or clustered calcifications that are new or increasing in number and extent are also worrisome (Box 6-4).

Fine Pleomorphic and Fine Linear/Fine-Linear Branching Calcifications

Among the different morphologic types in the BI-RADS lexicon, fine pleomorphic calcifications have the highest suspicion for malignancy (Fig. 6-25). If fine pleomorphic calcifications contain linear or branching forms, they are designated "fine linear" or "fine-linear branching" calcifications (Fig. 6-26).

Heterogeneous and pleomorphic mean essentially the same thing—calcifications of differing sizes and shapes. The main differentiating factor between fine pleomorphic and coarse heterogeneous is the *predominant size* of the calcifications: Fine pleomorphic calcifications are usually smaller than 0.5 mm, and coarse heterogeneous calcifications are generally larger than 0.5 mm (see Fig. 6-18)

The differential diagnosis of fine pleomorphic calcifications is similar to that for coarse heterogeneous, except that papilloma and fibroadenoma are less common. Both coarse heterogeneous and fine pleomorphic calcifications are often associated with high-grade DCIS (see Fig. 6-18). Comparison with previous mammograms will usually show progression.

When segmental in distribution, fine pleomorphic calcifications are highly suspicious for DCIS, usually high grade (see Fig. 6-26). Fine pleomorphic calcifications that

---

BOX 6-3 Differential Diagnosis of Amorphous Calcifications

- Fibrocystic change
- Sclerosing adenosis
- Columnar cell change
- DCIS, usually low or intermediate grade

BOX 6-4 Differential Diagnosis of Coarse Heterogeneous Calcifications

- Fibroadenoma
- Papilloma
- Fibrocystic change
- DCIS, usually high grade

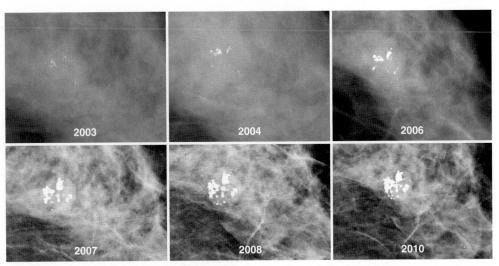

FIGURE 6-20 **Fibroadenoma: Evolution of Coarse Heterogeneous to Popcorn-like Calcifications.** A few coarse heterogeneous calcifications are initially seen near the periphery of a mass. Over several years, a few more calcifications fill in the ring. The calcifications become larger and more dense over time, but do not expand their distribution. Even with coarse, popcorn-like calcifications, a ring shape can often still be seen. Eventually, the calcifications may coalesce so that only one large calcification is visible.

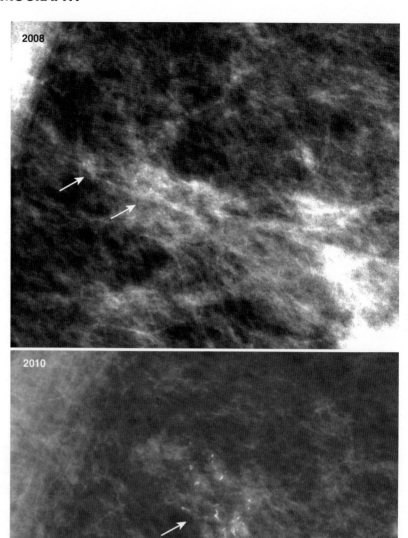

FIGURE 6-21 **Malignant Coarse Heterogeneous Calcifications.** Magnification views from a patient recalled from screening shows a small group of coarse heterogeneous calcifications (*arrow*). A few calcifications were present previously (about 1.5 years earlier), but they have increased in both number and area. They are also very sharp looking. If these items were on your kitchen floor, you would reach for the dustpan, not just a paper towel. BI-RADS 5: Malignant. Biopsy showed high-grade DCIS.

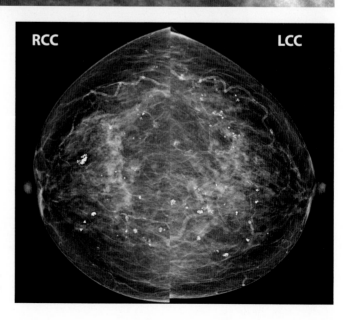

FIGURE 6-22 **Multiple Bilateral Coarse Heterogeneous and Popcorn-like Calcifications.** Multiple bilateral similar-appearing clusters of coarse heterogeneous calcifications are considered benign (BI-RADS 2).

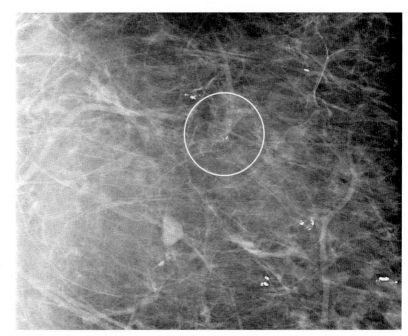

FIGURE 6-23 **Multiple Clusters of Coarse Heterogeneous Calcifications.** CC magnified view of the right breast shows multiple clusters of coarse heterogeneous calcifications. Stereotactic biopsy of a new cluster of fine pleomorphic calcifications (*circle*) revealed fibroadenomatous calcifications. The remaining calcifications are also consistent with multiple fibroadenomas.

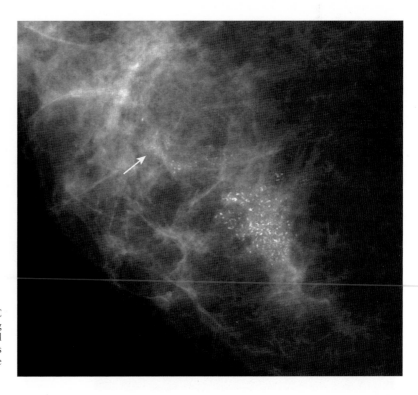

FIGURE 6-24 **Coarse, Heterogeneous Calcifications.** CC magnification view from a patient recalled from screening shows coarse heterogeneous calcifications in a segmental distribution in the medial breast. Note that calcifications are present between the primary group and the nipple (*arrow*). Biopsy showed high-grade DCIS.

are grouped or clustered are also suspicious, and biopsy is usually indicated. New or increasing calcifications of this type are very concerning.

Occasionally, it may be difficult to tell if fine linear calcifications represent early vascular calcifications or DCIS (Fig. 6-27). This may occur because the wall of the vessel is obscured by dense tissue and only partially calcified, so it does not have the characteristic "tram track" appearance. If you perform a significant number of stereotactic biopsies, you will encounter an occasional case

of calcifications within atherosclerotic arteries at histologic examination. If suspected, we try to schedule these women for their biopsy on our partner's day so that they can hold pressure afterward.

When a background of benign calcifications is present, it is easy to assume that all of the calcifications are benign. These mammograms are difficult. Remember to evaluate each group of calcifications individually (Fig. 6-28). Comparison with previous mammograms can also be very helpful in this setting.

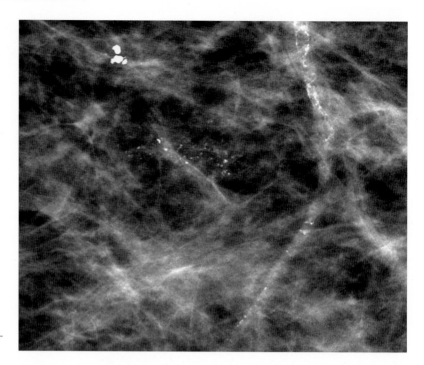

FIGURE 6-25 Fine Pleomorphic Calcifications. Stereotactic biopsy showed high-grade DCIS.

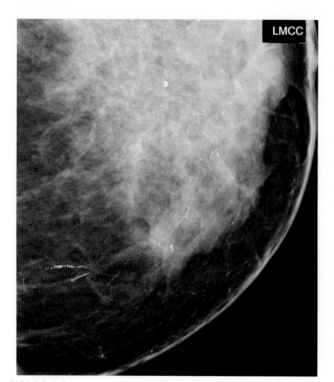

FIGURE 6-26 Fine Linear Branching Calcifications. CC magnification view showing fine, linear branching calcifications in a segmental distribution. Surgical biopsy revealed infiltrating ductal carcinoma and high-grade DCIS (comedo and cribriform types).

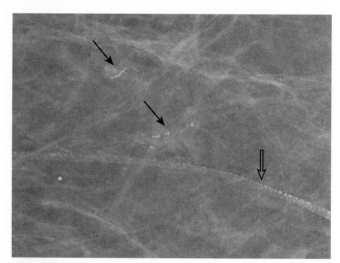

FIGURE 6-27 Vascular or DCIS? The answer is YES. There are two groups of fine, linear calcifications (*arrows*) that at first glance look much like the vascular calcifications (*open arrow*) in the same area.

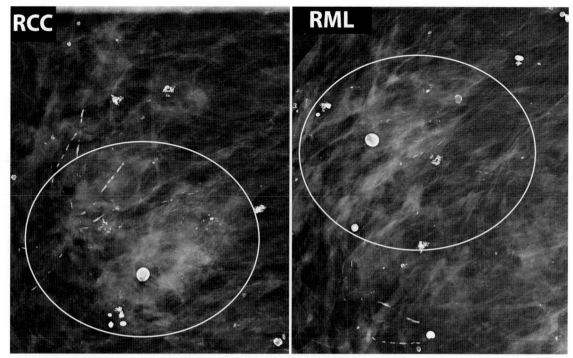

FIGURE 6-28 **Evaluating Multiple Types of Calcifications.** This 75-year-old woman was recalled from screening to evaluate new calcifications. The breast contains secretory, popcorn-like, and fat necrosis calcifications. The new calcifications (*ovals*) include particles with fine linear and coarse heterogeneous morphologic features. Biopsy revealed DCIS.

Factors That Increase Suspicion of Calcifications

Associated Focal Asymmetry

When calcifications are due to carcinoma, they typically represent an intraductal component (DCIS). Cancer can eventually invade through the wall of the duct and become IDC (also sometimes called "infiltrating" ductal carcinoma; the terms are synonymous). Increased tissue density either focally or diffusely around calcifications may indicate that there is invasive carcinoma associated with DCIS (Fig. 6-29). Think of this "puff of smoke" around the calcifications as a warning sign: when associated with malignant calcifications, an invasive component is present about 50% of the time. In these cases, ultrasound may be helpful to identify and guide biopsy of an associated suspicious mass; core biopsy of an invasive component is more valuable in treatment planning than diagnosis of the DCIS component alone. A focal asymmetry may also be associated with benign calcifications, such as those due to FCC or adenosis with enlargement of the lobules.

Associated Mass

When the invasive carcinoma is larger or the tissue less dense, a true mass (outwardly convex margins, seen in two views) may be associated with the calcifications on mammography. Ultrasound may also be used to identify an invasive component and to guide core biopsy when there is a visible mass associated with the calcifications or, in some cases, when extensive calcifications are present without a mammographically visible mass.

Calcifications in or Near a Lumpectomy Scar

These calcifications deserve special scrutiny. About 6% of women with breast conserving surgery for cancer will develop a local recurrence. However, benign calcifications are also very common after breast conservation. Please review Chapter 18, The Postoperative Breast, for special tips.

Final Comments

Calcifications should generally be judged by their worst features. Morphologically benign calcifications may be concerning if in a suspicious distribution (e.g., punctate calcifications in a segmental distribution), and morphologically suspicious calcifications should not be viewed more favorably if their distribution is of lower suspicion (e.g., fine pleomorphic calcifications in a regional distribution). New calcifications should be viewed with suspicion unless definitely benign in morphologic features and distribution (e.g., milk of calcium).

Magnification views may be needed to evaluate the morphology and distribution of calcifications and should definitely be obtained prior to recommending short-term follow-up or biopsy. See Chapter 2, Physics That WILL Improve Your Images, for tips on getting beautiful magnification views.

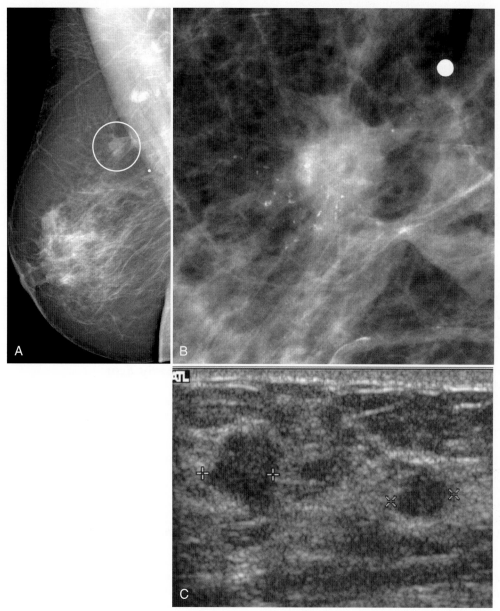

FIGURE 6-29 **Calcifications with an Associated Focal Asymmetry. A,** Right MLO view from screening mammogram shows calcifications and focal asymmetry in the posterior superior breast (*circle*). **B,** ML magnification view shows grouped fine, linear pleomorphic calcifications with an associated mass. **C,** US demonstrates a corresponding solid hypoechoic mass as well as an adjacent satellite lesion. Biopsy showed multifocal IDC with high-grade DCIS.

KEY POINTS

- Calcifications that are potentially suspicious should be evaluated on magnified views and described in terms of their distribution, morphology, and change over time.
- Round & punctate calcifications are usually benign, but biopsy may be needed if a new cluster develops or distribution is linear or segmental.
- Amorphous calcifications may be due to low-grade DCIS, so distribution is more helpful in assessment than stability.
- Coarse heterogeneous calcifications may be due to high-grade DCIS, which will usually show progression when compared with prior studies.
- Calcifications that are linear or segmental in distribution and do not have typically benign features should be viewed with suspicion.
- Calcifications should be judged by their worst features.

References

American College of Radiology. ACR BI-RADS: mammography. In ACR Breast Imaging Reporting and Data System, Breast Imaging Atlas, 4th ed. Reston, VA, American College of Radiology, 2003.

Bent CK, Bassett LW, D'Orsi CJ, Sayre JW. The positive predictive value of BI-RADS microcalcification descriptors and final assessment categories. AJR 2010;194:1378-1383.

Berg WA, Arnoldus CL, Teferra E, Bhargavan M. Biopsy of amorphous breast calcifications: Pathologic outcome and yield at stereotactic biopsy. Radiology 2001;221:495-503.

Burnside ES, Ochsner JE, Fowler KJ, et al. Use of microcalcification descriptors in BI-RADS 4th Edition to stratify risk of malignancy. Radiology 2007;242:388-395.

Haigh PI, Brenner RJ, Giuliano AE. Origin of metallic particles resembling microcalcifications on mammograms after use of abrasive cautery-tip cleaning pads during breast surgery: Experimental demonstration. Radiology 2000;216:539-544.

Sanders ME, Schuyler PA, Dupont WD, Page DL. The natural history of low-grade ductal carcinoma in situ of the breast in women treated by biopsy only revealed over 30 years of long-term follow-up. Cancer 2005;103(12):2481-2484.

Stomper PC, Geradts J, Edge SB, Levine EG. Mammographic predictors of the presence and size of invasive carcinomas associated with malignant microcalcification lesions without a mass. AJR 2003;181:1679-1684.

CASE 6-1. A 56-year-old woman presents for mammogram prior to radiation therapy after a recent diagnosis of DCIS. There are calcifications posterior to the lumpectomy bed that may be dermal in origin. What view may be helpful to confirm dermal origin? What approach would you use? Medial? Lateral? Top?

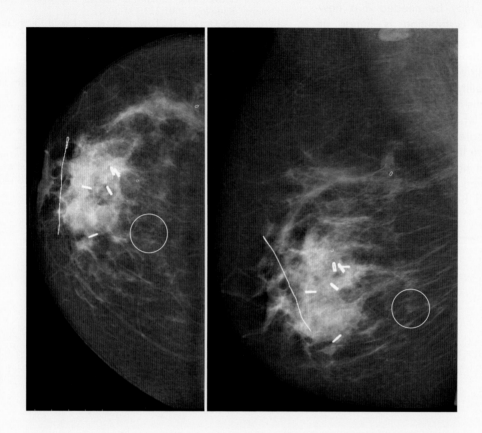

CASE 6-2. Magnification views of screening-detected calcifications in the left breast. How would you describe the calcifications? What is the most likely diagnosis? What are your BI-RADS assessment and recommendation?

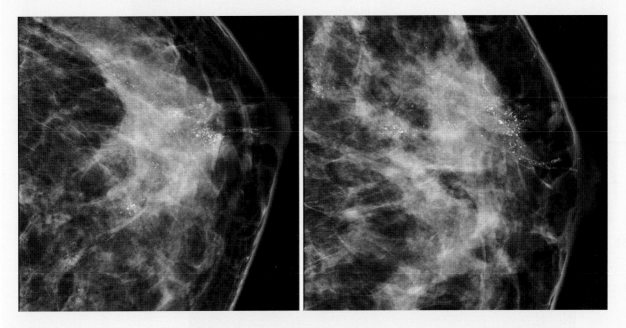

CASE 6-3. CC magnification view of the left breast in a patient with a history of lumpectomy and radiation therapy for left breast carcinoma 5 years ago. The scar is marked with a wire. How would you describe the findings? What are your BI-RADS assessment and recommendation?

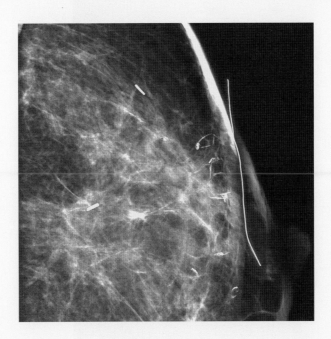

CASE 6-4. Magnification views of a palpable mass in the right breast. What is the most likely diagnosis? What is the next step in managing the patient?

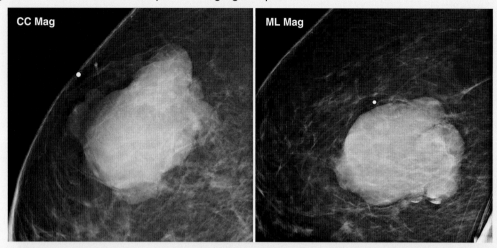

CC Mag   ML Mag

CASE 6-5. CC views from a screening mammogram (triangle marks a stable palpable lump with a previous negative workup) at top. A magnified CC view of the rectangular area marked on the left CC view is also shown at the bottom. How would you describe the calcifications? What is the most likely diagnosis? What are your BI-RADS assessment and recommendation for this case?

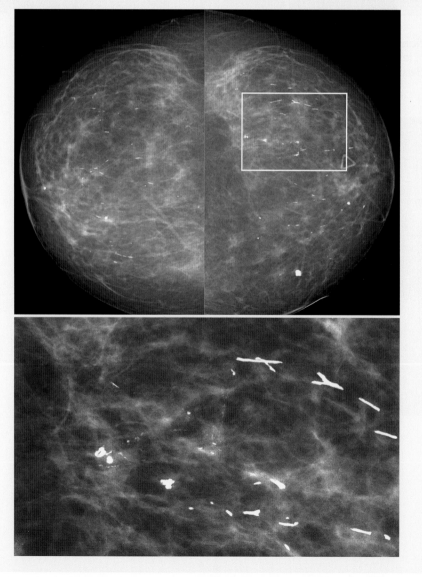

CASE 6-6. Screening mammogram in a 72-year-old woman. What is the most likely diagnosis? What are your BI-RADS assessment and recommendation?

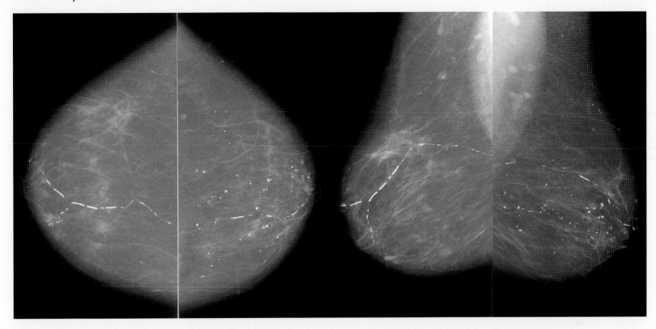

CASE 6-7. Magnification views for a patient recalled from screening. How would you describe the calcifications? What would be most helpful as the next step in management? What are your BI-RADS assessment and recommendation?

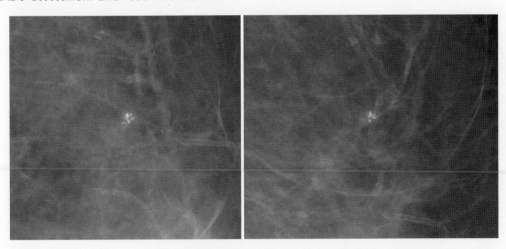

CASE 6-8. ML magnification view from a patient recalled from screening for new calcifications in the right breast. Describe the calcifications. What is your differential diagnosis? What are your BI-RADS assessment and recommendation?

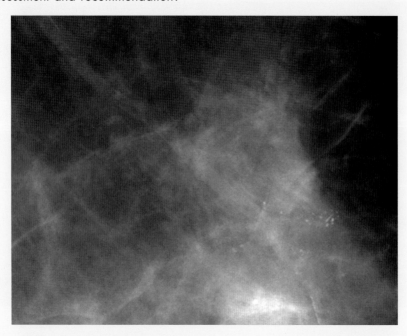

CASE 6-9. ML magnification view from a patient recalled from screening. Describe the calcifications (*circle*). What is the differential diagnosis? What are your BI-RADS assessment and recommendation?

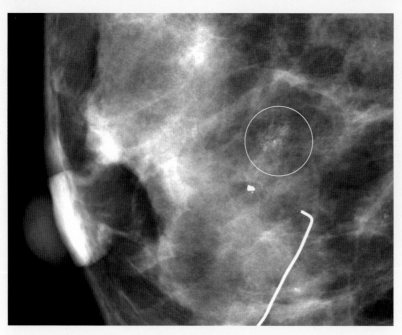

CASE 6-10. A 42-year-old woman is recalled to assess calcifications after her initial screening mammogram. How would you describe the findings? What are your BI-RADS assessment and recommendation?

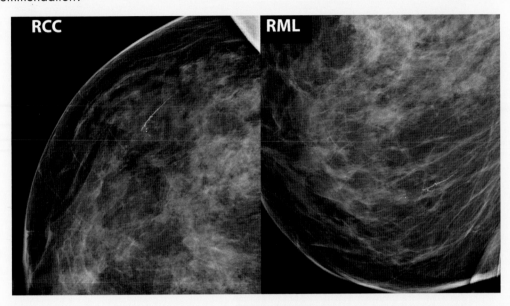

CASE 6-11. A 55-year-old patient was recalled from screening to assess calcifications, and an ML magnification view was performed. The calcifications are new compared with the prior mammogram. What are your BI-RADS assessment and recommendation?

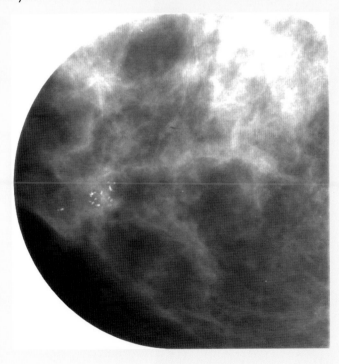

CASE 6-12. Close-up of right CC views over time. What are your assessment and recommendation for the calcifications?

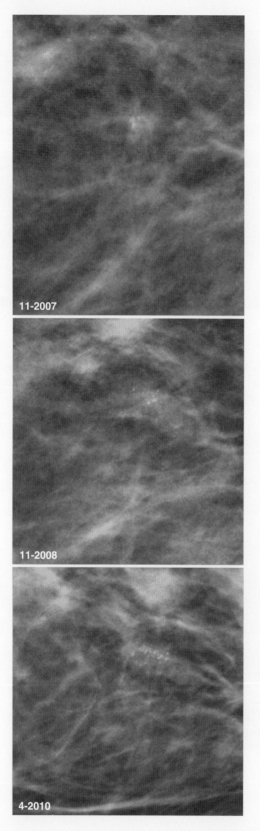

CASE ANSWERS

CASE 6-1. A tangential view would be used to confirm dermal origin. A medial approach was used. The breast was placed in a wire localization grid and a BB placed over the location of the calcifications. The BB was then rolled in profile to obtain the tangential view. The calcifications are dermal. BI-RADS 2. Recommend routine imaging after breast conserving therapy.

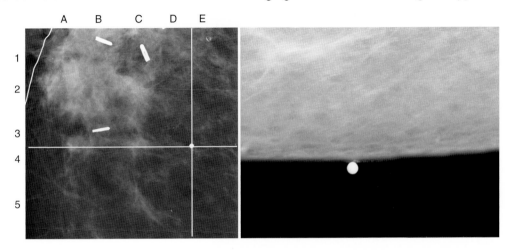

CASE 6-2. Magnification views show coarse heterogeneous and fine linear branching calcifications in a segmental distribution. BI-RADS 5: Malignant finding. Biopsy is recommended. Diagnosis: High-grade DCIS. The calcifications in this case have morphologic features and distribution that are both highly suspicious.

CASE 6-3. These are suture calcifications. BI-RADS 2: Benign finding. Recommend annual mammography. The oval shape of the calcifications, their regular distribution along the scar, and visibility of calcified knots are clues to this diagnosis.

CASE 6-4. There is calcific sediment that is difficult to visualize on the CC view and layers in the dependent portion of the mass on the ML view. US confirms a cyst. This is milk of calcium. BI-RADS 2: Benign finding. Recommend annual mammography.

Calcific sediment can form in cysts of any size, including macrocysts, as in this case. The change in shape of the calcifications in different projections and the characteristic "teacup" appearance on the lateral view indicate the diagnosis.

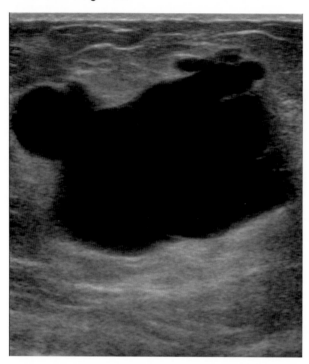

CASE 6-5. Bilateral, benign, large rod-like (secretory) calcifications are scattered in both breasts. However, there are also calcifications in the central left breast that are not typical of secretory calcifications. These fine linear branching calcifications in a linear distribution are highly suspicious for high-grade DCIS. BI-RADS 5: Malignant. Stereotactic biopsy is recommended. Biopsy confirmed high-grade DCIS. In cases with multiple calcifications, examine each region carefully for particles with morphologic features and distribution that are different from the others and potentially suspicious.

CASE 6-6. Unilateral fat necrosis calcifications are scattered throughout the left breast. The patient did not recall trauma. Nevertheless, these are benign. BI-RADS 2: Benign finding. Recommend routine annual mammography.

CASE 6-7. These are grouped coarse, heterogeneous calcifications. As such, previous mammograms would be very helpful for comparison. BI-RADS 0: Needs additional evaluation. Recommend comparison with prior mammogram.

Here are close-up views of her mammogram from 2 years earlier. The calcifications have become coarser and denser over 2 years, without an increase in extent. This change is characteristic of benign coarse heterogeneous calcifications. BI-RADS 2: Benign finding. Recommend annual mammography. Calcifications that enlarge individually and become more coalescent over time are usually benign. Those that increase in number and extent are more suspicious.

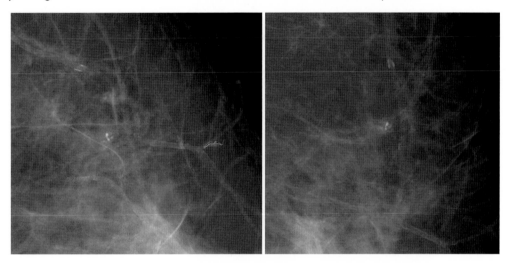

CASE 6-8. This view shows a cluster of fine pleomorphic calcifications. The differential diagnosis includes FCC, fibroadenoma, papilloma, and DCIS, often high grade. Because these calcifications are new, they are suspicious. BI-RADS 4: Suspicious finding. Stereotactic biopsy is recommended. Histologic examination showed high-grade DCIS. Calcifications should be judged by their most suspicious features. In this case the morphology, including at least one linear form, the fact that they are new by history, and their clustered distribution are suspicious.

CASE 6-9. This cluster of amorphous calcifications (you cannot count these!) in the central right breast was not significantly changed over the last 2 years. The differential diagnosis includes sclerosing adenosis, fibrocystic change, and DCIS, usually low grade. The morphology and distribution are concerning. BI-RADS 4: Suspicious. Stereotactic biopsy is recommended. Histologic findings showed low-grade DCIS. Stability over 2 years in this case does not help in the management of this patient because this appearance can represent low-grade malignancy.

CASE 6-10. There are fine pleomorphic calcifications in the lower outer quadrant. Distribution is linear, strongly suggesting that they are ductal in location. BI-RADS 4: Suspicious. Stereotactic biopsy is recommended. Diagnosis: IDC with high-grade DCIS.

Linear ductal calcifications are usually secretory or due to high-grade DCIS. The largest calcification is longer than that seen in most cases of DCIS. However, the calcifications are irregular and the patient is premenopausal, making DCIS much more likely than benign secretory calcifications.

CASE 6-11. A cluster of coarse heterogeneous calcifications is seen that is somewhat forming a ring. This may suggest a degenerating fibroadenoma. However, these are definitely dustpan material (e.g., very sharp), rather than paper towel, and *new* by history. Did you notice the very subtle linear calcification nearby (*arrow*)? This is another clue that should increase your concern. BI-RADS 4: Suspicious. Stereotactic biopsy showed DCIS, high-grade.

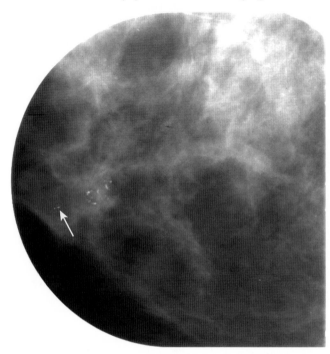

CASE 6-12. Fine pleomorphic calcifications are present that are increasing in number and area in a linear distribution, making them very concerning for DCIS. BI-RADS 4: Suspicious. Stereotactic biopsy confirmed DCIS, high-grade.

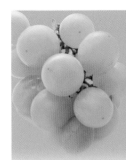

CHAPTER 7

Management of Masses: BI-RADS 2, 3, or 4?

Always a rush in the morning. Time to fix lunch for the kids. Did we go grocery shopping this week? Those grapes don't look so hot. I think they've been in the produce drawer too long. What about these other grapes? Oh no—they have seeds. The kids never eat those. I'd better find something else to send with my kids for lunch. There are often clues that a mass in the breast is a potential problem. Something about it doesn't look so great.

Lawyers have been known to ask a radiologist on the stand, "Shouldn't you do a biopsy if there is *any* chance of cancer?" The answer is plainly, "No." Reading mammograms is all about the odds. What are the odds that a particular finding represents cancer? If the odds are less than 2%, then biopsy is not usually indicated.

A primary role of the radiologist is to determine the likelihood of cancer and to base management decisions according to that level of risk. Mass characteristics and change over time are the primary determinants of management. The shape and margins are important features of masses on any modality. Additional characteristics include density on mammography; echotexture, heterogeneity, and posterior acoustic features on ultrasonography (US); and enhancement pattern on magnetic resonance imaging (MRI). The management of masses is relatively straightforward once the characteristics and behavior over time are determined.

Benign Masses (BI-RADS 2)

The ability to recognize masses that are characteristically benign provides a great service to our patients. Establishing a mass as benign (BI-RADS 2) by any modality provides immediate reassurance to the patient and can spare her the anxiety and discomfort of unnecessary follow-up studies or biopsy. Certain masses—specifically, the fat-containing circumscribed masses, most cystic masses, and solid circumscribed masses that are stable for at least 2 years—are considered benign.

Fat-Containing Circumscribed Masses

On screening mammography, a circumscribed fat-containing mass is considered benign BI-RADS 2, without the need for recall. These masses are virtually always benign (BI-RADS 2). Okay, yes, it is possible that a hamartoma could have a cancer develop within its

boundaries, but the odds of that are extremely small. Okay, and also a lymph node that is enlarged or has a thickened cortex could be due to metastatic disease or lymphoma/leukemia. But otherwise, fat-containing circumscribed masses are benign.

Why circumscribed? An invasive carcinoma that has engulfed fat can present as an irregular fat-containing mass, so those don't count. A fat-containing circumscribed mass seen on screening mammography does not need recall for diagnostic imaging. BI-RADS 2 at screening is fine. In fact, if you do bring the patient back for a diagnostic evaluation and end up performing US, the odd appearance of the mass may end up prompting a biopsy recommendation.

Fat-containing circumscribed masses are no problem. There are only five types, and they are pretty easy to tell apart (Box 7-1). Note that the first two masses, lipoma and oil cyst, are completely fat density with no soft tissue components on mammography. The last three have both fat and soft-tissue density and are therefore mixed radiodense and radiolucent on mammography.

Lipoma

These common masses may be asymptomatic or palpable as a soft mobile mass, and they may be multiple. They are completely fat containing (radiolucent) on mammography (Fig. 7-1). Occasionally, lipomas can contain central lucent-centered calcifications.

Elsewhere in the body, lipomas are hyperechoic. In the breast, however, lipomas on US are isoechoic to the fat or minimally hyperechoic (see Fig. 7-1). Sometimes it is difficult to tell whether a palpable lump represents a fat lobule or a lipoma. If it is just a fat lobule, the edges will blend into the next fat lobule. If it is a lipoma, rocking the transducer from side to side may demonstrate the well-defined margins. Note that fibroadenomas can also be isoechoic to fat, so correlation with mammography is important. A lipoma will be radiolucent, whereas a fibroadenoma will be radiopaque.

Oil Cyst

An oil cyst occurs when a fat lobule is devascularized and undergoes liquefaction necrosis, forming a lipid-containing mass. When an area of fat necrosis is larger than 1 cm, it is often referred to as an oil cyst. These cysts are usually due to significant trauma, such as a motor vehicle collision with seatbelt injury or an encounter with a surgeon (Fig. 7-2). The rim of oil cysts often calcifies. In the acute phase, the mass may be mixed fat and soft

BOX 7-1 *The Fat-Containing Circumscribed Masses*

- Lipoma
- Oil cyst
- Hamartoma
- Lymph node
- Galactocele

BOX 7-2 *Common Causes of Oil Cysts*

- Motor vehicle collision
- Reduction mammoplasty
- Benign surgical biopsy
- Lumpectomy ± radiation therapy

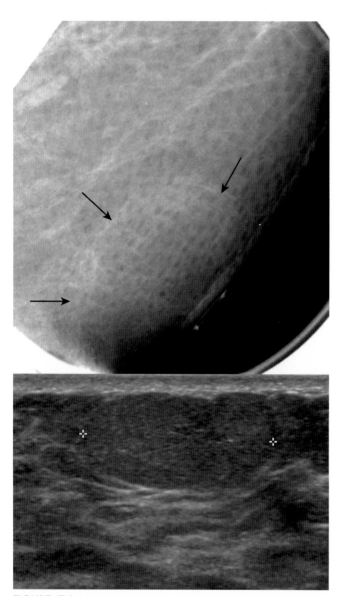

FIGURE 7-1 **Lipoma.** On mammography, there is an oval, circumscribed, radiolucent mass (*arrows*) under a triangle marker denoting a palpable mass. US shows a corresponding mass (*calipers*) that is isoechoic to fat.

tissue density, but will quickly evolve to fat density over a few months (Box 7-2).

The US appearance of oil cysts can be quite variable (Fig. 7-3). Remember that these are called oil *cysts*—their appearance is often similar to a fluid-filled cyst on US. The most common appearance is a round or oval circumscribed anechoic mass. Unlike fluid-filled cysts, though, oil cysts do not usually have increased through transmission and can even have some shadowing. Oil cysts can also have mixed echogenicity, mimicking a complex mass such as a papillary carcinoma. The lesions do not need aspiration or biopsy! Correlation with the mammogram is key. A papillary lesion would have to be white on the mammogram, whereas an oil cyst will be black.

In its earliest stage, fat necrosis may present as a palpable mass, often with tenderness. The patient may or may not recall trauma or bruising. The US appearance of an oval, circumscribed, very hyperechoic subcutaneous mass is quite characteristic (Fig. 7-4). If you are unsure about the cause, place a radiopaque marker over the finding and do a tangential view. The finding should correspond to a circumscribed fat-containing mass. If not, then biopsy should be considered.

Lymph Node
Lymph nodes are unmistakable with their C-shaped cortex and central fat. Intramammary lymph nodes may require recall with spot compression views or even US if the fatty hilum is not visualized on a screening mammogram. Lymph nodes with an abnormal appearance, such as loss of the fatty hilum, enlargement, rounding, or focal or diffuse cortical thickening, should be considered suspicious, however, because these may contain metastatic deposits or lymphoma.

Galactocele
These masses are seen exclusively in women who are lactating or are late in pregnancy (Fig. 7-5). Galactocele literally means "milk cyst," which explains why this finding is included with the fat-containing masses. Human milk has a very high fat content. The fatty component will rise above the solids. That said, the fat-fluid line of a galactocele is rarely sharp. It is more common that there are bubbles of fat at the superior aspect of the mass on mammography.

On US, galactoceles have mixed echogenicity. The contents often shift during scanning, similar to a complicated cyst.

Hamartoma
Let's say that you have found a mixed-density circumscribed mass on mammography. Because is it not completely radiolucent, it is not a lipoma or an oil cyst. It doesn't look like a lymph node, and the patients' not pregnant or lactating. Of the five fat-containing circumscribed masses, that leaves only hamartoma. Occasionally, acute fat necrosis that has not yet formed a perfect oil cyst can appear as a mixed-density fat-containing

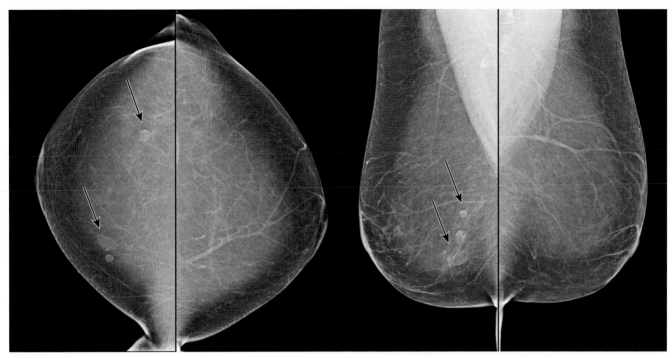

FIGURE 7-2 **Oil Cysts After Reduction Mammoplasty.** This 61-year-old woman had reduction mammoplasty more than 10 years ago. There are several oval or round circumscribed, fat-containing masses in the right breast (*arrows*) that are consistent with oil cysts. Two are developing rim calcifications.

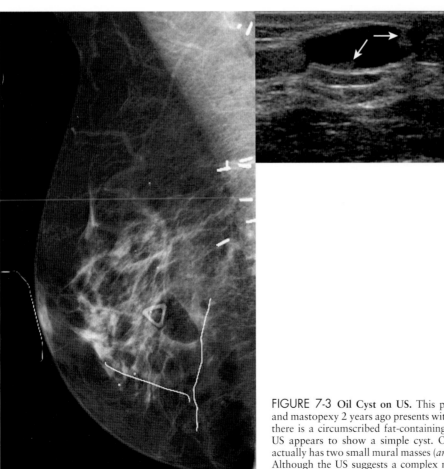

FIGURE 7-3 **Oil Cyst on US.** This patient with history of right breast lumpectomy and mastopexy 2 years ago presents with a palpable lump (*triangle*). On mammography, there is a circumscribed fat-containing mass diagnostic of an oil cyst. At first glance, US appears to show a simple cyst. On closer inspection, the mostly anechoic mass actually has two small mural masses (*arrows*) and lacks posterior acoustic enhancement. Although the US suggests a complex mass that would require biopsy, the appearance of the mass on mammography is pathognomonic for an oil cyst. BI-RADS 2. No intervention is required.

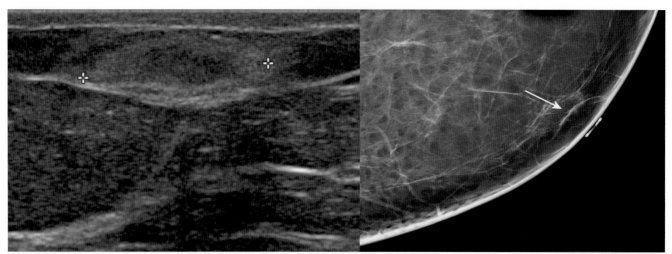

FIGURE 7-4 **US of Fat Necrosis.** This 32-year-old woman presented with a palpable lump in the medial left breast. US shows an oval, circumscribed, hyperechoic mass with a parallel orientation (*calipers*). The mass is more hypoechoic in the center. Eventually this will become anechoic (as in Figure 7-3). A clue to the diagnosis of fat necrosis is the subcutaneous location. She did not recall trauma or bruising, but a mammographic image confirms that this is a circumscribed fat-containing mass (*arrow*).

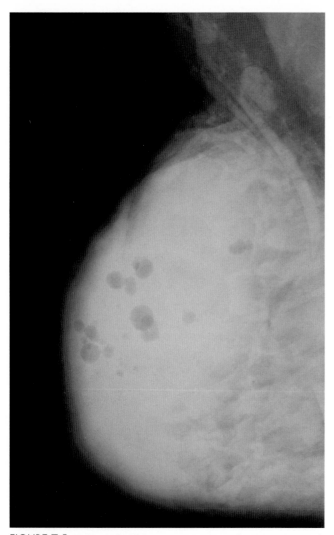

FIGURE 7-5 **Galactocele.** This woman was 3 months post partum with a large palpable lump. Right mediolateral oblique (MLO) view shows a large mass containing fat droplets, consistent with a galactocele. This was managed by observation and resolved after the completion of lactation. (*Image courtesy of Sandhai Agarwal.*)

mass on mammography. However, there is usually a history of trauma to help make that diagnosis.

Hamartomas are congenital masses with mixed fat and soft-tissue density and circumscribed margins (Fig. 7-6). The soft-tissue component is often slightly strange looking—a little denser than the rest of the tissue and perhaps slightly distorted. Think of a hamartoma as a fat and soft-tissue mass in which the components have been slightly swirled. Our eyes tend to rest on the odd appearing white soft-tissue component and do not always recognize the surrounding fat and capsule. Reviewing many cases of hamartomas will train your eye to spot them easily as they are an Aunt Minnie.

On US, hamartomas can also appear somewhat bizarre. Hyperechoic breast tissue is mixed with hypoechoic fat (Fig. 7-7).

Benign Cystic Masses

There are four types of cystic masses in the breast: simple, clustered microcysts, complicated, and complex (Box 7-3). Simple cysts, clustered microcysts, and most complicated cysts are benign. Complex masses have a moderate risk of malignancy.

The mammographic appearance of cystic masses is typically a round or oval, circumscribed, low- or equal-density mass. The margins may also be obscured on mammography, or the mass may be palpable but occult on mammography.

Simple Cysts
The cysts should have imperceptible walls, be completely anechoic (a little reverberation artifact is fine), and demonstrate posterior acoustic enhancement (Fig. 7-8). They may be multiple and wax and wane in size. Obviously a simple cyst needs no further intervention (BI-RADS 2). Or does it? What if she is 72 years old, not on hormones, and develops a new simple cyst? It's still okay! The ACRIN 6666 Screening US trial found that 39% of

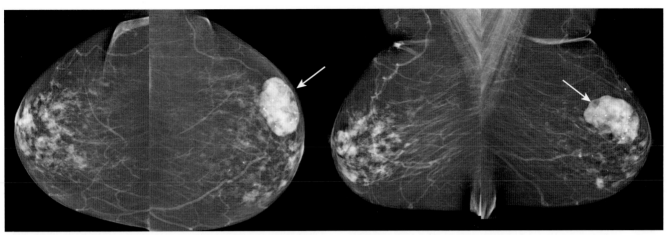

FIGURE 7-6 **Hamartoma.** There is an oval circumscribed mixed fat and soft-tissue density mass in the left breast at 2 o'clock (*arrows*). Because this is clearly not a lymph node and she is not pregnant or lactating, this is a hamartoma.

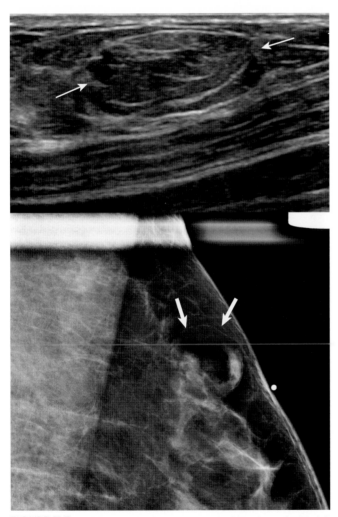

FIGURE 7-7 **Palpable Hamartoma.** A 25-year-old with a palpable left breast mass was initially evaluated by US, which showed a discrete mass-like lesion resembling normal breast tissue. A single mammographic view shows a mass with mixed fatty and fibroglandular tissue (*arrows*) confirming the diagnosis.

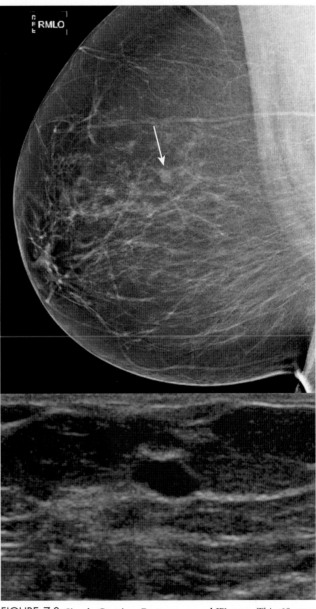

FIGURE 7-8 **Simple Cyst in a Postmenopausal Woman.** This 60-year-old woman had a new round mass on her mammogram (*arrow*). On US, this represented a simple cyst. BI-RADS 2. Routine screening is recommended. Aspiration is not needed.

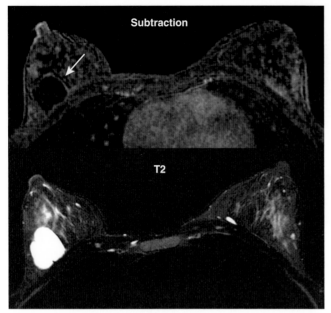

FIGURE 7-9 **Enhancing Benign Cyst.** There is only a thin rim of enhancement (*arrow*) and a corresponding hyperintense mass on T2.

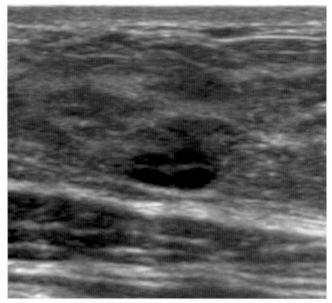

FIGURE 7-10 **Clustered Microcysts.** Each tiny cyst is simple. They are anechoic with thin walls. There are no intracystic masses. This looks like a nice cluster of grapes.

BOX 7-3   Cystic Breast Masses

- Simple cyst
- Clustered microcysts
- Complicated cyst (includes hemorrhagic cysts)
- Complex mass

---

postmenopausal women had simple breast cysts. Aspiration is not indicated unless the patient requests it because of pain. Routine screening is all that is needed (even if the mass is palpable).

On MRI, benign cysts may occasionally have a thin rim of enhancement around a T2 hyperintense mass (Fig. 7-9). This is a normal finding, and aspiration or biopsy is not necessary.

Clustered Microcysts

These microcysts are a common, benign variant of simple cysts (Fig. 7-10). They are essentially a lobule that is expanded with fluid. Think of them as a bunch of grapes. It's really hard to take a good picture of them on US because some of the microcysts will be in the scan plane and others will not. At real time US, each of the microcysts should be otherwise simple.

Of 203 women with clustered microcysts across four series, one cancer was detected, for an overall incidence of 0.5%. Clustered microcysts are BI-RADS 2, even in postmenopausal women. Just like simple cysts, microcysts may correspond to a new mammographic finding and are still BI-RADS 2. However, we need to look really closely. They should look like grapes that you would send with your child to school. If it looks like the grapes have been in your produce drawer too long—and you know what we mean—they have ill-defined margins, or if they

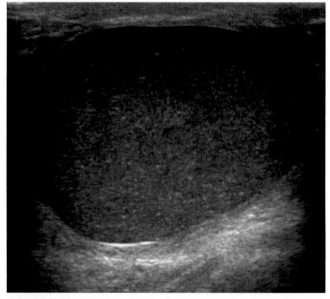

FIGURE 7-11 **Complicated Cyst.** At real time US, swirling debris was present throughout the cyst. No further evaluation was performed. BI-RADS 2.

look like grapes with seeds (which your children are not going to eat anyway), then biopsy should be considered. If the grapes have gone bad, they are no longer considered clustered microcysts but a complex cystic mass.

Complicated Cysts

These cysts contain diffuse low level echoes. If the echoes are seen swirling around inside the cyst or layer at real time US, then you know that it is a complicated cyst and not a solid mass (Figs. 7-11 and 7-12). As long as the wall is thin, these cysts are typically BI-RADS 2.

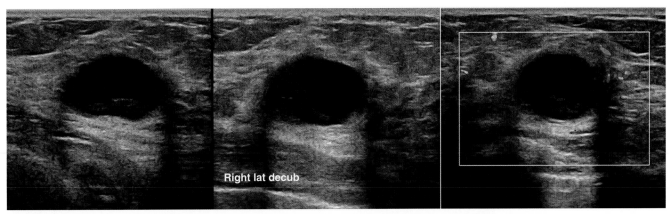

FIGURE 7-12 **Complicated Cyst with Layering Debris.** Layering debris in the dependent portion of the cyst shifts as the patient changes position and there is no flow on color Doppler. This finding is BI-RADS 2.

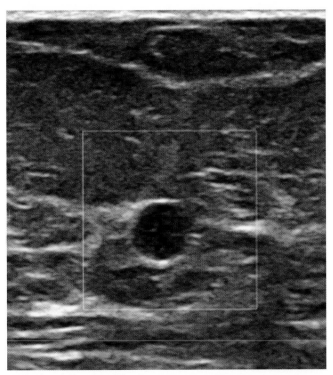

FIGURE 7-13 **Complicated Cyst Versus a Solid Mass.** Even if no blood flow is detected on Doppler, this mass should be managed as though it were solid. If new, sampling will be needed. Aspiration may be attempted first, but if unsuccessful then core biopsy is performed.

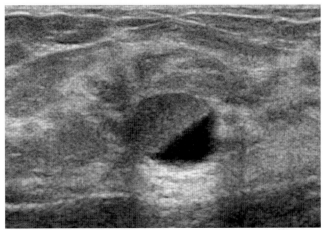

FIGURE 7-14 **Hemorrhagic Cyst.** There is a broad-based clot on the anterior wall of the cyst. The patient gave a history of prior cyst aspiration by her gynecologist. BI-RADS 2.

detected in seven series that included a total of 1343 patients with complicated cysts for an overall cancer incidence of 0.3%. When these are identified in a background of other simple cysts, BI-RADS 2 is reasonable. However, a solitary complicated cyst on a first study may be considered BI-RADS 3. Aspiration may be indicated for a new or enlarging complicated cyst (BI-RADS 4), particularly if it is a solitary finding or high-density appearance on mammography.

Hemorrhagic Cyst

These cysts are also included in the category of complicated cysts. Hemorrhagic cysts have a very distinctive appearance (Fig. 7-14). They look like the yin-yang symbol. These often occur following cyst aspiration. A small clot develops on the anterior wall and appears solid. These can be confused with complex masses. The solid clot, however, has a broad base along the wall rather than being exophytic within the cyst.

Do you see these a lot in your practice? If so, then you have someone who is aspirating the fluid out of cysts. This is easy to change. After aspiration, injection of air

Differentiating a complicated cyst with low level echoes that are not moving from a solid mass can be very challenging (Fig. 7-13). If blood flow is present within the mass, then it is solid. However, the absence of blood flow by Doppler interrogation does not exclude a solid mass. These masses must be assumed solid and managed as such. If the mass corresponds to a new or enlarging mass on mammography, then biopsy should be considered. An attempt can first be made to aspirate the lesion, followed by core biopsy if fluid is not obtained.

The risk of malignancy is very low for complicated cysts. Nearly all of them are benign. Four cancers were

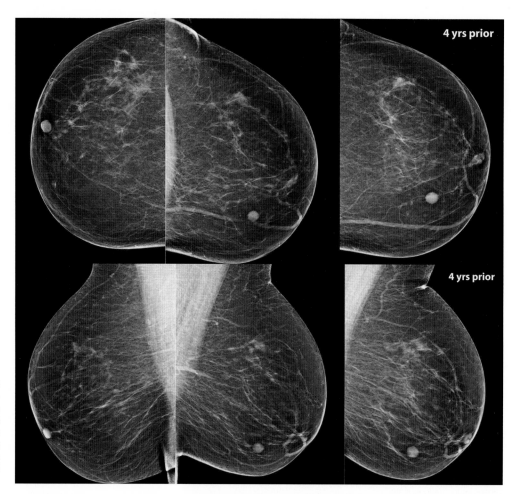

FIGURE 7-15 **Stable Mass with Benign Features.** Screening mammogram on a 52-year-old woman shows a well-circumscribed mass in her left breast that shows no concerning changes in its features and is slightly smaller than on a previous mammogram from 4 years prior. BI-RADS 2.

into the cyst will considerably lower the chance of recurrence of the cyst. If you inject an equal or slightly smaller volume of room air into a cyst following aspiration, the likelihood of recurrence is only about 15% compared with 80% if you simply remove the fluid.

Stable Solid Mass with Benign Features

Benign features for a solid mass include a round or oval shape, circumscribed margins, low or equal density on mammography (Fig. 7-15), and homogeneously hypoechoic with a parallel orientation on US. Benign features on MRI include smooth margin, oval or round shape, homogenous persistent enhancement, nonenhancing septations, and T2 hyperintensity (Fig. 7-16).

However, the presence of benign features does not automatically equal BI-RADS 2. Although most of the masses with these features are fibroadenomas, papillomas, or adenosis, cancer can certainly have this appearance. Therefore, we can only assume that these masses are benign when we have documented stability (see Fig. 7-15). Both mass size and characteristics should be stable over time, preferably for at least 2 years. When stability is not clear when comparing images that are 2 years old, pulling images from 3, 4, or 5 years earlier may make stability or change more apparent.

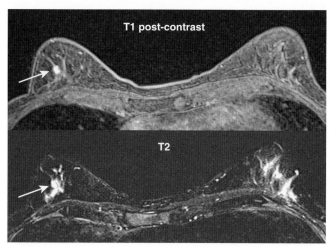

FIGURE 7-16 **Benign Mass on MRI.** There is a 6-mm oval mass with smooth margins in the right breast at 6 o'clock (*arrows*). The mass had slow initial and persistent delayed enhancement. There is a suggestion of nonenhancing septations. The mass is hyperintense on T2. This is likely a fibroadenoma and is BI-RADS 2. The mass has been stable for 4 years.

Multiple Bilateral Circumscribed Masses

Multiple bilateral circumscribed masses are also considered benign—BI-RADS 2. They usually represent multiple fibroadenomas or cysts. The risk of cancer is 0.14% over 2 years, which is lower than observed in the overall screening population. However, be careful about assuming that everything that you see on that mammogram is benign. See Chapter 8, Multiple Masses, for more advice on screening and managing patients with this finding.

Skin Lesions

These are also BI-RADS 2. Clinical examination can help you here. Sebaceous cysts have a characteristic feel on examination: they result in thickening of the dermis and do not roll freely under the skin. There is often a black dot on the skin that corresponds to a small neck on US (Fig. 7-17). The claw sign, which is echogenic skin wrapping around a lesion on US, also helps determine the dermal location. Epidermal inclusion cysts are another type of skin lesion that can form following surgery or other intervention. Their appearance is similar to that of sebaceous cysts. It is good to avoid biopsy of these lesions. Biopsy of sebaceous and epidermal inclusion cysts can result in a chemical dermatitis that resembles infection.

Moles and other skin lesions may present as a round or oval circumscribed mass on mammography. They often have a dark "halo" around their periphery due to air entrapped around an elevated dermal lesion. However, the "halo" sign is not very specific, so confirmation of the dermal location may be needed using a BB pellet.

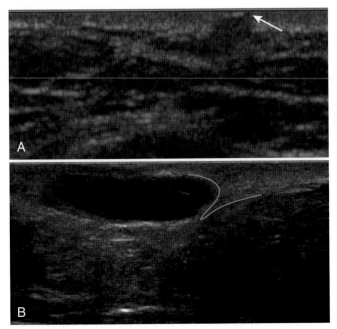

FIGURE 7-17 **Sebaceous Cysts.** US of these subcutaneous masses in two different patients demonstrate a small neck (**A**, *arrow*) and the "claw" sign (**B**, *blue line*) where the dermis wraps around the lesion.

One Last Point on BI-RADS 2

A potential source of confusion can arise when a mass has typically benign features by one modality but is suspicious on another. If the imaging features are diagnostic of a specific benign finding (e.g., oil cyst on mammography or lymph node on US), they are benign and biopsy is not indicated. Another example is a circumscribed mass with coarse popcorn-like calcifications, which is benign regardless of shadowing seen by US or suspicious enhancement characteristics on MRI.

However, if the mass has features that suggest but are not diagnostic of a benign cause on one modality and suspicious features on another, then the mass should be managed based on the worst features. For example, an oval, circumscribed, hypoechoic solid mass on US suggests a benign diagnosis, but if the mass also has a suspicious feature such as spiculated margins on mammography, then biopsy is indicated.

Probably Benign Masses (BI-RADS 3)

Let's say that you are reading a mammogram for a 42-year-old woman and it is her first (baseline) mammogram (Fig. 7-18). She has a well-circumscribed oval mass in her right breast. You recall her from screening and find a corresponding solid mass with benign features (see Fig. 7-18). This almost surely represents a fibroadenoma that has probably been there for decades. However, we don't know actually know that. There is a very small possibility that it is new, so short-term follow-up is indicated to document stability. We will follow the mass at 6, 12, and 24 months to document stability over time (BI-RADS 3).

In order for us to use BI-RADS 3, the mass should not be suspicious on US or another modality. The outcome of BI-RADS 3 masses does not vary by patient age or lesion size (Box 7-4).

Basis for BI-RADS 3

In 1991, Sickles published a study of 3184 mammographic lesions that he considered probably benign. At follow-up, there were 17 cancers for an overall malignancy rate of 0.5%. When these lesions did represent cancer, they were still of early stage at the time of diagnosis. Subsequent studies, including the Women's Health

---

BOX 7-4 Best Supported Use of BI-RADS 3

First mammogram (or priors not available and you tried to get them) with any of the following:
- Round or oval mass with circumscribed margins
- Group or cluster of round or punctate calcifications
- Focal asymmetry

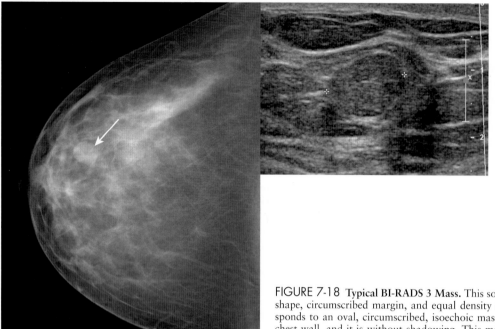

FIGURE 7-18 **Typical BI-RADS 3 Mass.** This solid mass has benign features: an oval shape, circumscribed margin, and equal density on mammography. On US, it corresponds to an oval, circumscribed, isoechoic mass with an orientation parallel to the chest wall, and it is without shadowing. This mass very likely represents a fibroadenoma. For this baseline mammogram, BI-RADS 3, with a follow-up unilateral mammogram or US in 6 months is appropriate. This mass has been stable for 5 years.

Initiative, DMIST, and the Breast Cancer Surveillance Consortium (BCSC), have confirmed cancer rates of 0.8% to 1.9% for BI-RADS 3 lesions. In the BI-RADS lexicon, lesions with a less than 2% probability of cancer are considered appropriate for short-term follow-up. Masses that are typical candidates for BI-RADS 3 are solid with benign features on a baseline mammogram following diagnostic evaluation.

Baseline (Initial) Mammogram

When a woman has her first mammogram, lesions with benign features have likely been present for decades but have never been imaged before. When prior mammograms are available, the BI-RADS category changes to either BI-RADS 2, because it is stable, or BI-RADS 4 because it is new or enlarging. Because old studies change management of these lesions, we need to make every reasonable effort to obtain them.

After Diagnostic Evaluation

In Sickles's 1991 study, all women underwent diagnostic imaging before a finding was categorized as probably benign. Are you tempted to use BI-RADS 3 from screening? Don't do it. What is the advantage? One less diagnostic patient on your schedule? That is *so* not worth it! What is the disadvantage? You may recommend short-term follow-up for masses that are definitely benign (e.g., simple cyst), so some women will experience needless anxiety. You may also recommend short-term follow-up for some malignancies that would have been characterized as suspicious by diagnostic mammography or US

(Fig. 7-19). Women with cancer may therefore have a delay in diagnosis.

A large study from the BCSC confirms the disadvantages of using BI-RADS 3 from screening. The study included more than 1 million mammograms showing a cancer incidence of 0.96% for women after diagnostic evaluation compared to 0.54% for women given BI-RADS 3 directly from screening. These results suggest that women with benign lesions underwent unnecessary short-term follow-up when BI-RADS 3 was used at screening. In addition, the percentage of women with cancers higher than stage II at diagnosis was higher for women given BI-RADS 3 from screening (34.7%), compared with women given BI-RADS 3 after diagnostic mammography (24.4%). These results also suggest that some women had cancers that may have been diagnosed earlier if diagnostic mammography had been performed.

Can we ever use BI-RADS 3 when prior mammograms are present? We all make exceptions to the rules now and then. There are times when the prior mammogram may not be very useful to assess stability because of differences in technique or positioning or interval involution of the parenchyma. A mass that looks like a fibroadenoma may have been there for a long time, but could have been obscured previously if her last mammogram was 8 years ago and the breast tissue then was very dense. A finding with benign features may be located in the far posterior breast, and if the prior mammograms were not positioned as well (mammography technologists just keep getting better!), it could have been excluded from the previous study. The area not visualized on the prior mammograms can potentially be considered as a "baseline" because that area has not been imaged previously (Fig. 7-20). Just be aware that there is little support in the literature for use of BI-RADS 3 when old films are present.

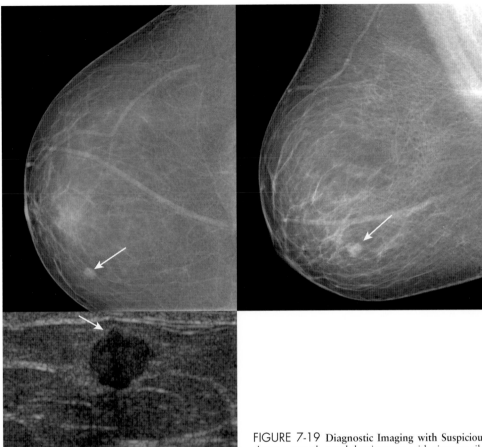

FIGURE 7-19 **Diagnostic Imaging with Suspicious Features.** The screening mammogram shows a round, equal density mass with circumscribed margins. On the screening views, this looks like a good candidate for BI-RADS 3. However, US reveals that the mass actually has a microlobulated border (*arrow*) shifting the finding to BI-RADS 4. Ultrasound-guided core biopsy showed IDC.

BI-RADS 3 Masses on Ultrasonography

The evidence for using BI-RADS 3 for masses seen on US is more recent. Short-term follow-up is a reasonable approach for managing solid masses with benign features and some complicated cysts on a first US.

The vast majority of solid masses with benign features on US are fibroadenomas and can be managed similarly to benign-appearing masses on mammography. If incidental on a first US of the area, then BI-RADS 3 is appropriate. Across six studies of both palpable and nonpalpable benign-appearing solid masses on US, only 8 cancers were found in 1910 women (0.4%). Short-term follow-up is appropriate.

Can I use BI-RADS 3 if the mass is palpable? If the mass has all of the characteristics of a fibroadenoma, then follow-up may be a reasonable alternative to biopsy (Fig. 7-21). The outcome of six series of benign-appearing masses on US were the same whether the mass was palpable or nonpalpable.

BI-RADS 3 Masses on Magnetic Resonance Imaging

There is considerable variability in the use and outcome of BI-RADS 3 on breast MRI. Liberman et al. (2003) found that 24% of breast MRI studies at their institution were assessed as BI-RADS 3, and 10% of these patients were subsequently diagnosed with carcinoma. A more recent multicenter study (the ACRIN 6667 contralateral breast MRI trial) showed that 11% of patients were given a BI-RADS 3 assessment and only 0.9% had subsequent cancer. The older studies largely included MRIs performed before the development of parallel imaging, which made high spatial and temporal resolution possible.

A difficulty with all of these studies is the lack of descriptions of the types of findings for which follow-up was recommended. Hence, there is wide variability in the use and indications for BI-RADS 3 for breast MRI. Some radiologists never use BI-RADS 3 for breast MRI owing to the lack of supporting evidence in the literature. As our experience with breast MRI evolves, so will our understanding of the role of short-term follow-up.

In our practices, we mainly use BI-RADS 3 for small masses that do not fulfill all of the criteria for benign masses (Fig. 7-22). Larger size is associated with a higher risk of malignancy. We'll talk more about MRI interpretation in Chapter 13, when we discuss the screening of high-risk women. In the diagnostic setting, a benign-appearing mass in the same quadrant as a known or suspected breast cancer has a higher risk of malignancy than if observed on a screening MRI. Tissue sampling is

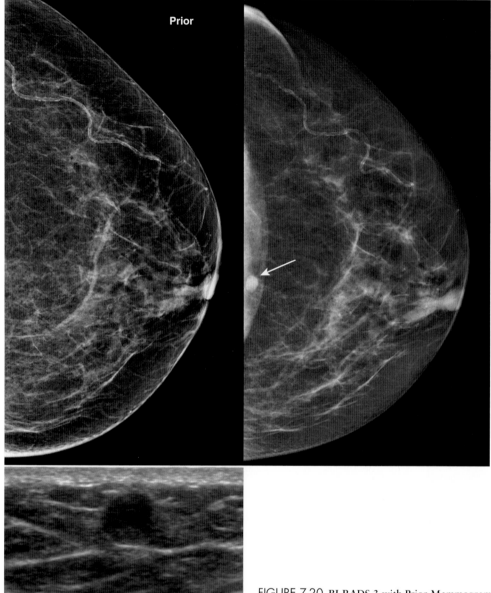

Prior

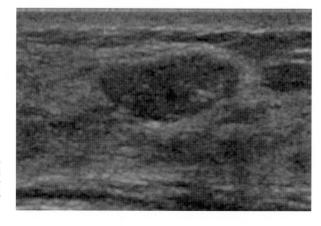

FIGURE 7-20 **BI-RADS 3 with Prior Mammograms.** A 56-year-old woman with a round circumscribed mass in the far posterior left breast, best seen on the craniocaudal (CC) view (*arrow*). Although this patient has prior mammograms, this posterior area was not included on the prior CC view. On US, the mass has benign features. The mass was given BI-RADS 3 and has been stable for more than 2 years.

FIGURE 7-21 **Palpable Mass with Benign Features.** This 28-year-old woman felt a lump in her right breast. On US, this mass is oval with well-defined margins, homogeneously hypoechoic, with no shadowing, and almost surely represents a fibroadenoma. There is support in the literature for using BI-RADS 3 in these cases, though some prefer BI-RADS 4.

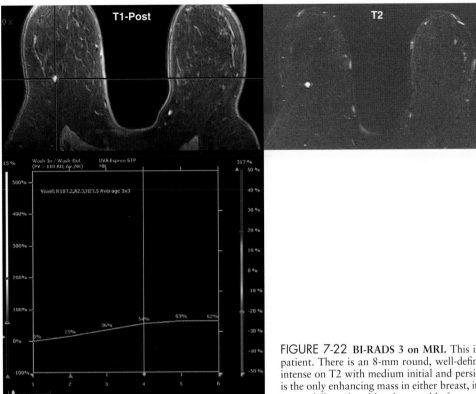

FIGURE 7-22 **BI-RADS 3 on MRI.** This is a baseline screening MRI in a high-risk patient. There is an 8-mm round, well-defined mass in the right breast that is hyperintense on T2 with medium initial and persistent delayed enhancement. Although this is the only enhancing mass in either breast, it almost surely represents a fibroadenoma. It was followed and has been stable for more than 2 years.

usually indicated if the patient is considering breast conservation.

If you are thinking that Figures 7-16 and 7-22 look very similar, you are correct. There are not well-defined criteria for deciding what should be considered BI-RADS 3 versus BI-RADS 2 for MRI. If a mass has benign shape and margins but has plateau enhancement or is not T2 hyperintense, then BI-RADS 3 may be a good idea. Likewise, short-term follow-up may be considered for a mass with otherwise benign features if it is the sole finding on a first screening MRI.

Short-Term Follow-up Protocol

The first follow-up study is usually performed at 6 months. Follow-up at an earlier interval, such as 2 or 3 months, is not typically recommended but may occasionally be helpful for findings that are likely due to either infection or trauma, where resolution or significant improvement in the finding is anticipated and will shift the assessment to a BI-RADS 2.

Imaging for BI-RADS 3 lesions is typically performed at 6, 12, 24, and sometimes 36 months following the initial evaluation. The 18-month examination is skipped because a lesion that is unchanged at 12 months is not likely to change significantly between 12 and18 months. About 70% of cancers in the BI-RADS 3 category will be diagnosed by the 12-month examination. An additional 24% of the cancers will be diagnosed by the 24-month examination. In Sickles's original article, only one cancer was not detected until the 36-month examination. Some

radiologists continue close follow-up for 2 years, although others continue for 3 years.

Women in the BI-RADS 3 category are typically evaluated with diagnostic mammography (or US or MRI if that is how the lesion is best seen) at each of these examinations. The mass is assigned BI-RADS 3 during the entire 2 to 3 years of follow-up. Stability at the conclusion of the 24- or 36-month follow-up period means that the lesion can now be assigned BI-RADS 2 and the patient can return to screening. The finding may also be downgraded to BI-RADS 2 if it becomes obviously benign (e.g., typical lymph node or decrease in size), and she can return to screening.

Remember that a few of these women will be diagnosed with cancer during the follow-up period. The 1% to 2% is a real number. Cancers in this population will typically be diagnosed at the 6- or 12-month imaging. Look for changes not only in the size of the mass but in its appearance (Fig. 7-23). Do the margins appear less distinct? Is the mass higher in density? Also, at the initial diagnostic evaluation, talk with the patient and remind her to return promptly if she notices a change on self-examination.

Immediate Biopsy

Sometimes the patient is too anxious to wait for 6 months. Maybe her good friend just died of breast cancer, or her mother had breast cancer at a young age. If she is going to lose sleep at night, please offer her a biopsy. Biopsy rather than follow-up should also be considered for women who may not be reliable or able to return in 6 months, such as migrant workers or the homeless. Women

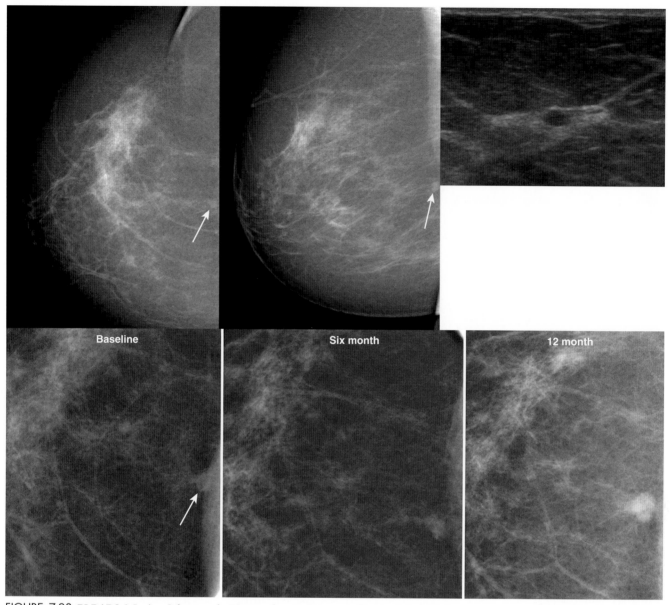

FIGURE 7-23 BI-RADS 3 Lesion Subsequently Diagnosed as Cancer. A small, round, low-density mass was identified in the right breast at 6 o'clock (*arrows*). On US, there was a corresponding hypoechoic mass. The mass was unchanged at 6 months, but had enlarged on the 12-month mammogram. Histologic diagnosis: medullary carcinoma.

who are being considered for organ transplant may require biopsy confirmation that the mass is benign in order to be considered eligible. If you perform biopsy rather than follow-up, the finding is still BI-RADS 3. The category is assigned based on the imaging findings rather than patient circumstances or desires.

Suspicious Masses (BI-RADS 4)

A mass with suspicious features on any modality or one that is new or enlarging is nearly always considered BI-RADS 4. On US, the BI-RADS 4 masses include complex and solid masses and complicated cysts that are a sole finding or a new or enlarging mass.

New or Enlarging Solid Mass with Benign Features

Despite benign features, any solid mass that is new or enlarging is suspicious for cancer (Fig. 7-24). Many of these round or oval masses still represent fibroadenomas that have enlarged because of hormonal fluctuation or menopausal hormone therapy. However, cancer can also present as a mass with benign features (Box 7-5).

Solid Mass with Suspicious Features

Suspicious features on mammography include an ill-defined or spiculated margin, irregular shape, or high

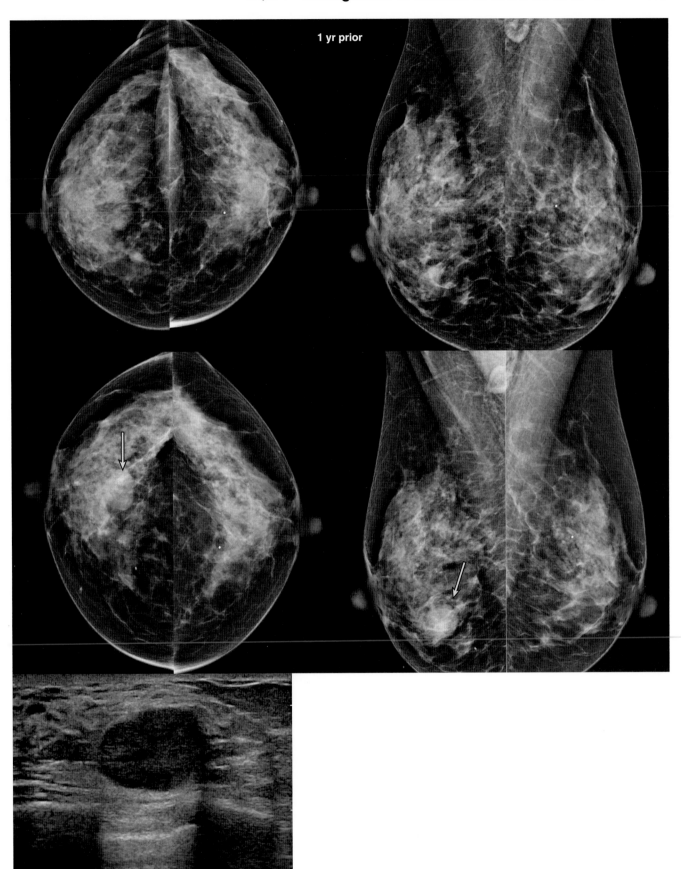

FIGURE 7-24 **New Mass with Benign Features (BI-RADS 4).** Screening mammogram on a 52-year-old woman shows a new obscured mass in her inferior central right breast (*arrow*). US shows a solid mass with benign features. Core biopsy revealed grade 3 IDC.

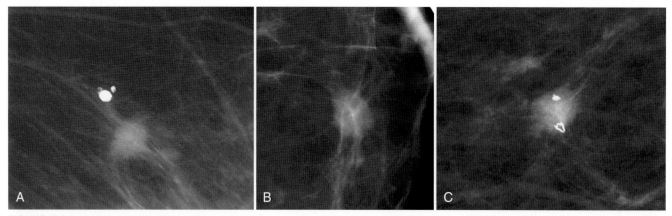

FIGURE 7-25 **Masses with Suspicious Features.** All of these small round masses are IDC. Their suspicious features include spiculated margin (**A**), ill-defined margin (**B**), and high density (**C**).

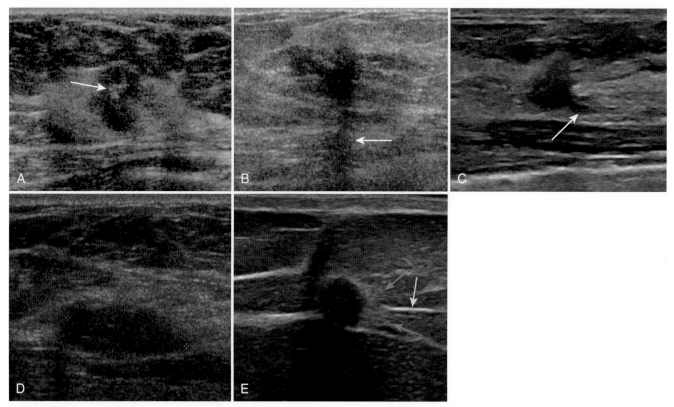

FIGURE 7-26 **Suspicious Features on US.** These masses are all IDC. Their suspicious features include nonparallel orientation (**A**), irregular shape (**B** and **C**), indistinct margin (**C** and **D**), echogenic rim (**E**, *blue arrows*), posterior acoustic shadowing (**B**, *arrow*), calcifications (**A**, *arrow*), and duct extension (**C**, *arrow*). Shadowing may be present deep to the entire mass or just a part of it. **E**, Did you notice that the Cooper ligament (*yellow arrow*) terminates at the echogenic margin?

BOX 7-5 Differential Diagnosis of Solid Mass with Benign Features

- Fibroadenoma
- Papilloma
- Adenosis
- Invasive ductal carcinoma—not otherwise specified (IDC-NOS)
- Ductal carcinoma in situ (DCIS)
- Medullary carcinoma
- Mucinous carcinoma
- Phyllodes tumor

density (Fig. 7-25). The presence of only one of these features pushes these masses to BI-RADS 4, and biopsy is indicated even if it is found on the first (baseline) mammogram. Stability is not useful in these cases, and biopsy is generally indicated even if US is negative.

On US, suspicious features (Fig. 7-26) include irregular shape; microlobulated, ill-defined, or echogenic margins; nonparallel orientation; posterior acoustic shadowing; duct extension; sonographic distortion; calcifications; and associated abnormal ducts.

On MRI, suspicious features include irregular shape; ill-defined, microlobulated, or spiculated margin; and heterogeneous or rim enhancement, and washout kinetics. Analysis of enhancement curves is only useful when the morphologic features are benign. Persistent enhancement in the setting of a mass with suspicious morphologic appearance is irrelevant. The morphologic appearance of the mass always trumps the enhancement pattern in deciding the level of suspicion (Fig. 7-27).

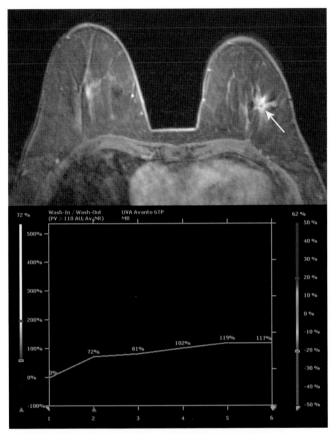

FIGURE 7-27 **Malignant Mass with Benign Enhancement Pattern.** There is an irregular mass with spiculated margins in the left breast (*arrow*). The mass has slow initial enhancement with persistent delayed enhancement. Diagnosis: invasive lobular carcinoma (ILC).

Complex Mass

These masses contain both solid and cystic components (Fig. 7-28) and are associated with a higher risk of malignancy, on the order of 20% to 30%. Complex cystic and solid masses are BI-RADS 4, and sometimes BI-RADS 5. There are three variations of complex mass: cyst with thick walls or septations, intracystic mass, and mixed cystic and solid components. Clustered microcysts that have ill-defined margins, thick walls or septations, or intracystic masses are also included in this category (Fig. 7-29). The majority of complex masses will still be due to fibrocystic change. Malignant causes include IDC, particularly with necrosis, DCIS, and papillary carcinoma.

Benign Morphologic Features with Suspicious Enhancement on MRI

Although morphologic features may suggests a benign mass, a suspicious enhancement pattern makes these

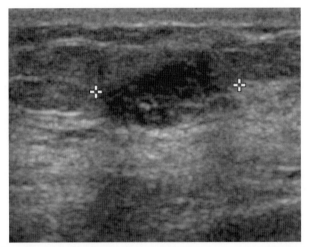

FIGURE 7-29 **Suspicious Microcysts.** The walls are ill defined, and the septations are thick. If these were grapes in your refrigerator, you would get rid of them! BI-RADS 4. Histologic diagnosis: DCIS.

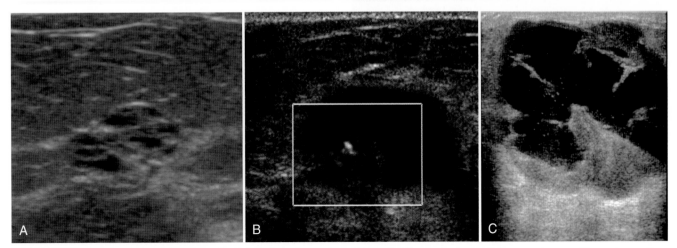

FIGURE 7-28 **Complex Masses. A,** Mass with thick walls and septations. Diagnosis: fibrocystic change. **B,** Intracystic mass. Diagnosis: papillary carcinoma. **C,** Mixed cystic and solid components. Diagnosis: necrotic IDC. All subtypes of complex masses are associated with a similar incidence of breast cancer.

TABLE 7-1   Breast Imaging Reporting and Data System (BI-RADS) Classification for Mass Characteristics by Modality

CATEGORY	Mammography	US	MRI (Evolving)
BI-RADS 2	Stable round or oval mass Multiple bilateral circumscribed masses Fat-containing circumscribed mass	Simple cyst Clustered microcysts Hemorrhagic cyst Most complicated cysts Lymph node Sebaceous cyst Fat necrosis	Mass with benign features, T2-hyperintense, and benign enhancement pattern, especially with multiple lesions
BI-RADS 3	Round or oval mass with benign features (first mammogram)	Solid mass with benign features (not new)	Round or oval mass with circumscribed margins and plateau enhancement or not T2-hyperintense Sole benign-appearing mass
BI-RADS 4	New or enlarging round or oval mass (not a cyst or lymph node on US) Mass with any suspicious features	New or enlarging mass with otherwise benign features Solid mass with any suspicious features Complex cystic and solid mass	Round or oval circumscribed mass with washout enhancement pattern Mass with suspicious shape or margins

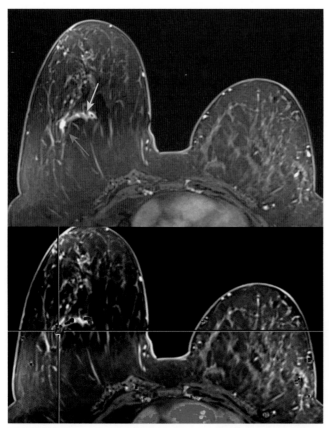

FIGURE 7-30 **Benign Morphology with Washout (BI-RADS 4).** This small round mass in the lateral right breast (*blue arrow*) has well-defined margins but a washout enhancement curve. This woman had a recent biopsy showing IDC. Note that the enhancing area in the transverse plane (*yellow arrow*) is due to the biopsy track.

lesions more concerning (Fig. 7-30). Rim or heterogeneous enhancement or washout kinetics may be suspicious despite a round or oval shape with well-defined margins. This appearance must be put into the context of the entire case, however. Some patients with high parenchymal enhancement may have enhancement of many benign masses, some with washout.

Final Comments

Comparison with the prior mammograms is very helpful in determining whether a round or oval mass requires recall from screening or, if the mass is solid, biopsy (Table 7-1). If stability is questionable, diagnostic evaluations using spot compression views and/or US will provide mass characteristics helpful in the decision-making process. As with calcifications, masses should be judged by their worst features.

KEY POINTS

- Circumscribed fat-containing masses, stable solid masses with benign features, simple cysts, many complicated cysts, multiple circumscribed masses, and sebaceous cysts are considered BI-RADS 2. Routine screening is recommended.
- Use of BI-RADS 3 is best validated for round or oval circumscribed solid masses, grouped round or punctate calcifications, and focal asymmetry on a baseline mammogram.
- BI-RADS 3 should be used after diagnostic workup, not from the screening mammogram.
- Solid benign-appearing masses on US can undergo short-term follow-up (BI-RADS 3) if they are not new or enlarging on mammography or US, and do not appear suspicious by another modality.
- Comparison with prior images changes most benign-appearing lesions from BI-RADS 3 to BI-RADS 2 (stable) or 4 (new or changing).
- BI-RADS 3 should *not* be used as an IDK (I Don't Know and my colleagues have left for the day).
- BI-RADS 4 should be considered for any new or enlarging solid mass despite benign features, a complex mass on US, or a solid mass with suspicious features by any modality. The exception to the last finding is a mass that has a pathognomonic benign appearance on one modality (e.g., oil cyst on mammography) but is suspicious on another (e.g., appears complex on US).

References

American College of Radiology. Breast Imaging Reporting and Data System (BI-RADS), 4th ed. Reston, VA, American College of Radiology, 2003.

Baum JK, Hanna LG, Acharyya S, et al. Use of BI-RADS 3 probably benign category in the American College of Radiology Imaging Network Digital Mammographic Imaging Screening Trial. Radiology 2011;260:61-67.

Bergwa WA, Sechtih AG, Marques H, et al. Cystic breast masses and the ACRIN 6666 experience. Radiol Clin North Am 2010;48:931-987.

Bowles EJA, Miglioretti DL, Sickles EA, et al. Accuracy of short-interval follow-up mammograms by patient and radiologist characteristics. Am J Roentgenol 2008;190:1200-1208.

Graf O, Helbich TH, Fuchsjaeger MH, et al. Follow-up of palpable circumscribed noncalcified solid breast masses at mammography and US: Can biopsy be averted? Radiology 2004;233:850-856.

Harvey JA, Nicholson BT, LoRusso AP, et al. Short-term follow-up of palpable breast lesions with benign imaging features: Evaluation of 375 lesions in 320 women. Am J Roentgenol 2009;193:1723-1730.

Liberman L, Morris EA, Benton CL, et al. Probably benign lesions at magnetic resonance imaging. Cancer 2003;98:377-388.

Mahoney MC, Gatsonis C, Hanna L, et al. Positive predictive value of BI-RADS MR imaging. Radiology 2012;264:51-58.

Shin JH, Han BK, Ko EY, et al. Probably benign breast masses diagnosed by sonography: Is there a difference in the cancer rate according to palpability? Am J Roentgenol 2009;192:W187-W191.

Sickles EA. Periodic mammographic follow-up of probably benign lesions: Results in 3184 consecutive cases. Radiology 1991;179:463-468.

Sickles EA. Nonpalpable, circumscribed, noncalcified solid breast masses: Likelihood of malignancy based on lesion size and age of patient. Radiology 1994;192:439-442.

Sickles EA. Probably benign breast lesions: When should follow-up be recommended and what is the optimal follow-up protocol? Radiology 1999;213:11-14.

Yasmeen S, Romano PS, Pettinger M, et al. Frequency and predictive value of a mammographic recommendation for short-interval follow-up. J Natl Cancer Inst 2003;95:429-436.

CASE 7-1. Asymptomatic 64-year-old woman for screening mammogram. What are your BI-RADS assessment and recommendation?

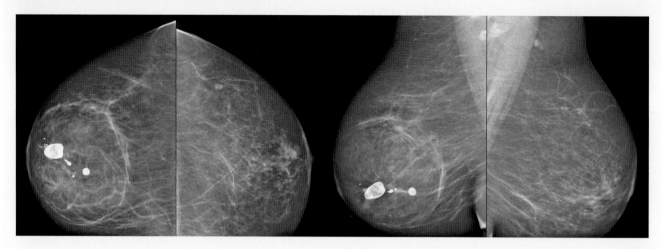

CASE 7-2. A 42-year-old woman is recalled from her initial screening mammogram for evaluation of a left breast mass. How would you characterize the mass? What is your BI-RADS assessment?

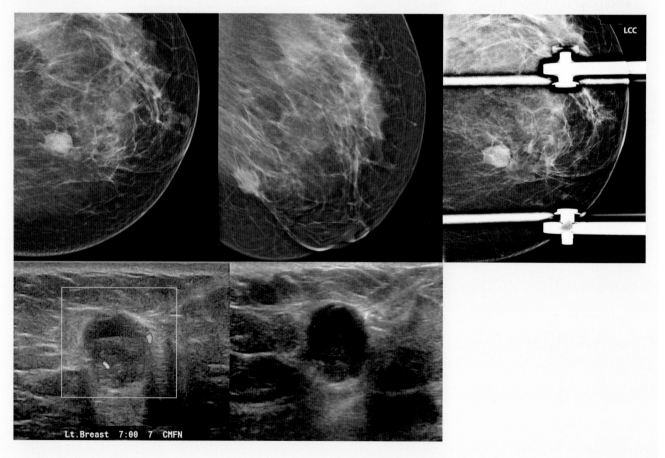

CASE 7-3. A 40-year-old woman recalled from baseline screening mammogram for a round mass in the right breast. Spot compression view, US and power Doppler US are provided. What is the lesion? What is your BI-RADS assessment category?

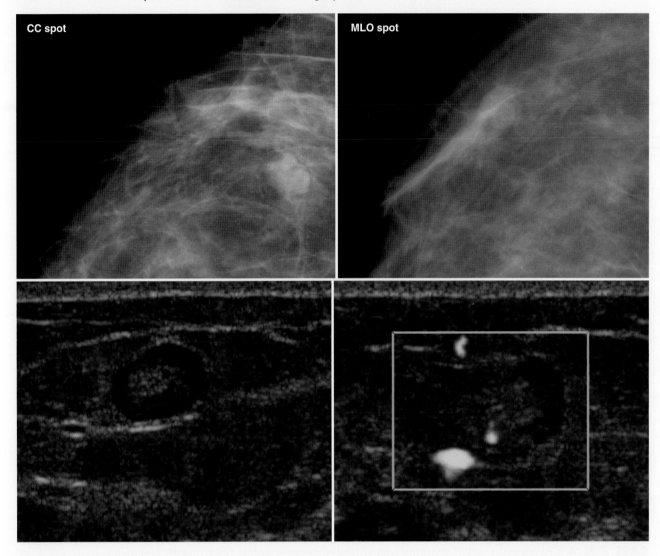

CASE 7-4. This 67-year-old woman noticed a palpable lump (marked by the *triangle*) in her left breast. What is the cause of her lump?

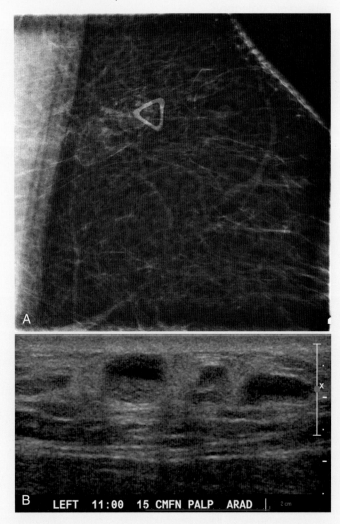

CASE 7-5. A 52-year-old woman presents with a palpable lump in her right breast. Her mammogram shows only dense tissue. What are the US findings? What are your BI-RADS category and recommendation?

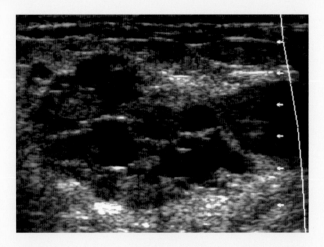

CASE 7-6. A 46-year-old woman is seen for evaluation of a palpable mass that is a simple cyst. Adjacent to the simple cyst is the mass shown here. There is no flow on power Doppler. What might you ask the patient? What are your BI-RADS assessment and recommendation?

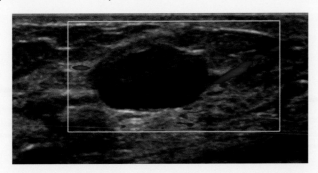

CASE 7-7. A 54-year-old woman is recalled from screening for a focal asymmetry. One of her spot compression views and US are shown. Can you describe the finding? What are your BI-RADS category and recommendation?

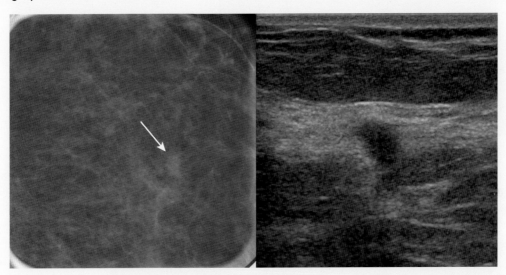

CASE 7-8. A 69-year-old woman is recalled from screening due to interval enlargement of a mass in the right breast. Her mammogram and US are presented. What is your differential diagnosis? What are your BI-RADS assessment and recommendation?

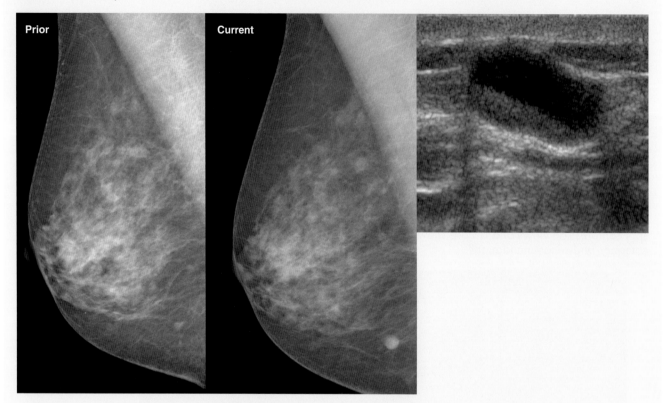

CASE 7-9. A 32-year-old woman presents with a palpable left breast mass. She had a fibroadenoma removed 4 years ago. What is your BI-RADS category for this patient based on US? Your recommendation?

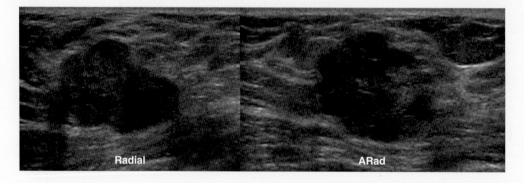

CASE 7-10. A 72-year-old woman is recalled from screening to evaluate a mass in her right breast. No previous mammograms were available for comparison. What are your BI-RADS assessment and recommendation?

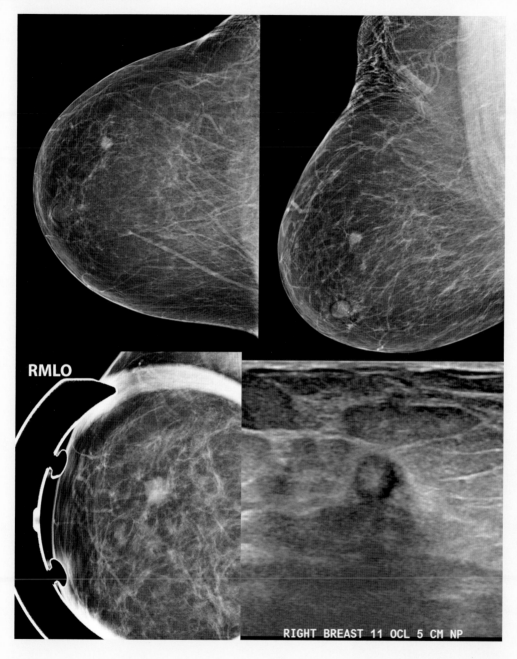

CASE 7-11. A 58-year-old woman is recalled from screening for evaluation of a mass in her right breast (*arrow*). No previous mammograms are available for comparison. Does the mass have benign features? What is your BI-RADS category?

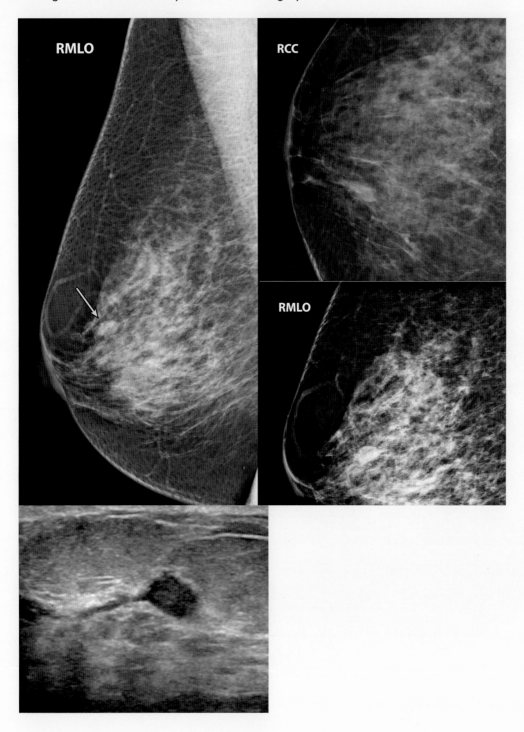

CASE 7-12. This 70-year-old woman is recalled from screening for evaluation of a right breast mass. What are your BI-RADS assessment and recommendation?

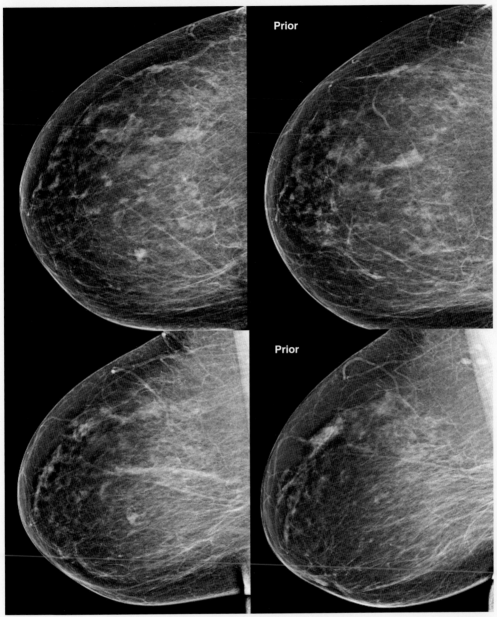

Figure continued on the next page.

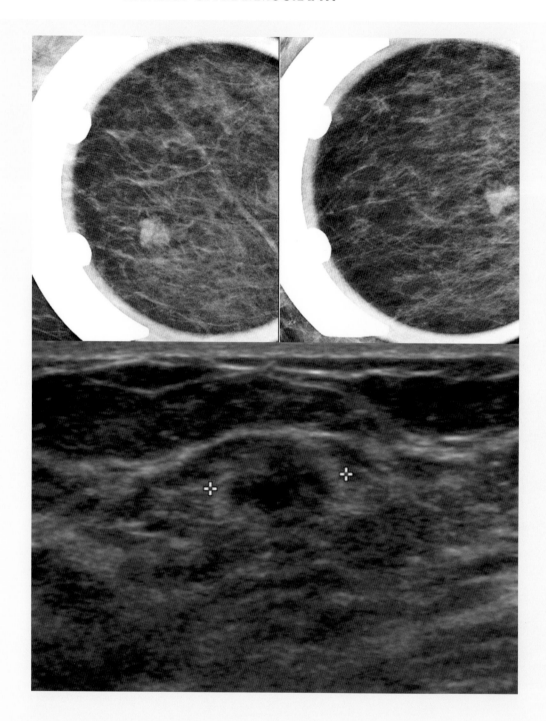

CASE ANSWERS

CASE 7-1. There is a large lipoma in the right breast with central lucent-centered calcifications. BI-RADS 2. Recommend routine annual screening.

CASE 7-2. The mass is oval and high density. Small spicules can be seen arising from the margins on both mammography and US. The mass has complex features on US with a fluid level. Flow is seen within the solid portion by Doppler. This mass is suspicious (BI-RADS 4). Aspiration yielded bloody fluid, and core biopsy of the remaining solid component revealed grade 3 IDC.

CASE 7-3. The spot compression views show a lobular, circumscribed mass, possibly fat-containing. US shows an oval, well-circumscribed mass with a hypoechoic rim and a central hyperechoic hilum, classic for an intramammary lymph node. Power Doppler shows vessels entering the hilum and arborizing toward the cortex. BI-RADS 2. Routine screening is recommended.

CASE 7-4. A, Mammography shows an oval, circumscribed, fat-containing mass corresponding to the palpable lump (*triangle*). **B,** US shows several complicated cysts. Two have dependent debris and another has diffuse low-level echoes. These had no Doppler flow. Because the mammogram shows completely fatty replacement in this area, there should be no confusion regarding the diagnosis of fat necrosis. The patient gave history of prior motor vehicle collision. The findings are consistent with a seatbelt injury.

CASE 7-5. At first glance, you might consider this to be clustered microcysts. However, the presence of small solid intracystic masses makes this a complex (cystic and solid) mass. In other words, the grapes have seeds! This is BI-RADS 4. Ultrasound-guided biopsy showed papillary DCIS.

CASE 7-6. There is a broad-based, hypoechoic, intracystic mass without Doppler flow. The appearance is consistent with a hemorrhagic cyst. She has probably had this cyst aspirated before, so this would be a good question to ask. BI-RADS 2. Return to screening. (Remember that you can avoid most of these recurrences by simply injecting room air into every cyst that you aspirate; the air dries out the lining, and there is a much lower incidence of cyst recurrence.)

CASE 7-7. There is an oval, homogeneously hypoechoic mass that corresponds with the mammographic finding. The US finding may represent a small, solid mass or complicated cyst. A concerning feature of this mass is that its orientation is not parallel. Doppler can be used to confirm that the mass is solid; however, the absence of flow does not exclude a solid mass. The differential diagnosis includes fibrocystic change, adenosis, fibroadenoma, and IDC. BI-RADS 4. Ultrasound-guided biopsy was recommended. Histologic diagnosis: IDC—not otherwise specified.

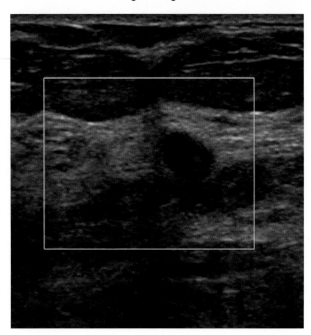

CASE 7-8. This is an enlarging, round, high-density mass. The only thing that will get this woman out of a biopsy is a specific benign finding on US such as a simple cyst or lymph node. Instead we find a cystic mass with dependent debris and a thick wall, making this a complex cystic and solid mass. BI-RADS 4. Histologic diagnosis: DCIS.

CASE 7-9. This mass is BI-RADS 4 based on the US features. On the radial image (*left*), the mass has a lobular shape and parallel orientation, posterior acoustic enhancement, and circumscribed margins, suggesting a possible fibroadenoma. However, the microlobulated margin on the antiradial image is suspicious. BI-RADS 4. Biopsy rather than short-interval follow-up is indicated. Her mammogram below confirms the ill-defined margin (*arrow*). Ultrasound-guided core biopsy showed IDC.

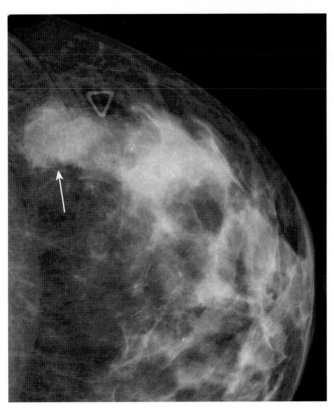

CASE 7-10. Mammography shows the mass to have indistinct margins. By US, the mass resembles a lymph node, but the location is unusual for a node: there is no fatty hilum on mammography, and the margin characteristics are suspicious. BI-RADS 4. Core biopsy revealed IDC with central necrosis.

CASE 7-11. The mass is oval and has fairly well-defined margins on mammography. However, by US, there is duct extension (*arrow*) and the mass has slightly angular margins. These features are suspicious (BI-RADS 4). Biopsy revealed IDC with DCIS.

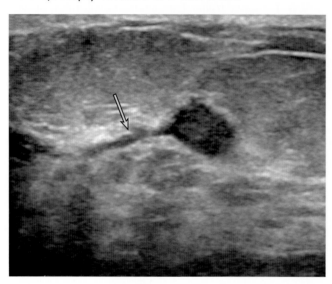

CASE 7-12. On the screening views, the mass looks like it might be fat containing, like a hamartoma. However, a hamartoma is congenital so should not be a new finding as it is in this case. The spot compression views and US reveal suspicious features. This is at least BI-RADS 4. Ultrasound-guided core biopsy showed IDC, grade II. This was a tricky case. Good job if you figured this one out!

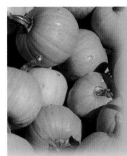

CHAPTER 8

Multiple Masses

Multiple masses. Sigh. Do you hate these? Take a deep breath and lean into it. These masses are really not that hard to assess. They are almost always benign, BI-RADS 2, representing multiple cysts or fibroadenomas. This is like a "Get Out of Jail Free" card in Monopoly. Before we use the card though, we need to carefully look at each one to ensure that a cancer is not masquerading as a benign mass. We'll give you our best tips for figuring out which patients actually need recall and which can be seen next year. Soon you will be thinking, "Bring it on!" instead of putting these cases on your partner's desk.

The rule of multiplicity in mammography is that multiple and bilateral similar-appearing findings with low-suspicion features have a very high probability of being benign. The basis for this rule is that the genetic, hormonal, and other influences that produce benign findings in one breast tend to produce similar findings in the other, and it is very uncommon for malignant lesions to present simultaneously as similar-appearing findings in multiple regions of both breasts.

When multiple bilateral masses with circumscribed margins are detected by mammography, the rule of multiplicity can be applied and the findings are considered benign. These women can be spared the discomfort, inconvenience, anxiety, and cost of diagnostic mammography, ultrasonography (US), and in some cases, aspiration or biopsy.

However, with multiple masses, it is important to avoid the pitfall of using the rule of multiplicity too soon. Don't play your "Get Out of Jail Free" card too early. These cases are complex and can be difficult to interpret. Benign masses may obscure other lesions or distract the radiologist from findings that need further evaluation.

Etiology of Multiple Bilateral Masses

Multiple bilateral masses may represent one type of lesion or more than one type. Cysts are the most common lesions contributing to multiple bilateral masses (Figs. 8-1 and 8-2). Cysts can develop at any age, but are most common in premenopausal women. Milk of calcium may be seen mammographically, providing clues to the cystic nature of one or more of the masses.

Fibroadenomas are the second most common lesion causing multiple bilateral masses. When coarse calcifications are seen within one or more of the masses, it suggests that other, noncalcified masses may represent fibroadenomas as well (Fig. 8-3).

Peripheral papillomas uncommonly present as multiple bilateral masses. Multiple papillomas are usually round or oval masses with circumscribed margins and are associated with an increased risk for breast cancer. Papillary carcinoma commonly presents as multiple circumscribed masses with segmental distributions on mammography.

Malignant multiple bilateral masses are very uncommon. Nevertheless, metastatic disease should still cross your mind when evaluating multiple bilateral breast masses (Fig. 8-4). Most women with breast metastases have a known history of malignancy. Unfortunately, breast involvement may be the first sign of recurrent disease in a woman thought cured of a malignant disease. Melanoma is the most common nonbreast primary neoplasm to metastasize to the breast. The appearance of the mammogram is usually different from that seen in the benign causes of multiple masses. The masses are typically denser than cysts or fibroadenomas, and the margins are often ill defined. Metastatic lesions of the breast are typically located throughout the organ, including the fatty tissue in the inframammary fold and axilla, whereas cysts and fibroadenomas are located within breast tissue. Metastatic disease to the breast is often associated with axillary adenopathy, and some of the breast masses may represent metastatic intramammary lymph nodes. Lymphoma, leukemia, and rhabdomyosarcoma are rare in the breast and will be covered in more detail in Chapter 11, Expanding the Differential Diagnosis.

Intramammary lymph nodes typically demonstrate a lucent notch representing the fatty hilum. However, if the lucent notch is not visible, lymph nodes may contribute to the pattern of multiple bilateral masses. When lymph nodes have a characteristically benign appearance, we do not consider them one of the multiple bilateral masses. For example, if there are two indeterminate circumscribed masses in one breast and a typical intramammary lymph node in the other, the findings are not considered as multiple bilateral masses.

Skin lesions, such as nevi or neurofibromas, can mimic multiple bilateral breast masses. Ideally, your technologists will help you by noting them on the clinical history sheet (Box 8-1).

Management of Multiple Bilateral Masses

"Multiple bilateral masses" refers to asymptomatic women whose mammograms show a minimum of three

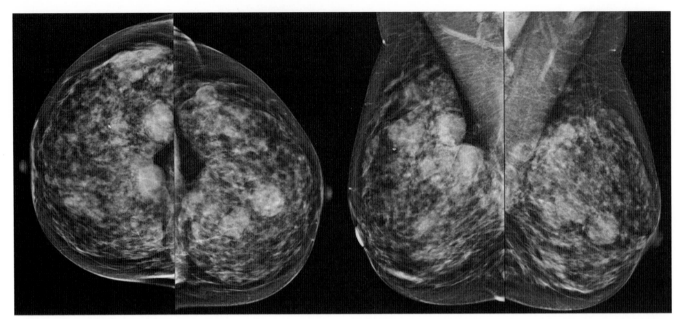

FIGURE 8-1 **Multiple Bilateral Benign Masses.** Screening mammogram on a 48-year-old woman showing multiple bilateral similar-appearing masses with partially circumscribed margins. This woman had bilateral cysts previously demonstrated by US. There were no suspicious changes compared with previous mammograms. The patient was assigned BI-RADS 2, and no suspicious changes have occurred in over 2 years on subsequent mammography.

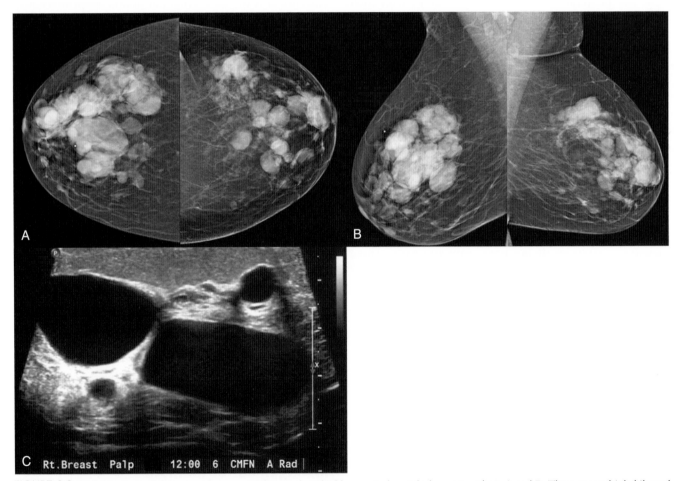

FIGURE 8-2 **Multiple Cysts.** A 55-year-old woman with a newly palpable mass in her right breast (*marker*). **A** and **B,** There are multiple bilateral similar-appearing masses with circumscribed margins. When compared with previous mammograms, some masses had decreased in size while others showed enlargement. US targeted to the region of the newly palpable mass reveals multiple cysts (**C**). Sonographic evaluation of the remaining masses was considered unnecessary, and the patient was assigned BI-RADS 2.

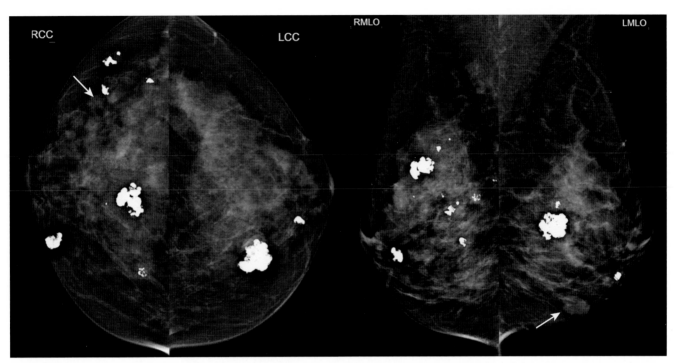

FIGURE 8-3 **Multiple Fibroadenomas.** Screening mammogram on a 50-year-old woman. There are multiple bilateral masses, most with coarse calcifications typical of fibroadenomas. The noncalcified masses (*arrows*) likely represent fibroadenomas as well. The findings showed no suspicious changes for over 4 years.

BOX 8-1 Differential Diagnosis of Multiple Bilateral Masses

- Cysts
- Fibroadenomas
- Papillomas
- Metastatic disease or lymphoma (really uncommon!)
- Skin lesions (mimic)

masses, with at least one mass in each breast. These findings occur in 0.5% to 1.7% of patients in a screening population.

Management recommendations for multiple bilateral masses with benign features differ among radiologists. Many assign BI-RADS 2 and recommend annual screening mammography. Some radiologists recommend bilateral US after the initial mammogram, to serve as a baseline for future studies, while others assign BI-RADS 3 on the initial mammogram and recommend a 6-month bilateral follow-up study to evaluate stability. Our preference is to assign BI-RADS 2 and recommend annual mammographic screening. However, if any of the masses has suspicious features, we have a low threshold for recalling the patient for targeted diagnostic evaluation, as we demonstrate in some of the cases in this chapter.

Why not bring them all in for US? The use of US to evaluate multiple bilateral masses with benign mammographic features yields frequent false-positive findings. As a group, these women do not appear to be at increased risk for developing breast cancer. In women with fibrocystic changes, complicated cysts or complex masses are frequently detected. Benign solid masses, which also frequently occur in these patients, often have indeterminate sonographic features. A degenerating fibroadenoma may have shadowing on US. When masses other than simple cysts are identified by US, they often prompt a recommendation for aspiration, biopsy, or short-term follow-up studies. In addition, when a mass is seen by US, it may be difficult or impossible to identify a corresponding mammographic finding with certainty, unless a localizing intervention is performed.

What Is the Evidence?

There is strong support in the literature, when certain criteria are met, to consider multiple bilateral masses benign, even when there are no previous mammograms for comparison. Leung and Sickles (2000) studied 1440 women with multiple bilateral masses, with circumscribed margins, whose mammograms were prospectively interpreted as benign, irrespective of the availability of prior mammograms. In fact, no comparison studies were available in almost half of the cases. The interval cancer rate for women with multiple bilateral masses was 0.14%, which is similar to previously reported interval cancer rates for the general population and lower than the incident cancer rate in the United States. In an earlier study (Sickles, 1991), 1 cancer was found at follow-up of 253 women (0.4%) with multiple bilateral well-defined solid masses. In the ACRIN 6666 trial, none of 39 women with multiple bilateral circumscribed masses on mammography had cancer. Likewise, none of 48 women with

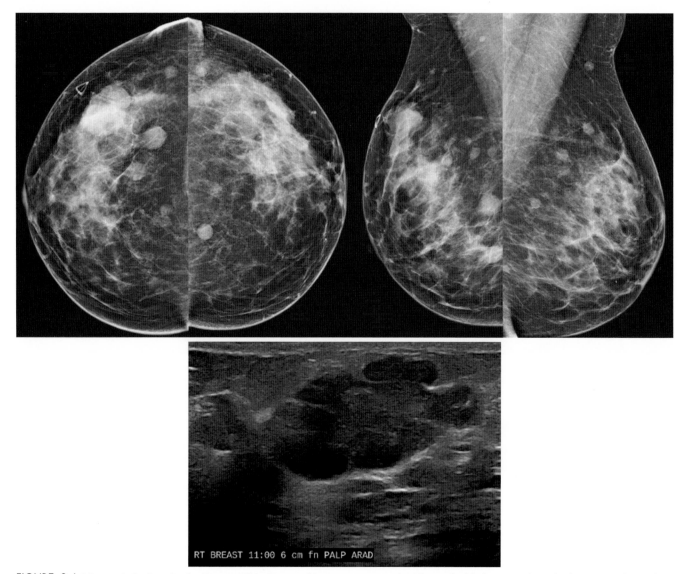

FIGURE 8-4 **Metastatic Lesions in the Breasts.** This 47-year-old woman presented with a palpable lump in the right breast (*marker*). There are multiple circumscribed masses in both breasts. Note that the masses are primarily located in the retromammary fat and even in the axillary fat. US shows a solid hypoechoic mass with microloculated margins. Ultrasound-guided core biopsy samples were black in appearance. The patient subsequently gave a history of ocular melanoma 5 years earlier. Biopsy showed metastatic melanoma.

multiple solid masses with benign features on whole breast US had cancer.

Criteria for Assigning BI-RADS 2 Category to Multiple Masses

The Masses Must Be Bilateral

Multiple circumscribed masses in one breast do not fulfill the multiplicity rule and cannot be considered benign at screening. Unilateral masses with benign features are still most likely to represent cysts or fibroadenomas, and sometimes papillomas. However, the risk of carcinoma is higher than when the masses are bilateral (Fig. 8-5). Suspicion for malignancy is increased if the masses are in a segmental distribution.

The Masses Must Be Multiple

Because the masses must be bilateral, the minimum number of masses present is three; two in one breast and one in the other breast.

The Margins Must Be Circumscribed

A circumscribed margin is a benign feature. When multiple masses are present, some of the mass margins may be obscured. The BI-RADS lexicon defines "circumscribed" as having at least 75% of the margin visible as circumscribed. If a mass is not obscured and most of the mass is circumscribed but the remainder of the margin is ill defined, irregular, or spiculated, then diagnostic evaluation is needed.

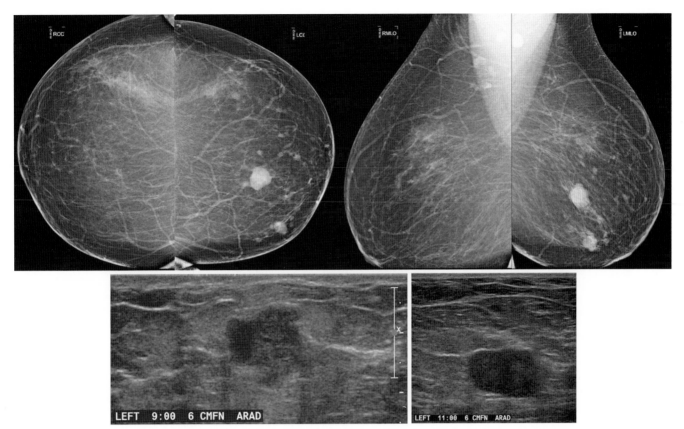

FIGURE 8-5 **Unilateral Circumscribed Masses.** Several masses are present in the left lower inner quadrant. On US, these are solid hypoechoic masses. Some have irregular shapes. Diagnosis: multifocal invasive ductal carcinoma (IDC).

Evaluating Multiple Bilateral Masses

The presence of multiple bilateral masses can often be appreciated on an overview of the case images. Are you finished? Sorry, but no. You can't use the "Get Out of Jail Free" card until you *really* look! There is no evidence that the presence of multiple bilateral circumscribed masses reduces the chance that a malignant lesion will also develop. To find her cancer, look for mass features that distinguish one from the others. Next, ignore all those masses and look at everything else. Last, be aware of new or changing clinical findings described by the patient or her health care provider.

Which One of These Is Not Like the Others?

Do you remember playing that game when you were a kid? You had to figure out which of several very similar objects was different. We'll bet that you were really good at that game because you are a radiologist now!

When multiple bilateral masses are present, their size, shape, density, and margins should be individually examined. Is one mass substantially larger than the others (dominant)? Search for masses that stand out from others, such as those that are very dense, irregular in shape, or have indistinct, microlobulated, or spiculated margins (Figs. 8-6 to 8-8, and Box 8-2). Search for associated suspicious findings such as calcifications, architectural

---

BOX 8-2 When to Consider Diagnostic Imaging in the Setting of Multiple Bilateral Benign-Appearing Masses

- Palpable mass (one or more)
- One mass is dominant (larger or denser)
- A new or enlarging mass
- Multiple new masses when no masses are seen on previous mammograms
- Suspicious features: irregular shape, spiculation, calcifications that are not obviously benign

---

distortion, adenopathy, skin thickening, or nipple retraction.

New or Enlarging Masses

When prior mammograms are available, assess how the masses have changed over time. In cases with multiple bilateral circumscribed masses, it is common to observe that some masses are stable while others have decreased or increased in size. Provided the masses have no suspicious characteristics that distinguish them from the others, these cases can still be assigned BI-RADS 2.

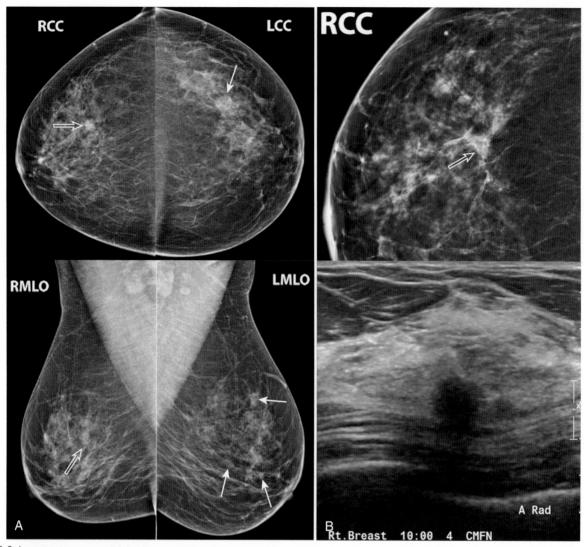

FIGURE 8-6 **Multiple Masses with Malignancy.** Screening mammogram of a 40-year-old woman (**A**). Multiple masses are seen bilaterally (*arrows*). A right breast mass is dense for its size (*open arrow*). The patient was recalled and this mass is shown to have spiculated margins on a craniocaudal (CC) spot compression view (*open arrow*; **B**, *top*). US shows a corresponding hypoechoic solid mass with indistinct margins (**B**, *bottom*). Two left breast cysts were also seen. Diagnosis: IDC and ductal carcinoma in situ (DCIS) in the right breast.

Cysts commonly fluctuate in size; they wax and wane (Fig. 8-9). Over half of new cysts will regress within 1 year. After 5 years, about 85% of cysts will either resolve or decrease in size. If a mass has increased dramatically in size, we therefore perform US, even if the patient has a history of cysts.

Fibroadenomas often enlarge or fluctuate slightly in size in premenopausal women. Aside from the very rapid growth of juvenile fibroadenomas in some young patients, enlarging fibroadenomas usually show fairly gradual increases in size. In postmenopausal women, fibroadenomas regress; it is rare for new fibroadenomas to develop and uncommon for existing fibroadenomas to enlarge. The exception is that fibroadenomas can enlarge significantly in postmenopausal women who are using menopausal hormone therapy.

Because cysts and fibroadenomas account for most multiple bilateral masses, search for findings that do not

> ### BOX 8-3   When BI-RADS 2 Still Applies in the Setting of Multiple Bilateral Benign-Appearing Masses
>
> - All are getting smaller
> - All are a little bigger
> - Some are a little bigger and some are smaller

fit well with these diagnoses (Box 8-3). Look for one mass that has increased rapidly or substantially in size, especially if enlargement has occurred while other masses have been stable or have regressed. These masses warrant diagnostic evaluation. US is also indicated for patients of

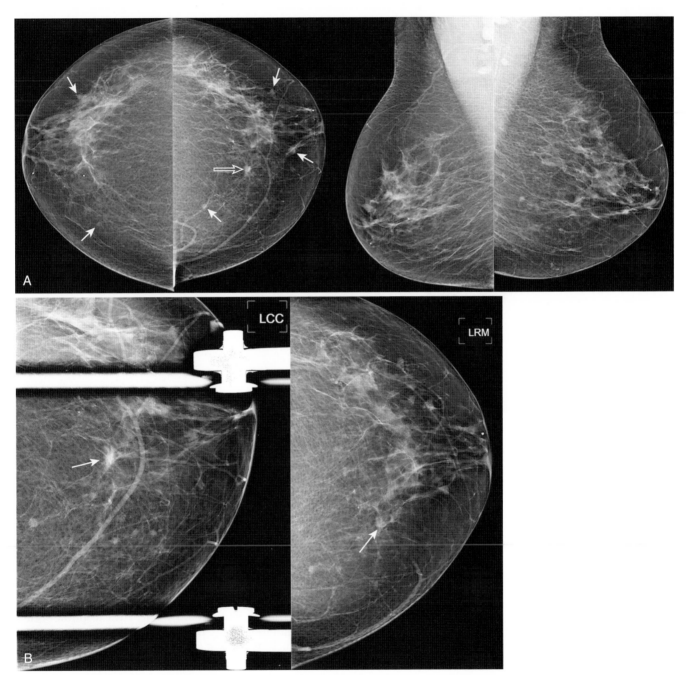

FIGURE 8-7 **Multiple Masses and IDC.** Screening mammogram of a 75-year-old woman shows multiple bilateral less-than-1 cm masses (*arrows*). **A,** One mass (*open arrow*), in the medial left breast, is denser than the others and has spiculated margins. **B,** The appearance remains suspicious on CC spot and CC rolled medial views (*arrows*). Diagnosis: infiltrating carcinoma with ductal and lobular features and DCIS.

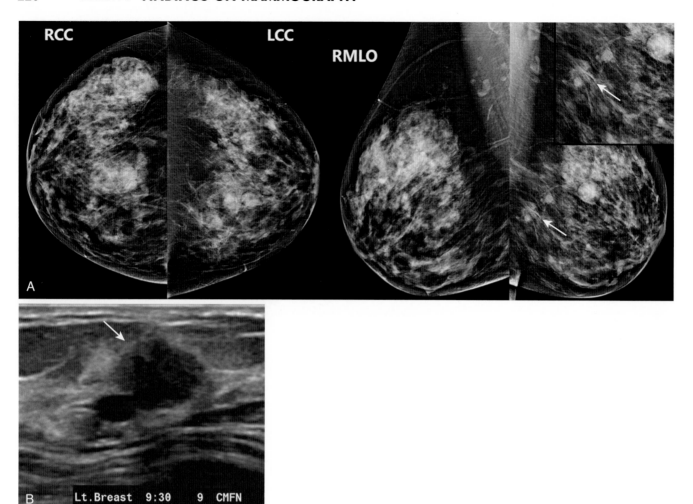

FIGURE 8-8 **Multiple Masses and One-View Asymmetry Due to IDC. A,** Screening mammogram on a 64-year-old woman shows multiple bilateral masses. There is an irregular one-view asymmetry in the posterior left breast (*arrows*). **B,** US reveals a corresponding solid mass with microlobulated margins (*arrow*). Multiple cysts were also seen. Core biopsy revealed IDC.

any age who have not had masses on prior mammograms and now have multiple masses. When new or enlarging masses are shown to be solid or complex by US, biopsy is indicated.

Clinical Factors

History can be very helpful in evaluating multiple bilateral masses. If previous US, aspiration, or biopsy has been performed, these studies should be reviewed. The use of hormone replacement therapy predisposes to cyst formation and enlargement. When there is a history of malignancy, the possibility of bilateral metastatic lesions should be considered.

When a clinically suspicious palpable abnormality develops in a woman with multiple bilateral masses on mammography, it should be evaluated by US even if the mammographic findings are stable. An exception occurs when mammography demonstrates a typically benign lesion, such as a calcified fibroadenoma or hamartoma, which corresponds to the palpable finding.

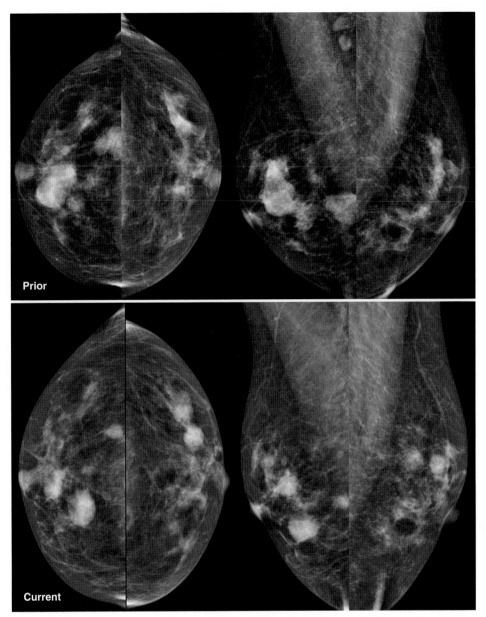

FIGURE 8-9 **Waxing and Waning Cysts.** Some masses have enlarged while some have decreased in size. As long as the masses all have benign features and none are dramatically larger, recall is not necessary. This is BI-RADS 2.

KEY POINTS

- Multiple masses (a minimum of three masses with at least one mass in each breast) that have benign features, are similar in appearance, and show no suspicious changes from previous studies are considered benign and can be assigned BI-RADS 2.
- If any of the masses appear different from the others (dominant in size, higher density) or have suspicious features (ill-defined margin, associated concerning calcifications), then further evaluation should be considered.

- The presence of multiple masses makes these mammograms more complex. After looking at the masses, force yourself to look at everything else to identify other abnormalities such as calcifications or architectural distortion.
- At follow-up, BI-RADS 2 can still be used if some or all of the masses are a little bigger. If one mass is enlarging while the rest are stable or regressing, recall should be considered.

References

Berg WA, Zhang A, Adams A, Mendelson E. Multiple Bilateral Similar Findings on Mammography: Results of ACRIN 6666 Trial. Presented at Radiological Society of North America Meeting, 2010.

Berg WA, Zhang A, Adams A, Mendelson E. Multiple Bilateral Similar Masses on Ultrasound: Results of ACRIN 6666 Trial. Presented at Radiological Society of North America Meeting, 2010.

Brenner RJ, Bein ME, Sarti DA, Vinstein AL. Spontaneous regression of interval benign cysts of the breast. Radiology 1994;193:365-368.

Cardenosa G, Eklund GW. Benign pap illary neoplasms of the breast: Mammographic findings. Radiology 1991;181:751-755.

Chung SY, Oh KK. Imaging findings of metastatic disease to the breast. Yonsei Med J 2001;42:497-502.

Fornage BD, Lorigan JG, Andry E. Fibroadenoma of the breast: Sonographic appearance. Radiology 1989;172:671-675.

Gordon PB, Gagnon FA, Lanzkowsky L. Solid breast masses diagnosed as fibroadenoma at fine-needle aspiration biopsy: Acceptable rates of growth at long-term follow-up. Radiology 2003;229:233-238.

Kopans D. Breast Imaging, 2nd ed. Philadelphia, Lippincott Williams & Wilkins, 1998, p 311.

Leung JW, Sickles EA. Multiple bilateral masses detected on screening mammography: Assessment of the need for recall imaging. AJR 2000;175:23-29.

Liberman L, Giess CS, Dershaw DD, et al. Non-Hodgkin lymphoma of the breast: Imaging characteristics and correlation with histopathologic findings. Radiology 1994;192:157-160.

McCrae ES, Johnston C, Haney PJ. Metastases to the breast. AJR 1983;141:685-690.

Meyer JE, Frenna TH, Polger M, et al. Enlarging occult fibroadenomas. Radiology 1992;183:639-641.

Mitnick JS, Vazquez MF, Harris MN, et al. Invasive papillary carcinoma of the breast: Mammographic appearance. Radiology 1990;177:803-806.

Muttarak M, Lerttumnongtum P, Chaiwun B, Peh WCG. Spectrum of papillary lesions of the breast: Clinical, imaging, and pathologic correlation. AJR 2008;191:700-707.

Rahbar G, Die AC, Hansen GC, et al. Benign versus malignant solid breast masses: US differentiation. Radiology 1999;213:889-894.

Sickles EA. Periodic mammographic follow-up of probably benign lesions: Results in 3,184 consecutive cases. Radiology 1991;179:463-468.

Toombs BD, Kalisher L. Metastatic disease to the breast: Clinical, pathologic, and radiographic features. AJR 1977;129:673-676.

CASE QUESTIONS

CASE 8-1. A 40-year-old woman has her first screening mammogram. What are the findings? What BI-RADS category would you assign?

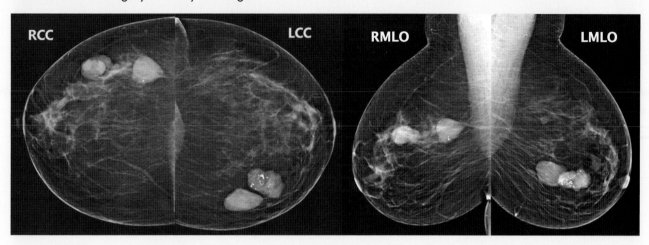

CASE 8-2. Screening mammogram of a 55-year-old woman. What are the findings? What is your BI-RADS assessment? The right *clip* is from previous core biopsy of a benign mass.

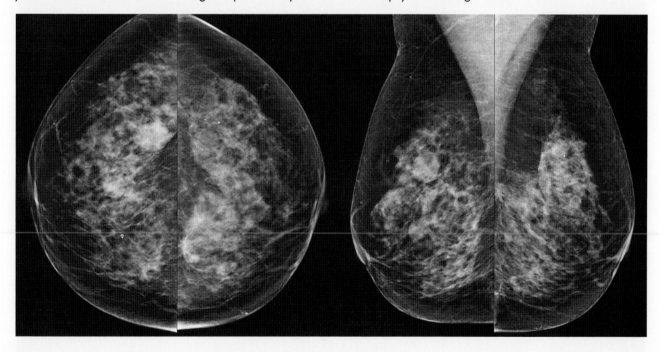

CASE 8-3. Screening mammogram on a 55-year-old woman. On comparison with previous mammograms, some of the masses were bigger and some were smaller. Can the rule of multiplicity be applied? What is the most likely cause of the findings? BI-RADS assessment?

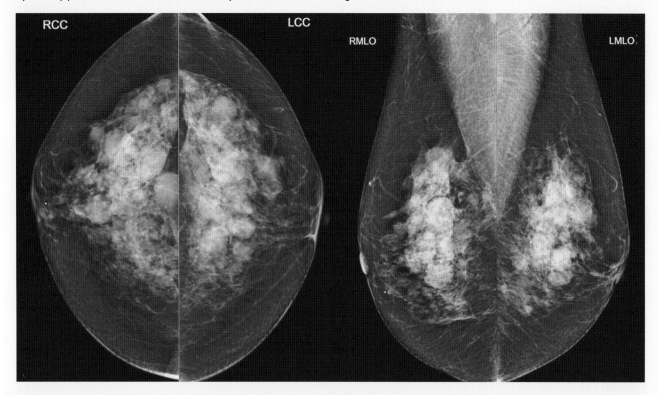

CASE 8-4. Screening mammogram of a 62-year-old woman. No previous mammograms are available. What are the significant findings? What management do you recommend? Can the rule of multiplicity be applied?

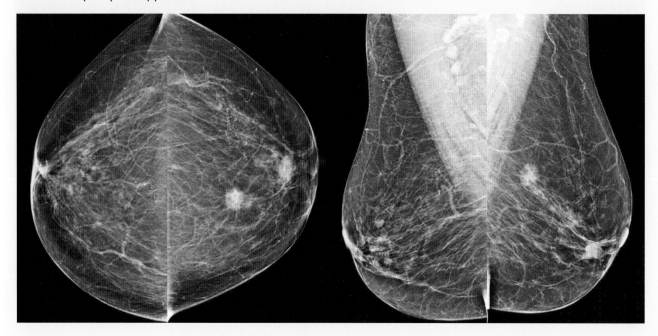

CASE 8-5. Screening mammogram of a 49-year-old woman with a comparison study from 1 year prior. A left breast cyst (C) was diagnosed by previous US. Can the rule of multiplicity be applied? What do you recommend?

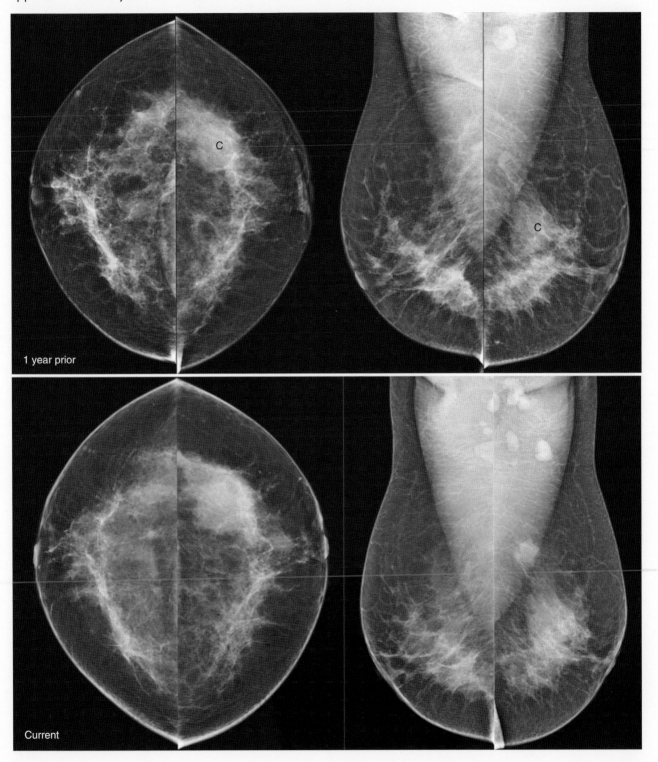

CASE 8-6. A screening mammogram on an 80-year-old woman is compared with a previous mammogram from 1 year ago. The patient has a history of multiple bilateral cysts diagnosed by US and core biopsy of a left breast mass revealing fibroadenoma. Can the rule of multiplicity be applied?

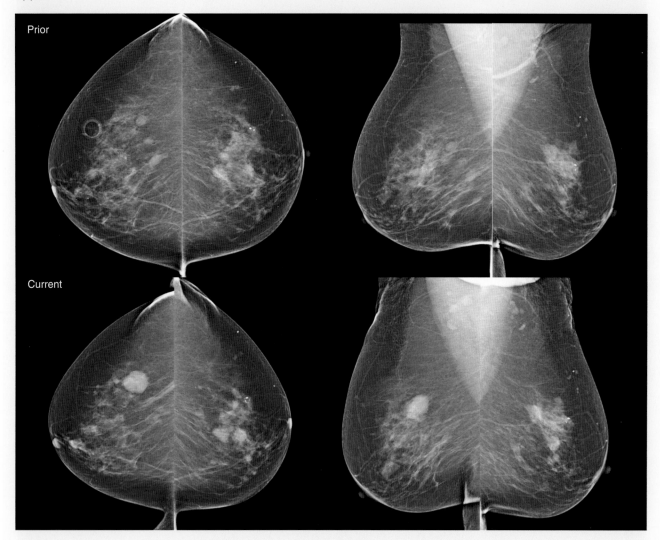

Prior

Current

CASE 8-7. Screening mammogram of a 72-year-old woman with a history of lumpectomy and radiation therapy for right breast carcinoma. What are the findings? What do you recommend?

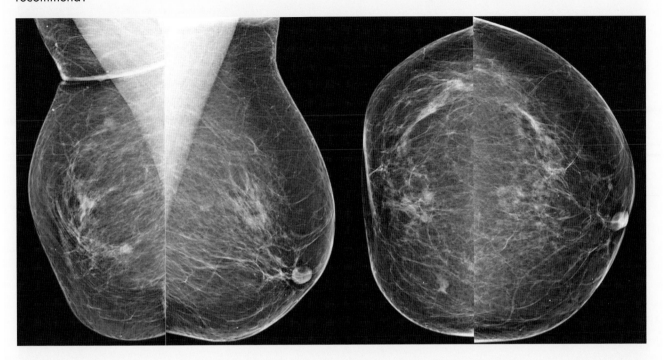

CASE 8-8. Screening mammogram on a 68-year-old woman with a comparison study from 2 years prior. What are the findings? What are your BI-RADS assessment and recommendation?

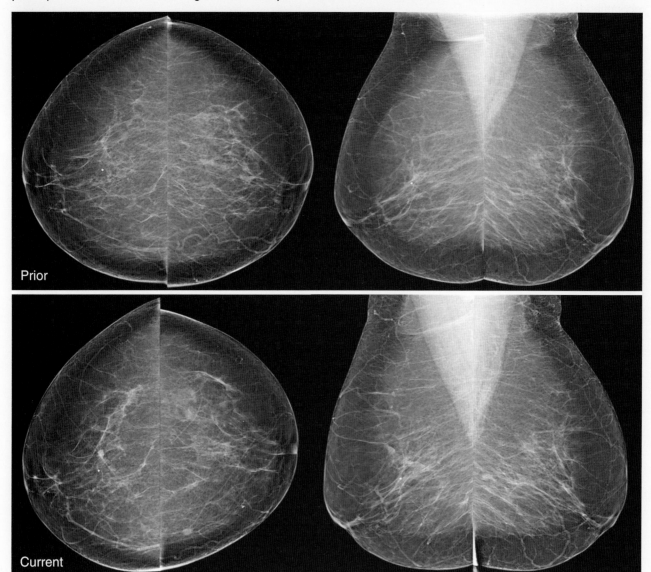

Prior

Current

CASE 8-9. A 41-year-old woman with a history of bilateral cysts had screening mammography performed 2 months ago that showed extremely dense tissue with multiple bilateral benign-appearing masses. There were no suspicious findings (BI-RADS 2).

She now presents with a new palpable mass in her upper right breast and is referred for US. Your sonographer brings you the following images from the palpable region. What do you recommend?

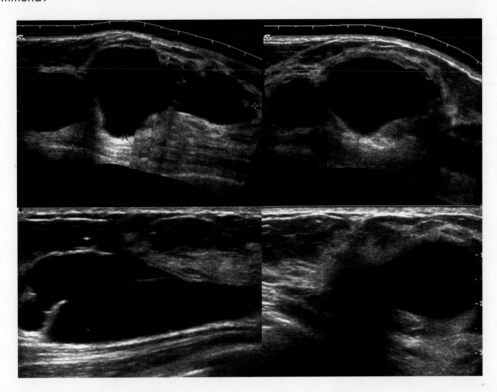

CASE 8-10. Screening mammogram showing the left breast of a 64-year-old woman. There are known multiple bilateral masses. The *clip* is from remote benign core biopsy. What significant change has occurred since the previous study?

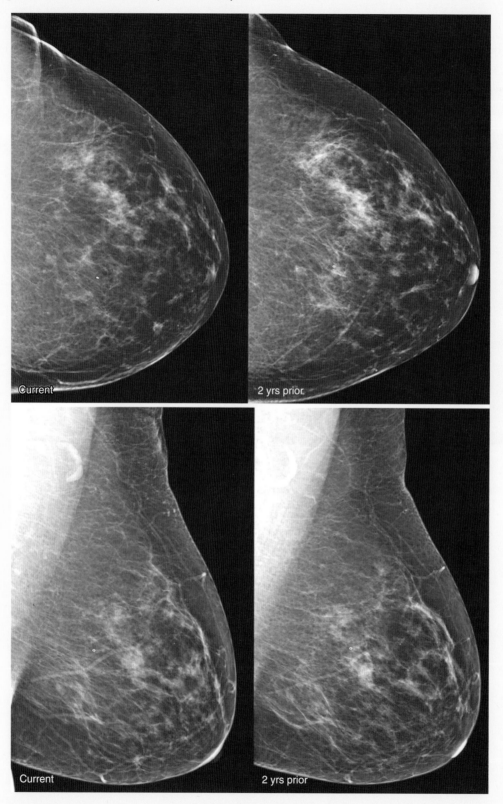

CASE ANSWERS

CASE 8-1. There are multiple bilateral similar-appearing masses with benign features. There are coarse fibroadenomatous calcifications within masses in each breast, and the remaining masses most likely represent fibroadenomas as well. These findings are benign (BI-RADS 2), and the patient can be recommended for annual screening mammography.

CASE 8-2. The tissue is heterogeneously dense, and there are multiple bilateral masses. There is an irregular focal asymmetry in the posterior medial left breast (arrows; **A** and **B**). BI-RADS 0. Recommend diagnostic views and ultrasonography.

On diagnostic views a spiculated mass is confirmed in the retroglandular fat (arrows; **C**). US shows a corresponding irregular hypoechoic mass with indistinct margins (**D**). An adjacent oval hypoechoic circumscribed mass is also seen (arrow). Core biopsy of the irregular mass revealed invasive lobular carcinoma with pleomorphic features. Core biopsy of the circumscribed mass showed fat necrosis and LCIS.

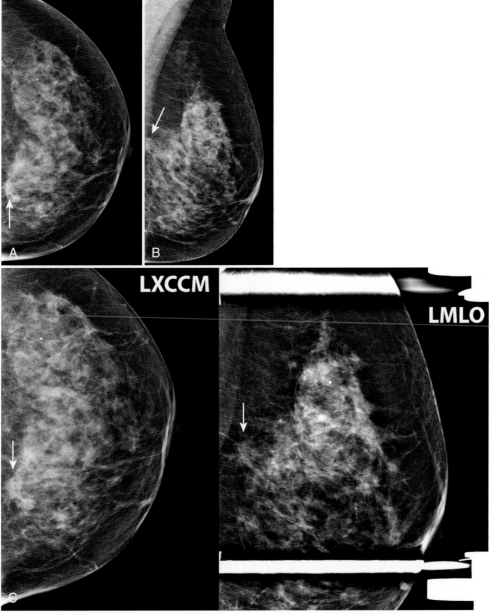

Figure continued on next page.

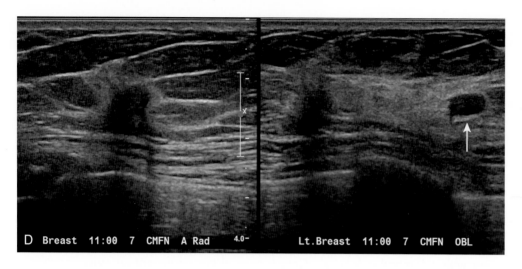

CASE 8-3. There are multiple bilateral similar-appearing masses. No single mass is more suspicious than the others. Fluctuation in size is usually indicative of cysts. Yes, we can use the rule of multiplicity. The findings are considered benign (BI-RADS 2).

CASE 8-4. There are two masses in the left breast (upper inner quadrant and subareolar) and at least two much smaller masses in the anterior right breast (*arrows; A* and **B**). The rule of multiplicity cannot be applied because the 11 o'clock mass on the left has spiculated margins (*circle*).

These findings are better seen on spot compression views (*arrows; C*). US of the left breast reveals a mass with indistinct margins in the 11 o'clock position and a circumscribed mass in the subareolar region (**D**). US of the anterior right breast shows one hypoechoic solid mass with indistinct margins and one simple cyst (**E**).

Diagnoses: Left breast: 11 o'clock mass, IDC and DCIS; left subareolar mass, infiltrating carcinoma with mucinous features. Right breast: 11 o'clock mass, multifocal DCIS.

See figure on the next page.

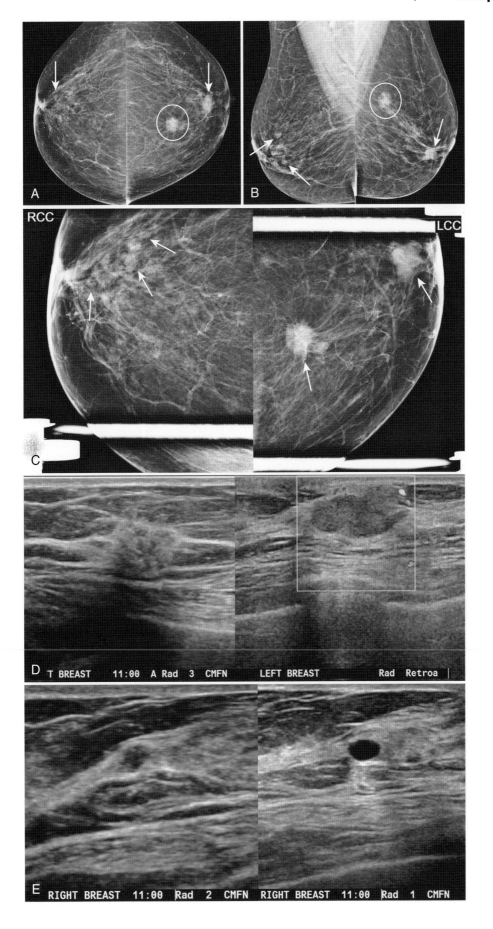

CASE 8-5. There are two masses in the left breast, including the previously documented cyst (*C*), which has obscured margins. The more posterior mass is excluded from the screening CC view but is confirmed on the exaggerated craniocaudal lateral (XCCL) and mediolateral views (*arrows*). It has enlarged since the previous mammogram.

The rule of multiplicity should not be applied. The masses are unilateral. The posterior left breast mass has suspicious features (irregular shape, indistinct margins) and has clearly enlarged. There is a dense left axillary lymph node. US shows the known cyst and an adjacent, irregular hypoechoic mass, which was biopsied. Diagnosis: IDC grade 2.

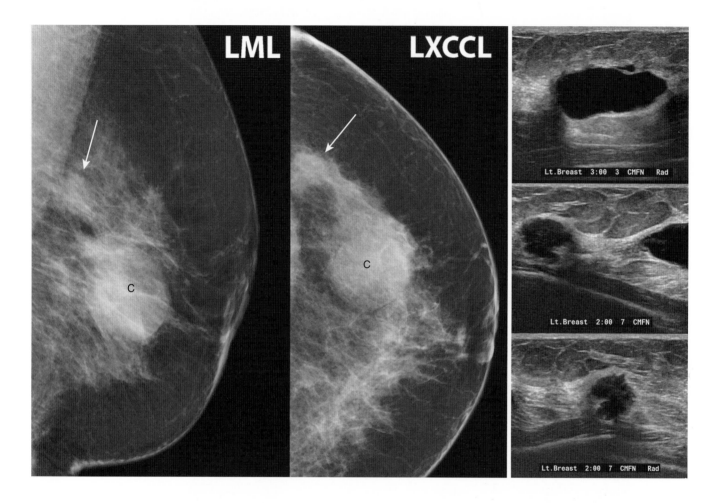

CASE 8-6. There are multiple bilateral masses. However, the findings cannot be considered benign because one mass, in the upper-outer quadrant of the right breast (*arrows*), has enlarged markedly since the previous mammogram and, therefore, warrants diagnostic evaluation. US shows an oval, circumscribed, solid mass with parallel orientation in the 10 o'clock position. Biopsy is indicated because of the rapid enlargement of the mass. Core biopsy revealed benign phyllodes tumor associated with lobular carcinoma in situ with the same diagnosis at excision.

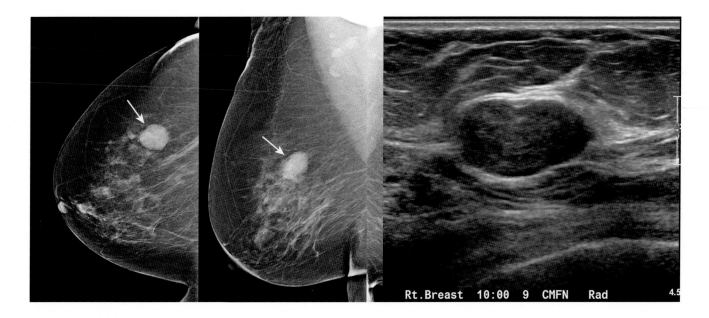

CASE 8-7. There is postsurgical deformity of the anterior right breast. Multiple masses are present in the right breast. Some of the masses (*arrows*) have indistinct margins. The findings are suspicious for recurrent carcinoma. Diagnostic views and US are recommended.

Magnification views confirm multiple masses, one with spiculated margins (*arrow*). US reveals three solid masses. Core biopsies of two masses both revealed IDC and DCIS.

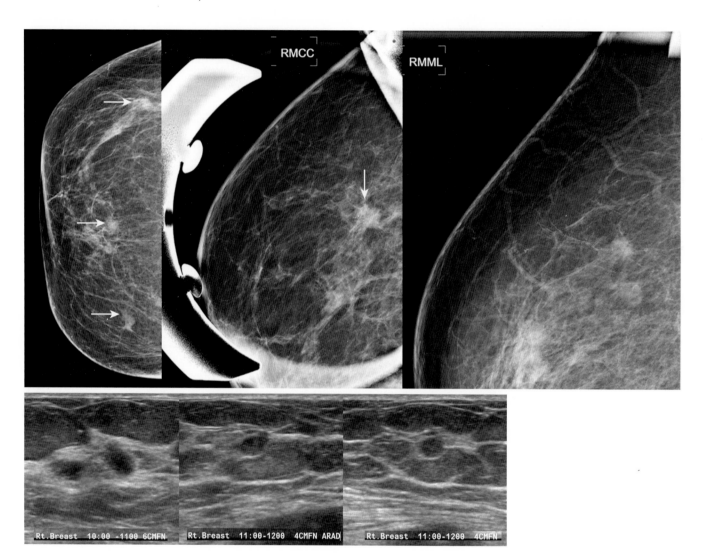

CASE 8-8. There are at least three new bilateral isodense masses with circumscribed margins (*arrows*). There were no masses on prior mammograms; therefore, diagnostic views and US were performed. CC spot compression views show circumscribed margins. US reveals bilateral oval solid masses. Core biopsy of masses in the 12 o'clock position of the right breast and the 10 o'clock position of the left breast both revealed previously unsuspected extranodal marginal zone B-cell lymphoma.

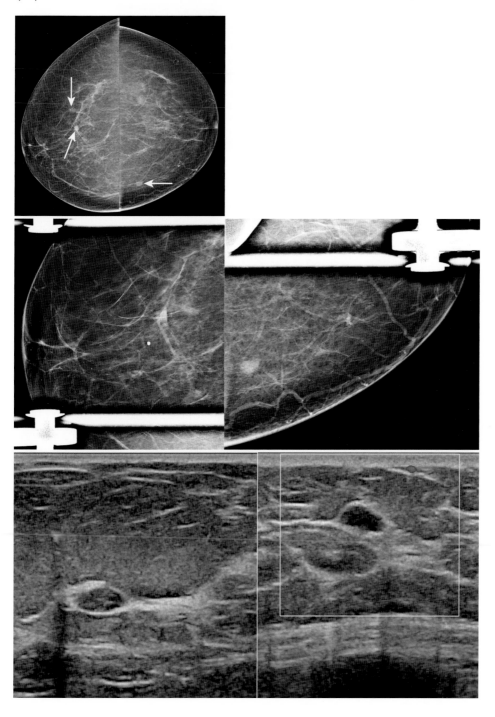

CASE 8-9. There are multiple cysts. Did you notice the hypoechoic shadowing region on the lower right image? You rescan this region and find a hypoechoic solid shadowing mass with spiculated margins, adjacent to cysts. This is highly suspicious. Diagnosis: IDC.

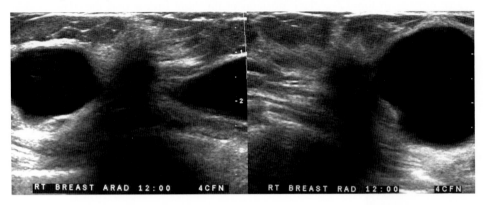

CASE 8-10. There are multiple masses. One, in the lower inner quadrant of the breast, stands out from the others (*arrow*). It is irregular in shape and has enlarged.

Spot compression views and US were performed. The mass has spiculated margins. US shows a round mass with an echogenic halo. These features are highly suspicious (BI-RADS 5). Diagnosis: IDC.

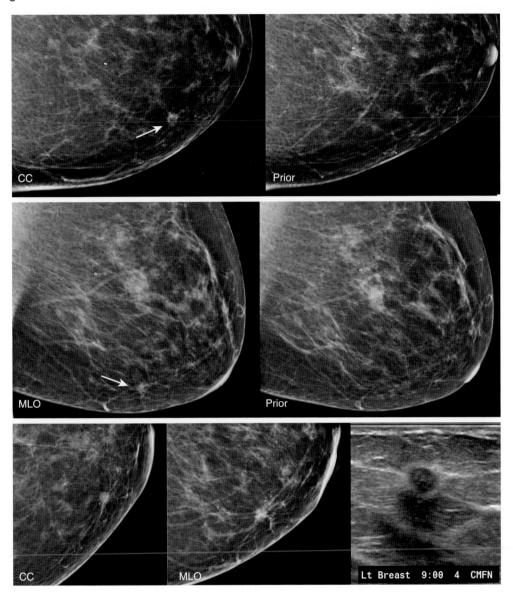

CHAPTER 9

Architectural Distortion

A radiologist friend from another city called one day and asked for a review of his wife's mammogram. She had been recalled from screening, told that the findings were probably benign, and asked to return in 6 months for a follow-up mammogram. He thought that there might be some architectural distortion present and wanted a second opinion. After review and a few additional images, architectural distortion was indeed identified. Biopsy showed invasive lobular carcinoma. She was stage I. They send a case of champagne every year on the anniversary of her diagnosis. Joie de vivre!

Architectural distortion (AD) is often a subtle sign of malignancy with a high positive predictive value of approximately 60% on diagnostic mammography. Detection of AD is challenging because it is often similar in density to the surrounding parenchyma and it may contain fat. It is often changeable in appearance in different projections or visible on only a single view. For these reasons, AD is a common cause of false-negative screening mammograms and is also frequently missed by computer-aided detection (CAD).

How to Recognize Architectural Distortion

AD can appear as radiating lines, alteration of the normal tissue contours, or both. It is described in the BI-RADS Atlas as follows:

> The normal architecture is distorted with no definite mass visible. This includes thin lines or spiculations radiating from a point and focal retraction or distortion of the edge of the parenchyma. AD can also be associated with a mass, asymmetry, or calcifications.
>
> AD can be the primary finding or an associated finding (e.g., a mass or calcifications with associated AD).

Radiating Lines

The classic appearance of AD is radiating lines without a visible central mass (Fig. 9-1). If a central mass is visible, the finding is more accurately described as a mass with spiculated margins rather than AD. Imagine you are looking at the flight map in an airline magazine: looking for AD is like looking for hub cities. Normal overlapping structures (fibrous bands, ducts, and blood vessels) create patterns resembling intersecting flight paths.

The lines of AD may not radiate in all directions or be symmetric about a central point. Only a portion of the distorted area may be visible. Think of these as a coastal hub such as LaGuardia airport in New York City. Most of the incoming flights arrive from the West, with many fewer arriving from the East (Fig. 9-2). Detection of even a few lines that appear to radiate from a central point or are associated with tissue retraction warrants careful examination and often diagnostic evaluation.

Abnormal Tissue Contours

Another presentation of AD results from tethering or retraction of tissue, causing abnormal tissue contours (see Fig. 9-1). These findings can appear mammographically as straightening of the Cooper ligaments, focal retraction, or angulation of tissue contours. It is as though a crochet hook had been dragged through the tissue at that spot.

Distorted tissue contours are often detected at the interface between the parenchymal tissue and the subcutaneous or retroglandular fat (see Fig. 9-1). During mammographic interpretation, it is important to evaluate these borders and to compare the tissue contours with previous studies.

Differentiating Architectural Distortion from Summation Artifact

Overlapping Cooper ligaments, ducts, and vessels may mimic the pattern of AD. However, these overlapping structures never actually radiate from a central point. What may appear at first glance to be AD on screening mammography may often be dismissed after close inspection without the need for additional imaging.

Normal lines extend through and beyond the center of the questioned finding, rather than ending at the central point, as occurs with true AD (Fig. 9-3). If we use our airline route map analogy, normal structures represent overlapping flight paths rather than the hub city.

One technique that can be used to analyze questioned AD is to deconstruct the finding by visually subtracting the definitely normal structures, then imagining what it would look like without those structures. If the resulting appearance would no longer be suspicious, it is consistent

240

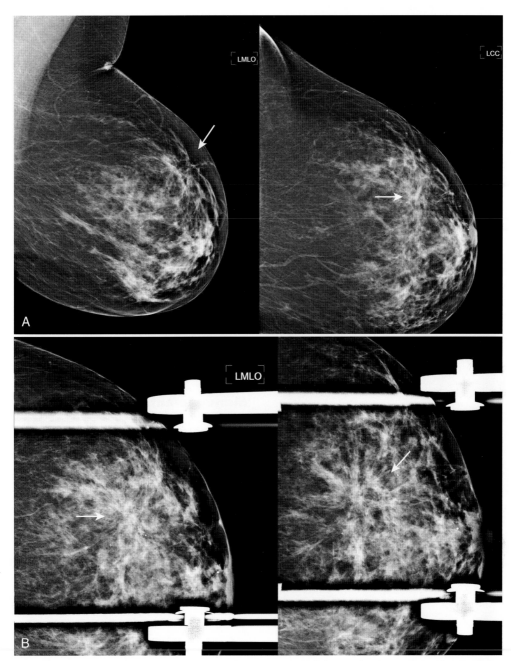

FIGURE 9-1 **Architectural Distortion. A,** Screening mammogram shows retraction of the interface between the fibroglandular tissue and subcutaneous fat (*arrow*) on the mediolateral oblique (MLO) view. **B,** Spot compression MLO and craniocaudal (CC) views more clearly demonstrate AD with radiating lines and no central mass. Diagnosis: multifocal infiltrating carcinoma with ductal and lobular features and ductal carcinoma in situ.

with summation artifact (Fig. 9-4). If you believe normal structures cannot fully account for the suspected distortion, additional evaluation is needed.

Diagnostic Evaluation of Suspected Architectural Distortion

When AD is suspected on screening mammography, it should be evaluated in greater detail on diagnostic views (Fig. 9-5). True AD will usually persist and appear more pronounced on spot compression views. Associated

masses, asymmetries, or calcifications may also become apparent on these views.

Ultrasonography (US) is often useful in confirming, characterizing, and localizing lesions presenting as AD (see Fig. 9-5) and in detecting associated masses that may be mammographically occult. Harmonic tissue imaging improves conspicuity of some lesions presenting as AD. However, the use of compound imaging can eliminate the posterior acoustic shadowing often seen with AD—particularly when due to invasive lobular carcinoma (ILC)—and may make these lesions more difficult to detect (Fig. 9-6). The lack of a US correlate should not eliminate the consideration of biopsy if distortion is present on the mammogram.

Magnetic resonance imaging (MRI) can be useful in a problem-solving role for occasional cases of questioned AD that are not resolved by diagnostic mammography or US (Fig. 9-7). Keep in mind that even MRI does not have sufficiently high negative predictive value to avoid biopsy of AD that is mammographically suspicious.

Differential Diagnosis of Architectural Distortion

Malignancies presenting as AD usually represent either infiltrating ductal or infiltrating lobular carcinoma. Ductal carcinoma in situ (DCIS) uncommonly presents with this appearance (Box 9-1).

The presence of suspicious calcifications associated with AD is suggestive of invasive ductal carcinoma (IDC)

with DCIS. AD—typically without calcifications—is the presenting finding for ILC in approximately 25% of cases (Fig. 9-8). Masses, asymmetries, or retraction of the skin or nipple may also be associated with AD. A new or enlarging palpable finding in the region of AD also increases suspicion, even if no changes are appreciated on mammography.

Radial scar/complex sclerosing lesions usually present as AD (Fig. 9-9). Typically, the spicules of this lesion are long and thin and there is no central mass, producing a "dark star" appearance. These lesions are not typically palpable, and may be planar, resulting in a variable appearance in different projections.

Among benign causes of AD, postsurgical change is the most common (Fig. 9-10). The distortion due to postsurgical scarring decreases in prominence over time. Enlargement of an area of AD in the region of previous surgery is suspicious and warrants further evaluation. In patients who have had lumpectomy for breast cancer, MRI can be useful in distinguishing postsurgical scarring from recurrent carcinoma. AD may also be caused by fat necrosis in a patient who has had surgery or trauma to the breast; associated oil cysts or dystrophic calcifications support this diagnosis (Fig. 9-11).

Management of Architectural Distortion

Mammography cannot reliably distinguish AD due to benign entities from AD due to those that are malignant. Therefore, AD that is not explained by prior surgery is almost always coded BI-RADS 4 or 5, and core or excisional biopsy is indicated. The use of short-term follow-up (BI-RADS 3) for AD has no supporting basis in the literature. Remember the vignette at the beginning of this

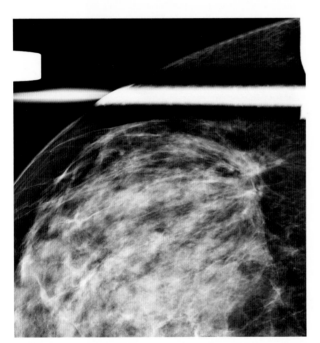

FIGURE 9-2 **Asymmetric AD.** CC spot compression view showing AD with asymmetric radiating lines. The spicules extend mainly anteriorly, into the fibroglandular tissue. Biopsy revealed infiltrating ductal carcinoma.

> ### BOX 9-1   **Differential Diagnosis of Architectural Distortion**
>
> - Infiltrating ductal carcinoma
> - Infiltrating lobular carcinoma
> - Radial scar/complex sclerosing lesion
> - Postsurgical change
> - Fat necrosis

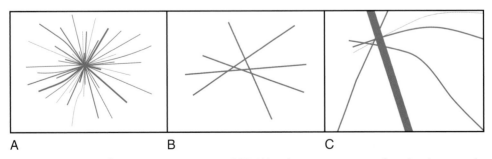

A   B   C

FIGURE 9-3 **Schematic Representation of AD.** Intersecting pattern of AD (**A**) and common patterns of overlapping normal structures (**B** and **C**). With normal structures, note the off-center intersections and continuous visualization of individual lines as they extend through the questioned finding.

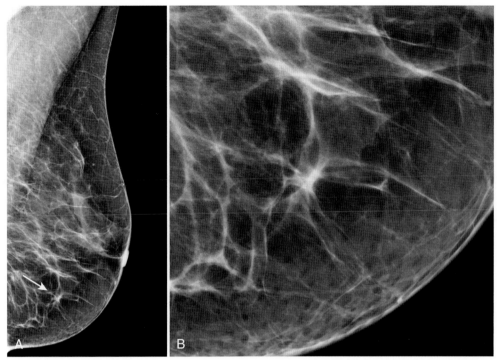

FIGURE 9-4 **Summation Artifact.** Screening MLO (**A,** full image and **B,** enlargement) views showing a finding marked by CAD (*arrow*) that at first glance appears to represent AD. However, on close inspection the lines extend through the finding, rather than radiating from its center. Subtracting these normal tissue lines, there would be no residual finding, and the appearance is therefore summation artifact rather than true AD.

chapter: AD has a high positive predictive value for malignancy, and when there is uncertainty about whether it is benign, biopsy is usually indicated.

There are several pitfalls in managing AD that can contribute to a delay in diagnosis of malignancy. One is to assume that AD represents scar tissue in a patient who has had prior surgery. A simple way to resolve this uncertainty is to mark all visible scars with wires and obtain additional mammographic views, which will determine whether the AD corresponds to the surgical site (Fig. 9-12). If the patient gives you a history of removal of a fibroadenoma at age 26 and she is now of screening age, the AD is not likely due to a benign scar. Benign surgical scars typically become difficult to see after 5 to 10 years, so be cautious in assuming that the finding represents a remote scar. Scarring from lumpectomy is typically visualized much longer after surgery than scarring from benign biopsy.

Another pitfall is to be overly reassured by history or associated mammographic findings. A history of trauma in the region of AD can be particularly misleading (Fig. 9-13). The presence of benign calcifications near an area of AD or of fat within AD should also not alleviate concern for AD that would otherwise be considered suspicious.

A third pitfall is to assume that unexplained AD that is stable is benign. ILC in particular often grows slowly. Biopsy should be considered even if AD is visible in retrospect and appears stable—even for several years.

Text continued on p. 250

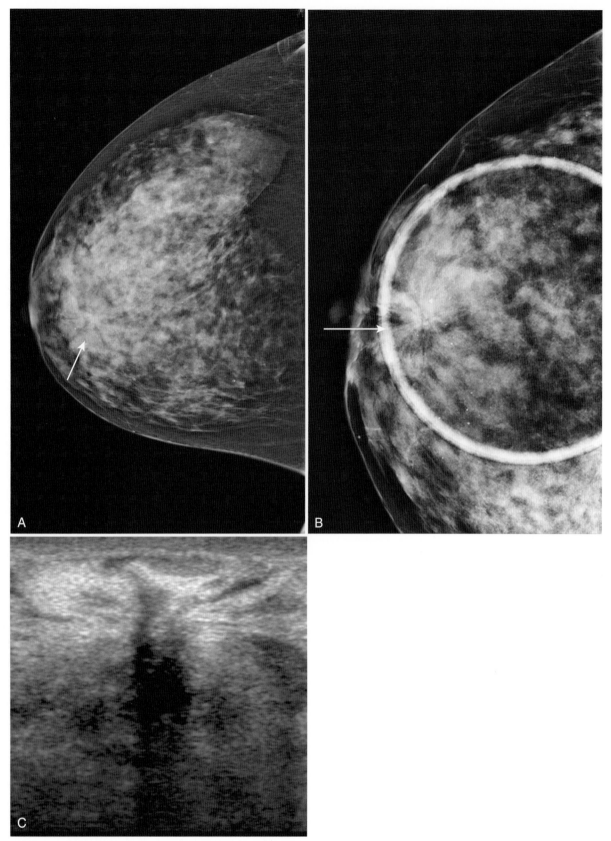

FIGURE 9-5 **AD with Abnormal Finding on US.** Screening mammogram (**A**) shows extremely dense tissue with subtle radiating lines of AD (*arrow*) in the subareolar region that is visualized on the CC view only. This finding is confirmed on a CC spot view (**B**). On US, there is an irregular hypoechoic shadowing mass in the 6 o'clock position (**C**). Biopsy revealed infiltrating ductal carcinoma.

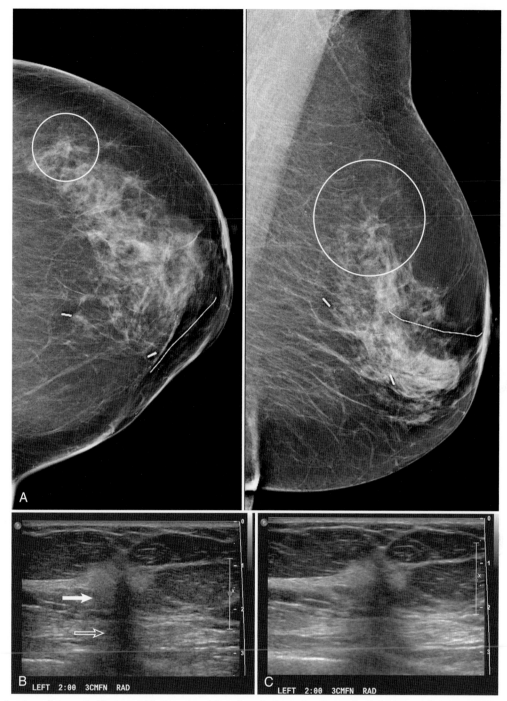

FIGURE 9-6 **Reduction of Acoustic Shadow with Compound Imaging. A,** Screening detected subtle AD (*circles*) in a woman with a history of lumpectomy. **B,** On US, there is a corresponding hypoechoic solid mass (*arrow*) with irregular margins, echogenic halo, and posterior acoustic shadowing (*open arrow*). **C,** With compound imaging, the shadowing is much less obvious, making the lesion less conspicuous. This is most problematic with smaller lesions. Biopsy showed mixed IDC and ILC.

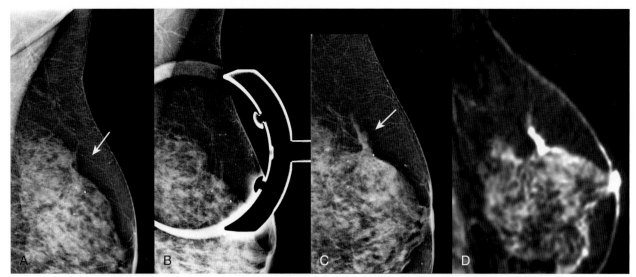

FIGURE 9-7 **MRI in Evaluation of AD. A,** AD with slight retraction and spiculation were questioned on a screening MLO view (*arrow*). This finding was suspicious on MLO spot (**B**) and mediolateral (ML) (**C**) views, but no abnormalities were seen on the CC view or by US. **D,** Sagittal postcontrast fat-suppressed MRI shows intense linear enhancement in the area of mammographic suspicion. Diagnosis: high-grade DCIS.

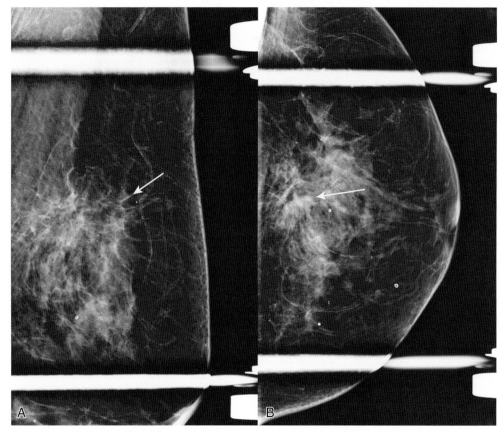

FIGURE 9-8 **Invasive Lobular Carcinoma.** AD in the superior left breast (*arrows*) due to infiltrating lobular carcinoma (**A,** MLO and **B,** CC spot compression views).

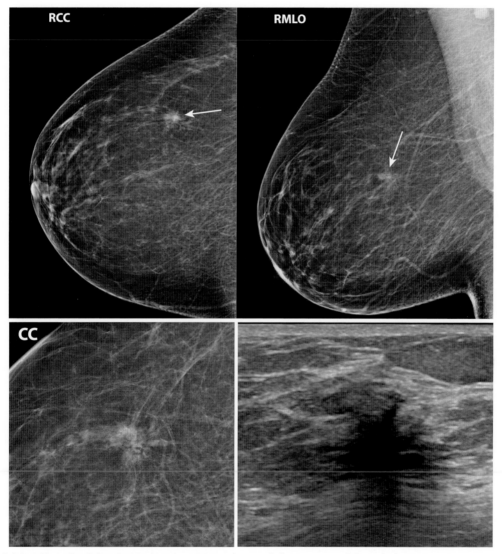

FIGURE 9-9 **Radial Scar/Complex Sclerosing Lesion.** Screening and magnified CC images of the right breast in a 42-year-old woman show AD with fine radiating spicules (*arrows*). US with harmonic imaging shows a corresponding irregular hypoechoic lesion.

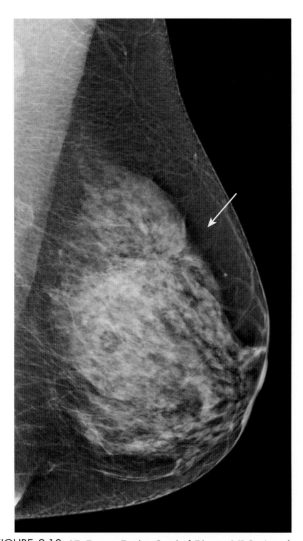

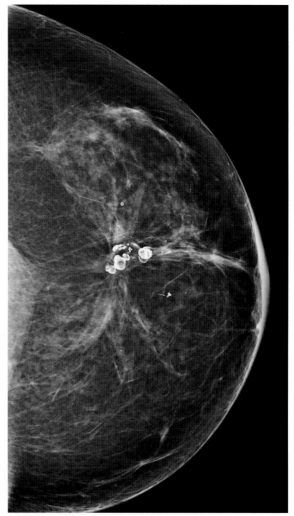

FIGURE 9-10 **AD Due to Benign Surgical Biopsy.** MLO view shows radiating lines within dense tissue in the superior left breast with indentation of the edge of the fibroglandular tissue (*arrow*).

FIGURE 9-11 **AD Due to Lumpectomy.** A 52-year-old woman with a history of lumpectomy and radiation therapy for left breast cancer. AD and lucent-centered calcifications at the lumpectomy site are due to scarring and fat necrosis.

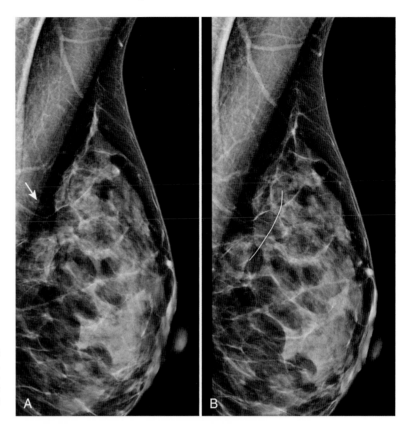

FIGURE 9-12 **Postsurgical Scarring. A,** AD in a woman with a history of benign surgical biopsy of the left breast. There is retraction of the posterior border of the fibroglandular tissue (*arrow*). **B,** The MLO view was repeated after marking the scar, showing that it corresponds to the distortion.

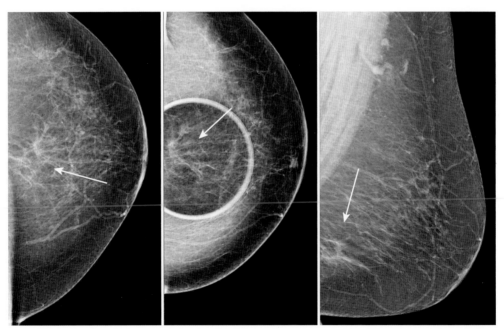

FIGURE 9-13 **AD Due to Invasive Lobular Carcinoma.** AD (*arrows*) in the inferior left breast in a woman with a recent history of trauma to this region. US revealed no abnormalities. Short-interval follow-up mammography was performed, and the finding became more prominent. Biopsy revealed infiltrating lobular carcinoma.

KEY POINTS

- AD is often subtle but frequently malignant with a positive predictive value of approximately 60%.
- AD can appear as radiating lines, retraction or straightening of tissue, or both.
- Unexplained AD is almost always assigned BI-RADS 4 or 5 and warrants biopsy. It is almost never assigned BI-RADS 3.
- Pitfalls in the assessment and management of AD include incorrectly assuming that it is caused by previous surgery or that the lesion is benign because of history, associated findings, or stability.

References

American College of Radiology. ACR BI-RADS: Mammography. In ACR Breast Imaging Reporting and Data System, Breast Imaging Atlas, 4th ed. Reston, VA, American College of Radiology, 2003.

Baker JA, Rosen EL, Lo JY, et al. Computer-aided detection (CAD) in screening mammography: Sensitivity of commercial CAD systems for detecting architectural distortion. AJR 2003;181:1083-1088.

Jacobs TW, Byrne C, Colditz G, et al. Radial scars in benign breast-biopsy specimens and the risk of breast cancer. N Engl J Med 1999;340:430-436.

Krecke KN, Gisvold JJ. Invasive lobular carcinoma of the breast: Mammographic findings and extent of disease in 184 patients. AJR 1993;161:957-960.

Lopez JK, Bassett LW. Invasive lobular carcinoma of the breast: Spectrum of mammographic, US, and MR imaging findings. Radiographics 2009;29:165-176.

Sickles EA. Mammographic features of 300 consecutive nonpalpable breast cancers. AJR 1986;146:661-663.

Venkatesan A, Chu P, Kerlikowske K, et al. Positive predictive value of specific mammographic findings according to reader and patient variables. Radiology 2009;250:649-657.

CASE QUESTIONS

CASE 9-1. Screening mammogram on a 50-year-old woman. What is the significant finding? What do you recommend?

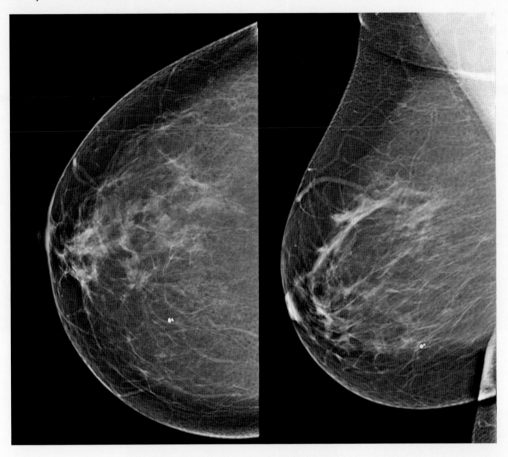

CASE 9-2. Screening views of the left breast in a 50-year-old woman. Images from 4 years prior are provided for comparison. The patient had a benign surgical biopsy of the left upper outer quadrant 10 years ago. What is your BI-RADS assessment and recommendation?

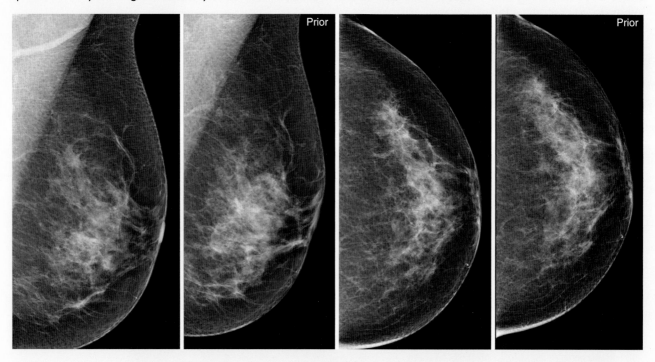

CASE 9-3. A 56-year-old woman presents for screening. What is the finding? BI-RADS category? Recommendation?

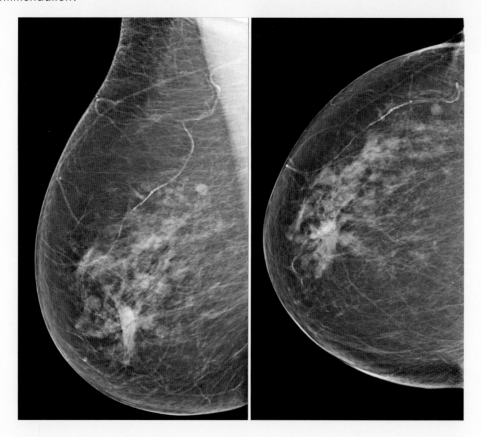

CASE 9-4. A 42-year-old woman is recalled after her initial screening mammogram for evaluation of the area marked by the *arrows*. Diagnostic views and US of the right breast are obtained. How would you describe the findings? What are your BI-RADS assessment and management recommendations?

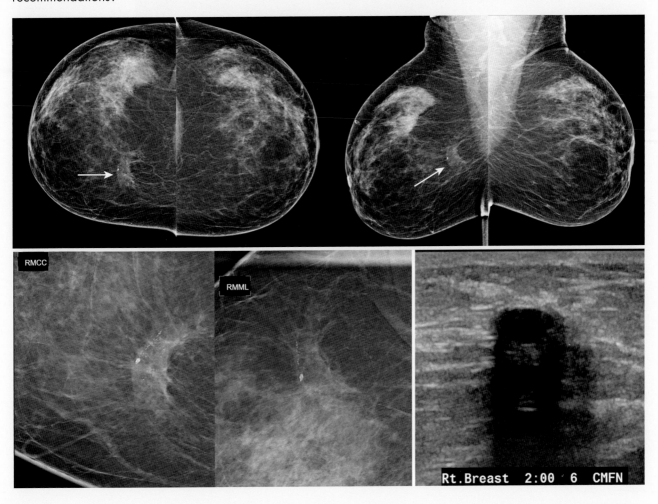

CASE 9-5. Screening views of the left breast in a 66-year-old woman with prior history of benign biopsies. What is the finding? What would you recommend?

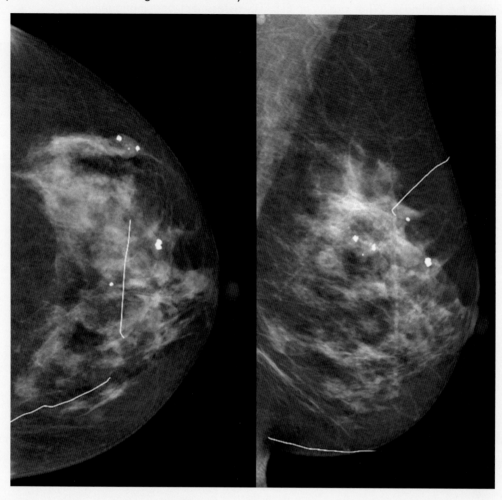

CASE 9-6. A 43-year-old woman is recalled after screening to further evaluate the findings indicated by the *arrows*. CC and MLO spot compression views and US are shown. How would you describe the findings? What are your BI-RADS assessment and recommendation?

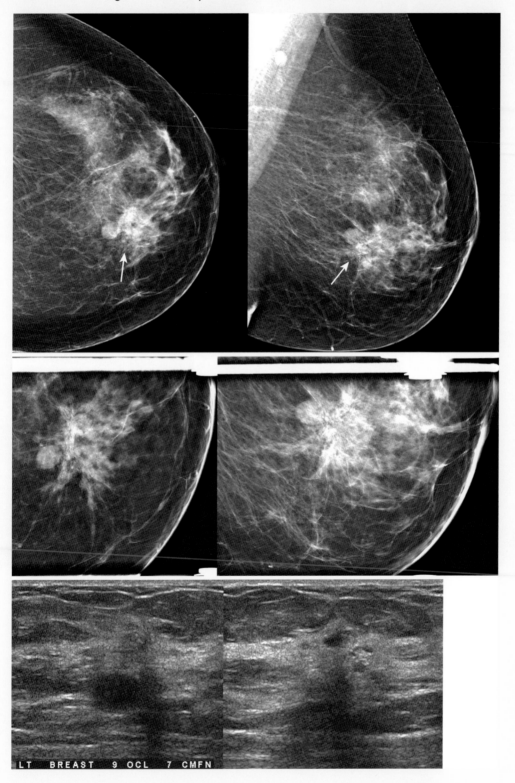

CASE 9-7. These images are from three patients. Which one is most likely to represent true AD?

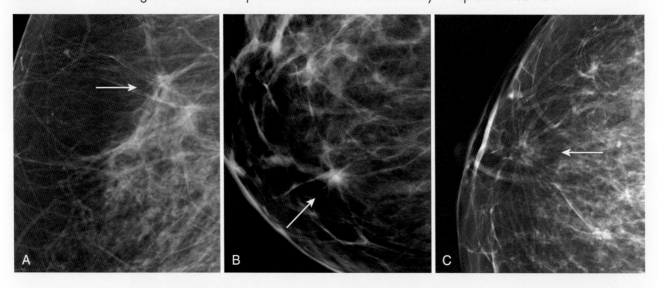

CASE 9-8. Here are three images from three additional cases. Which one most likely represents true AD?

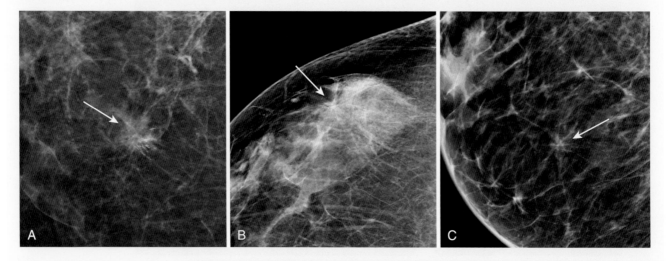

CASE 9-9. Screening mammogram on a 58-year-old woman. What is the finding? What is your BI-RADS assessment, and what do you recommend?

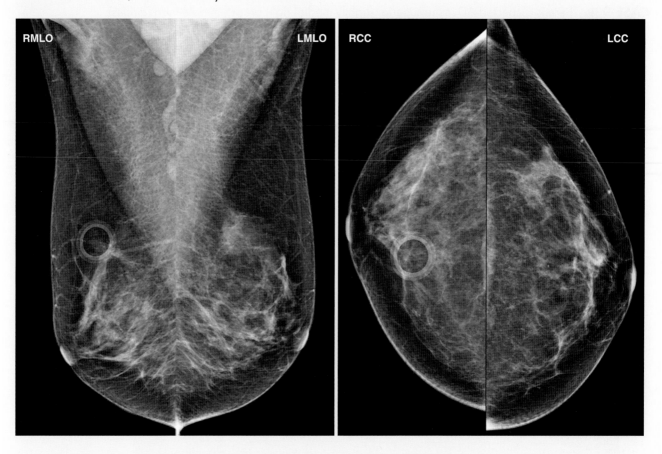

CASE 9-10. A 62-year-old woman with a history of left mastectomy has a screening mammogram. What is the finding?

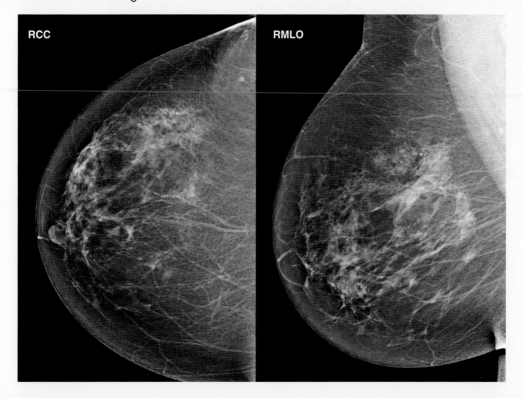

CASE ANSWERS

CASE 9-1. There is suspected AD in the superior slightly medial right breast, middle third (*circles*). Here are the diagnostic images and US.

Distortion is confirmed on CC spot compression and ML views (*arrows*). Fat is seen centrally. US shows an irregular hypoechoic shadowing mass. The findings are highly suspicious (BI-RADS 5). Diagnosis: IDC and DCIS. Fat can become entrapped within or project into malignant lesions presenting as AD and should not be viewed as a reassuring finding.

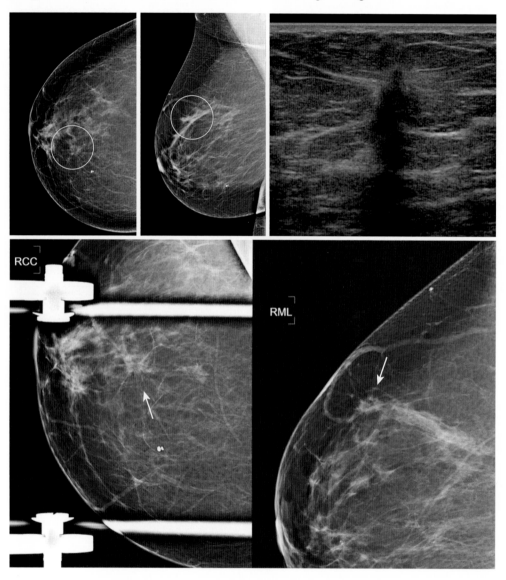

CASE 9-2. There is subtle AD (*circles*) in the left upper outer quadrant that is slightly larger and denser than on the previous mammogram, especially as seen on the MLO view. Diagnostic views and US are shown.

Spot compression views with a wire marking the scar show the AD to persist (*arrows*) and to lie in the region of previous surgery. US shows an irregular hypoechoic mass. Biopsy revealed invasive carcinoma with both ductal and lobular features. AD in the region of prior surgery that increases in size or density should be viewed with suspicion.

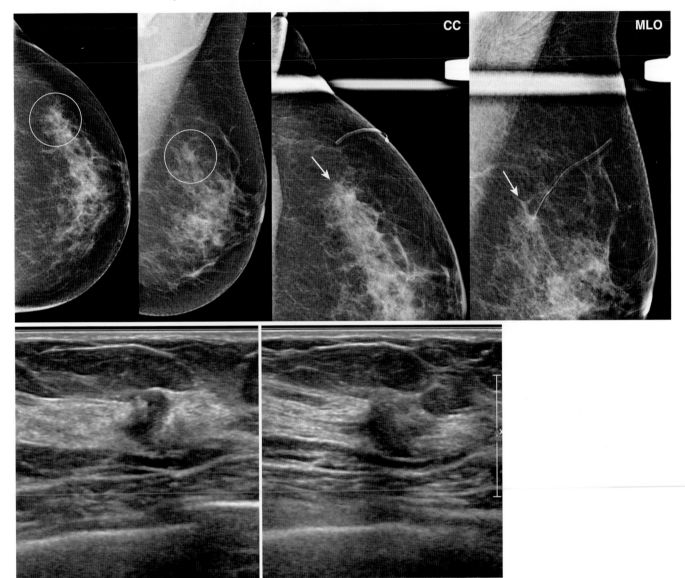

CASE 9-3. There is AD with straight lines visible on the MLO view and radiating lines on the CC view (*circles*). BI-RADS 0. Recommend spot compression views.

ML magnification and CC spot compression views confirm AD (*arrows*) and show associated skin retraction. Diagnosis: infiltrating lobular carcinoma.

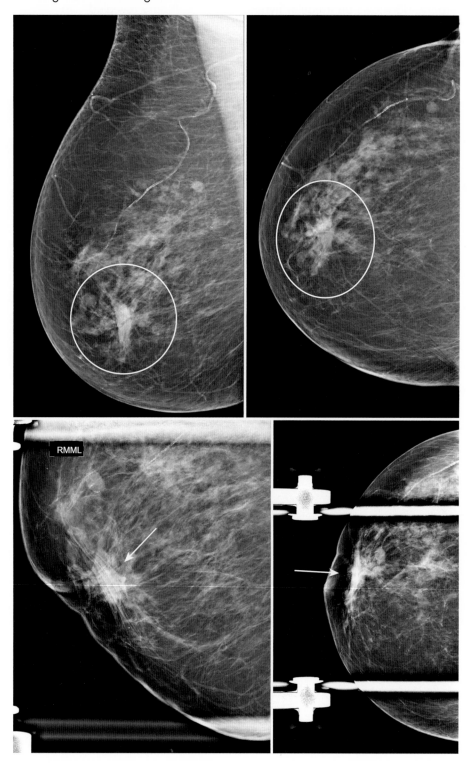

CASE 9-4. There is an irregular mass with associated AD and fine pleomorphic calcifications in a linear distribution in the medial right breast. US shows a corresponding hypoechoic shadowing mass. BI-RADS 4. Recommend biopsy.

Ultrasound-guided core biopsy revealed dense stromal fibrosis with calcifications. Additional history revealed that 10 years prior, the patient had been in a motor vehicle accident with seat belt injury to this region.

CASE 9-5. AD is seen at two locations in the left breast: 12 o'clock, anterior third, and 11 o'clock, middle third, best seen in the CC view. Here are the diagnostic views and US. Note that the AD on the CC view is too far anterior to be the same lesion seen on the MLO view. On the CC view, the AD represents the 12 o'clock anterior lesion. On the MLO view, the AD represents the 11 o'clock middle third lesion. US confirms two lesions (*arrows*). Ultrasound-guided core needle biopsy showed IDC at both sites.

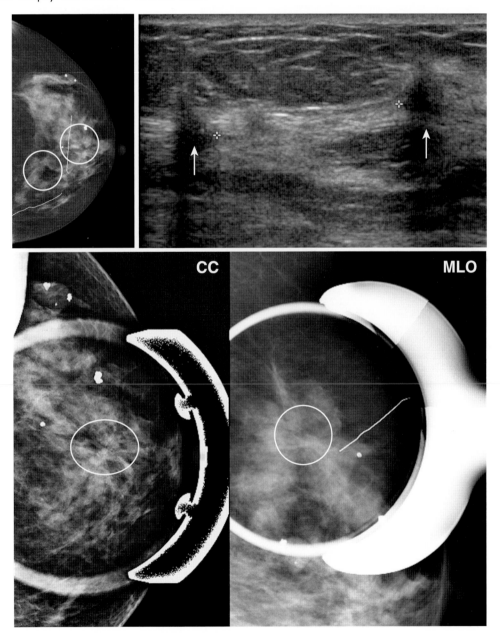

CASE 9-6. There is a large area of AD in the medial breast that persists on spot compression views. An oval mass is seen posterior to the distortion. US shows a complicated cyst with adjacent subtle shadowing that corresponds to the mass and distortion seen on mammography. BI-RADS 4. Recommend biopsy. Core biopsy revealed a complex sclerosing lesion, and excision showed associated LCIS and ALH.

CASE 9-7. Images A and B reveal summation artifact. **A,** Note off-center line intersections and lines extending through "lesion." **B,** Finding produced by vessel and lines extending through the area. **C,** True AD in the subareolar region with multiple converging lines with slight skin retraction.

Spot compression magnification view of Case 9-7C is shown here. Diagnosis: grade 3 IDC.

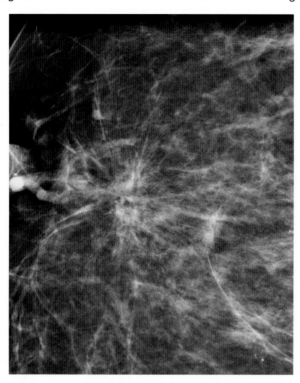

CASE 9-8. A, A few lines appear to pass through the lesion but most do not. This is true AD. There are associated calcifications. **B,** Vessel and fibrous lines extend through the area. **C,** Off-center intersections caused solely by lines that extend through the region.

CC magnification view of Case 9-8A is shown here, confirming AD with fine linear calcifications. Diagnosis: IDC and DCIS.

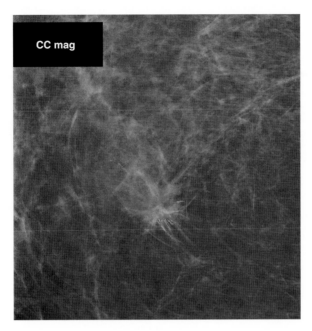

CC mag

CASE 9-9. AD is suspected in the upper right breast, under the mole marker (*circle*). BI-RADS 0. Recommend spot compression views.

On spot compression views the area continues to appear distorted. US was recommended. Based on the position of this finding on MLO and ML views, where is the lesion located?

The lesion moved down on the ML view and, therefore, it lies in the lateral breast. US of the 10 o'clock position shows an irregular hypoechoic mass. Diagnosis: infiltrating carcinoma (tubulolobular).

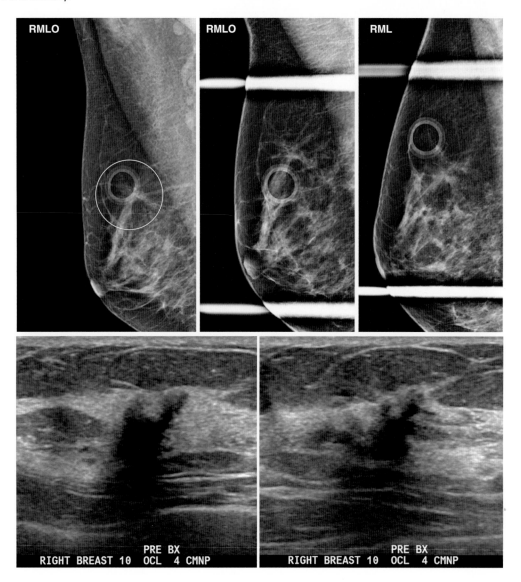

CASE 9-10. There is subtle AD with radiating lines and retraction of adjacent tissues (*arrows* and *circle*). The distortion is much more apparent on the CC and MLO magnification views (*below*). BI-RADS 4. Diagnosis: grade 1 IDC with tubular features and DCIS. If you found this one, you have a very good eye. Congratulations!

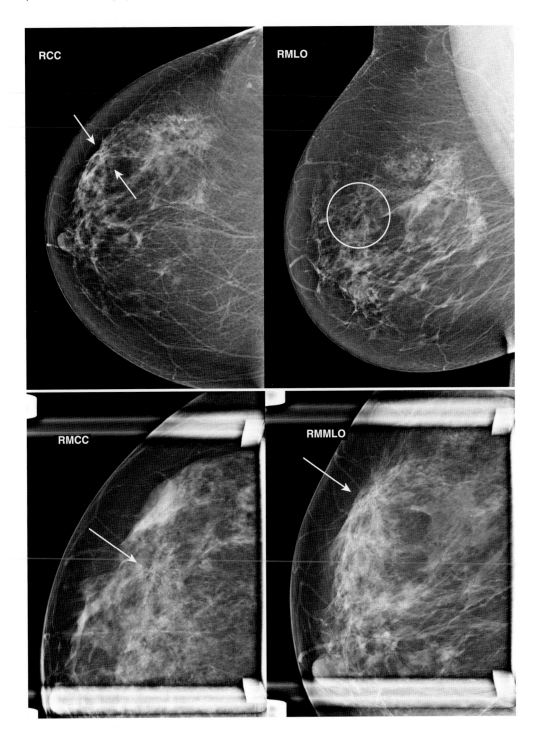

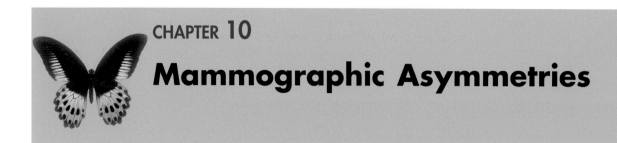

CHAPTER 10

Mammographic Asymmetries

Almost lunchtime. Need to finish the screening board first. Could that little area on the left craniocaudal (CC) be new? I don't see anything on the mediolateral oblique (MLO). I'll give her a 6-month follow-up and then we'll know if it is important or not.

This is not a good approach to asymmetries! Malignant asymmetry is often subtle and can appear identical to normal fibroglandular tissue. In one study nearly half (47%) of interval cancers that were visible in retrospect appeared as an asymmetry. If we want to detect early breast cancer, then we need to pay attention to asymmetries.

The distribution of fibroglandular tissue, ducts, and adipose tissue in the right and left breasts usually produces a fairly symmetric pattern on mammography. Asymmetry in this pattern most commonly represents normal variation, but it may also be the sole presenting sign of breast cancer.

Differentiating between the two is one of the most challenging aspects of mammographic interpretation. Careful right-to-left comparison and comparison with previous mammograms are vital in this process. Detection and analysis of asymmetric soft tissue density findings are important components of mammographic interpretation that will increase the breast cancer detection rate and provide many women with an opportunity for earlier diagnosis.

Terminology and Significance of Types

There are four types of asymmetries: global asymmetry, focal asymmetry, developing asymmetry, and one-view asymmetry (Box 10-1). Differentiation between the types is important because the positive predictive value for malignancy and management differs according to type. Asymmetry may be global (diffuse) or focal (one or more areas). If an asymmetry is new compared with old mammograms, it is considered a developing asymmetry. If an asymmetry is only seen on a single projection, it is a one-view asymmetry.

Asymmetries do not fulfill the criteria for the other soft tissue density findings described in the BI-RADS Atlas. They lack the convex borders of masses and are often interspersed with fat (Fig. 10-1). They also lack the radiating lines or tissue retraction of architectural distortion

(AD) and the tubular branching appearance of a dilated duct.

Global Asymmetry

Global asymmetry is asymmetric tissue that occupies at least one breast quadrant (Fig. 10-2) and is visualized on two or more projections. Global asymmetry is not uncommon; the prevalence is about 3%. Because the asymmetric tissue extends over a large region, a malignancy of this size is almost always associated with a palpable mass or other clinical abnormality.

Global asymmetry usually represents a normal variant. Therefore, provided there are no associated clinical abnormalities or suspicious changes on mammography, it is typically benign and is given BI-RADS 2 category. Global asymmetry associated with a palpable finding may indicate an underlying invasive cancer or noncalcified ductal carcinoma in situ (DCIS). When global asymmetry is encountered, it is important to ensure that the patient has had a recent clinical breast examination; when there is a corresponding palpable abnormality, the chance of malignancy increases to about 8%.

One malignant cause of global asymmetry is the "shrinking breast" that may be caused by invasive lobular carcinoma (ILC). In these cases, one breast appears smaller and denser than the contralateral side on mammography. This is not a clinical finding; the clinical examination may be underwhelming. The "shrinking breast" is discussed in more detail in Chapter 11, Expanding the Differential Diagnosis. If the breast that is denser is also *larger* and associated with the clinical finding of erythema or edema, the patient may have mastitis or inflammatory breast cancer. Likewise, associated mammographic findings of increased density in one breast with AD or suspicious calcifications may be due to underlying cancer. (Box 10-2).

Focal Asymmetry

Focal asymmetries are localized findings that have a similar shape on at least two views and occupy less than one breast quadrant (see Fig. 10-1); they lack the borders and conspicuity of a true mass. A finding detected at screening may be considered a focal asymmetry, but then it may be shown to be a mass on diagnostic mammography or ultrasonography (US).

Most focal asymmetries represent islands of normal tissue. Provided there are no associated clinical, mammographic, or sonographic abnormalities, then focal asymmetries on a baseline mammogram are probably benign findings (BI-RADS 3) with a less than 2% chance of malignancy. Short-term follow-up is reasonable after diagnostic evaluation.

Developing Asymmetry

Developing asymmetry is a type of focal asymmetry (visualized on two or more projections) that has increased in size or density since a previous mammogram (Figs. 10-3 and 10-4). It is the only type of asymmetry that, by

definition, has undergone a suspicious change and it is therefore the most likely to be malignant. About 13% of developing asymmetries are malignant when detected at screening, and 27% are malignant based on diagnostic findings. Developing asymmetries detected on screening nearly always warrant diagnostic evaluation.

Over half of developing asymmetries are explained by summation artifact, which is resolved on diagnostic evaluation. Benign causes that may be suggested by the patient's history include hormone-replacement therapy, trauma, surgery, and mastitis.

If a developing asymmetry persists on diagnostic views or there are suspicious findings on US, biopsy is indicated (BI-RADS 4). Importantly, US is negative in about 25%

BOX 10-1 Types of Asymmetries

- Global asymmetry
- Focal asymmetry
- Developing asymmetry
- One-view asymmetry

BOX 10-2 When to Worry about Global Asymmetry

- Palpable
- Associated breast erythema or edema
- Associated AD or calcifications
- One breast appears smaller and denser than the other (the "shrinking breast")

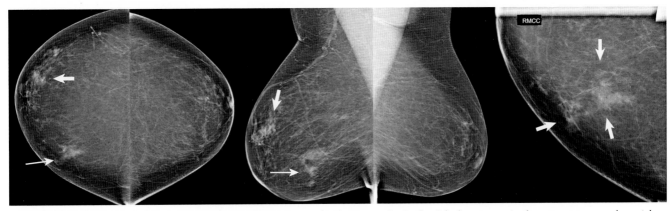

FIGURE 10-1 **Typical Appearance of Asymmetries.** There are two focal asymmetries in the right breast, one in the upper outer quadrant (*short arrow*) and the second in the central medial breast (*long arrow*), which is also evaluated on a CC magnification view (*arrows*). Note interspersed fat and absence of a convex border, radiating lines, or a tubular branching shape. BI-RADS 3 would be acceptable on a baseline mammogram. These findings were stable for over 4 years and considered benign (BI-RADS 2).

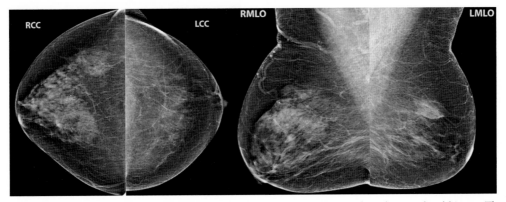

FIGURE 10-2 **Benign Global Asymmetry.** Screening mammogram on a 72-year-old woman with no breast-related history. There is global asymmetry in the right breast, stable for 10 years (BI-RADS 2).

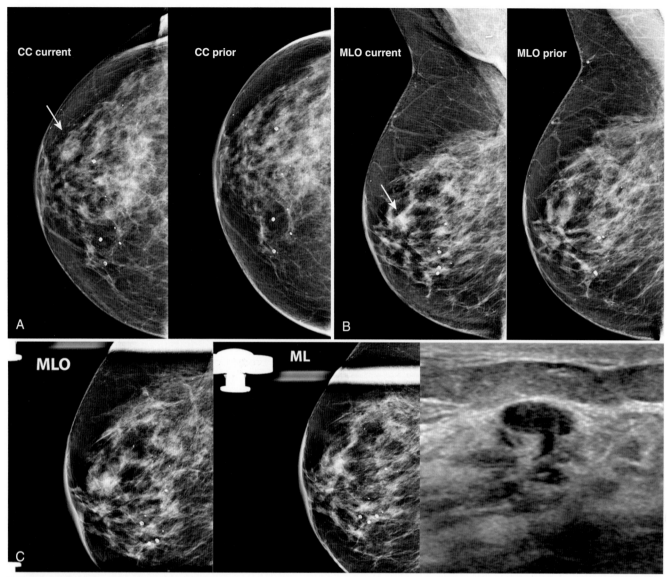

FIGURE 10-3 **Malignant Developing Asymmetry.** A 62-year-old woman with a history of lumpectomy for right breast carcinoma 12 years ago. There is a developing asymmetry in the anterior lateral right breast that is visible on both the CC (**A**) and MLO (**B**) projections (*arrows*). C, The finding persists on spot compression views, and a hypoechoic irregular solid mass is visualized by US. Diagnosis: invasive ductal carcinoma (IDC).

of malignant developing asymmetries, so the absence of findings on US does not justify follow-up rather than biopsy (Box 10-3).

One-View Asymmetry

The old adage in radiology, "one view is no view," doesn't necessarily apply to mammographic screening. Single-view asymmetries are potential abnormalities detected in about 3% of mammograms (Fig. 10-5). Fewer than 2% are found to be malignant. Most one-view asymmetries represent superimposed normal tissues (summation artifact). When asymmetries are not due to summation artifact, 10% prove to be malignant.

So how do we decide if a one-view asymmetry is important? An asymmetry that has been stable for at least

---

BOX 10-3   Differential Diagnosis of Developing Asymmetries

Benign
- Summation artifact
- Fibrocystic changes
- Pseudoangiomatous stromal hyperplasia (PASH)
- Hormone-replacement therapy
- Trauma

Malignant
- Infiltrating ductal carcinoma
- Infiltrating lobular carcinoma
- Noncalcifying DCIS

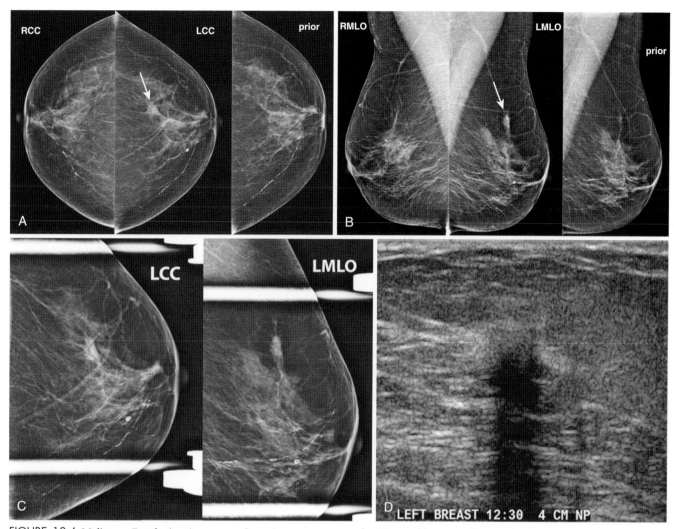

FIGURE 10-4 **Malignant Developing Asymmetry.** Screening mammogram of a 59-year-old woman shows a developing asymmetry in the upper left breast (*arrows*; **A** and **B**). It has features of a mass on spot compression views (**C**), and by US (**D**), there is a corresponding irregular shadowing mass with spiculated margins. Diagnosis: infiltrating lobular carcinoma.

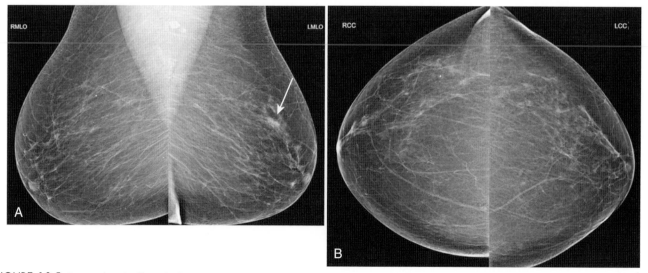

FIGURE 10-5 **Summation Artifact. A,** One-view asymmetry (*arrow*) in the superior left breast on the screening MLO view. **B,** No corresponding abnormality is seen on the CC view, and the tissue consists almost entirely of fat. A true lesion of this size could not have been obscured on this view. The appearance is therefore consistent with summation artifact. Recall is not needed. BI-RADS 1.

several years is unlikely to be significant. If not, we need to figure out why the asymmetry is only seen in one view. An asymmetry that is in the posterior third of the breast may have been excluded from the other projection (Fig. 10-6). A one-view asymmetry that is not in the posterior breast would usually have been included on the other view. In that case, the asymmetry is either due to summation artifact (see Fig. 10-5) or is obscured on the other view (Fig. 10-7). So look at the other view closely, keeping in mind the size, density, and depth of asymmetry.

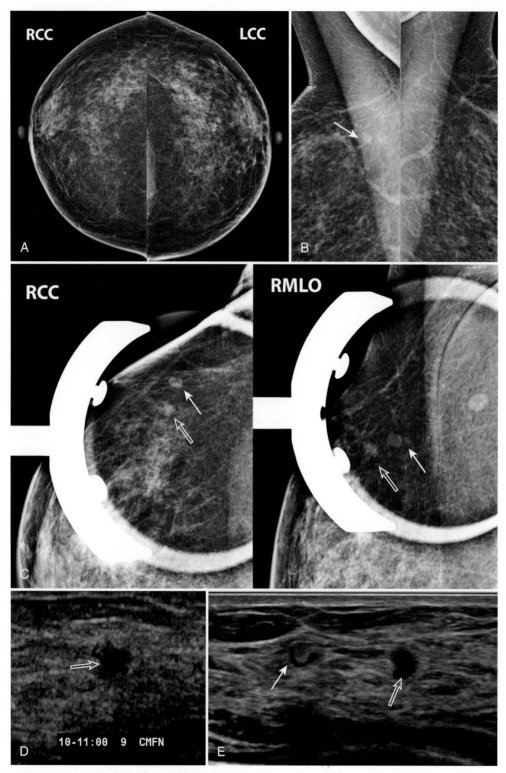

FIGURE 10-6 **One-View Asymmetry Excluded from the Other View.** Small asymmetry on the screening MLO view of the right breast (*arrow*; **B**), overlying the pectoralis muscle. This new finding was excluded from the CC view (**A**) due to the far posterior location. **C,** Spot compression views show that the finding represents a mass (*open arrows*) in the upper outer breast, adjacent to a normal-appearing lymph node (*closed arrows*). **D** and **E,** US shows an irregular hypoechoic mass (*open arrows*) adjacent to the node (*arrow*). Diagnosis: IDC.

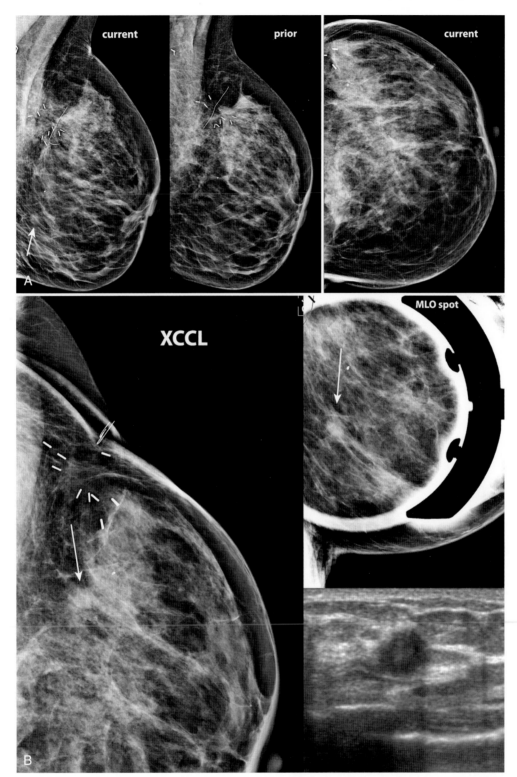

FIGURE 10-7 **One-View Asymmetry Obscured in the Other View. A,** Screening mammogram of a woman with a history of lumpectomy for left breast carcinoma. There is a new one-view asymmetry in the posterior inferior breast visualized on the MLO view only. Based on its small size and the large amount of dense fibroglandular tissue, a mass could easily be obscured on the CC view. **B,** Spot compression MLO and exaggerated CC views reveal a mass with obscured margins (*arrows*) in the 4 o'clock position, which was confirmed by US (*lower right*). Diagnosis: IDC.

If the asymmetry may have been excluded or obscured on the other projection, diagnostic evaluation is often necessary.

Malignancies detected on a single view include invasive ductal carcinoma (IDC) (50%), ILC (33%), and DCIS (17%). Single-view detected IDC and DCIS are most commonly seen on the MLO view, and ILC is most commonly seen on the CC view. Infiltrating lobular carcinoma is overrepresented among malignancies detected on a single view, presenting in 33% of such cases compared with its prevalence of 7% to 10% among breast cancers.

Detection of Asymmetries on Screening Mammography

Asymmetries are a unique class of mammographic findings because their detection may depend on the distribution of tissues in the contralateral breast. To detect potentially malignant asymmetries it is therefore helpful to review the images of the right and left breast in mirror-image display. A stepwise search pattern comparing the same regions in both breasts aids in the detection of asymmetric findings. Although asymmetries in any region of the breast may represent malignancy, particular attention should be paid to the retromammary fat, the inferior breast on the MLO view, and the medial breast on the CC view. This is discussed in more detail in Chapter 3, Screening Mammography 101 and Beyond.

If an asymmetry is seen with the suggestion of an associated finding (calcifications, mass, or AD) recall should be considered, even if individually, the findings may not have warranted diagnostic evaluation.

Although identification of asymmetries involves comparing the right and left images from the current study, determining whether the finding is a *developing* asymmetry involves a different skill—detecting changes in the tissue pattern over time. Because developing asymmetries may appear identical to normal tissue, these changes may be quite subtle. For example, they may appear as a soft tissue density that is "filling in" a region that was previously fat, focally increasing density within fibroglandular tissue, or new soft tissue density protrusion that causes

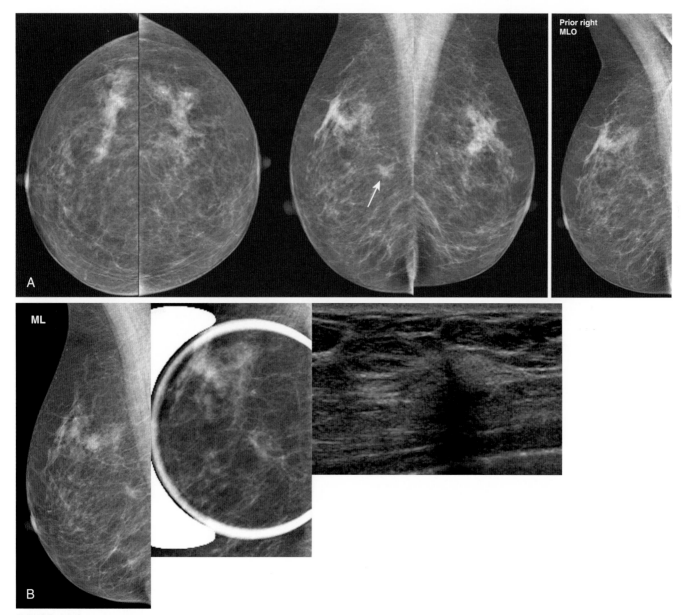

FIGURE 10-8 **US in Evaluation of Developing Asymmetry. A,** A new one-view asymmetry is present on the right, seen only on the MLO view (*arrow*). **B,** The asymmetry appears to disperse on the MLO spot compression view but is still concerning on the ML view. A highly suspicious mass is identified on US. Diagnosis: IDC.

a change in tissue contour. Apparent changes may also be due to differences in positioning, compression, or technique, which can make detection of such changes even more difficult. This may be challenging, but you probably chose radiology because you are really good at visual assessment. You can totally do this!

Comparison with prior mammograms is obviously required in order to assess whether the asymmetry is developing. Comparison with a mammogram that is about 2 years older is routine in most practices. But what if you aren't sure? Keep going! Comparison with multiple priors and with mammograms that are 3 to 5 years older will usually answer the question of change. The development of the asymmetry will be more obvious when compared with the older studies, or the asymmetry will be

reproduced on a prior study, probably due to similar positioning of the patient. Using older prior studies thereby increases confidence that the asymmetry is truly developing or that recall is unnecessary.

Diagnostic Evaluation of Asymmetries

Women with potentially suspicious asymmetries detected on screening mammography should be recalled for additional mammographic views and possibly US.

During diagnostic evaluation, spot compression with or without magnification, rolled CC, and mediolateral (ML) views are frequently obtained. When an asymmetry is shown to represent summation artifact, it is considered

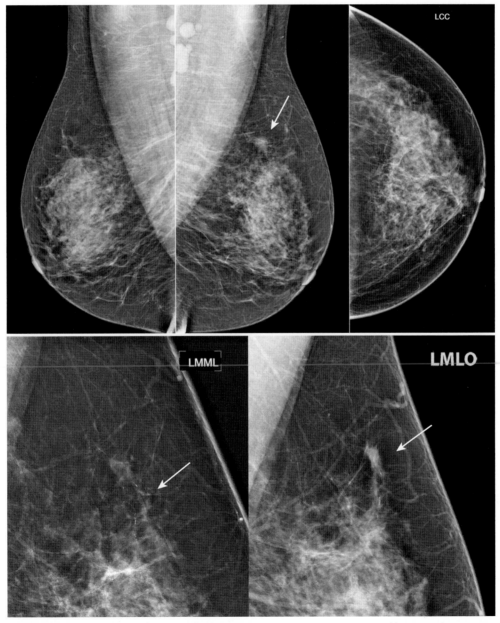

FIGURE 10-9 **One-View Asymmetry with Calcifications.** Initial screening mammogram on a 44-year-old woman shows a one-view asymmetry in the superior left breast (*arrow*). MLO and ML magnified views show persistent asymmetry with associated fine-linear calcifications (*arrows*). Diagnosis: IDC and DCIS.

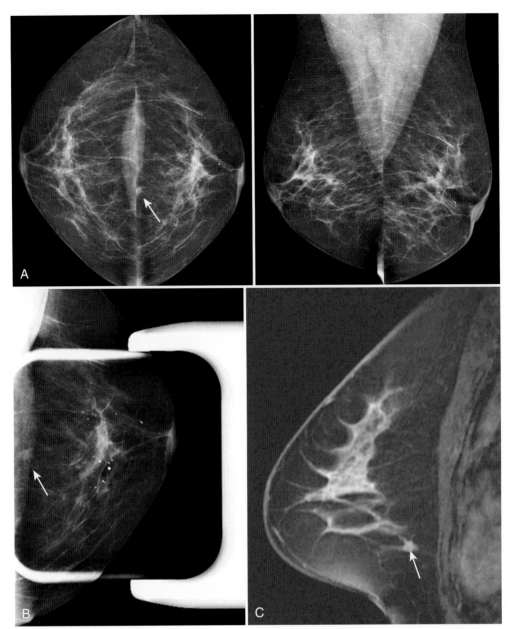

FIGURE 10-10 **Malignant One-View Asymmetry. A,** On screening mammography, a one-view asymmetry is seen in the far posterior left breast on the CC view only (*arrow*). **B,** The finding persists on CC spot compression view (*arrow*), but could not be identified on any other view. US was negative. **C,** Because the lesion appeared suspicious, problem-solving magnetic resonance imaging (MRI) was performed. A corresponding 6 mm irregular enhancing mass is seen in the left breast at about 7 o'clock (*arrow*). Targeted US identified a very small irregular isoechoic mass. Ultrasound-guided core biopsy showed IDC.

BI-RADS 1 and the patient can return to normal screening. If an asymmetry only partially effaces or could be obscured by dense tissue on diagnostic views, remember that US can be your (and the patient's) best friend! A malignant lesion may become less apparent on diagnostic views, and it is wise to have a low decision threshold for performing US (Fig. 10-8, page 272).

During diagnostic evaluation, asymmetries may be found to fulfill the criteria of a mass or other finding. For example, a one-view asymmetry detected on screening may be shown to represent a mass. Associated findings such as calcifications or AD may become apparent (Fig. 10-9, page 273). An asymmetry should be judged in the context of all imaging and clinical findings together, and management should be based on the most suspicious features.

Diagnostic evaluation with mammography and, in some cases, US, will guide appropriate management of the vast majority of patients with asymmetries. Occasionally, MRI can be used in a problem-solving role if the significance of an asymmetry is unresolved by conventional modalities (Fig. 10-10).

KEY POINTS

- Asymmetries are usually benign but may represent a subtle malignancy.
- There are four types of asymmetries: global asymmetry, focal asymmetry, developing asymmetry, and one-view asymmetry.
- Developing asymmetry is the most suspicious type with a 13% to 27% chance of malignancy.
- Detection of developing asymmetries requires careful comparison with previous mammograms to detect changes in the tissue pattern. If it is unclear whether the asymmetry is changing, keep going and compare further back.
- US is negative in about 25% of malignant developing asymmetries. Negative US should not deter biopsy of a suspicious developing asymmetry.
- Management of asymmetries should be based on the type, its evolution over time, and the presence of any associated imaging or clinical findings.

References

American College of Radiology. ACR BI-RADS: Mammography. In ACR Breast Imaging Reporting and Data System, Breast Imaging Atlas, 4th ed. Reston, VA, American College of Radiology, 2003.

Harvey JA, Nicholson BT, Cohen MA. Finding early invasive breast cancers: A practical approach. Radiology 2008;248:61-76.

Kopans DB, Swann CA, White G, et al. Asymmetric breast tissue. Radiology 1989;171:639-643.

Leung JWT, Sickles EA. Developing asymmetry identified on mammography: Correlation with imaging outcome and pathologic findings. AJR 2007;188:667-675.

Martin JE, Moskowitz M, Milbrath JR. Breast cancer missed by mammography. AJR 1979;132:737-739.

Shetty MK, Watson AB. Sonographic evaluation of focal asymmetric density of the breast. Ultrasound Q 2002;18:115-121.

Sickles EA. Findings at mammographic screening on only one standard projection: Outcomes analysis. Radiology 1998;208:471-475.

Sickles EA. Mammographic features of 300 consecutive nonpalpable breast cancers. AJR 1986;146:661-663.

Sickles EA. The spectrum of breast asymmetries: Imaging features, work-up, management. Radiol Clin North Am 2007;45:765-771.

Tabar L, Tot T, Dean PB. Breast cancer: The art and science of early detection with mammography. New York, Thieme, 2005.

Venkatesan A, Chu P, Kerlikowske K, et al. Positive predictive value of specific mammographic findings according to reader and patient variables. Radiology 2009;250:648-657.

Youk JH, Kim EK. Asymmetric mammographic findings based on the fourth edition of BI-RADS: Types, evaluation and management. RadioGraphics 2008;10:11.

CASE QUESTIONS

CASE 10-1. Screening mammogram on a 45-year-old woman is compared with previous from 2 years prior. What is the significant finding? What is the most appropriate management recommendation?

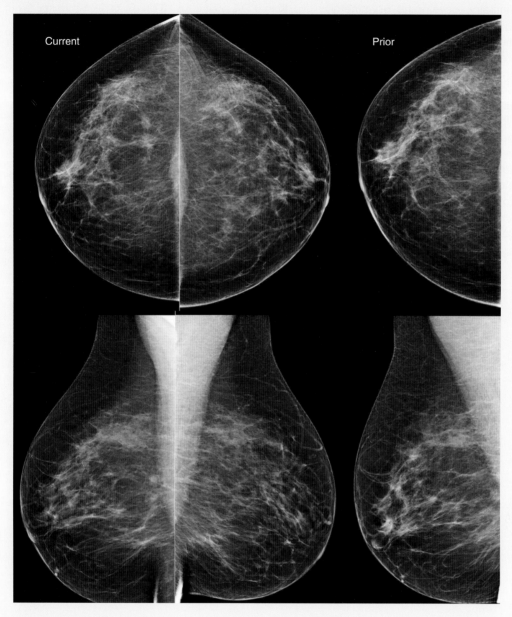

CASE 10-2. Screening mammogram on a 69-year-old woman. How would you describe the abnormality? What are your BI-RADS assessment category and recommendation?

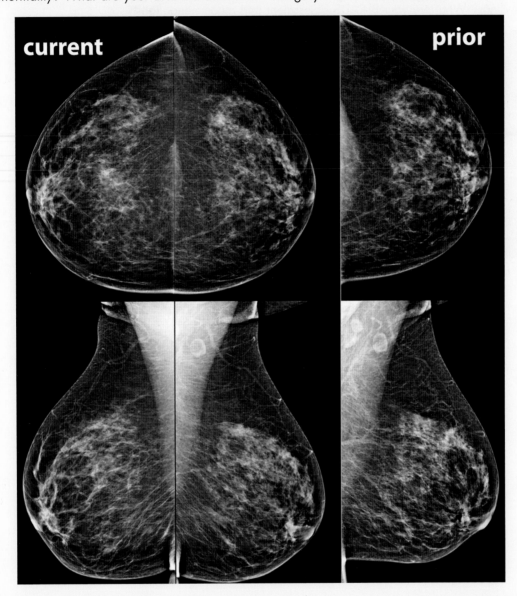

CASE 10-3. Screening mammogram on a 58-year-old woman with no breast-related history. Comparison with previous mammograms from 4 years earlier revealed no changes. How would you describe the findings? What are your BI-RADS assessment and recommendation?

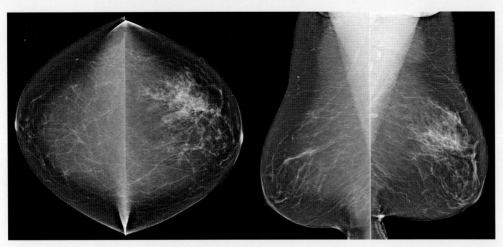

CASE 10-4. A 65-year-old woman was recalled from screening because of a focal asymmetry in the left breast (*arrows*). Here are images from her screening and diagnostic mammograms. What are your BI-RADS assessment and recommendation?

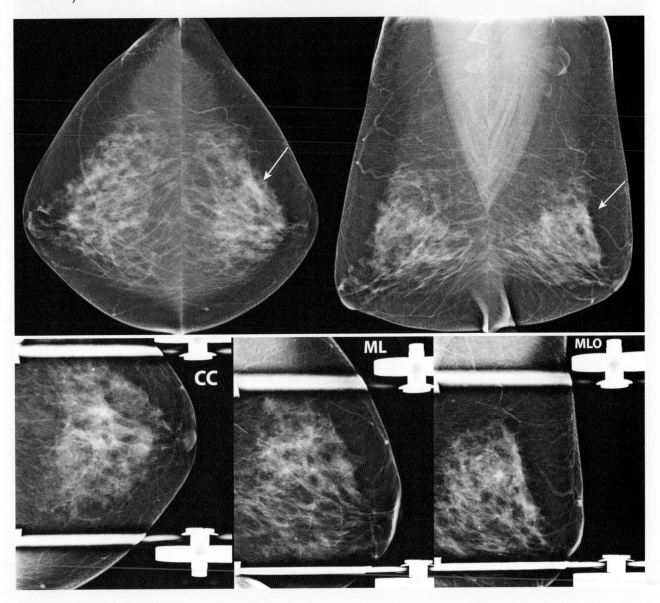

CASE 10-5. Screening mammogram of a 46-year-old woman. How would you describe the abnormality? What are your BI-RADS assessment and recommendation?

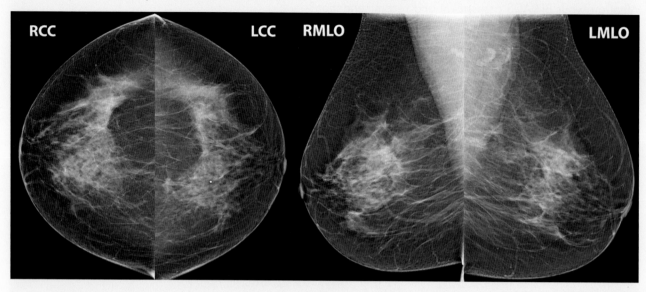

CASE 10-6. Screening mammogram on a 62-year-old woman. How would you describe the abnormality? What are your BI-RADS assessment and recommendation?

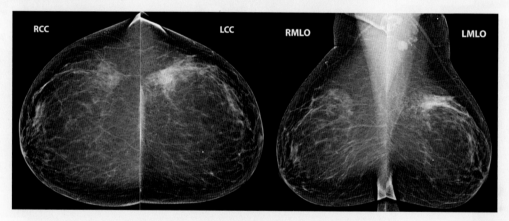

CASE 10-7. Screening mammogram on a 52-year-old woman. Compared with prior mammograms, what change has occurred? What are your BI-RADS assessment and recommendation?

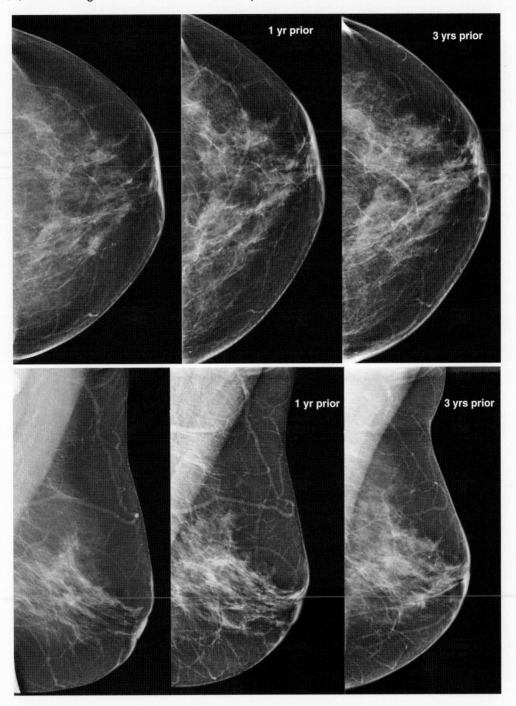

CASE 10-8. Screening mammogram on a 49-year-old woman with a history of benign stereotactic biopsy of calcifications in both breasts 9 years ago. Comparison with a mammogram from 1 year prior revealed no changes. How would you describe the findings? What are your BI-RADS assessment and recommendation?

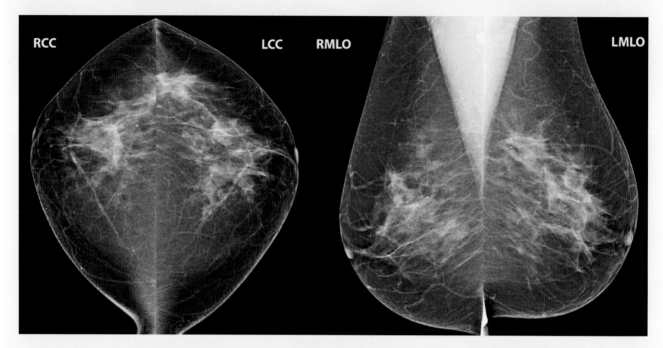

CASE 10-9. Screening mammogram of a 58-year-old woman. What are your findings and BI-RADS assessment?

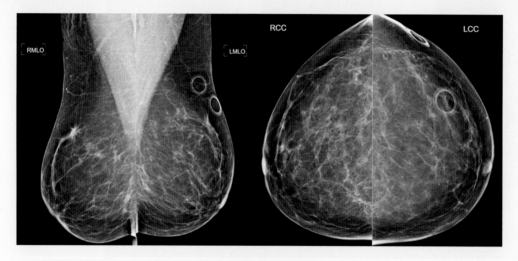

CASE 10-10. Screening mammogram on a 61-year-old woman. The region indicated by the arrow is not seen on the previous mammogram from 1 year ago. Is recall for diagnostic imaging warranted?

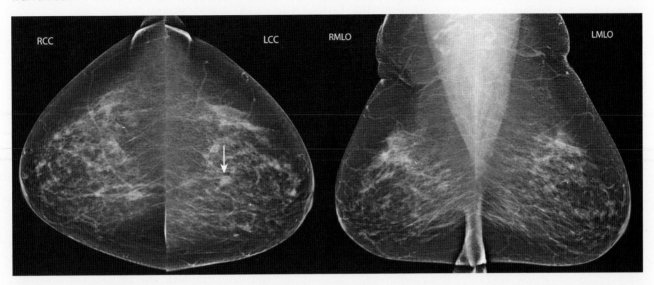

CASE 10-11. Screening mammogram on a 66-year-old woman. What are your BI-RADS assessment and recommendation?

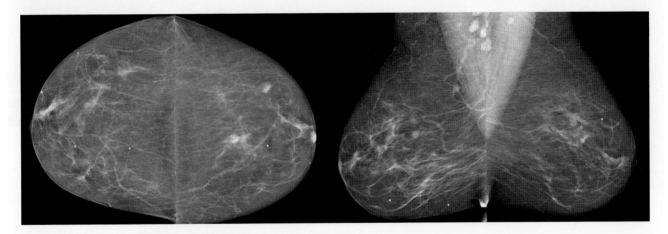

CASE 10-1. A, On the CC view of the right breast, there is a new asymmetry in the retroglandular fat in the posterior lateral breast (*circle*). This finding is not well seen on the MLO view. (Also note one-view asymmetry (*arrow*) in the right subareolar region on the CC view that was stable and not concerning.)

On diagnostic images (**B–D**), the asymmetry is shown to represent an irregular mass with spiculated margins (*arrows*); **E,** a corresponding shadowing, nonparallel mass is seen by US. BI-RADS 4. Ultrasound-guided core biopsy is recommended. Diagnosis: IDC. This case highlights the importance of careful comparison with previous mammograms.

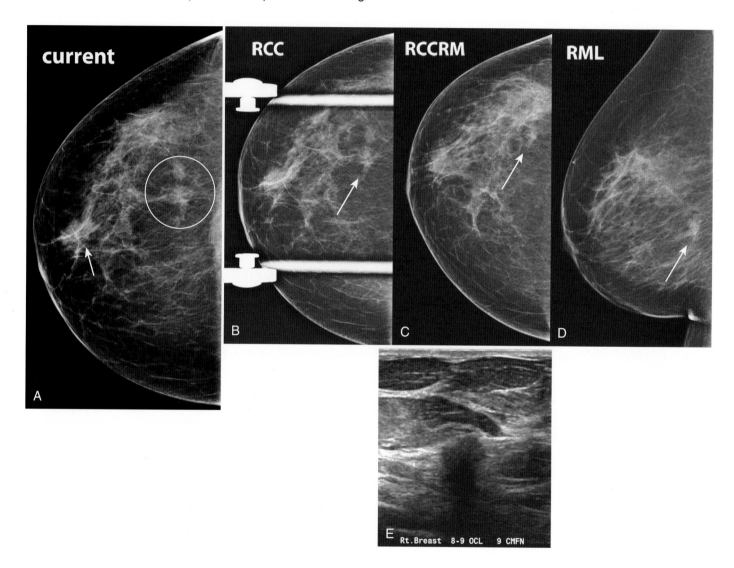

CASE 10-2. There is a developing asymmetry at the edge of the fibroglandular tissue in the upper-outer quadrant of the left breast (*circles*). BI-RADS 0. Recommend spot compression views, ML, with possible US.

On diagnostic images, the finding is confirmed and is shown to represent a mass with obscured margins (*arrows*). US shows a solid mass with indistinct margins in the 1 o'clock position. The central echogenic focus on the lower US image corresponds to a calcification visualized on the mammogram. BI-RADS 5. Ultrasound-guided biopsy is recommended. Diagnosis: IDC. A mass that develops within dense tissue may present as an asymmetry on screening, as in this case.

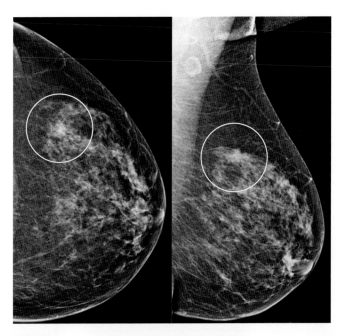

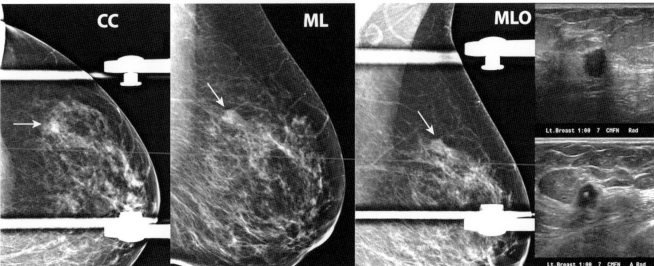

CASE 10-3. There is a large focal asymmetry in the superior lateral quadrant of the left breast, middle third. There is no evidence of associated mass, AD, or calcifications. Because this finding has been stable for 4 years and there are no palpable abnormalities (screening examination), it is considered benign (BI-RADS 2) and no additional evaluation is indicated.

CASE 10-4. The focal asymmetry is partially obscured by dense tissue but does not completely efface on spot compression views. A mass of this size could easily be obscured by dense tissue. There is associated AD with radiating lines best seen on the CC spot view. There are a few associated calcifications. US reveals an irregular hypoechoic mass with angular margins within the echogenic fibroglandular tissue. BI-RADS 4. Ultrasound-guided core biopsy recommended. Diagnosis: IDC and DCIS.

If you are uncertain whether an asymmetry effaces on spot compression views or if your level of concern is high based on the appearance on the screening views, US should be performed.

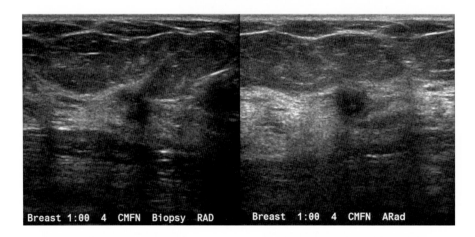

CASE 10-5. A focal asymmetry in the upper inner quadrant of the left breast is best seen on the CC view, protruding from the posterior edge of the fibroglandular tissue into the retroglandular fat (*circle*). On the MLO view, several possible corresponding findings are seen in the upper breast. BI-RADS 0. Recommend diagnostic mammography.

The finding persists on diagnostic views as an irregular mass with spiculated margins. It moves medially on the rolled medial view, confirming its location in the upper breast. A sonographic correlate was seen in the 11 o'clock position. Even if the US were negative, the mammographic findings warrant biopsy. BI-RADS 4. Recommend image-guided biopsy. Diagnosis: IDC.

Protrusion of tissue from the edge of the fibroglandular tissue into the adjacent fat should be examined carefully and considered for diagnostic imaging.

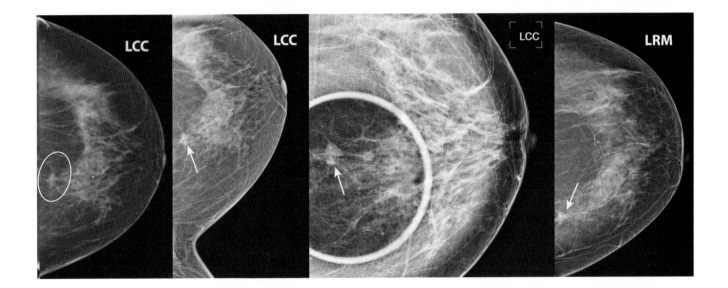

CASE 10-6. A focal asymmetry is seen in the upper outer quadrant of the left breast. A round dense lymph node is present in the left axilla. BI-RADS 0. Recommend spot compression views.

The focal asymmetry persists with subtle spiculation of the posterior edge of tissue. Put her in ultrasound! There is a hypoechoic mass with indistinct margins. Diagnosis: IDC and DCIS with axillary lymph node metastases. The asymmetric density of breast tissue was the key to diagnosis in this patient.

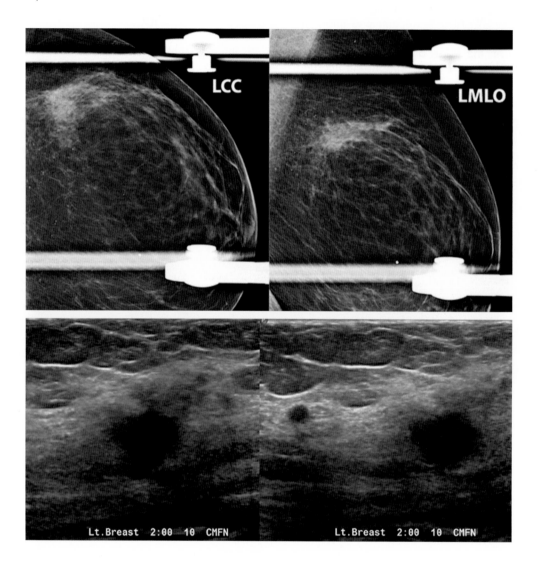

CASE 10-7. There is a new one-view asymmetry in the medial left breast seen only on the CC view (*circle*). BI-RADS 0. Recommend spot compression views.

CC spot compression views were obtained, including a CC rolled medial view.

The asymmetry persists. The finding was not seen on the true lateral. The rolled view projects the finding off the adjacent dense tissue. There is little change in position of the finding on this view so the lesion is likely in the central breast. Recommend US. A hypoechoic solid mass with angular margins is seen in the 9 o'clock position. BI-RADS 4. Recommend ultrasound-guided core biopsy. Diagnosis: IDC. One-view asymmetries usually represent summation artifacts but may also be the sole presenting sign of malignancy.

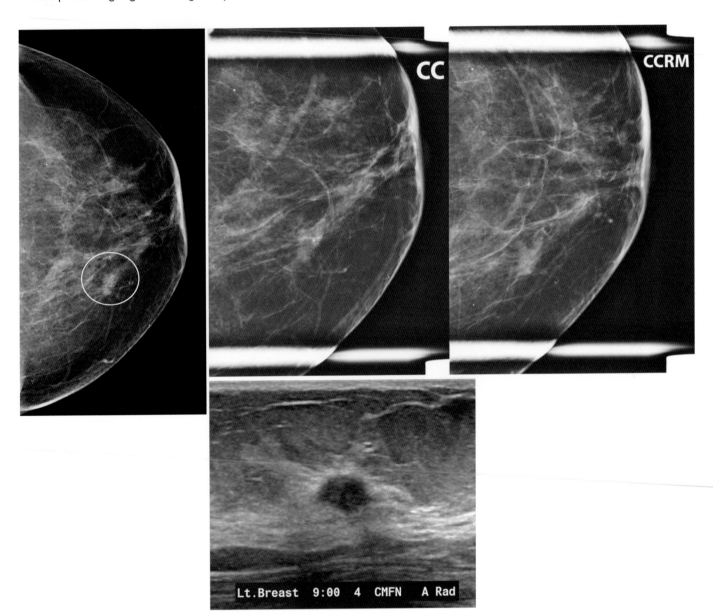

CASE 10-8. Mammography shows a focal asymmetry with associated AD near the marker *clip* in the upper outer left breast. Stability for only 1 year and remote history of benign core biopsy are not reassuring. BI-RADS 0. Recommend spot compression views.

Spot compression views reveal focal asymmetry with AD near the *clip* from benign biopsy. Prior stereotactic biopsy cannot account for these findings. US shows an ill-defined hypoechoic shadowing mass. Postcontrast MRI (see the next page) showed an enhancing mass (*arrow*) adjacent to the clip (signal void). BI-RADS 4. Recommend biopsy. Diagnosis: IDC at the site of previous benign stereotactic biopsy.

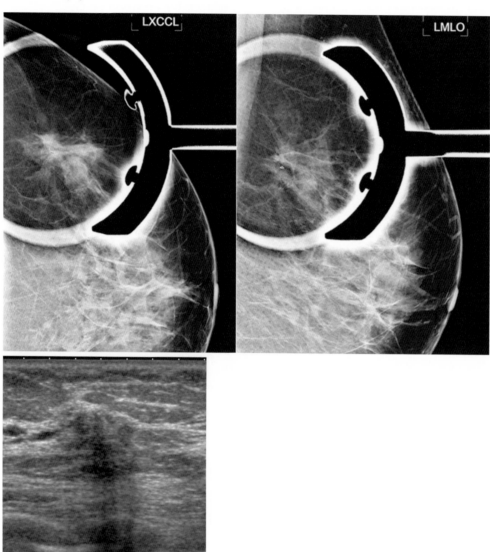

Figure continued on next page.

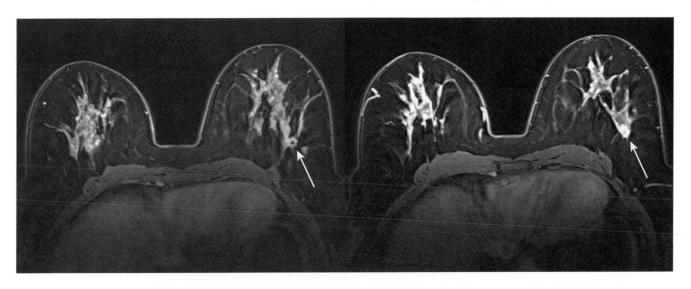

CASE 10-9. There is an irregular one-view asymmetry in the upper right breast (*circle*). The tissue consists almost entirely of fat. A true finding of this size and this far forward in the breast could not have been obscured on the CC view or excluded from the field of view. Therefore, the finding represents summation artifact. BI-RADS 1.

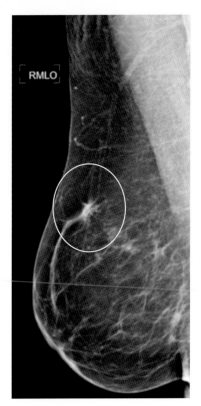

CASE 10-10. Yes! There is oval asymmetry on the CC view. A corresponding finding is not well seen on the MLO view; there is enough dense tissue to obscure a small mass. On the diagnostic views and US a mass is confirmed (*arrows*). Diagnosis: IDC.

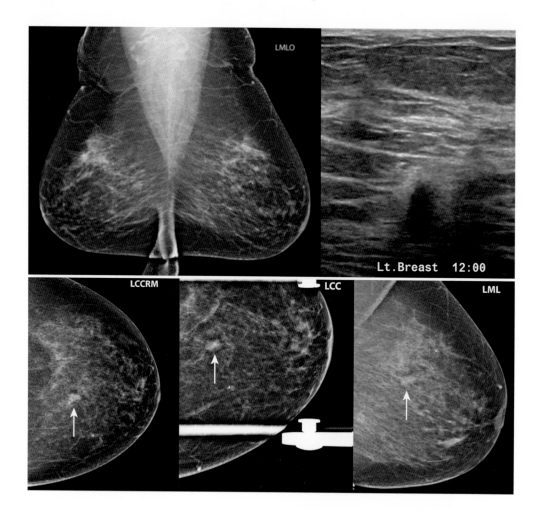

CASE 10-11. There is a one-view asymmetry located centrally on the left CC view (*circle*) and a small low-density circumscribed mass in the left breast at 3 o'clock (*arrow*). This is BI-RADS 0.

We were able to obtain a prior mammogram from 2 years earlier; the mass was stable, but the central asymmetry was new. The asymmetry persists on the CC spot compression view, but it is not well seen on the MLO spot view. It is probably in the superior breast. US of the area was negative.

Because the finding is new, stereotactic biopsy was performed using a CC from above approach. Histologic findings: DCIS, high grade. This case highlights the need to pursue biopsy of asymmetries if the finding is new, even when US is negative.

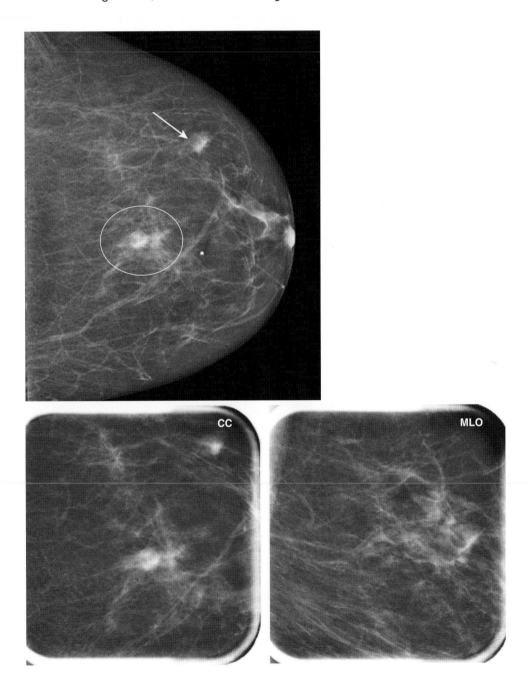

CHAPTER 11

Expanding the Differential Diagnosis: Going Beyond IDC-NOS

So you found the architectural distortion on her screening mammogram. She had a diagnostic workup and you found a small abnormal area, no more than 1 or 2 cm. Ultrasound-guided core biopsy showed invasive lobular carcinoma (ILC). She opted for mastectomy even though she looked like a good breast conservation candidate. The pathologist found 7 cm of tumor! How could I have underestimated the size by so much? How could we not have seen such a big invasive cancer last year?

This scenario is actually quite common with ILC, which invades the breast in thin strands of cells much like a spider web. In this chapter we will review the less common breast cancers, including some pathology correlation that may help you expand your differential diagnosis beyond invasive ductal carcinoma (IDC).

Invasive ductal carcinoma–not otherwise specified (IDC-NOS) and ductal carcinoma in situ (DCIS) are by far the most commonly diagnosed breast cancers, making up about 85% of new cases. The remaining 15% of breast cancers often have features that suggest that the diagnosis is something less common.

IDC-NOS simply means that the cancer is differentiated enough to form ducts but does not display other differentiating features, such as making mucin (as in mucinous carcinoma) or papillary formations (as in papillary carcinoma). IDC-NOS typically presents as a spiculated mass or developing asymmetry. DCIS, the nonobligatory predecessor to IDC, typically presents as either coarse heterogeneous or fine pleomorphic calcifications.

The "other" breast cancers can be broadly divided into ILC, the well-differentiated subtypes of IDC, tumors of stromal origin, and metastatic carcinomas. Some rare types of breast malignancies also display characteristic features that suggest the diagnosis. An understanding of these less common breast malignances will improve skills in detection and diagnosis.

Invasive Lobular Carcinoma

ILC is very different from IDC. On histologic examination, it is characterized by a lack of e-cadherin. Why are we boring you with pathology? Although the study of Latin among premedical students is less common these days, e-cadherin sounds rather like "adhere," which explains ILC in a nutshell. The cells in ILC lose their

ability to adhere to one another, resulting in cancers that are very infiltrative in the breast, like a spider web. ILC is characterized by lines and sheets of cells invading into the breast tissue (Fig. 11-1). This insidious growth pattern and failure to elicit a desmoplastic reaction can make ILC difficult to detect on clinical examination and mammography.

Let's think about how a spider web of tumor cells in the breast (ILC) is going to be different from IDC, where a mass of adherent tumor cells is more characteristic. How would a web of tumor cells feel on clinical examination? Although IDC typically presents as a firm palpable mass on clinical examination, ILC more often presents with an ill-defined mass or thickening of the tissue, or with nipple retraction if the web becomes tethered to the subareolar tissues. If the web of tumor cells is dense enough, ILC can also present as a firm palpable lump.

How would a web of tumor cells look on a mammogram or ultrasonography (US)? The mammogram may show only very subtle findings or be completely normal, even in the setting of extensive ILC (Fig. 11-2). Only the densest part of the tumor will be visible on mammography. ILC may appear as a mass with ill-defined or spiculated margins or as architectural distortion with or without a central mass. When a central mass is present, then it is considered a spiculated mass. When there is architectural distortion without a central mass, these lesions are often called the "dark star." Calcifications are uncommon, though ILC can have associated DCIS. ILC is often seen in only one view, most commonly the craniocaudal (CC) view. This makes sense because the CC view has better compression of the breast tissue than does the mediolateral oblique (MLO) view. Greater compression can bring out the subtle distortion to better advantage. The extent of disease of ILC is not easily assessed on mammography because the edges of that web are not well defined.

When the tumor is very large, the breast affected with ILC can appear to be getting smaller on mammography—the "shrinking breast" (Fig. 11-3). This is not due to the breast becoming physically smaller, but to the decreased compressibility of the breast tissue that is full of webs of cancer cells. If the contralateral breast compresses to a thickness of 5 cm, a breast with extensive ILC may only compress to 8 cm. Although this results in the appearance of a smaller breast on mammography, breast size is typically symmetric on clinical examination.

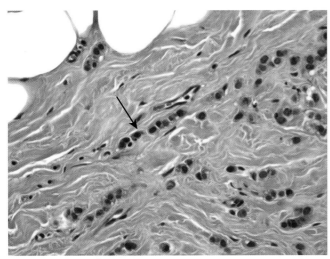

FIGURE 11-1 **Histology of ILC.** ILC is characterized by single file sheets of cells (*arrow*). Note that there is little lymphocytic response or edema. (*Reprinted with permission from Harvey JA. Unusual breast cancers: Useful clues to expanding the differential diagnosis. Radiology 2007;242:683-694.*)

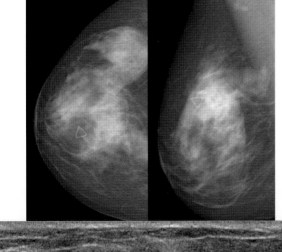

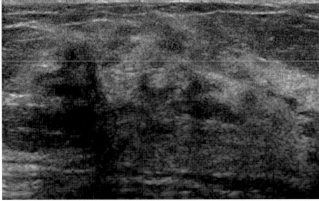

FIGURE 11-2 **ILC.** A 49-year-old woman with a firm palpable lump in the right breast. Mammogram is normal in the palpable area that is marked by a *triangle*. US shows multiple hypoechoic areas with shadowing but no discrete mass, which is characteristic of ILC. (*Reprinted with permission from Harvey JA. Unusual breast cancers: Useful clues to expanding the differential diagnosis. Radiology 2007;242:683-694.*)

On US, ILC may present as a defined mass (see Fig. 11-3) but more often presents as ill-defined areas of shadowing without a distinct mass (see Fig. 11-2). The lines and arcs of tumor can produce bands of shadowing, like the edges of a spider web. Although tumor size is often underestimated by US, this modality is more accurate than clinical examination or mammography in assessing extent of disease.

Magnetic resonance imaging (MRI) is helpful in evaluating the extent of disease with ILC, showing more extensive disease than does mammography in 39% of cases. A cautionary note—ILC may show only faint enhancement with progressive kinetics on MRI. The washout pattern is much less common for ILC than IDC. Remember—when interpreting breast MRI and deciding on your management recommendation, the morphologic appearance always trumps the curve.

ILC is often larger at diagnosis than IDC and is often multifocal. Likewise, ILC is more commonly associated with positive margins and more often treated with mastectomy than IDC. Axillary metastasis is less common, however, so overall ILC has a similar prognosis to IDC. The most evil variant of ILC is pleomorphic ILC. These tumors show more variability of the nuclear size and less uniform cell size. A few recent studies suggest that pleomorphic ILC may have a higher predisposition to metastasis and a worse prognosis compared with usual ILC.

When ILC metastasizes, it may spread to strange places like peritoneal surfaces, the stomach, uterus, ovaries, and bladder. ILC may therefore present with ascites, hydronephrosis, or pelvic masses.

As might be expected, fine-needle aspiration (FNA) of ILC is less sensitive than for IDC. This is logical because FNA of ILC attempts to obtain material from single-file sheets of tumor cells with intervening normal tissue, rather than from a more easily targeted mass of adherent tumor cells that is seen with IDC.

Lobular carcinoma in situ (LCIS) is characterized by a monomorphic population of cells expanding lobules. It is typically mammographically occult and, as such, is an incidental finding on biopsy. However, proliferative lesions such as LCIS are common on biopsy of MRI-detected lesions.

Pleomorphic LCIS is characterized by increased cellular atypia compared with usual LCIS. Some small series suggest a higher incidence of associated invasive carcinoma when core biopsy shows pleomorphic LCIS (Boxes 11-1 and 11-2).

Radial scar can mimic ILC on mammography. Both frequently present as distortion without a central mass (the "dark star"). Radial scar is not actually a scar; it is not due to trauma or surgery, but does look somewhat like a scar at histologic examination. Benign lobules and ducts are entrapped by dense central fibrosis and elastosis, which results in the appearance of architectural distortion on the mammogram (Fig. 11-4). The cause is unclear, but these are proliferative lesions. Hyperplasia, atypical ductal hyperplasia, and papillomas are common in the surrounding tissue. From 10% to 30% of radial scars are associated with DCIS or IDC. Multiple small foci of carcinoma are not uncommon. A history of biopsy showing radial scar is also associated with a higher risk

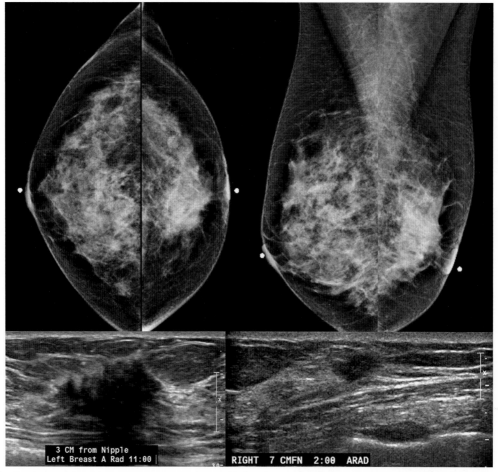

FIGURE 11-3 **Shrinking Breast.** A 52-year-old woman noted thickening in her left breast. On clinical examination, the breasts are symmetric in size but the texture of the left breast is diffusely thickened. On mammography, the left breast appears to be smaller than the right. Biopsy showed ILC. Did you also notice the one-view asymmetry in the right medial breast? US of this area shows a small hypoechoic mass. Biopsy of the right breast showed IDC.

BOX 11-1 Is LCIS Simply a Marker of Increased Breast Cancer Risk or a Premalignant Lesion?

- Prior to the mid-1990s, LCIS was treated aggressively as a premalignant condition, often resulting in bilateral mastectomy.
- In the mid-1990s, studies suggested that LCIS was not a premalignant neoplasm but a marker of high risk, elevating the risk of breast cancer four- to sevenfold in either breast, and for either ILC or IDC.
- Studies now show that LCIS and ILC have similar genetic mutations, suggesting that LCIS is indeed a premalignant lesion.
- LCIS appears to be a nonobligate precursor of ILC. The risk for subsequent invasion may be very low or delayed in onset compared with the risk of IDC developing from DCIS.

BOX 11-2 Differential Diagnosis of Architectural Distortion without a Central Mass ("the Dark Star")

- IDC-NOS
- ILC
- Radial scar
- Surgical scar

of breast cancer (relative risk of two times that of women without this history).

Radial scar may also mimic an invasive cancer, particularly tubular carcinoma, at both gross and histopathologic examination. A myosin stain is sometimes used to identify myoepithelial cells in the basement membrane, which will be present in radial scar but not in invasive carcinoma.

Radial scar is a general term that may refer to any of these pathologic entities: *radial sclerosing lesion, sclerosing papillary proliferation,* and *complex sclerosing lesion.* Radial scar/complex sclerosing lesion is characterized by a dense central fibrotic nidus surrounded by

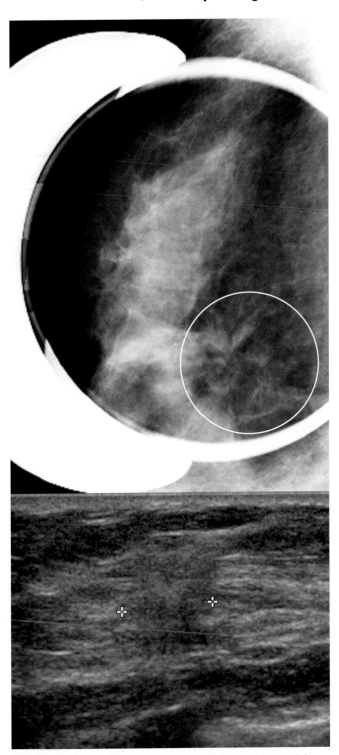

FIGURE 11-4 **Radial Scar with Associated DCIS.** Architectural distortion is present in the right breast (*circle*). On US, there is a corresponding hypoechoic, irregular mass. Ultrasound-guided core biopsy showed radial scar. Excisional biopsy showed radial scar with associated DCIS.

carcinoma. At initial mammographic interpretation, either core biopsy or diagnostic surgical biopsy can be performed. Core biopsy showing a benign result will often result in a recommendation for excision of the area due the underlying distortion. On the other hand, surgeons may prefer to know before surgery if the pathologic finding is consistent with radial scar, requiring only a small volume excision, or invasive carcinoma, which requires a larger volume excision and nodal sampling. Hence, core biopsy can aid in biopsy planning (Box 11-3).

If a core biopsy is performed for a different type of BI-RADS 4 lesion, such as calcifications or a focal asymmetry, and shows an incidental minute radial scar that was completely contained within the core sample, excisional biopsy is probably not necessary.

Subtypes of IDC

IDC-NOS is the most common type of breast cancer. Essentially, the carcinoma is differentiated enough to form ducts, but that is all. There are several subtypes of IDC that are better differentiated—they make mucin, form tubules, etc. Because these cancers are more differentiated, they tend to grow slowly (except medullary carcinoma) and be circumscribed (except tubular). They are typically grade I and have a better prognosis than IDC-NOS overall (Boxes 11-4 and 11-5).

Tubular carcinoma is characterized by the formation of tubules or small ductules. It typically presents as a small mass, often with long spicules (Fig. 11-5) like cat whiskers, and is often multifocal. Tubular carcinoma has an excellent outcome with a cause-specific survival

circumferentially radiating ducts and lobules. Complex sclerosing lesions are similar, but larger (usually > 10 mm) and less organized. Sclerosing papillary proliferation is a sclerosing lesion with associated papillomas.

Management of architectural distortion having the dark star appearance on mammography is somewhat controversial. Up to 29% of these women will have invasive

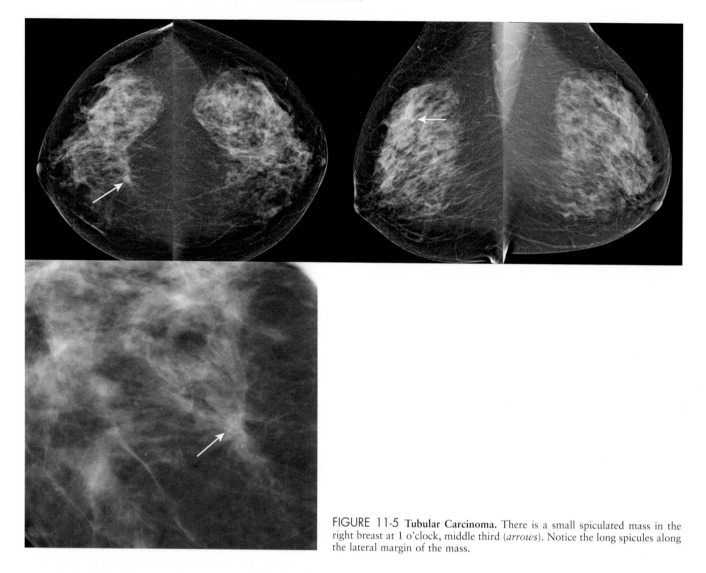

FIGURE 11-5 **Tubular Carcinoma.** There is a small spiculated mass in the right breast at 1 o'clock, middle third (*arrows*). Notice the long spicules along the lateral margin of the mass.

BOX 11-5   The "Round" Cancers

- IDC-NOS
- Medullary
- Mucinous
- Papillary
- Phyllodes

rate of 98% at 10 years. Axillary metastasis is very uncommon, and distant disease is even less common. If you could pick your type of invasive cancer to be diagnosed with, this is the one.

One of our prior fellows (a "Valley Girl" from California), pointed out that "tubular" was synonymous with "cool" during the 1980s. So think, "Like, tubular, man!" and you'll remember that this is the cool, easy-going invasive cancer despite the appearance of a spiculated mass. A word of caution—if you have teenage kids, we don't recommend using this language (or related terms like "nifty") in their presence unless you really want to see their eyes roll!

Histologically, tubular carcinoma can mimic a radial scar and vice versa. The pathologist may use actin stain to check for myoepithelial cells that are present in the basement membrane of tubules associated with radial scar, but absent in tubular carcinoma.

Medullary carcinoma is a very rapidly growing cancer that typically presents as a palpable mass in young or middle-aged women (Fig. 11-6). The median age of diagnosis is 51. "Medulla" means marrow. Like basal cell (triple negative) IDC, medullary carcinoma is characterized by a brisk lymphocytic response, absence of fibroglandular differentiation, and pleomorphic nuclei. There is usually little or no associated DCIS. So at first glance under the microscope medullary carcinoma resembles an aggressive IDC. There is considerable interobserver variability in the pathologic diagnosis of medullary carcinoma that may explain the variable patient outcomes reported across different series. The prognosis for women with this cancer is better than for typical IDC in most series.

On mammography, medullary carcinoma typically presents as a round or oval, circumscribed mass without calcifications. It is often palpable.

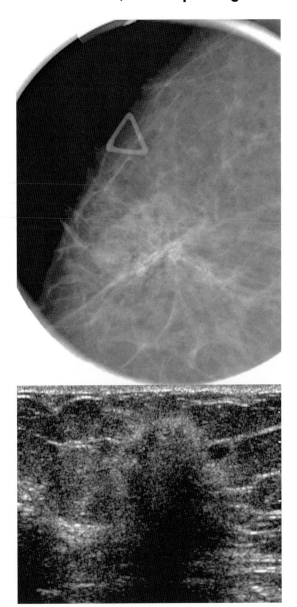

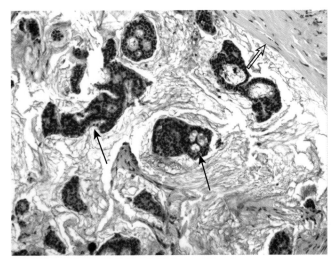

FIGURE 11-7 **Histologic Appearance of Mucinous Carcinoma.** Islands of cancer cells (*arrows*) are floating in mucin. Note the abrupt margin with normal breast tissue (*open arrow*). *(Reprinted with permission from Harvey JA. Unusual breast cancers: Useful clues to expanding the differential diagnosis. Radiology 2007;242:683-694.)*

FIGURE 11-6 **Medullary Carcinoma.** This 44-year-old woman presented with a palpable mass (*triangle*) that corresponds to an oval, relatively circumscribed, high-density mass. US demonstrates a hypoechoic, solid, oval mass with posterior acoustic shadowing.

Mucinous (colloid) carcinoma is characterized by tumor cells floating in a pool of mucin (Fig. 11-7). This lesion presents most commonly in older women with a median age of 71. Your last experience with an upper respiratory infection should remind you that mucin is a soft semiliquid. As a result, the mammographic appearance is usually a *low-density* mass rather than a dense clump of cells like most cancers (Fig. 11-8). The margins are typically fairly well-circumscribed. The US appearance can be relatively isoechoic, and often there is posterior acoustic enhancement. Like proliferative fibroadenomas, these masses are very T2 hyperintense on MRI, but tend to be more heterogeneous on T1 postcontrast sequences.

There may be a paucity of neoplastic cells in mucinous carcinoma. For this reason, a core biopsy containing mucin may represent either a benign mucocoele or mucinous carcinoma and should be excised even in the absence of neoplastic cells.

Papillary carcinoma represents 1% to 2% of breast cancers. Papillary carcinoma shares some similarities with benign papillomas. Both most commonly present as intraductal or intracystic masses (Fig. 11-9), may be associated with nipple discharge, and are frequently located in the subareolar region. Papillary carcinoma often presents as a palpable mass. On mammography, papillary carcinoma is usually a round or oval, circumscribed, equal- to high-density mass. On US, the most common finding is an intraductal or intracystic mass. These cancers are termed *encapsulated (or intracystic) papillary carcinoma*. Because the cancer is largely confined to the contents of the cyst, these lesions behave and are treated in a manner similar to DCIS. If the cancer invades through the wall of the cyst, the size and degree of invasion determine management and outcome. So, a woman with a 3-cm palpable intracystic papillary carcinoma may only have a 5-mm invasive component, and is treated and staged based on the 5-mm measurement. The prognosis for these tumors is excellent.

Solid papillary carcinoma is a rare variant of DCIS that occurs in older women. *Invasive papillary carcinoma* that is not intracystic is extremely rare.

A Few Other Lesions

This section is for the detail-oriented people.

Invasive cribriform carcinoma, like tubular carcinoma, presents as a spiculated mass but has an excellent prognosis.

Invasive micropapillary carcinoma represents less than 2% of breast cancers and has no specific imaging or clinical features. About 70% have associated cribriform or micropapillary DCIS. About 75% of patients have

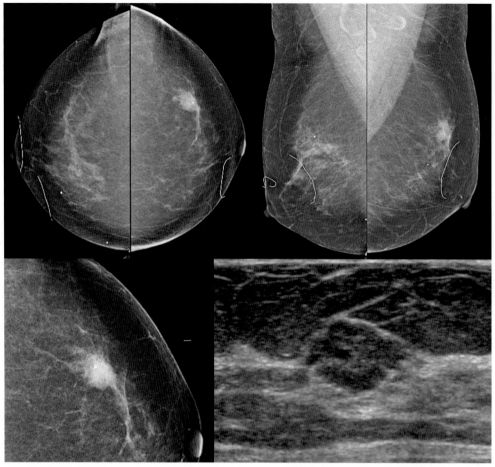

FIGURE 11-8 **Mucinous Carcinoma.** A 67-year-old woman with a round mass with ill-defined margins in the left breast at 1 o'clock. On US, there is an isoechoic lobular mass with abrupt defined margins.

metastatic adenopathy at diagnosis; this tumor has a poorer prognosis than the other ductal subtypes.

Invasive apocrine carcinoma is an uncommon lesion that has a similar mammographic appearance and prognosis as IDC-NOS.

Granular cell tumor is most commonly seen in the tongue, but may present as a subcutaneous spiculated mass in the breast (Fig. 11-10). It is more common in African-American women. These tumors are benign but may be locally aggressive, so they require wide local excision.

Adenoid cystic carcinoma represents 0.1% of breast cancers. These tumors are typically seen in the salivary glands, so why in the breast? Remember way back to your embryology class? The breast and salivary glands are both modified sweat glands. Adenoid cystic carcinomas are most common in older women and present as a mammographic or palpable mass that is relatively well circumscribed (Fig. 11-11). These patients have an excellent prognosis; axillary metastasis is rare.

Metaplastic carcinoma (carcinosarcoma) contains both epithelial (carcinoma) and sarcomatous elements. The nonfibroglandular component may be epithelial (e.g., squamous) or mesenchymal (e.g., chondroid, spindle cell, osseous). These lesions typically grow rapidly and present as a palpable mass. On imaging, the appearance

BOX 11-6   Fibroepithelial Lesions

- Fibroadenoma
- Juvenile fibroadenoma
- Lactating adenoma
- Tubular adenoma
- Apocrine adenoma
- (Ductal adenoma)
- (Pleomorphic adenoma)
- Phyllodes tumor

is nonspecific, though they often present as a mass with partly circumscribed and partly spiculated margins without calcifications (Fig. 11-12). Prognosis is similar to that for other high-grade invasive breast carcinomas. *Spindle cell carcinoma* is a subtype of metaplastic carcinoma.

The Fibroepithelial Lesions: Phyllodes to Fibroadenoma (Box 11-6)

Phyllodes tumor is a very rapidly growing tumor that typically occurs in middle-aged or older women. It usually

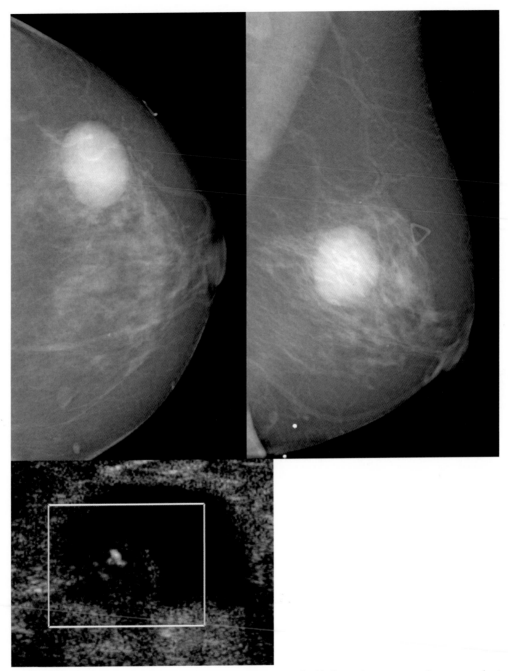

FIGURE 11-9 Intracystic Papillary Carcinoma. This patient presented with a palpable lump that corresponds to an oval, circumscribed, high-density mass on mammography and a complex mass on US. At histologic examination, only a few millimeters of invasive tumor were present. *(Reprinted with permission from Harvey JA. Unusual breast cancers: Useful clues to expanding the differential diagnosis. Radiology 2007;242:683-694.)*

presents as a very large but defined oval mass (Fig. 11-13). Phyllodes tumor is classified with a group of masses known as fibroepithelial lesions that originate from the lobule. The old name for phyllodes tumor is "cystosarcoma phyllodes," which hints at the behavior of this tumor. Like all sarcomas, wide excision is the primary and most effective treatment. Even low-grade phyllodes tumors can be locally aggressive. High-grade phyllodes tumor can metastasize hematogenously, most frequently to the lungs. Sentinel lymph node biopsy is not indicated for phyllodes tumor because lymphatic metastasis is rare.

These tumors can undergo sarcomatous degeneration, in which cartilage or bone can be seen within the tumor. The prognosis is then poor. *Spindle cell sarcoma* in the breast most commonly represents a subtype of phyllodes tumor.

Benign fibroadenomas are also fibroepithelial lesions. They are the most common breast lesion, occurring in 25% of asymptomatic women. You may run across certain descriptive pathologic terms for fibroadenomas, including pericanalicular, intracanalicular, and complex. These descriptions refer to growth patterns of

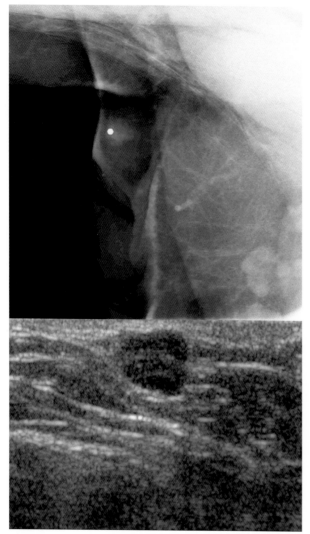

FIGURE 11-10 **Granular Cell Tumor.** There is a small spiculated mass in a subcutaneous location. This would be an uncommon location for IDC-NOS. Wide excision is indicated.

fibroadenomas that contain cysts, adenosis, or other hyperplastic changes. The bottom line is that all of these histologic subtypes are managed similarly.

When small, phyllodes tumor can mimic a fibroadenoma on imaging (Table 11-1). Phyllodes tumors tend to arise in older women and to be faster growing than fibroadenomas. Ill-defined margins and internal cystic spaces on imaging are also suggestive of phyllodes tumor.

On histologic examination, phyllodes tumor is very similar to fibroadenoma, but with considerably more proliferation. They are two ends of the same spectrum of disease. Phyllodes means "leaf," and the histologic appearance of the tumor is characterized by leaf-like growth of cells. It may be difficult to differentiate a proliferative fibroadenoma from a low-grade phyllodes tumor, and there are no special stains to tell the two apart. Occasionally, a core biopsy result may read "proliferative fibroadenoma versus phyllodes," and excision is then needed to make the diagnosis.

Juvenile fibroadenoma is a variant of fibroadenoma that typically presents in adolescents and young women

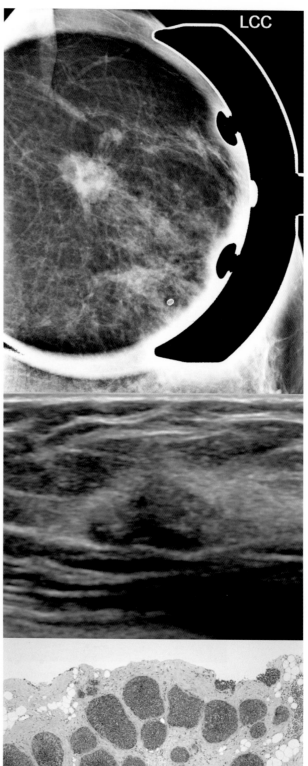

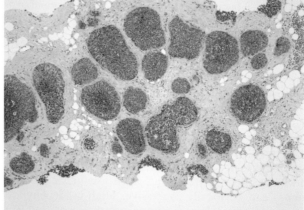

FIGURE 11-11 **Adenoid Cystic Carcinoma.** This 46-year-old woman's screening detected an oval mass that has mixed echogenicity by US. Core biopsy (hematoxylin-eosin) showed solid nests of tumor cells that lack a myoepithelial cell layer.

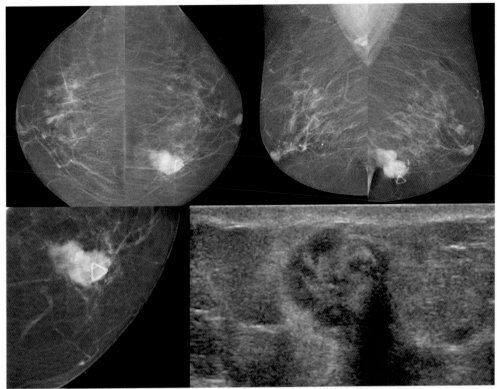

FIGURE 11-12 **Metaplastic Carcinoma.** The presentation of a palpable mass *(triangle)* that is partly circumscribed and partly spiculated is typical of metaplastic carcinoma. On US, a heterogeneous solid mass is seen with cystic areas representing tumor necrosis.

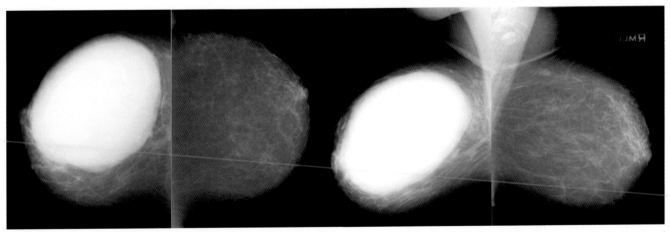

FIGURE 11-13 **Phyllodes Tumor.** Large rapidly growing mass in a 56-year-old woman. The mass is oval and relatively circumscribed. *(Reprinted with permission from Harvey JA. Unusual breast cancers: Useful clues to expanding the differential diagnosis. Radiology 2007;242:683-694.)*

as a rapidly growing and often very large mass. When very large (over 5-10 cm), they are referred to as *giant fibroadenomas.* Histologically, these lesions show hypercellular stromal proliferation. A very large mass in a young woman typically represents a giant fibroadenoma. Because phyllodes tumor and giant fibroadenoma both grow rapidly, patient age can usually suggest the correct diagnosis. Both are usually managed by excision.

Tubular adenoma and *lactating adenoma* are also fibroepithelial lesions with histologic and imaging features similar to those of fibroadenoma, but with a paucity of stroma and a greater epithelial component at histologic examination. Lactating adenomas present in women who are pregnant or lactating. Some pathologists believe that these are literally fibroadenomas on steroids—that they may represent preexisting fibroadenomas that are stimulated by the hormones of pregnancy and lactation. Tubular adenomas and lactating adenomas are managed the same as run-of-the-mill fibroadenomas.

Ductal adenoma and *pleomorphic adenoma* are actually considered variants of intraductal papilloma rather than fibroadenoma. Nevertheless, they are benign and can be managed like fibroadenomas.

TABLE 11-1	Differentiation between Fibroadenoma and Phyllodes Tumor	
FEATURE	**FIBROADENOMA**	**PHYLLODES TUMOR**
Patient age at diagnosis	Young	Middle age or older
Size	1-3 cm	Very large
Growth	Mild or none	Very rapid
Margins	Circumscribed	Ill-defined
Ultrasound findings	Internal septations	Cleft-like spaces

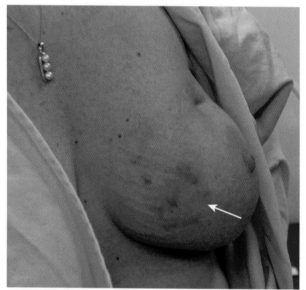

FIGURE 11-14 Cutaneous Angiosarcoma. This 57-year-old woman had lumpectomy with radiation therapy 7 years ago and now notes bruising of her breast (*arrow*), though she does not recall trauma.

Breast Sarcomas

Yes, these neoplasms are rare, but there are some cases in which you really should think about them, so read on!

All of the breast sarcomas are more common after radiation therapy to the breast. Sarcomas in general are characterized by rapid growth, hematogenous metastasis most frequently to the lungs, and poor prognosis. Lymphatic metastasis is rare, so sentinel lymph node sampling is not typically performed.

The primary treatment for sarcoma is wide local excision. The surgeon will often try to have a 1 cm margin around the lesion. Radiation therapy and chemotherapy are less effective than for carcinomas.

Angiosarcoma is the most common breast sarcoma. In the irradiated breast, cutaneous presentation (Fig. 11-14) is more common than within the breast parenchyma (Fig. 11-15). A diagnosis of cutaneous angiosarcoma should be considered for women with prior lumpectomy treated with radiation therapy who present with apparent breast bruising but no recallable trauma.

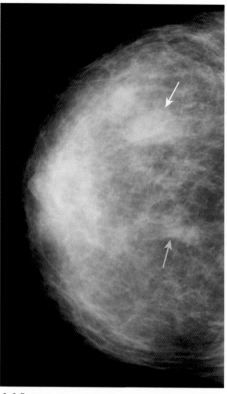

FIGURE 11-15 Parenchymal Angiosarcoma. This 54-year-old woman developed a new mass (*white arrow*) in a different location than her prior lumpectomy scar (*yellow arrow*) from 10 years earlier. Clinically, she presented with a warm, red breast that was suspicious for inflammatory recurrence. (*Reprinted with permission from Harvey JA. Unusual breast cancers: Useful clues to expanding the differential diagnosis. Radiology 2007;242:683-694.*)

Pseudoangiomatous stromal hyperplasia (PASH) is a benign myofibroblastic proliferation that can mimic angiosarcoma at histologic examination (hence, the pseudoangiomatous designation). PASH is uncommon and most frequently presents as an asymmetry rather than a mass or calcifications. A core biopsy showing PASH is benign, so excision is not indicated if the imaging findings are concordant.

Osteosarcoma presents as a really strange looking calcification almost anywhere in the body (Fig. 11-16). The primary and metastatic lesions may show increased activity on bone scintigraphy.

Sarcomas other than angiosarcoma and osteosarcoma are rare and typically associated with phyllodes tumor.

Metastasis to the Breast

Metastatic lesions in the breast are usually a late finding of malignancy. They typically present as multiple round bilateral breast masses (Fig. 11-17), and may also be present in the subcutaneous tissues of the axilla. The mass margins are usually ill-defined compared with those of multiple cysts or fibroadenomas. Metastasis can also present as axillary or intramammary adenopathy (Fig. 11-18).

Melanoma is the most common nonbreast primary neoplasm to metastasize to the breast (Box 11-7).

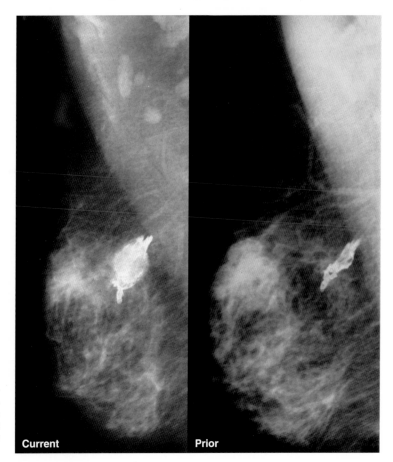

FIGURE 11-16 **Osteosarcoma of the Breast.** The calcification appears lucent-centered, although not typical for dystrophic calcification. It increased in size and became palpable since the mammogram from 6 months earlier. *(Reprinted from Harvey JA, Fondreist JT, Smith MM. Densely calcified breast mass. Invest Radiol 1994;29:516-517.)*

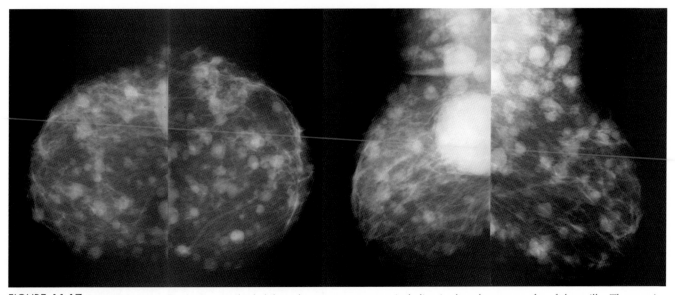

FIGURE 11-17 **Metastatic Lung Carcinoma.** Multiple bilateral masses are present, including in the subcutaneous fat of the axilla. The margins of the masses are ill-defined. This mammographic appearance should not be confused with multiple benign masses, which are discussed in Chapter 8, Multiple Masses. *(Reprinted with permission from Harvey JA. Unusual breast cancers: Useful clues to expanding the differential diagnosis. Radiology 2007;242:683-694.)*

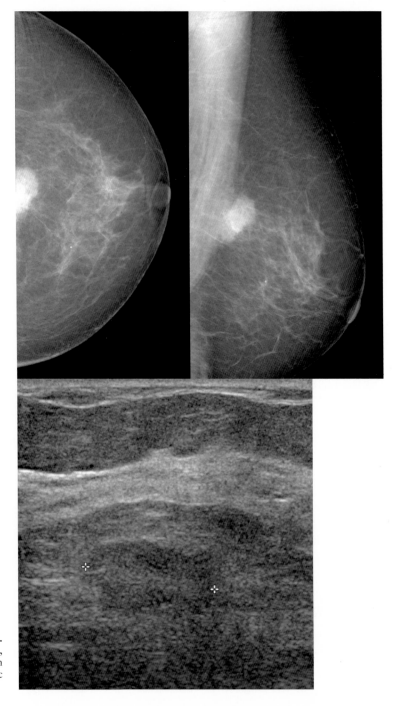

FIGURE 11-18 **Metastatic Intramammary Lymph Node.** Although the mammographic appearance is nonspecific, the location and US appearance are consistent with an abnormal intramammary lymph node. Diagnosis: metastatic melanoma.

Non-Hodgkin lymphoma (NHL) rarely involves the breast. Breast involvement usually occurs in women with known extramammary disease. NHL of the breast most commonly presents as a solitary mass, and multiple masses are less common. Primary breast lymphoma is very rare (Fig. 11-19).

Rhabdomysarcoma and leukemic infiltrates can present as palpable thickening with asymmetry on mammography and poorly defined areas of hyperechogenic breast tissue on US (Fig. 11-20). Fat necrosis differs in appearance; it is typically subcutaneous and better defined.

BOX 11-7 Primary Carcinomas That Metastasize to the Breast

- Breast
- Melanoma
- Lung
- Ovarian
- Cervical
- Renal

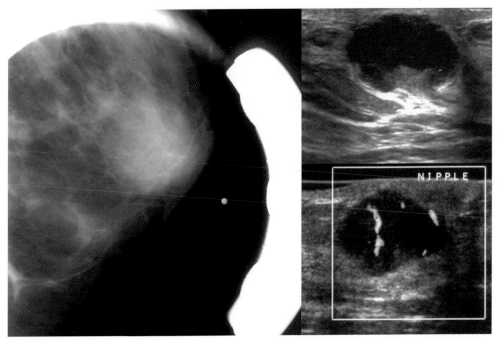

FIGURE 11-19 **Primary Breast Lymphoma.** A middle-aged woman presents with a palpable retroareolar mass. Mammography shows an obscured mass that is markedly hypoechoic and vascular by US. Core biopsy revealed non-Hodgkin lymphoma (diffuse large B cell). There was no evidence of extramammary disease and the patient was treated with chemotherapy and radiation therapy.

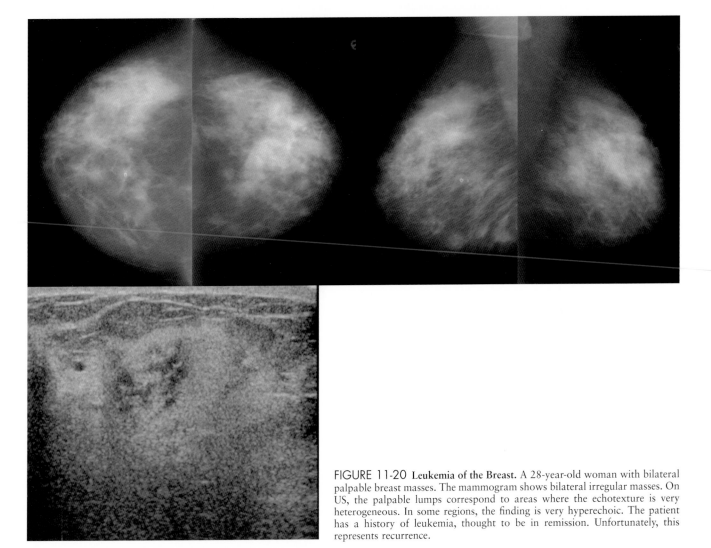

FIGURE 11-20 Leukemia of the Breast. A 28-year-old woman with bilateral palpable breast masses. The mammogram shows bilateral irregular masses. On US, the palpable lumps correspond to areas where the echotexture is very heterogeneous. In some regions, the finding is very hyperechoic. The patient has a history of leukemia, thought to be in remission. Unfortunately, this represents recurrence.

KEY POINTS

- ILC invades the breast like a spider web. It is more difficult to detect on mammography and clinical examination, tends to be larger at diagnosis, and has a higher association with positive margins at excision compared with IDC.
- ILC often presents as architectural distortion without a central mass. This appearance can also be due to radial scar, post-surgical scar, or IDC.
- The subtypes of IDC (medullary, mucinous, tubular, and papillary carcinomas) tend to be slow growing (except medullary), round with relatively well-circumscribed margins (except tubular), and have a better prognosis than IDC-NOS.
- Tubular carcinoma presents as a small mass with long spicules and is a very low-grade ("cool") neoplasm with a very high survival rate.
- Medullary carcinoma is rapidly growing and often presents as a palpable mass. Although this looks aggressive under the microscopic, the prognosis is generally favorable.
- Mucinous carcinoma presents as a low-density round mass. It is very T2 hyperintense on breast MRI, but the heterogeneous enhancement pattern should be a clue that it is not a fibroadenoma.
- Papillary carcinoma is the most common intracystic carcinoma.
- Fibroadenoma and phyllodes tumor are two ends of the spectrum of fibroepithelial lesions. A malignant phyllodes tumor behaves like a sarcoma with hematogenous spread.
- A very large, rapidly growing, circumscribed oval mass is likely to be a giant fibroadenoma in a young woman, but a phyllodes tumor in a middle aged or older woman.
- Breast sarcomas are most commonly seen in women previously treated with radiation therapy. Angiosarcoma is most common.

References

Anderson WF, Chu KC, Chang S, Sherman ME. Comparison of age-specific incidence rate patterns for different histopathologic types of breast carcinoma. Cancer Epidemiol Biomarkers Prev 2004;13:1128-1135.

Harvey JA. Unusual breast cancers: Useful clues to expanding the differential diagnosis. Radiology 2007;242:683-694.

Harvey JA, Fechner RE, Moore MM. Apparent ipsilateral decrease in breast size on mammography: A sign of infiltrating lobular carcinoma. Radiology 2000;213:883-889.

Harvey JA, Fondreist JT, Smith MM. Densely calcified breast mass. Invest Radiol 1994;29:516-517.

Kawashima M, Tamaki Y, Nonaka T, et al. MR imaging of mucinous carcinoma of the breast. Am J Roentgenol 2002;179(1):179-183.

Lagrange JL, Ramaioli A, Chateau MC, et al. Sarcoma after radiation therapy: Retrospective multiinstitutional study of 80 histologically confirmed cases. Radiology 2000;216(1):197-205.

Lam WWM, Chu WCW, Tse GM, Ma TK. Sonographic appearance of mucinous carcinoma of the breast. Am J Roentgenol 2004;182(4):1069-1074.

Livi L, Paiar F, Meldolesi E, et al. Tubular carcinoma of the breast: Outcome and loco-regional recurrence in 307 patients. Eur J Surg Oncol 2005;31(1):9-12.

Lopez JK, Bassett LW. Invasive lobular carcinoma of the breast: Spectrum of mammographic, US, and MR imaging findings. Radiographics 2009;29:165-176.

McGhan L, Wasif N, Gray R, et al. Use of preoperative magnetic resonance imaging for invasive lobular cancer: Good, better, but maybe not the best? Ann Surg Oncol 2010;17(0):255-262.

Mercado CL, Hamele-Bena D, Oken SM, et al. Papillary lesions of the breast at percutaneous core-needle biopsy. [see comment]. Radiology 2006;238(3):801-808.

Mylonas I, Janni W, Friese K, Gerber B. Unexpected metastatic lobular carcinoma of the breast with intraabdominal spread and subsequent port-site metastasis after diagnostic laparoscopy for exclusion of ovarian cancer. Gynecol Oncol 2004;95(2):405-408.

Sabate JM, Gomez A, Torrubia S, Flotats A. Osteosarcoma of the breast. Am J Roentgenol 2002;179(1):277-278.

Schnitt SJ, Collins LC. Biopsy Interpretation of the Breast. Philadelphia, Lippincott Williams & Wilkins, 2009.

Sheppard DG, Whitman GJ, Fornage BD, et al. Tubular carcinoma of the breast: Mammographic and sonographic features. Am J Roentgenol 2000;174(1):253-257.

Shin HJ, Kim HH, Kim SM, et al. Papillary lesions of the breast diagnosed at percutaneous sonographically guided biopsy: Comparison of sonographic features and biopsy methods. Am J Roentgenol 2008;190(3):630-636.

Sinclair DS, Olsen J, Spigos DG, Freedy L. Phyllodes (phylloides or cystosarcoma phyllodes) tumor: Wide local excision is the preferred method of treatment. Am J Roentgenol 2000;175(3):859-861.

CASE QUESTIONS

CASE 11-1. A 62-year-old woman with screening MRI. What is the most likely diagnosis of the left breast mass?

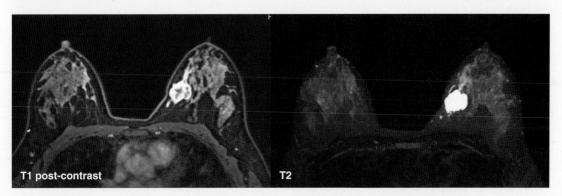

CASE 11-2. A 47-year-old woman for screening. What are your BI-RADS assessment and differential diagnosis for the mass in the right breast at 10 o'clock? *(Reprinted with permission from Harvey JA. Unusual breast cancers: Useful clues to expanding the differential diagnosis. Radiology 2007;242:683-694.)*

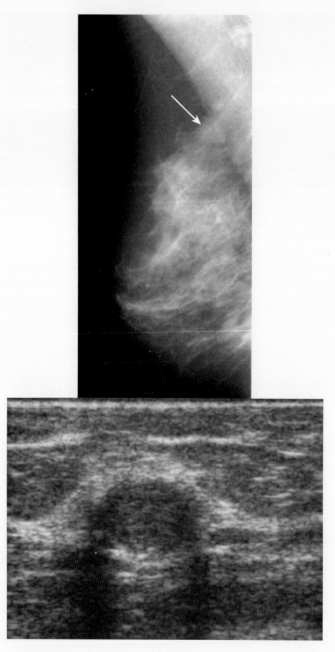

CASE 11-3. A 58-year-old woman with rapidly growing mass noted about 6 months earlier. What might you consider in the differential diagnosis?

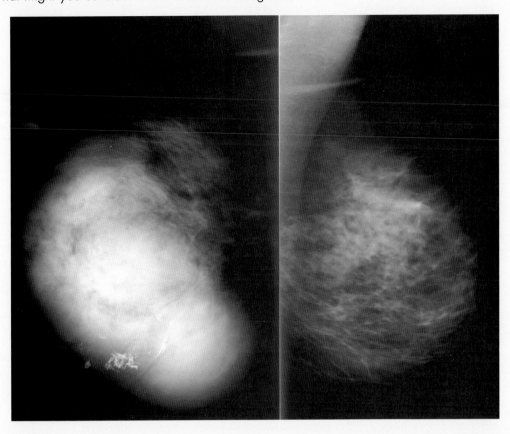

CASE 11-4. A 22-year-old woman presents with a rapidly growing mass in the left breast. What is the most likely diagnosis?

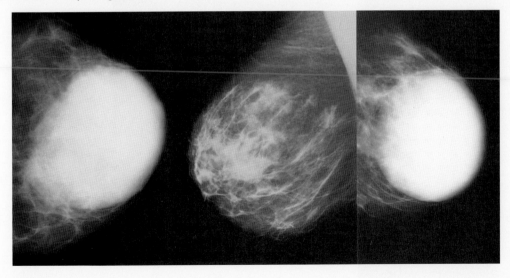

CASE 11-5. A 20-year-old woman who is 8 months pregnant presents for evaluation of several palpable lumps in both breasts. What is the most likely diagnosis given her US below? The other palpable lumps all looked similar. How would you manage her?

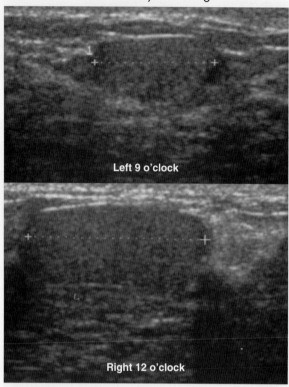

CASE 11-6. Ultrasound-guided core biopsy of the mass below (*arrow*) shows tubular adenoma. What is your recommendation given the imaging findings and result?

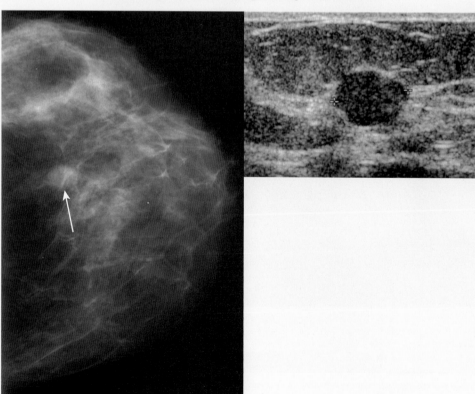

CASE 11-7. A 64-year-old woman with a history of left mastectomy is recalled from screening for diagnostic mammography and US. Which subtype of invasive ductal carcinoma is the most likely diagnosis?

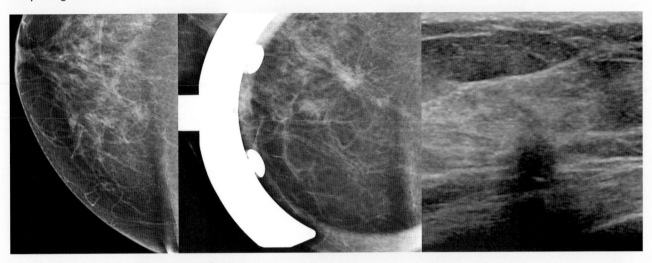

CASE 11-8. A 73-year-old woman presents with a palpable mass in her right breast. What is the most likely diagnosis based on the diagnostic mammogram and US?

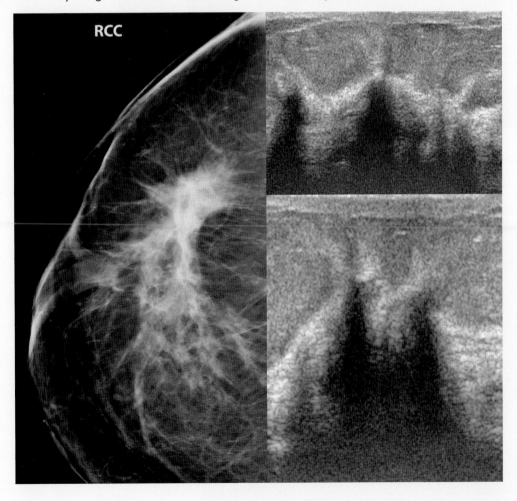

CASE 11-9. This 69-year-old woman was recalled from screening to evaluate a developing asymmetry (*arrow*). US was negative. Stereotactic biopsy shows pseudoangiomatous stromal hyperplasia. What do you recommend?

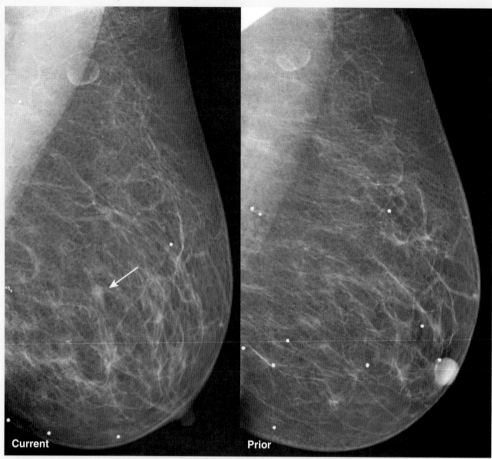

CASE 11-10. A 31-year-old woman at high risk due to family history of breast cancer has a suspicious enhancing mass on screening MRI. It is hyperintense on T2. The MRI-guided biopsy shows stromal fibrosis and focal mucin deposition. What is your recommendation for this biopsy result?

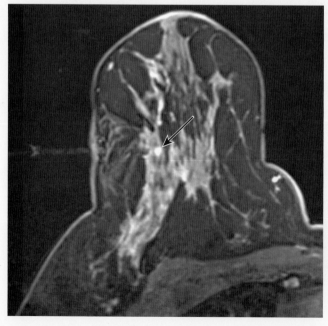

CASE 11-11. This 41-year-old woman is recalled due to architectural distortion (*arrows*) on her baseline screening mammogram. A corresponding mass is identified on US (*arrows*). What is your differential diagnosis? Ultrasound-guided core biopsy shows florid hyperplasia without atypia. What is your recommendation?

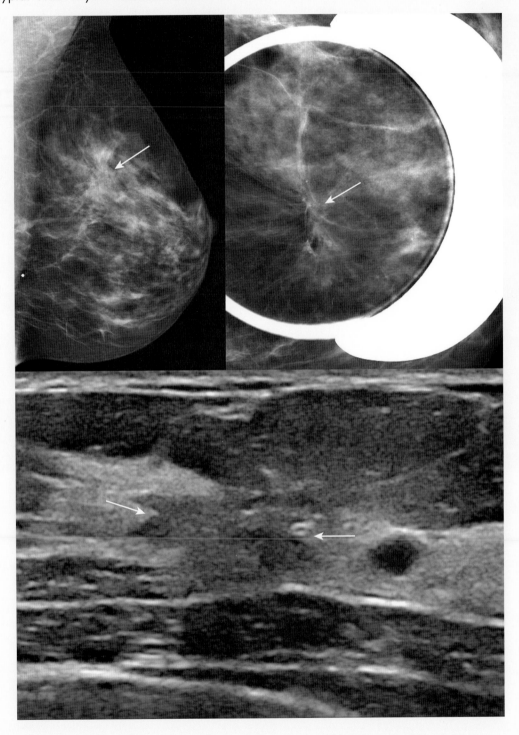

CASE 11-12. This 52-year-old woman has a very firm palpable lump measuring about 5 cm in the lower inner quadrant of her right breast (marked by the *triangle*). Below are her diagnostic mammogram and US. What are the findings? What is your differential diagnosis? BI-RADS assessment?

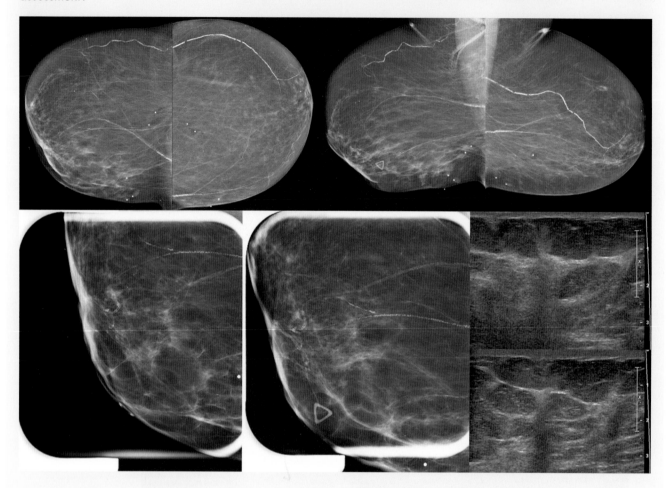

CASE ANSWERS

CASE 11-1. This is suspicious for a mucinous carcinoma. The mass is hyperintense on T2, but has heterogeneous enhancement and ill-defined margins. This should not be mistaken for a fibroadenoma.

CASE 11-2. This mass resembles a fibroadenoma, but the margins are ill-defined, and there are some internal cleft-like cystic spaces. This is concerning for phyllodes tumor, BI-RADS 4. USCNB confirmed the diagnosis. Although phyllodes tumor typically presents as a rapidly growing palpable mass in a middle-aged or older woman, these tumors may occasionally be detected at screening.

CASE 11-3. A rapidly growing mass should always be concerning for either a very poorly differentiated IDC, carcinosarcoma, or phyllodes tumor. Did you notice the coarse calcifications? The diagnosis in this case is phyllodes tumor with osteosarcomatous and chondrosarcomatous degeneration. The prognosis is poor when sarcomatous elements are present within a phyllodes tumor.

CASE 11-4. A large, rapidly growing, round or oval mass in a middle-aged or older woman would be most concerning for phyllodes tumor. However, this is a young woman, and giant fibroadenoma—which this represents—would be most likely.

CASE 11-5. The masses are all oval, circumscribed, and homogeneously hypoechoic with a parallel orientation. The findings suggest lactating adenomas.

Biopsy is tricky here. Doing an ultrasound-guided core biopsy may result in a milk fistula this late in pregnancy. A fine-needle aspiration may be reasonable with a smaller risk of fistula. The surgeons will not want to excise anything until after she delivers her baby.

   If these were multiple circumscribed masses on mammography and all similar in appearance, you would most likely give her BI-RADS 2. Instead of biopsy, we elected to see her back in 4 months; she was 3 months post partum and did not choose to breastfeed her infant. The masses decreased considerably in size, consistent with lactating adenomas. No further evaluation was needed.

CASE 11-6. The biopsy result of tubular adenoma is concordant. Tubular adenomas can be managed similarly to fibroadenomas. A follow-up mammogram or US can be performed in 6 to 12 months. Excision is not indicated.

CASE 11-7. Among the major subtypes of IDC, tubular carcinoma is most likely to appear as a small spiculated mass and is the diagnosis in this case. There was DCIS associated with the invasive tumor.

CASE 11-8. Mammography shows a large area of architectural distortion with skin retraction. US reveals extensive shadowing at the edge of the fibroglandular tissue. Diagnosis: ILC.

CASE 11-9. Pseudoangiomatous stromal hyperplasia (PASH) is a concordant result for this developing asymmetry. A mammogram in 6 months is reasonable to ensure stability.

CASE 11-10. The finding of mucin on a core biopsy may be due to a benign mucoceole, but may also be due to mucinous carcinoma. Excision should be recommended. Diagnosis: mucinous carcinoma.

CASE 11-11. There is persistent architectural distortion without a central mass on mammography ("the dark star"). On US, there is an irregular hypoechoic mass with spiculated margins. The echogenicity of the mass on US is higher than that of most breast cancers, and there is no echogenic margin. The appearance on mammography and US suggests that this may represent a radial scar. ILC, IDC-NOS, or tubular carcinoma is also possible. The patient has no history of prior breast surgery, so this is not a surgical scar. Excisional biopsy showed radial scar/complex sclerosing lesion. Core biopsy often does not result in a diagnosis of radial scar because a larger sample is often needed to display the diagnostic morphologic appearance of this lesion. A benign result should be considered discordant, and likely to be a radial scar.

CASE 11-12. There is mild asymmetry in the area of the palpable region in the right breast. There is no distortion or discrete mass on mammography. On US, there are areas of shadowing with sonographic distortion. The presence of a clinically suspicious mass with asymmetry and sonographic shadowing suggests the diagnosis of ILC, which was the diagnosis. Congratulations if you were thinking ILC. Good job!

SCREENING DETECTION

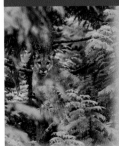

CHAPTER 12

Finding Cancers in Dense Tissue

A blind date: Things are going well, but really, this person could be a serial killer for all you know. How do you get to know him? Sometimes it's easy, but more often it takes time and attention to look for telling signs about his personality and values. Reading mammograms for women with dense breast tissue is likewise a process. Relax. Take your time. Dig in and find that little cancer that will save her life.

Women with dense breast tissue have two strikes against them. They are more likely to be diagnosed with breast cancer, and we are less likely to detect it. Dense tissue is a moderate independent risk factor for breast cancer and is associated with a four- to sixfold increase in breast cancer risk compared with that of women with fatty replaced breasts. The sensitivity of mammography for women with dense tissue is reduced to about 60%. Cancers are most likely to develop within the dense fibroglandular tissue rather than in the surrounding fat, where they might be easier to detect. Our level of concern as radiologists must be heightened for these women because they are at higher risk and have more difficult mammograms to interpret.

Factors Associated with Dense Tissue

In this chapter, "dense" tissue refers to heterogeneously dense and extremely dense fibroglandular tissue composition, as defined in the ACR BI-RADS Atlas. Mammographically dense tissue typically occurs in slightly less than half of screened populations. Younger age is strongly associated with increased mammographic density. In one study, 55% of women under 50 had dense tissue, compared with about 30% of women who were age 50 and older (Box 12-1).

Limitations of Mammography

All of the mammographic signs of malignancy tend to be more difficult to detect in dense tissue, and the reduced sensitivity of mammography in these women has been well established. In a series of over 460,000 women, the sensitivity of screening mammography was 62% when the tissue was extremely dense and 88% when it was almost entirely fatty. Other studies have even worse results, with sensitivity ranging from 29% to 50% for women with dense breast tissue.

Interpreting these dense mammograms is difficult but not impossible. We need to work really hard for these women to find their cancers! Keep in mind that many nonpalpable cancers remain detectable even when the tissue is extremely dense. For example, cancers that develop within the retromammary fat, are located at the border of the fibroglandular tissue, or are associated with calcifications are often readily perceived.

Detection of malignant lesions by ultrasonography (US) and magnetic resonance imaging (MRI) is less limited by dense tissue, and their use, according to established indications, will also provide your patients with dense tissue the chance for earlier cancer detection (Fig. 12-1).

Evaluating Findings in Dense Tissue

Technical Considerations

You can't get to know someone if you never meet the person. When the tissue is dense, it is particularly important to insist on a study of at least good technical quality, with proper exposure, compression, and absence of significant motion. The signs of cancer are often subtle even with the highest quality imaging; they may become undetectable on a technically limited study. Of course, poor positioning also reduces our ability to find cancer. As the saying goes, "If it's not on the image, you can't make the diagnosis." Don't let your ability to interpret a study be compromised by positioning or other technical factors. Recall the patient to have the limited views repeated.

Digital mammography has been shown to be superior to film-screen mammography in diagnostic accuracy in a screened population of women with heterogeneously dense or extremely dense tissue. Therefore, for facilities with both digital and film-screen mammography equipment, triaging women with dense tissue for imaging using the digital equipment may be beneficial.

Tomosynthesis is a digital mammographic technique that acquires multiple images from different angles that are processed for three-dimensional review. The first commercial unit received Food and Drug Administration (FDA) approval in 2011. This technique overcomes many of the limitations caused by tissue overlap. Although the most appropriate clinical use of this technology remains to be defined, it shows particular promise in improving the detection and characterization of soft tissue density lesions within dense tissue.

Screening US detected 3 additional cancers per 1000 high-risk women also screened with mammography in the ACRIN 6666 trial. Because of low specificity, the use of screening US remains controversial for women with the indication of dense breasts without other risk factors. The positive predictive value for cancer when biopsy was recommended was only 7% in the ACRIN 6666 trial and may be lower for women of moderate risk. We will focus on mammography in this chapter. For more information on nonmammographic screening, please see Chapter 13, Measuring and Managing Breast Cancer Risk.

Callback Threshold

In dense tissue, masses are often obscured and calcifications may be less conspicuous. The findings that are visualized may represent the "tip of the iceberg"—part of a more extensive lesion that is mostly obscured. It therefore makes sense to lower your threshold for recalling screening patients for diagnostic evaluation, to more fully evaluate subtle findings that are not well characterized on the screening views alone.

Getting to Know You

Let's think about that first date again. What are your techniques for getting to know someone? What is your first impression? Are there any apparent red flags? If not, then you are probably going to do the easy stuff, like finding out about common interests. What is his job? What are his hobbies? Things are going well. We've made it to the second date. Now you are going to dig deeper by assessing personality traits. Is he going to make you crazy by leaving off the toothpaste top? Or is he going to make you arrange 18 pillows on the couch correctly? Assuming that he makes it past that point, now you really need to know if he is a "keeper." You need to go very deep by understanding his values. Is family important? Is he honest and kind? Oh my, did he really just damage that person's car and keep driving?

Interpretation of dense mammograms is similar (Fig. 12-2). We'll start with that first impression. Lean back in your chair and get the big picture. Next, start with the easy stuff—the retroglandular fat (one of the "wrong neighborhoods" discussed in the Chapter 3, Screening Mammography 101 and Beyond). Then we dig in deeper. Look at the border between the fibroglandular tissue

---

BOX 12-1 Factors Associated with Higher Density Tissue on Mammography

- Younger age
- Lower body mass index
- Later menarche
- Later age of first birth
- Lower parity
- Genetic tendency
- Use of hormone replacement therapy

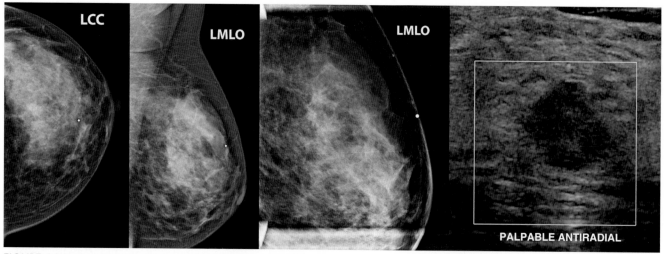

FIGURE 12-1 **Negative Mammogram with Suspicious US Findings.** A 37-year-old woman with a palpable mass in her left breast (marked with a BB). Mammography shows dense tissue with no detectable abnormalities on routine or magnified views. US reveals a hypoechoic mass with indistinct margins within the echogenic fibroglandular tissue. Diagnosis: invasive ductal carcinoma (IDC), grade III.

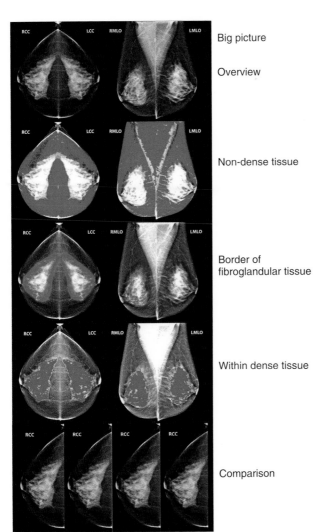

FIGURE 12-2 **Search Pattern for Dense Tissue Mammograms.** Work your way in. Using this search pattern is a good way to develop your approach to reading a dense tissue mammogram that will thoroughly evaluate these difficult studies. As your reading style matures, your approach will become less formal.

and fat. Then comes the really hard part: focus on the dense tissue, looking for subtle masses, calcifications, distortion, and asymmetries. Finally, compare the study carefully with mammograms that are at least 2 years older.

While interpreting these studies, remember to keep using all of the good habits you have already developed (reviewed in Chapter 3); minimize interruptions and use consistent hanging protocols and search patterns. The use of computer-aided detection is also a good strategy for reviewing these difficult mammograms.

First Impressions

Let's look at each step in a little more detail. We'll start with the first impression. At our biopsy review conference, we sometimes have a case in which the resident cannot see the lesion to save his soul. His face is inches from the screen as he searches and sweats. Meanwhile, the resident in the back of the room immediately sees the finding and wonders why her colleague is struggling.

Start the review of every mammogram by looking at the big picture. Findings that may be easier to see when leaning back in your chair include abnormalities of the skin and nipples (Figs. 12-3 and 12-4), differences in breast size and compressibility, and large asymmetries. Asymmetry of breast size on mammography—reflecting reduced compressibility of the tissue—is a sign of invasive lobular carcinoma (ILC) that may be detected on the overview interpretation of the images (see Fig. 12-4).

The Easy Part (What Do You Like to Do in Your Spare Time?)

The easy areas of the dense mammogram are those that are fatty. Even when the fibroglandular tissue is extremely dense, there are usually regions that contain enough fat to allow detection of small lesions (Fig. 12-5). These areas include the subcutaneous and retroglandular tissues, the axillary tail, and the axilla. Asymmetries in the posterior breast that are outside the fibroglandular tissue deserve careful scrutiny, since they are frequently found to

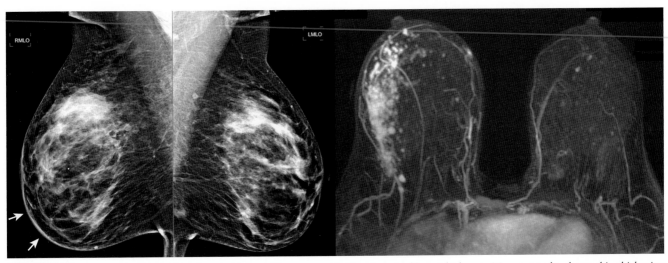

FIGURE 12-3 **Asymmetric Skin Thickening.** A 39-year-old woman with "heaviness" of her right breast. Mammography shows skin thickening on the right (*arrows*). No other mammographic or sonographic abnormalities were seen. MRI (maximum intensity projection) shows extensive non-mass enhancement in the lateral right breast. Diagnosis: ILC.

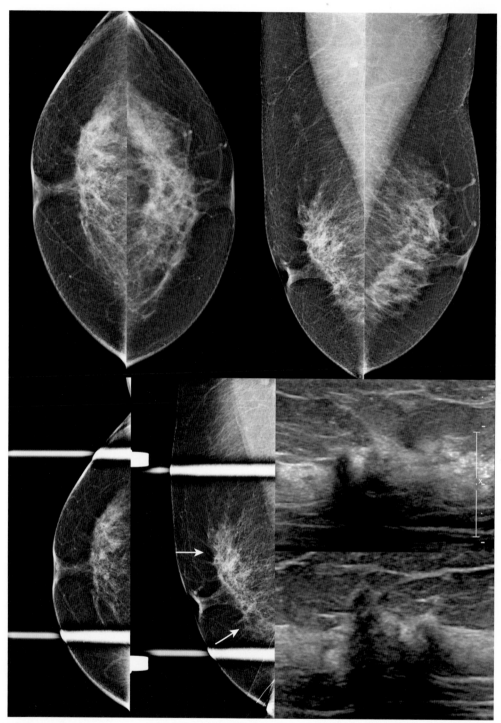

FIGURE 12-4 **Nipple Retraction with a Suspicious US.** Screening mammogram on a 50-year-old woman. The overview review of the mammogram shows right nipple retraction. There is also straightening of the anterior edge of the fibroglandular tissue (best seen on the mediolateral oblique view). The right breast is slightly smaller than the left. Spot compression views show architectural distortion with spicules extending into the subcutaneous fat (*arrows*). US with harmonic imaging shows ill-defined hypoechoic shadowing lesions within the echogenic fibroglandular tissue. Diagnosis: ILC.

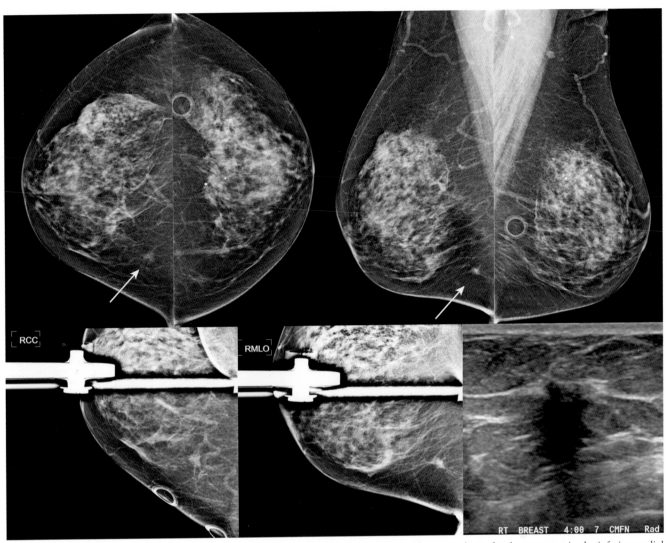

FIGURE 12-5 **Lesion in the Retromammary Fat.** Screening mammogram on a 68-year-old woman shows focal asymmetry in the inferior medial right breast lying outside the dense fibroglandular tissue (*arrows*). An irregular mass with spiculated margins is seen on spot compression views and US. Diagnosis: IDC.

be malignant. Axillary masses or adenopathy are often well visualized in women with dense fibroglandular tissue.

Going a Little Deeper (What Kind of Personality and Values Does He Have?)

Now we are going to dig in a little. Let's work our way into the tissue by looking at the fibroglandular border—the interface of the dense tissue with the subcutaneous and retroglandular fat. The fat adjacent to this border provides contrast that can make malignancies that develop in this region more conspicuous. The contour of this border should be closely examined and compared with the contralateral breast and with previous mammograms as part of the standard routine.

Although the mammographic appearance of the fibroglandular border varies greatly among patients and is affected by positioning, abrupt changes in this contour can be a sign of malignancy. Look at this border as though it were a road (Box 12-2). Are there potholes?

BOX 12-2 Border Patrol

- Retraction (pot hole)
- Protrusion (speed bump)
- Straightening or spicules (road hazard)

Retraction of the fibroglandular border can be caused by desmoplastic reaction that is commonly associated with invasive malignancies (Fig. 12-6). Are there speed bumps? Soft tissue density protrusions into the fat that alter the contour of the fibroglandular border can also signify the presence of a partially obscured mass (Fig. 12-7). A fallen tree in the way? Even if a cancer is mostly obscured by dense tissue, spicules may be visible extending from the fibroglandular border into the adjacent fat (Figs. 12-8 and 12-9).

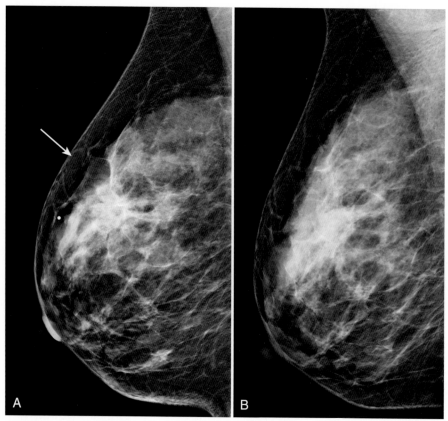

FIGURE 12-6 **Abnormal Tissue Contour with Retraction of the Fibroglandular Border.** A 52-year-old-woman presenting with a palpable right breast mass (**A**). There is architectural distortion with radiating lines within the dense tissue and retraction of the edge of the fibroglandular tissue (*arrow*). These findings are new since the previous mammogram (**B**). Diagnosis: ILC.

Evaluation of the apex of the breast—the most superior aspect of the triangular edge of tissue on the mediolateral oblique (MLO) view—can be challenging, especially in the case of women with dense tissue. The fibroglandular tissue often overlaps in this region, resulting in summation that may mimic a mass. Side-to-side right/left comparison and comparison with prior mammograms can be helpful in deciding whether or not to recall the patient.

As we work our way a little deeper into the peripheral breast tissue, the tissue is often still not extremely dense. This is a zone where cancers are commonly detected in women under 50. In this region, cancers may appear as an area that is a little more dense than the surrounding tissues (Figs. 12-10 and 12-11).

Finding Cancers Within the Dense Fibroglandular Tissue

Okay, the easy stuff is over. Good first impression. He flosses. He was nice to the server at the restaurant. You've gotten to know him. He seems kind of compulsive but hopefully that means there won't be dirty dishes left lying around. Now comes the hard part. Does he have a heart of gold? Will he be good to you and your family and friends? Will he stick around when life gets hard?

We have to stick around and keep our focus if we're going to find cancers within dense tissue. Finding these cancers is a challenge that directly confronts the primary limitation of mammography. It has been likened to finding a snowman in a snow storm. However, a complete white-out is rare. Even extremely dense tissue usually isn't *homogeneously* dense, especially with the higher contrast provided by digital mammography. Finding cancers in dense tissue is more like finding your kids when they are hiding in the yard. They are only partially camouflaged by the trees and shrubs. Likewise, there are almost always oval fat lobules of variable size scattered throughout the dense tissue, or bands of fat extending through it. This fatty tissue may provide enough contrast to allow visualization of small cancers. Look for areas that are more dense or appear different from the rest of the tissue. Check closely for associated findings that may increase the level of suspicion, and tilt your decision in favor of recall for diagnostic evaluation.

Masses

Portions of a mass margin may be detectable even when it is mostly obscured by dense tissue (Figs. 12-12 and 12-13). Keep in mind, however, that even large masses can be mostly or completely obscured by dense tissue.

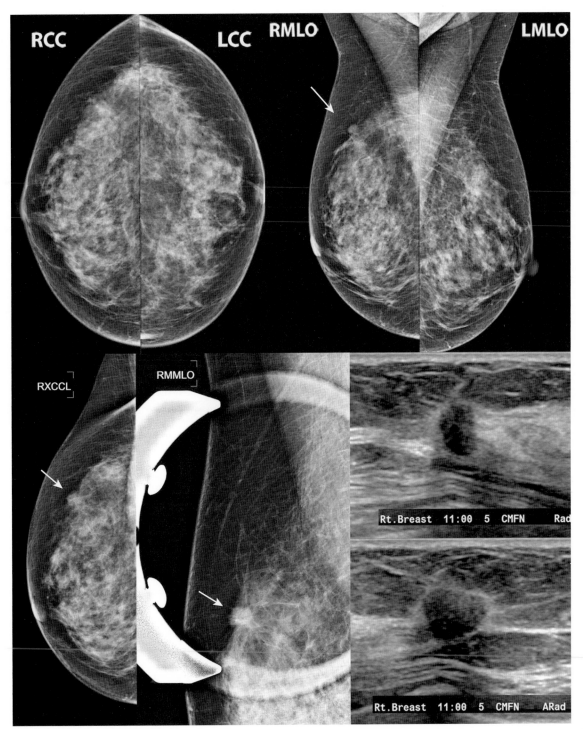

FIGURE 12-7 **Contour Abnormality with Protrusion at the Fibroglandular Border.** Screening mammogram on a 41-year-old woman with heterogeneously dense tissue. On the MLO view, there is oval asymmetry at the edge of the fibroglandular tissue in the superior right breast protruding into the adjacent fat. Laterally exaggerated craniocaudal (CC) and spot magnification MLO views show an irregular mass with small spicules arising from its margins (*arrows*). US shows the mass to be solid with nonparallel orientation in the radial plane. Diagnosis: IDC.

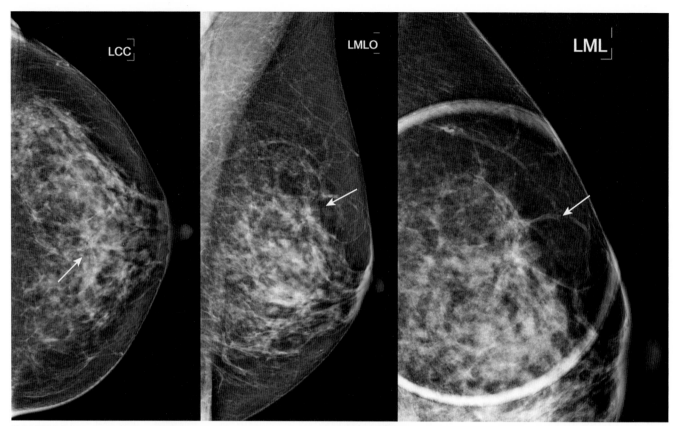

FIGURE 12-8 **Spicules at the Fibroglandular Border.** Screening mammogram of a 51-year-old woman shows architectural distortion at the superior edge of the fibroglandular tissue (*arrows*) with spicules extending into the adjacent fat. Diagnosis: IDC.

Women with dense tissue often have very lumpy breast tissue, resulting in difficult clinical and breast self-examination. Large cancers that are palpable may be considered part of the background lumpiness of a woman's examination. Clinicians need our help as much as we need theirs with these patients.

Calcifications

Calcifications attenuate x-rays more effectively than any other normal structures in the breast. However, they are often less conspicuous in dense tissue because of reduced contrast between the calcifications and the background tissue. Coarse heterogeneous calcifications are usually large enough to be readily visualized in dense tissue; fine pleomorphic and amorphous calcifications may be quite subtle and difficult to detect.

Frequently, many more calcifications can be seen on magnification views than are evident on screening, and their morphologic appearance and distribution are often more accurately assessed (Fig. 12-14). Magnification views should always be obtained before recommending short-interval follow-up or biopsy of calcifications.

When calcifications are detected within dense tissue, associated masses, architectural distortion (AD), and asymmetries are more likely to be obscured. These soft tissue density components often become apparent on diagnostic mammographic views or US.

Malignant lesions may be much larger than suggested by the calcifications; even a few sparse calcifications may be an indication of extensive disease. If linear calcifications are seen that are not typically secretory or vascular, consider recall for magnification views. These are particularly suspicious in premenopausal women, who are much less likely than older women to develop secretory or vascular calcifications (Fig. 12-15).

Architectural Distortion

There may be sufficient fat to visualize some of the radiating lines of AD, even within extremely dense tissue (Fig. 12-16). Masses with spiculated margins may appear as AD in dense tissue, when the central mass is obscured. In such cases, the mass-like nature of the lesion will usually be demonstrated on additional mammographic views and US.

Asymmetries

In dense tissue, masses are more likely to have obscured margins and to present with the more subtle findings of focal asymmetries or single-view asymmetries (Fig.

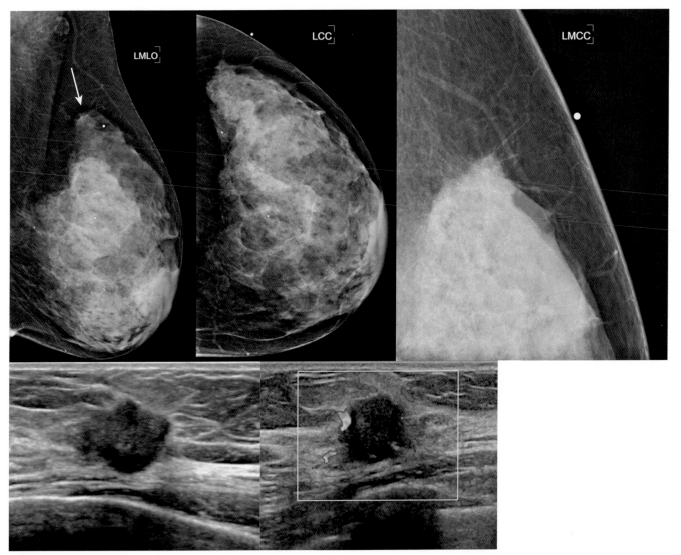

FIGURE 12-9 **Abnormal Density at Breast Apex.** A 60-year-old woman with extremely dense tissue presents with a palpable mass in her left breast. There is a subtle increased density with fine pleomorphic calcifications at the edge of the fibroglandular tissue. On the CC magnification view, fine spicules radiate from the mass, which is mostly obscured, into the subcutaneous fat. US reveals a hypoechoic mass with angular margins. Diagnosis: ILC.

12-17). Interpretation of mammograms with dense tissue should include careful examination of asymmetries, especially those that are most dense. Asymmetries should be closely examined for radiating spicules, calcifications, and other associated findings. They should also be compared with previous mammograms to determine whether they are new or have increased in size or density over time (i.e., represent developing asymmetries).

Even large masses may present as one-view asymmetries in dense tissue due to obscuration of the lesion on one view. One-view asymmetries detected at screening are more difficult to dismiss as summation artifacts when the tissue is dense because deconstruction of overlapping tissue is not always possible. When an asymmetry is new or enlarging, recall for diagnostic evaluation is generally warranted.

Use of Other Modalities

US and MRI are powerful modalities in breast imaging that are less impeded by dense tissue than is mammography. It is important to be familiar with the established indications for these modalities and to recognize clinical circumstances where their use is appropriate. The value of these modalities in detecting potentially curable cancers will be greatest in your patients with dense tissue, for whom mammography is most limited. The American Cancer Society and Society of Breast Imaging do not currently recommend for or against either screening MRI or screening US for women with dense breast tissue who are otherwise at average risk for breast cancer. However, this is an evolving issue that varies by locality and practice.

Text continued on p. 334

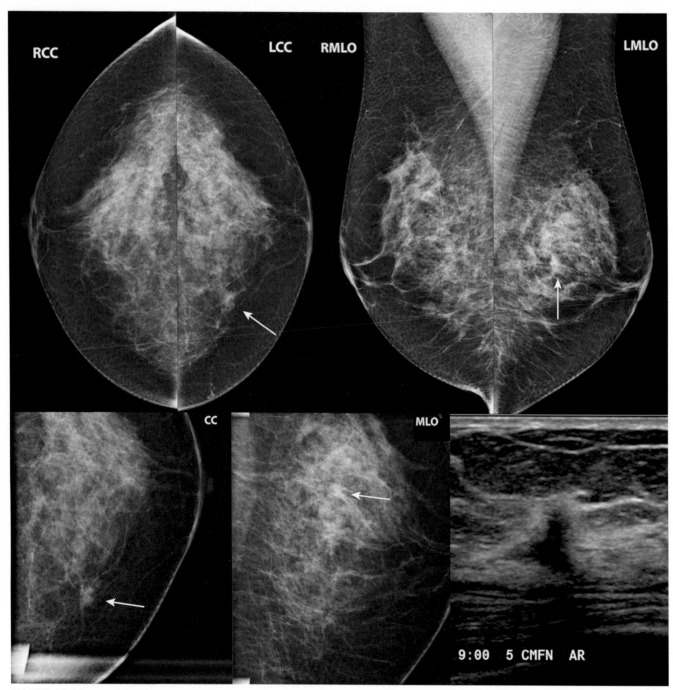

FIGURE 12-10 **Subtle Mass That Is Denser Than the Surrounding Tissue.** Screening mammogram on a 56-year-old woman shows focal asymmetry associated with faint amorphous calcifications in the medial left breast, at the edge of the fibroglandular tissue (*arrows*). US shows an irregular hypoechoic mass with angular margins. Diagnosis: IDC.

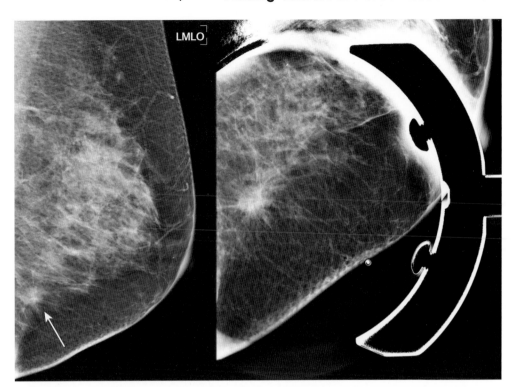

FIGURE 12-11 **Subtle Distortion and Increased Density with a Small Cancer.** A 60-year-old woman with a screening-detected mass in the inferior left breast, at the edge of the fibroglandular tissue (*arrow*). The lesion is higher in density than the adjacent tissue. A spot compression MLO view demonstrates spiculated margins. Diagnosis: infiltrating lobular carcinoma.

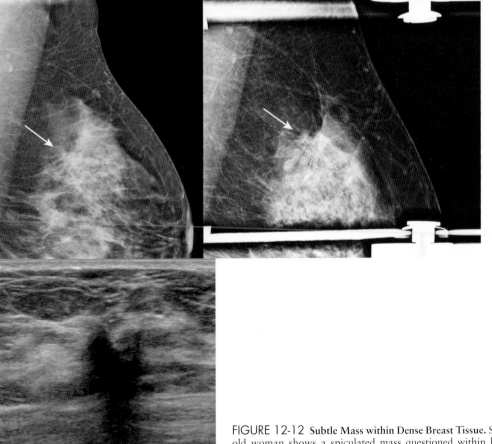

FIGURE 12-12 **Subtle Mass within Dense Breast Tissue.** Screening mammogram of a 54-year-old woman shows a spiculated mass questioned within heterogeneously dense tissue in the superior left breast on the screening MLO view (*arrow*). This finding is confirmed on a spot compression mediolateral (ML) view (*arrow*), and an irregular hypoechoic mass is seen by US. Diagnosis: infiltrating carcinoma with ductal and lobular features with high-grade ductal carcinoma in situ (DCIS).

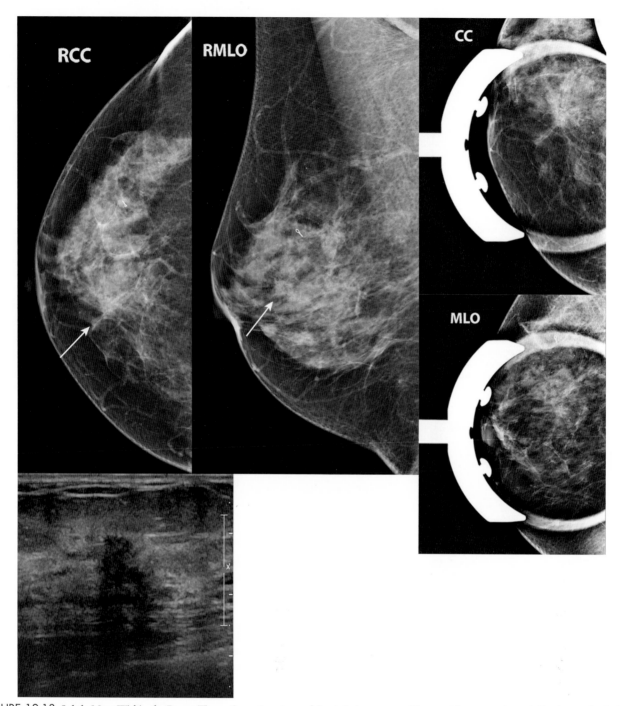

FIGURE 12-13 **Subtle Mass Within the Breast Tissue.** Screening views of the right breast on a 52-year-old woman. A partially obscured spiculated mass is questioned within dense fibroglandular tissue (*arrows*). The finding persists on spot compression views, and US shows a corresponding irregular shadowing mass. Diagnosis: IDC and DCIS.

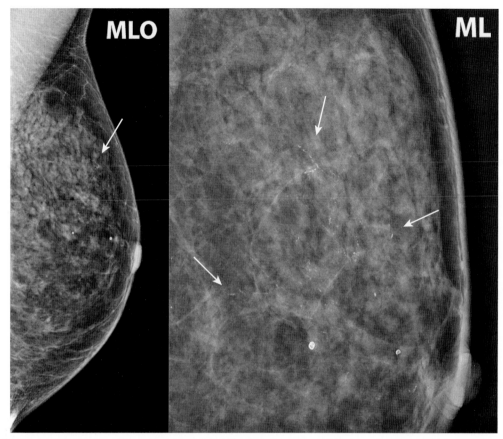

FIGURE 12-14 **Malignant Calcifications More Obvious on Magnification.** Screening MLO view of a 46-year-old woman shows heterogeneously dense tissue with faint calcifications in the superior left breast. Magnified ML view shows fine linear calcifications with segmental distribution. The morphologic appearance and distribution of the calcifications are much more accurately assessed with magnification. Diagnosis: high-grade DCIS.

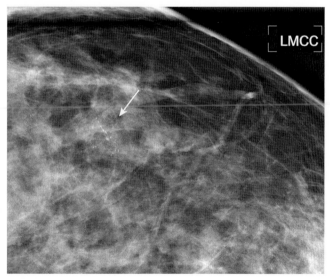

FIGURE 12-15 **Malignant Calcifications in Dense Tissue.** Magnified CC view of a 49-year-old woman showing a small cluster of fine linear calcifications within dense tissue. She is rather young to have vascular calcifications and has none elsewhere. These are suspicious and warrant biopsy (BI-RADS 4). Diagnosis: DCIS.

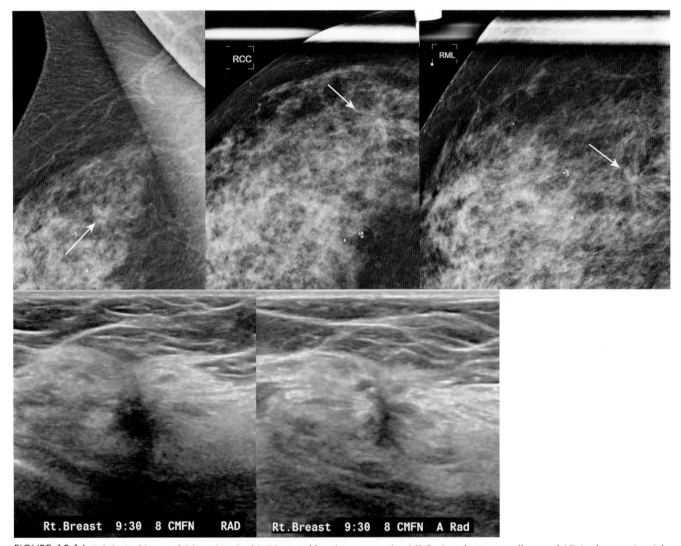

FIGURE 12-16 **Subtle Architectural Distortion.** In this 75-year-old patient a screening MLO view shows a small area of AD in the superior right breast that persists on spot compression views (*arrows*). US shows an irregular hypoechoic mass with spiculated margins within the fibroglandular tissue. Diagnosis: IDC.

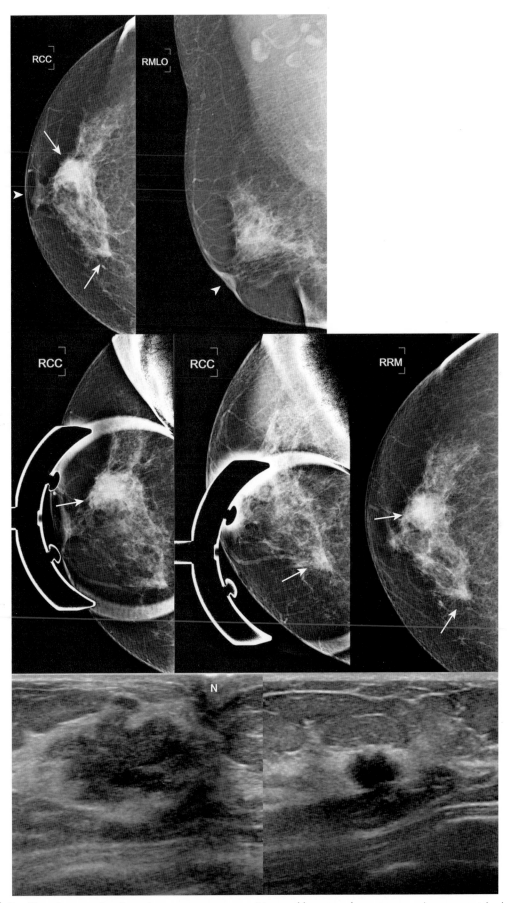

FIGURE 12-17 **One-View Asymmetries.** Screening mammogram on a 74-year-old woman shows two one-view asymmetries in the right breast visible on the CC view (*arrows*). The right nipple is retracted (*arrowheads*). Diagnostic views reveal two masses with ill-defined margins, and US shows corresponding masses in the 12 o'clock and 2 o'clock positions (N = nipple). Biopsy of both masses revealed IDC with DCIS.

KEY POINTS

- The sensitivity of mammography is lower when the tissue is dense; however, many cancers remain detectable. These women are also at moderately increased risk for breast cancer.
- Working from the outside in is an effective search pattern for dense breasts—big picture, fatty areas, fibroglandular tissue border, and finally the very dense tissue.
- Questioned abnormalities on screening should be further evaluated on diagnostic mammography and frequently US. Malignant findings are more likely to be partially obscured and underestimated in extent when the tissue is dense.
- US (and sometimes MRI) is particularly useful in women with dense tissue, where mammography is most limited.

References

ACR Practice Guidelines for the Performance of a Breast Ultrasound Examination. Reston, VA, American College of Radiology, 2007.

ACR Practice Guidelines for the Performance of Contrast-Enhanced Magnetic Resonance Imaging (MRI) of the Breast. Reston, VA, American College of Radiology, 2008.

American College of Radiology. ACR BI-RADS: Mammography. In ACR Breast Imaging Reporting and Data System, Breast Imaging Atlas, 4th ed. Reston, VA, American College of Radiology, 2003.

Berg WA, Blume JD, Cormack JB, et al. Combined screening with ultrasound and mammography vs. mammography alone in women at elevated risk of breast cancer. JAMA 2008;299:2151-2163.

Boyd NF, Dite GS, Stone J, et al. Heritability of mammographic density, a risk factor for breast cancer. N Engl J Med 2002;347:886-894.

Buist DSM, Porter PL, Lehman C, et al. Factors contributing to mammography failure in women aged 40-49 years. J Natl Cancer Inst 2004;96:1432-1440.

Carney PA, Miglioretti DL, Yankaskas BC, et al. Individual and combined effects of age, breast density, and hormone replacement therapy use on the accuracy of screening mammography. Ann Intern Med 2003;138:168-175.

Harvey JA, Fechner RE, Moore, MM. Apparent ipsilateral decrease in breast size at mammography: A sign of infiltrating lobular carcinoma. Radiology 2000;214:883-889.

Pisano ED Gatsonis C, Hendrick E, et al. Diagnostic performance of digital versus film mammography for breast-cancer screening. N Engl J Med 2005;1773-1783.

Saslow D, Boetes C, Burke W, et al. American cancer society guidelines for breast screening with MRI as an adjunct to mammography. CA Cancer J Clin 2007;57:75-89.

Stacey-Clear A, McCarthy KA, Hall DA, et al. Mammographically detected breast cancer: Location in women under 50 years old. Radiology 1993;186:677-680.

Stomper PC, D'Souza DJ, DiNitto PA, Arredondo MA. Analysis of parenchymal density on mammograms in 1353 women 25-79 years old. AJR 1996;167:1261-1265.

Taplin SH, Rutter CM, Finder C, et al. Screening mammography: Clinical image quality and the risk of interval breast cancer. AJR 2002;178:797-803.

Ursin G, Hovanessian-Larsen L, Parisky YR, et al. Greatly increased occurrence of breast cancers in areas of mammographically dense tissue. Breast Cancer Res 2005;7:605-608.

CASE QUESTIONS

CASE 12-1. Screening mammogram on a 51-year-old woman with heterogeneously dense tissue. What are the findings? What are your BI-RADS assessment and recommendation?

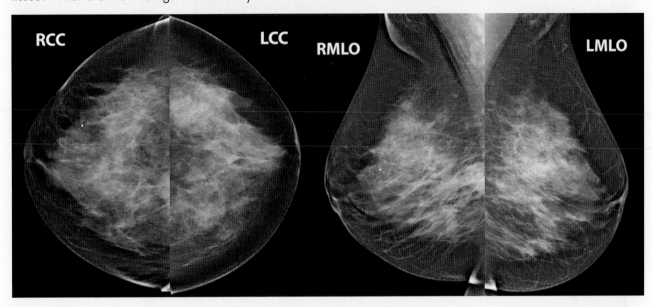

CASE 12-2. Screening mammogram on a 69-year-old-woman. What is the finding? Your BI-RADS assessment and recommendation?

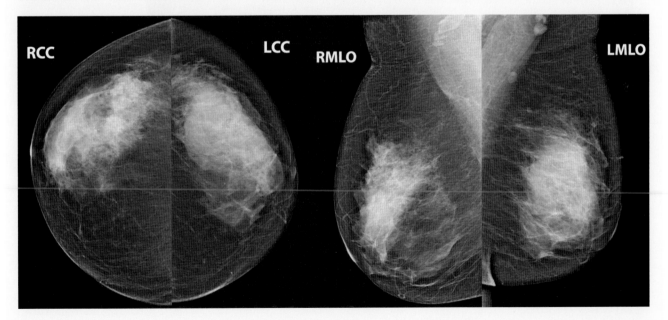

CASE 12-3. Screening mammogram on a 49-year-old-woman with extremely dense tissue. What are your assessment and recommendation?

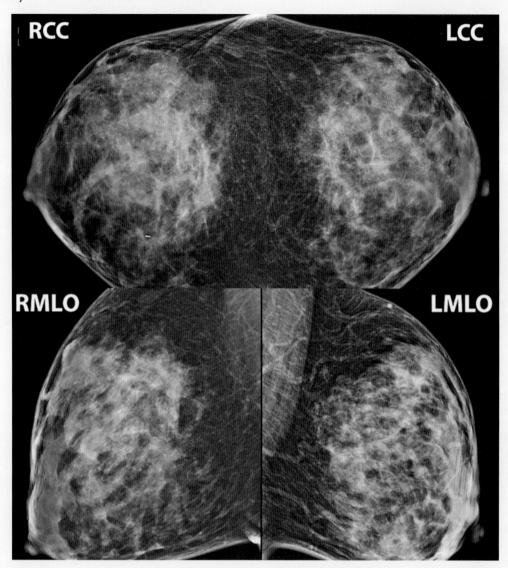

CASE 12-4. Screening mammogram on a 42-year-old-woman. One-view asymmetry in the central left breast on the CC view was stable. What is the abnormal finding? What are your BI-RADS assessment and recommendation?

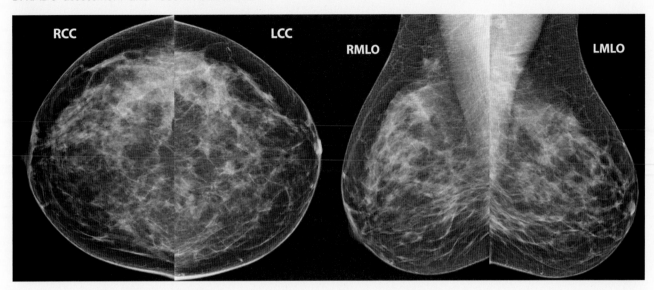

CASE 12-5. Screening mammogram on a 56-year-old-woman with heterogeneously dense tissue. Let's look through those tree branches. Anything catch your eye?

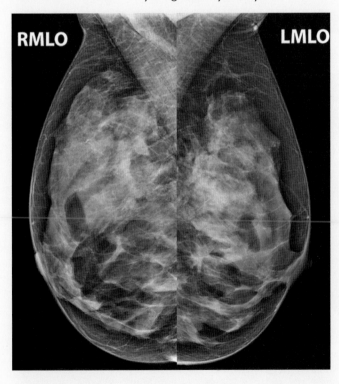

CASE 12-6. Screening mammogram on a 56-year-old woman. It's time for border patrol! What is the significant finding? Your BI-RADS assessment and recommendation? The low-density mass in the medial right breast was stable and can be disregarded.

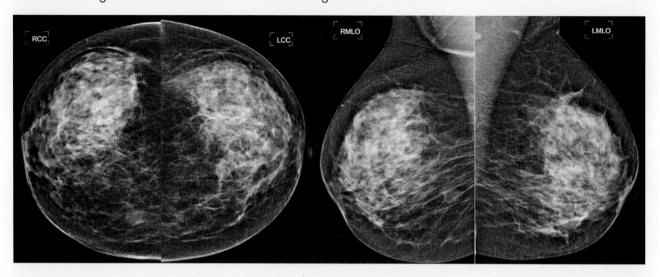

CASE 12-7. A 70-year-old woman is recalled for evaluation of new calcifications in her left breast. How would you describe the findings? What are your BI-RADS assessment and recommendation?

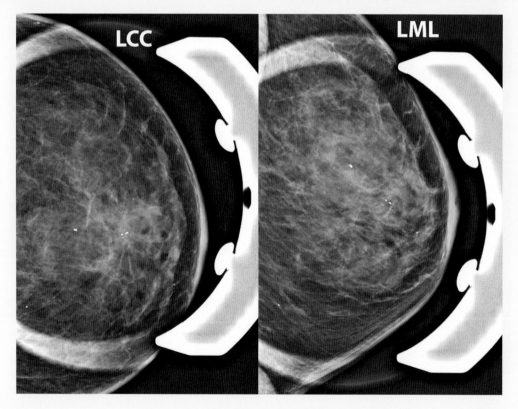

CASE 12-8. Screening mammogram of a 43-year-old woman. Anything catch your eye?

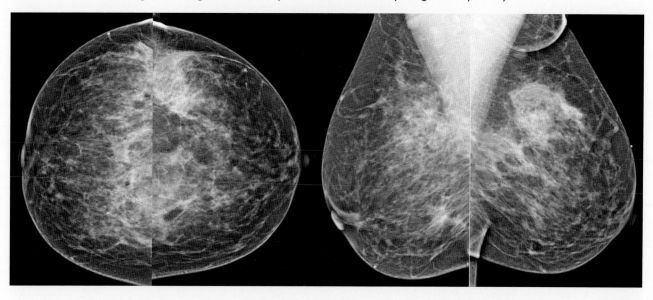

CASE 12-9. Screening mammogram on a 45-year-old woman. What is the finding? What do you recommend?

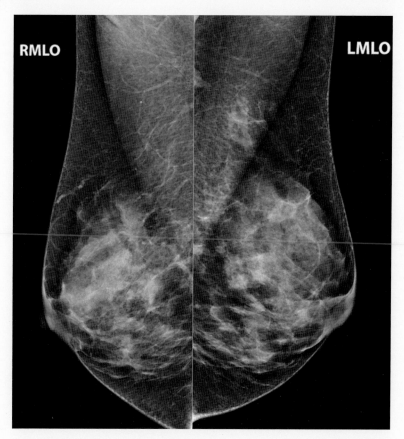

CASE 12-10. Initial screening mammogram on a 47-year-old woman. How would you describe the abnormality? What are your BI-RADS assessment and recommendation?

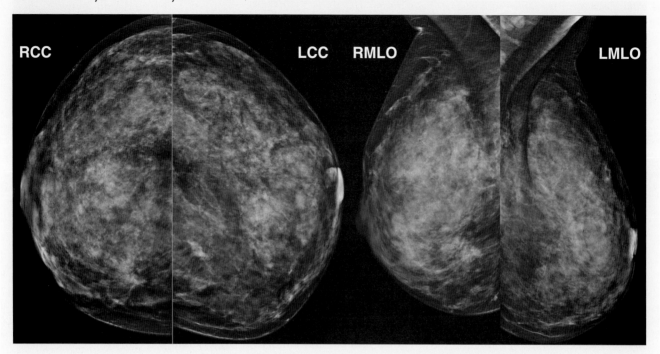

CASE ANSWERS

CASE 12-1. BI-RADS 0: Recall for diagnostic mammography and US. There is a partially visualized mass in the retroglandular fat of the right breast. On spot compression views, the margins of the mass are shown to be spiculated. Postcontrast MRI with fat saturation shows the mass abutting the pectoralis major. There is no pectoralis muscle enhancement to indicate invasion. Diagnosis: IDC grade III. Masses and asymmetries in the retroglandular fat should be viewed with suspicion because normal fibroglandular tissue is unusual in this region.

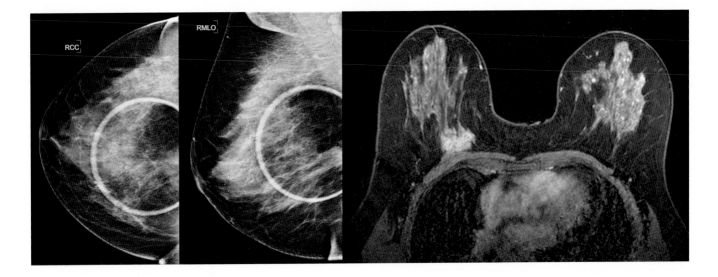

CASE 12-2. BI-RADS 0: Recall for diagnostic mammogram and possible US. There is one-view asymmetry in the lateral left breast on the CC view with a convex margin extending into the retroglandular fat. An obscured mass may be present.

A mass was confirmed on rolled CC and ML views. US shows a complex mass in the 3 o'clock position with flow in the solid component on Doppler examination. Diagnosis: IDC, grade III. Even large masses may be mostly obscured in dense tissue. A portion of a convex margin may be the only visible finding.

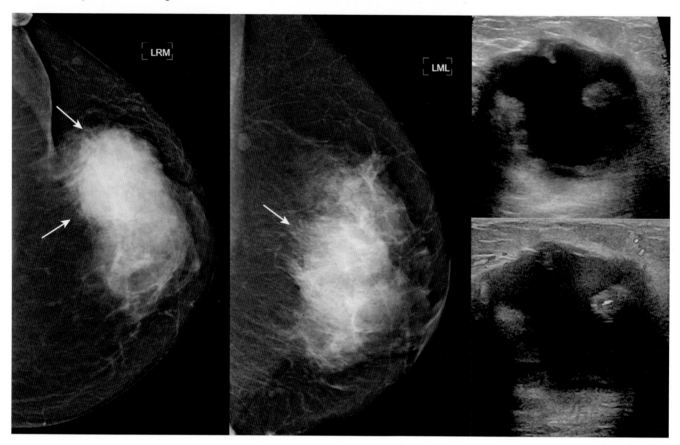

CASE 12-3. There is a 4 mm mass in the retroglandular fat of the left breast (*arrows*). The finding persists on rolled and spot magnified CC views. US shows a solid mass with indistinct margins. BI-RADS 4. Ultrasound-guided core biopsy revealed IDC, grade II.

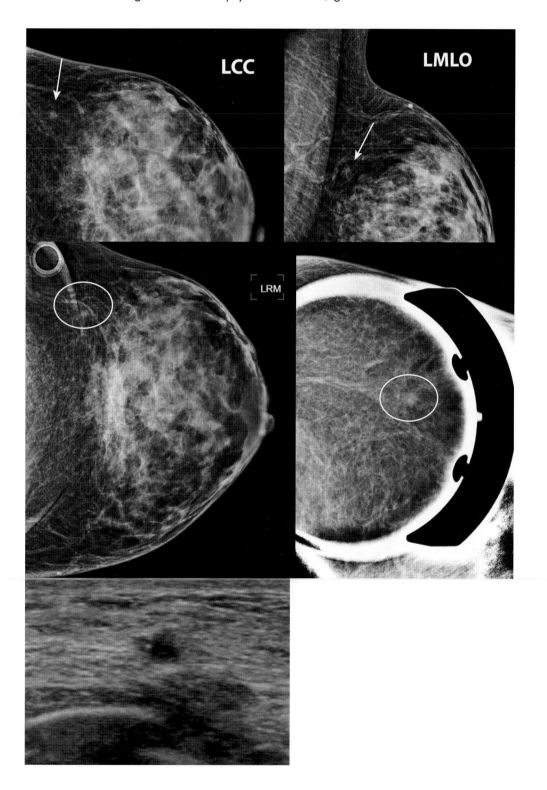

CASE 12-4. BI-RADS 0: Recall for diagnostic mammogram and possible US. There is a one-view asymmetry on the right MLO view protruding from the superior fibroglandular tissue into the adjacent fat. The finding persists on MLO and ML spot compression views but is not seen with certainty on the exaggerated CC view. US reveals an irregular hypoechoic mass in the axillary tail and a second smaller mass in the same quadrant. BI-RADS 5. Diagnosis: multifocal IDC with DCIS. Malignant asymmetries may closely resemble normal fibroglandular tissue, as in this case.

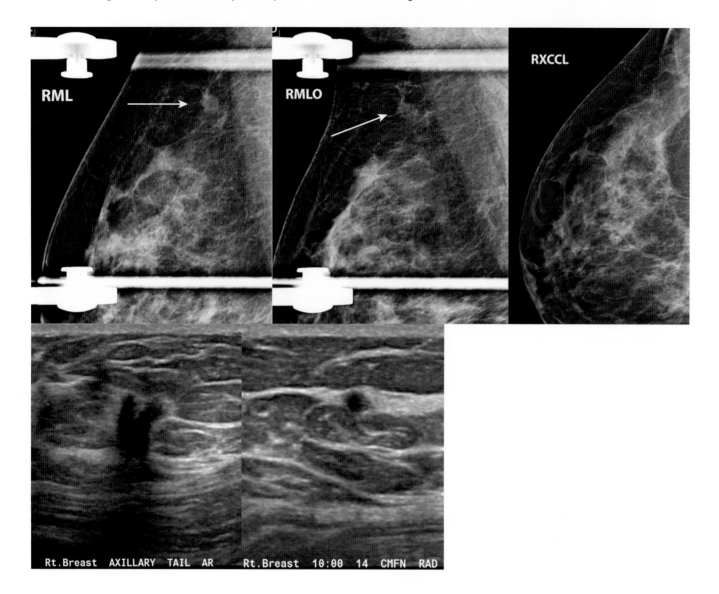

CASE 12-5. There is sufficient fat within the dense fibroglandular tissue to visualize an isodense spiculated mass, which is confirmed on MLO spot compression and ML views (*arrows*) and US. Diagnosis: IDC.

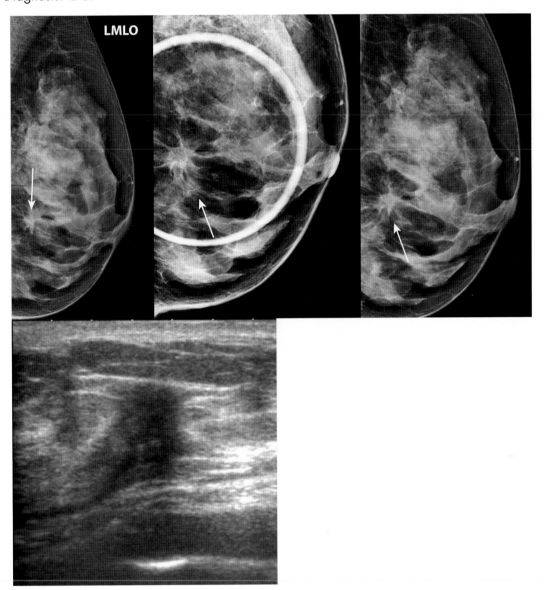

CASE 12-6. BI-RADS 0: Recall for diagnostic imaging. There is AD at the fibroglandular border in the posterior lateral right breast. The posterior fibroglandular border is straightened on the CC view compared with the appearance on the left. Spot compression views confirm AD at 10 o'clock, posterior third, right breast (*arrows*). US shows a corresponding irregular hypoechoic mass. BI-RADS 4. Diagnosis: IDC. In this case, straightening and spiculation at the edge of the fibroglandular tissue should raise a red flag during border patrol.

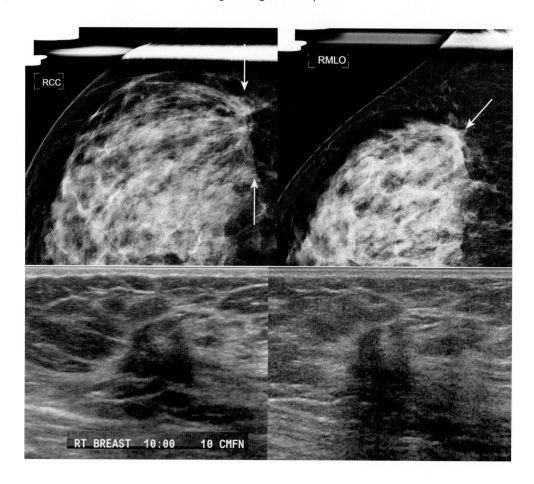

CASE 12-7. There are mostly coarse and mildly heterogeneous calcifications in a segmental distribution. BI-RADS 4. Diagnosis: IDC with high-grade DCIS. Even a few calcifications can signify extensive disease, particularly when the tissue is dense.

CASE 12-8. There is a one-view asymmetry on the right MLO view inferiorly (*arrow*). On the CC view it is probably present centrally. Let's spot those areas.

A spiculated mass is evident on the spot compression views. On US, there is a corresponding hypoechoic solid, highly suspicious mass. BI-RADS 5. Ultrasound-guided core biopsy showed IDC. Although this is scary on the diagnostic views, the screening findings are relatively subtle. Good job if you found this one!

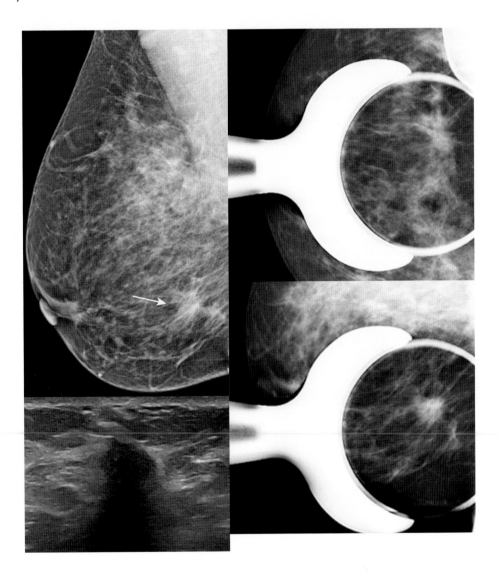

CASE 12-9. There is irregular asymmetry suspicious for a mass in the superior right breast (*arrow*). On spot compression MLO and ML views the finding persists (*arrows*). US shows an irregular hypoechoic mass in the 9:30 position. Diagnosis: infiltrating carcinoma with ductal and lobular features. If you got this one, you are awesome! This was a hard card.

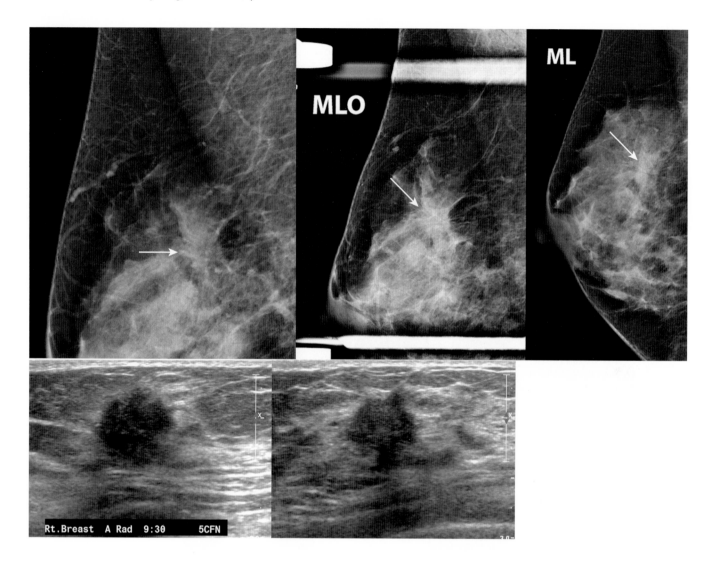

CASE 12-10. The tissue is extremely dense. There is focal asymmetry in the lower inner quadrant of the right breast, at the edge of the fibroglandular tissue (*arrows*). Recommend spot compression views and US.

MLO spot compression view shows a mass with spiculated margins. US reveals a corresponding irregular hypoechoic shadowing mass. Diagnosis: IDC. Great job if you found this one! Keep up the good work.

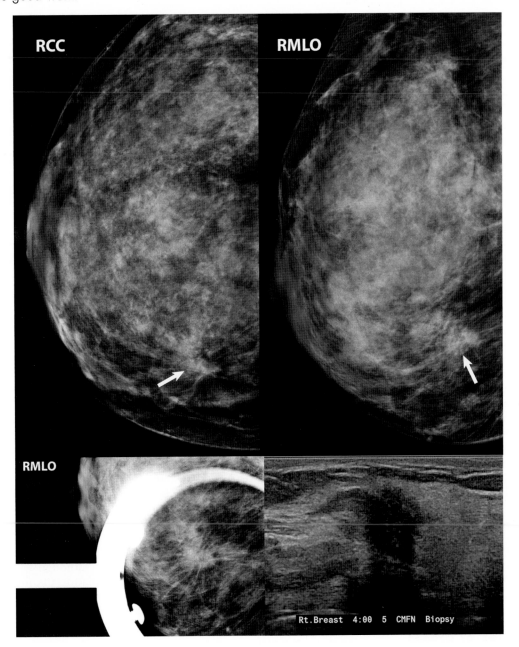

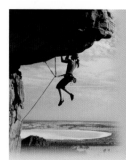

CHAPTER 13

Measuring and Managing Breast Cancer Risk

You're about to sign off on a negative screening mammogram when her history catches your eye. She's only 32 years old. Her sister was just diagnosed with breast cancer at age 40. Two of her paternal aunts have also had breast cancer. She should probably get mammograms every year, but does she also need a screening magnetic resonance imaging (MRI)? What if she were 72 years old with a similar family history?

It used to be so easy. Every woman age 40 and older got a mammogram every year, and that was it. If a woman had a mother or sister with breast cancer at a young age, then you could start screening with mammography early. We had little else to offer these patients, and the radiologist's role was much more limited.

Radiologists are now playing an increasingly active role in assessing breast cancer risk and making recommendations regarding risk reduction strategies. It can be very rewarding to empower women who are at high risk for breast cancer to manage their risk.

We have all experienced the worried well—women who are convinced that they will be diagnosed with breast cancer. About 28% of average-risk women overestimate their risk. Unfortunately, 57% of women who are actually high risk *underestimate* their personal risk of breast cancer. Although some gynecologists and other health care providers are very knowledgeable, radiologists are often considered the experts on this topic. This is not to say that radiologists will start running breast cancer risk clinics. However, we do see large numbers of women for mammographic screening and routinely collect much of the history needed to estimate risk. We are therefore in a great position to identify women who may need to have a more significant conversation about their breast cancer risk and to recommend the steps that can be taken to manage it.

The Three Categories of Breast Cancer Risk

Breast cancer risk factors can be divided into three categories: personal, breast-related, and genetic risk factors (Table 13-1). The pillars are not equal.

Personal Risk Factors

These are the best known risk factors. We tend to ask women most of these questions prior to mammography.

Although we know these well, no single personal risk factor increases lifetime risk to even a moderate level.

The personal risk factors are largely related to hormone exposure. Women who start menstruating at a young age or complete menopause at an older age have a greater duration of exposure to estrogen and progesterone and increased risk. Childbearing results in maturation of the lobules, so early parity is associated with lower breast cancer risk, and nulliparity and late parity are associated with a higher risk.

Women using menopausal hormone therapy (MHT) with estrogen alone (usually with hysterectomy) are not at elevated risk for breast cancer, but the use of estrogen with progesterone increases breast cancer risk by about 1.7 times. The risk occurs even in the first few years, so there is no "safe" period under which MHT can be used without considering breast cancer risk. That said, many women in perimenopause would rather cut off their right arm than not use hormone therapy. The symptoms of menopause can be severe. Sleep disruption and mood disorders make these women (and sometimes their families and friends) desperate. Women must find a balance between breast cancer risk and a reasonable lifestyle. Newer MHT regimens using lower doses and combining estrogens with a selective estrogen receptor modulator may reduce the associated breast cancer risk.

Fatty tissue contains an enzyme (aromatase) that converts circulating steroids to estrogens. Obesity is associated with a 30% to 50% increase in breast cancer risk in postmenopausal women. A 20-lb weight gain after age 18 is associated with a 50% to 100% increase in breast cancer risk. Sadly, the incidence of obesity in the United States has doubled since the 1960s. Although we mammographers are often accused of inflating the incidence of breast cancer, the incidence has also increased in women who are not engaged in screening. Certainly part of this may be related to the increasing incidence of obesity.

Alcohol consumption also increases breast cancer risk. Every 10 g of alcohol consumed per day (about one drink) increases breast cancer risk by 9%. This is likely mediated through interference with liver metabolism of estrogen products.

Breast-Related Risk Factors

A breast biopsy showing one of the high-risk lesions (atypical ductal hyperplasia [ADH], atypical lobular

TABLE 13-1 Breast Cancer Risk Factors

PERSONAL	BREAST	GENETIC
Young age at menarche	Biopsy with ADH, ALH, LCIS	BRCA1 or BRCA2
Older age at menopause	Radiation therapy to the chest	Li-Fraumeni syndrome
Nulliparity	Breast density	Cowden syndrome
Late parity		Bannayan-Riley-Ruvalcaba syndrome
Menopausal hormone therapy		
Obesity		

BOX 13-1 Comments About Genetic Testing

- Genetic testing is recommended when the risk of mutation is at least 10%.
- Mutation testing is separate for each gene (BRCA, Li-Fraumeni, Cowden).
- The relative with breast cancer ideally should be tested first.
- If the patient has a primary relative who is a known genetic mutation carrier, her negative genetic test is considered a true negative. For example, Mom is a known BRCA2 mutation carrier. If your patient tests negative, then she did not inherit that gene. She is not high risk and can have routine screening.
- It's not a perfect test. A negative genetic test does not change her high-risk status if there is not a known mutation in the family.

hyperplasia [ALH], lobular carcinoma in situ [LCIS]) is associated with an increase in lifetime risk of breast cancer. LCIS and ALH together are considered lobular neoplasia, which is associated with a 7- to 10-fold increase in breast cancer risk. If there is also a family history of breast cancer, then the risk associated with LCIS is doubled. A biopsy showing ADH is associated with a 3- to 4-fold increase in breast cancer risk.

Breast density is a moderate risk factor for breast cancer independent of other risk factors including age, parity, and family history. Women with very dense breast tissue have a 4-fold increase in breast cancer risk compared with women whose breast tissue is fatty-replaced. The risk is dose-dependent; compared with women with fatty breasts (relative risk [RR] 1.0), women who have scattered, heterogeneous, and extremely dense breast tissue have a 2.2-, 3.4-, and 5.3-fold increase in breast cancer risk. The reason some women have dense tissue and others do not is not known, but may reflect hormone metabolism, collagen deposition patterns, or growth hormones. At least 30% of breast density is genetically mediated.

Women who have had mantle radiation therapy to the chest, usually for treatment of lymphoma, are at high risk. The risk is increased about 5-fold compared to average-risk women. The younger the age of exposure, the higher the subsequent risk of breast cancer. The increased risk of breast cancer begins about 7 to 8 years and peaks at about 15 years after the radiation exposure. For patients who received 20 Gy or more to the chest/mediastinum, the Children's Oncology Group recommends annual mammography and MRI beginning at age 25 or 8 years after the exposure, whichever is later. Mantle radiation is being phased out—most women who receive radiation therapy for Hodgkin disease now undergo a more graded radiation dose across the chest, resulting in a lower dose to the breast tissue. It remains to be seen if this may lower breast cancer risk enough to forgo MRI screening.

Genetic Risk Factors

Family history of breast cancer increases risk. If a woman has one primary relative (mother, sister, daughter, father, brother, son) with breast cancer, her lifetime risk

is 13% compared to 8% for women without a first-degree relative with breast cancer. She becomes high risk (lifetime risk 21%) when two first-degree relatives have breast cancer.

There are several genetic mutations that increase the risk of being diagnosed with breast cancer. The most common mutations are in the BRCA1 and BRCA2 genes, but there are other less common mutations that are also associated with increased risk.

All of the genes that are associated with breast cancer risk are DNA repair (tumor suppressor) genes. We all have a little bit of damage to our DNA on a daily basis. Maybe you sat in the sun during lunch and an ultraviolet ray hit the DNA in your skin cells. Your body repairs these little hits using tumor suppressor genes. When these genes, like the BRCA1 gene, for example, have a mutation and don't work so well, the person carrying that mutated gene has a higher likelihood of developing breast and other cancers. The types of cancers depend upon the mutation type and gene affected.

We often call women "BRCA carriers" but in reality they are "BRCA mutation carriers." These genetic mutations actually occur with equal frequency in both men and women and are autosomal dominant. They are not located on the X or Y chromosome. Each of us has two sets of DNA, one inherited from our father and one from our mother. Therefore, if Dad has a BRCA2 mutation, you have a 50:50 chance of inheriting that copy of his gene. If you do get that gene, you will inherit an increased risk for cancer. Incidentally, if Dad is a BRCA2 mutation carrier, he is at increased risk for cancer of the pancreas, prostate, colon, and, yes, breast (Boxes 13-1 and 13-2).

Hereditary breast and ovarian cancer (HBOC) syndrome is a term applied to carriers of mutations in either *BRCA1 or BRCA2*. Alterations occur on chromosome 17q in *BRCA1* and 13q in *BRCA2*. These mutations are much more common in the Ashkenazi Jewish population (Eastern European Jewish ancestry). Most of the Jewish population in the United States is of Ashkenazi descent.

BOX 13-2 Guidelines for Genetics Referral*

Personal history of breast cancer (BC) and at least one of these:
- Diagnosed ≤ age 45
- Diagnosed ≤age 50 and:
  - Close relative with BC < age 50 OR
  - Close relative with ovarian cancer (any age)
- Two breast cancers , one ≤ age 50
- Two close relatives with BC at any age
- Two close relatives with pancreatic cancer
- Ashkenazi Jewish ancestry

First- or second- degree relative (not cousin) with breast cancer who was:
- Diagnosed ≤ age 45
- Diagnosed < age 50 and:
  - Close relative with BC < age 50 OR
  - Close relative with ovarian cancer (any age)
- Diagnosed with two BCs, one ≤ age 50
- Diagnosed at any age and has two close relatives with breast or ovarian cancer, any age
- Diagnosed at any age and has two close relatives with pancreatic cancer, any age

Primary relative with known genetic mutation but not yet tested.
Breast cancer in a close male family member
Ashkenazi Jewish ancestry and a first- or second-degree relative with BC

Note: Close relative (first-, second-, third-degree relative): mother, sister, half-sister, daughter, aunt, grandmother, cousin, brother, father, uncle.
*Based on National Comprehensive Cancer Network (NCCN).

TABLE 13-2 Risk Factors Associated with Moderate and High Lifetime Risk

RISK LEVEL	LIFETIME RISK	ASSOCIATED RISK FACTORS
Average risk	<15%	
Moderate risk	15-20%	LCIS, ADH, ALH Dense breast tissue Intermediate family history Previous breast cancer
High risk	>20%	Hereditary breast and ovarian cancer (HBOC) syndrome (e.g., *BRCA*) Other genetic mutations Chest irradiation at a young age Combination of risk factors

Bannayan-Riley-Ruvalcaba syndrome is a rare disorder associated with developmental disorders that are apparent at a young age.

Neurofibromatosis (NF1) is also likely associated with an increase in breast cancer risk. It may be associated with moderate risk rather than the high risk due to the preceding genetic syndromes.

Breast Cancer Risk Models

We know that women who are genetic mutation carriers are at high lifetime risk for breast cancer, but what about women with a combination of risk factors? For example, what if a woman has a mother with breast cancer and she had a biopsy showing LCIS? Breast cancer risk models combine risk factor information to yield a woman's lifetime and either 5- or 10-year risk of developing breast cancer (Table 13-2).

Gail Model

The Gail model is the oldest and best validated breast cancer risk model. It was developed using data from the Breast Cancer Detection Demonstration Project (BCDDP), which was conducted in the 1980s. This model primarily focuses on personal risk factors. It also includes biopsy showing ADH and family history of breast cancer in primary relatives (mother, sister, daughter).

This model is short and quick. It is only seven questions. Unfortunately, the accuracy of the Gail model is only about 50%. This model was developed before the *BRCA* mutations were discovered and does not include the paternal side of the family. It is the only model validated in African-American women.

Claus, BODICEA, and BRCAPro Models

Claus, BODICEA, and BRCAPro models target identification of genetic mutation carriers. These models do not

About 2% of those of Ashkenazi Jewish descent carry a mutation of *BRCA1* or *BRCA2* compared with about 0.5% of the United States population overall.

The lifetime risk of breast cancer is highest for women with a *BRCA1* mutation. These women have a 55% to 85% lifetime risk of breast cancer; *BRCA2* mutation is associated with a 25% to 60% lifetime risk of breast cancer. Mutation carriers of *BRCA1* and *BRCA2* also differ in the incidence of other cancers. *BRCA1* mutation carriers are at very high risk for ovarian cancer in women (21 times more likely than for average-risk women!), testicular cancer in men, and stomach, renal, bladder, liver, gallbladder, and pancreatic cancer in both sexes. *BRCA2* mutation carriers are at elevated risk for ovarian cancer in women, prostate cancer in men, and stomach, liver, gallbladder, and pancreatic cancer in both sexes.

Li-Fraumeni syndrome is associated with alteration of chromosome 17p. These mutation carriers have a 60% to 90% lifetime risk of breast cancer. These men and women also have an increased risk of rare cancers, including sarcomas, brain cancer, leukemia, and adrenal cancer.

Cowden syndrome is associated with alterations in chromosome 10q. These mutation carriers have a lifetime risk of breast cancer of 30% to 50%. Benign thyroid disease and thyroid cancers are common in these families. Multiple hamartomas occur on mucosal surfaces. Lipomas are also common.

include personal or breast-related risk factors. These models are based on family pedigree, including both maternal and paternal history. These models are great for identifying women with a strong family history of breast cancer. The last two models also predict the risk of a woman carrying a *BRCA* mutation. Genetic counseling and testing are recommended for women who have at least a 10% risk of being a *BRCA* mutation carrier. The accuracy of these models for predicting breast cancer risk in the general population is only about 56% (Box 13-3).

Tyrer-Cuzick Model

The Tyrer-Cuzick model is the most comprehensive, including personal risk factors, biopsy showing ADH or LCIS, and a family cancer pedigree. This model is more time intensive, but readily available. The accuracy is about 80%.

Breast Density Is Missing from the Models

When breast density is added to a comprehensive risk model, risk is slightly overestimated. Several investigators, including Dr. Harvey, are working on the development of a comprehensive risk assessment model that includes breast density.

Breast Cancer Risk Reduction

Reducing the risk of breast cancer includes both steps that make it less likely that a woman will develop the disease as well as screening efforts that allow earlier detection, with the goal of reducing the mortality rate.

All women can reduce their risk of developing breast cancer by limiting alcohol consumption (including red wine...sorry!), breastfeeding, controlling weight, exercising regularly, and not using MHT. Women age 40 and younger who spend at least 4 hours per week exercising reduce breast cancer risk by 60%. The effect is not as strong for postmenopausal women. Women ages 50 to 65 years who partake in moderate-to-strenuous exercise reduce breast cancer risk by 30%. Screening mammography reduces breast cancer mortality rate rather than incidence.

Options for risk reduction for women who are at high risk (>20% lifetime risk) include intensive screening, chemoprevention, and prophylactic surgery. Intensive screening may result in earlier detection and a reduction in breast cancer mortality rate. Chemoprevention with tamoxifen or raloxifene reduces breast cancer incidence by 50% to 60%, but primarily for ER/PR (estrogen receptor/progesterone receptor) positive cancers. Reduction in mortality rate may or may not be significant. Prophylactic mastectomy reduces breast cancer incidence by about 98%.

Let's remember that these women are at risk for many other cancers besides breast cancer. Offering screening MRI is the first step, but these patients need much more. Many women will opt for prophylactic

oophorectomies. Screening with colonoscopy is often also recommended.

Screening Breast MRI

Screening breast MRI is indicated for women who have at least a 20% to 25% lifetime risk of breast cancer. The vast majority of women with this level of risk are known or suspected genetic mutation carriers, although a combination of risk factors such as a biopsy showing LCIS and a primary relative with breast cancer may result in a similar lifetime risk.

Screening breast MRI detects about 30 cancers per 1000 women screened. This is a lot of cancers! For comparison, mammography finds 3 to 8 cancers per 1000 average-risk women screened. There are no trials that study mortality rates for screening breast MRI, but the majority of cancers detected are small invasive cancers that are node negative. The mean size of invasive cancers detected on screening MRI is 0.7 to 2.0 cm, and 65% to 100% are node negative (Fig. 13-1). This implies that many of the cancers detected by MRI are likely found at a lifesaving point in time.

What about women with fatty breasts? Do they *really* need screening breast MRI? Actually, yes. In a study of

507 high-risk women, MRI detected 3 of 3 and 14 of 15 cancers in fatty and scattered-density breasts, respectively, although mammography detected only 1 and 5 of those cancers. We used to think we were really good at reading fatty mammograms until we started reading breast MRI (Fig. 13-2).

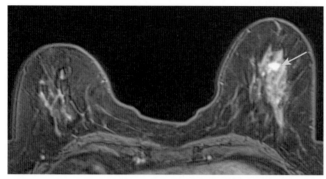

FIGURE 13-1 **Small Node Negative Invasive Ductal Carcinoma (IDC) on Screening MRI.** This 66-year-old woman has a history of ductal carcinoma in situ (DCIS) in her right breast 7 years ago. She now has a new 1.0-cm mass in the left breast (*arrow*). The mass was not seen on US. MRI-guided biopsy showed IDC, grade 2, node negative.

Screening Ultrasonography

The ACRIN 6666 Screening US Trial (Berg et al., 2008, 2012) included 2809 women at moderate or high risk with at least heterogeneously dense breast tissue. These women underwent annual mammography and screening ultrasonography (US) as well as MRI if these screens were negative at year 3. Of these, 2662 women underwent 7472 screening examinations detecting 111 cancers in 110 women; 33 cancers were detected by mammography only, 32 by US only, 26 by both, 9 by MRI, and 11 were not detected by any modality. Supplemental US added 5.3 cancers per 1000 women in the first year and 3.7 cancers per 1000 women in years 2 and 3 (incident screens); supplemental MRI added 14.7 cancers per 1000 women.

The cancer detection rate of screening US is considerably lower than the typical 30 cancers per 1000 attained in most screening MRI trials. If the results of the nine major high-risk screening trials are combined, mammography with screening US detects 52% of cancers, but mammography with MRI detects 93%. The cancers that are not detected by mammography with MRI largely present as interval cancers. If women are undergoing annual mammography and MRI, adding US will not increase cancer detection significantly.

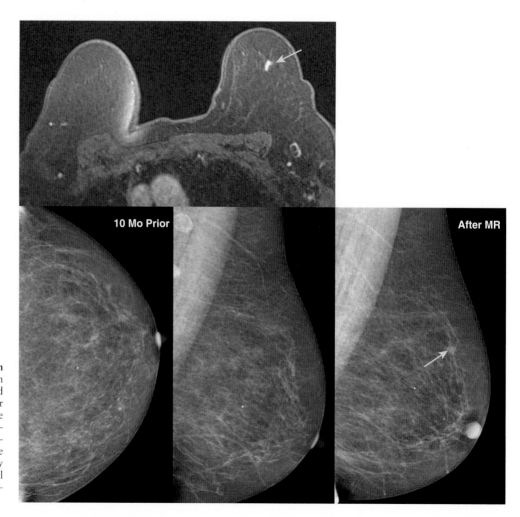

FIGURE 13-2 **Screening MRI in Fatty Breast.** A 64-year-old woman with a family history of breast and ovarian cancer. A small irregular enhancing mass is present on the MRI (*arrow*). Her last mammogram was negative. A mammogram performed following the MRI shows a subtle asymmetry seen only on the mediolateral oblique (MLO) view. Ultrasound-guided biopsy showed IDC.

A big problem with screening US is the low specificity. In the ACRIN 6666 Trial, the positive predictive value (PPV) for biopsy recommendation was only 8.9%. In comparison, the PPV for mammographic findings is generally 20% to 40%. This means that at least twice as many biopsies must be performed to diagnose the same number of cancers. For every 100 women undergoing mammography, 2.8 underwent biopsy due to an abnormal mammogram and 7.8 due to an abnormal first US. This figure decreased only to 7.0% on subsequent abnormal incident US in years 2 and 3 of the trial. This means that 10% of women undergoing mammography and their first US screening will have a biopsy recommended. However, if a woman who is at high risk for breast cancer cannot undergo screening MRI, then US would be a good second choice. US is also considerably less expensive than breast MRI.

Breast-Specific Gamma Imaging

Cellular mitochondria take up sestamibi labeled with technetium-99m. Cells that are more active, like cancer cells, take up more tracer. Small studies suggest that gamma imaging of the breast may have performance similar to that of breast MRI. Although the radiation dose to the breasts is similar for mammography and breast-specific gamma imaging (BSGI), the dose from BSGI is systemic with exposure to the intestine and other organs, making the whole body dose quite high for a screening examination. Newer dual-headed cameras may allow lower radiation doses that may eventually be similar to those of a mammogram.

Moderate-Risk Women

Women at moderate risk for breast cancer include those with a biopsy-proven high-risk lesion (LCIS, ADH, ALH), heterogeneous or dense breast tissue, or a personal history of breast cancer, including DCIS.

Legislation has been passed in at least four states requiring women to be notified about the impact of dense tissue on mammographic interpretation; 12 additional states have legislation pending, and a similar federal bill has been introduced. These efforts have led to an increase in the use of screening US. The cancer detection rate has been reported as 3% in these patients (Hooley, 2012; Weigert, 2012), which is higher than would be anticipated in women who are at moderate risk. As we discussed previously, the downside of screening US is the very low specificity: 7% to 8% of women will be recommended to have a biopsy after their first screening US, and fewer than 10% of those will have breast cancer. Screening US would certainly be more widely embraced if the specificity were higher and the test were less time intensive and operator dependent. This is an active area of change.

If you have or are planning to initiate a screening breast US program, you will need to have the mindset that the vast majority of examinations should be negative and that your goal is to find invasive cancer (Fig. 13-3). This approach is different from when you are performing a targeted US after an abnormal mammogram or to evaluate a clinical finding. Ignore those 2- to 3-mm round hypoechoic masses that are so commonly seen in fibrocystic change! In the ACRIN 6666 Trial, a complicated cyst that was seen in the background of simple cysts was also considered benign.

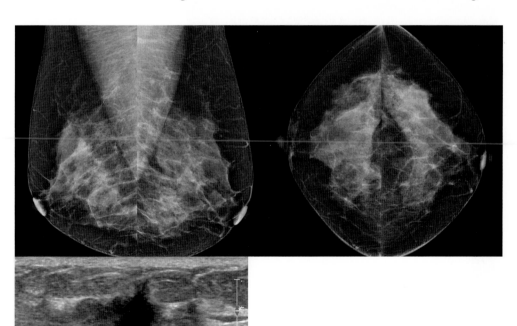

FIGURE 13-3 **Invasive Carcinoma on Screening US.** A 48-year-old moderate-risk woman underwent screening US 1 month after a normal mammogram. A highly suspicious irregular mass measuring 12 mm was found in the right lower inner quadrant. Biopsy revealed infiltrating carcinoma with ductal and lobular features.

Interpretation of Screening Breast Magnetic Resonance Imaging

Many of the same principles of interpretation of screening mammography apply to screening MRI. For example, a solid mass that is new or enlarging compared with a prior screening study is suspicious whether seen on mammography or MRI.

Parenchymal enhancement is normal and common. This is somewhat similar to breast density and is classified as minimal, mild, moderate, or marked. It is most common in the posterior breast, in the upper outer quadrants (Fig. 13-4). To reduce the effects of parenchymal enhancement, premenopausal women undergoing screening MRI should be scheduled during days 7 to 20 of their menstrual cycle.

Foci are defined as round or oval circumscribed areas of enhancement that are smaller than 5 mm (Fig. 13-5). Foci are generally benign, with a cancer risk of 2% to 3%. If one seems different than others because it has a suspicious enhancement pattern or ill-defined margins, then biopsy may be indicated.

Masses are typically at least 5 mm. Shapes are round, oval, or irregular. Margins are circumscribed/smooth, indistinct, irregular, or spiculated. Internal mass characteristics include heterogeneous, homogeneous, or rim enhancement and nonenhancing septations.

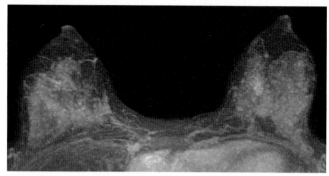

FIGURE 13-4 **Typical Parenchymal Enhancement.** This maximum intensity projection (MIP) image shows a bilateral symmetric pattern. Note that the enhancement is most pronounced in the posterior upper outer quadrants, which is very common.

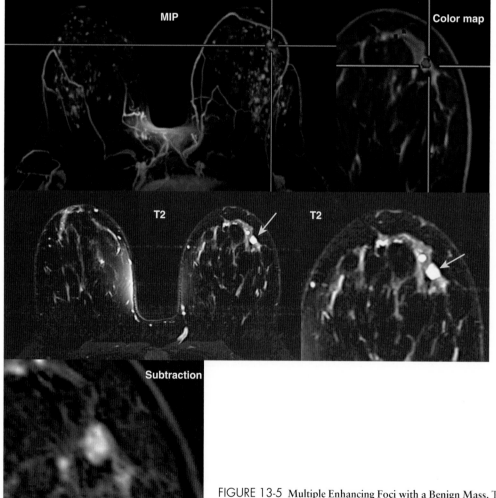

FIGURE 13-5 **Multiple Enhancing Foci with a Benign Mass.** There are multiple bilateral enhancing foci. On the color map these had persistent enhancement. In the left breast, there is a 6-mm oval mass with well-defined margins and plateau enhancement. It is T2 hyperintense (*arrow*). The subtraction sequence shows nonenhancing septations.

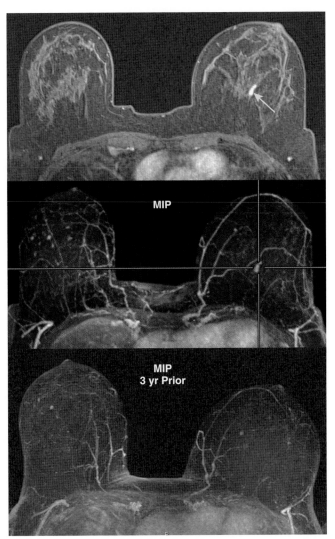

FIGURE 13-6 **New Mass with Benign Features.** There is an oval mass in the central left breast (*arrow*). On the MIP, the mass is clearly new compared with 3 years earlier. Mammography and US were negative. MRI-guided biopsy showed invasive carcinoma with ductal and lobular features.

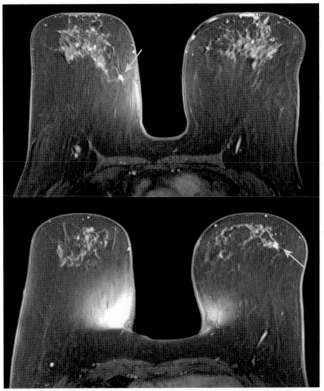

FIGURE 13-7 **Suspicious Masses.** A 48-year-old woman with a family history of breast cancer and lifetime risk of 28%. In the right breast, there is a 6-mm irregular mass with spiculated margins (*arrow*), BI-RADS 5. In the left breast, there is an 8-mm irregular mass with ill-defined margins (*arrow*), BI-RADS 4. The enhancement curves showed washout and plateau delayed enhancement, respectively. However, the curve type does not have any influence on the recommendation for biopsy since the morphology is suspicious. Diagnosis: bilateral IDC.

Benign mass features are round or oval, with a circumscribed margin, and are often T2 hyperintense (see Fig. 13-5). The most common benign mass, fibroadenoma, often has nonenhancing septations (see Fig. 13-5), though this is not a very specific finding. Just like mammography, biopsy will usually be indicated for a new solid mass on MRI even if it has benign features (Fig. 13-6).

Size does matter when it comes to evaluating breast masses on MRI. In a study of 666 masses seen on breast MRI (Liberman, 2006), the risk of malignancy was 3% for masses less than 5 mm (i.e., foci), 17% for masses 5 to 9 mm, 25% for masses 10 to 14 mm, 28% for masses 15 to 19 mm, and 31% for masses 20 mm or larger.

Suspicious features of masses on MRI are not dissimilar to those on mammography or US. If a mass has an irregular shape, spiculated margins, or shows heterogeneous or rim enhancement, biopsy is usually indicated (Fig. 13-7). If a mass has suspicious morphologic appearance, the enhancement kinetics should not influence a decision to recommend biopsy.

Enhancement pattern really only helps in the evaluation of masses that have benign features. These features include round shape, well-defined margins, and homogeneous enhancement. If the mass is alsoT2 bright and has nonenhancing septations, it is likely a fibroadenoma. However, masses with benign features that have a suspicious enhancement pattern are more concerning. Invasive cancers frequently have leaky blood vessels resulting in rapid initial enhancement followed by washout of the contrast in the delayed phase. A mass with benign morphologic appearance that displays suspicious enhancement may represent cancer (Fig. 13-8).

Nonmass enhancement (NME) is defined as an area of enhancement that is less defined than a mass or focus. NME is described by distribution (focal area, linear, ductal, segmental, regional, diffuse), enhancement pattern (homogeneous, heterogeneous, stippled/punctuate, clumped, reticular/dendritic), and symmetry (asymmetric or symmetric). Ductal or linear distribution and clumped or reticular enhancement have the highest associations with malignancy. NME may be due to parenchymal enhancement, fibrocystic change, or other proliferative process, but can also be due to DCIS. The positive predictive value for suspicious NME is lower than that of a

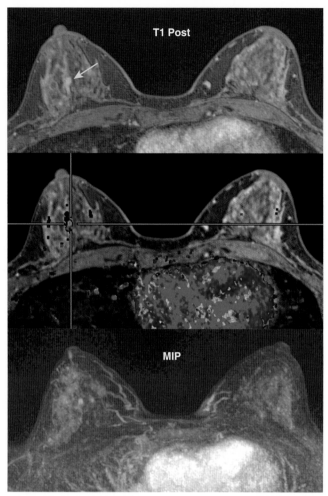

FIGURE 13-8 **Mass with Suspicious Enhancement.** Although this 6-mm mass is round and has well-defined margins (*arrow*), it has rapid initial enhancement with washout (*red* on color map). In addition, this is a dominant finding on the MIP. US was negative. MRI-guided biopsy showed DCIS, high grade.

mass. Just as in mammographic density, asymmetry in enhancement should be scrutinized (Fig. 13-9).

BI-RADS for Magnetic Resonance Imaging

With few exceptions, BI-RADS 0 should not be used for screening breast MRI. Occasionally, an indeterminate mass on MRI may represent a mass that is documented as stable on mammography (Fig. 13-10). Unless comparison with a prior MRI or correlation with mammography is needed, then a final BI-RADS category should be made based on the MRI finding. The BI-RADS assessment of a suspicious MRI finding should not be based on the characteristics of a presumptive US correlate, which may or may not be found on subsequent examination.

Localization for Biopsy

When a suspicious finding is identified on MRI, biopsy may be easier for the patient and radiologist if there is a

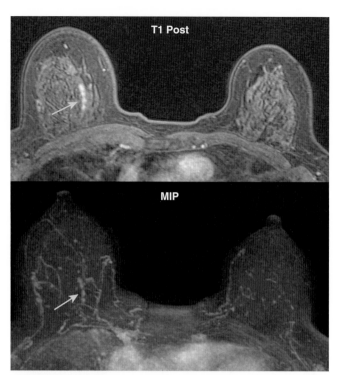

FIGURE 13-9 **NME Due to Malignancy.** This 53-year-old woman had a biopsy in her right breast 2 years ago that showed ADH. Her mother had breast cancer at age 51. According to the Gail model, her lifetime risk is 33%. The MIP shows asymmetric enhancement in her medial right breast (*arrows*). The T1 postcontrast image shows clumped linear enhancement in the medial right breast. MRI-guided biopsy showed DCIS.

mammographic or sonographic correlate. The BI-RADS category for the MRI should be 4 (suspicious) or 5 (malignant), not 0 (needs additional imaging). If mammography and US are negative, an MRI-guided biopsy is indicated.

US can identify a suspicious MRI finding in about 50% of cases (Fig. 13-11). Success is higher for masses than NME. This is often called "second look US," but is often really the first US performed, so the term "targeted US" may be preferable. We usually think of doing a targeted US after abnormal MRI, but often forget about a possible mammographic correlate (Fig. 13-12). Be very sure that you have identified the correct US (or mammographic) correlate to the suspicious MRI finding. One study found that 14% of US findings did not actually correlate to the MRI lesion. If the biopsy returns as benign, will you be confident that the correct area was biopsied? If not, MRI-guided biopsy would be the preferred approach.

Pitfalls of Screening Magnetic Resonance Imaging

Just like screening mammography, breast MRI will result in false-positive and false-negative examinations.

Although the sensitivity of breast MRI is at least 95% for invasive carcinoma, the specificity is lower. The positive predictive value for biopsy recommended due to a breast MRI is 20% to 40%, which is similar to that for screening mammography. False-positive results are more

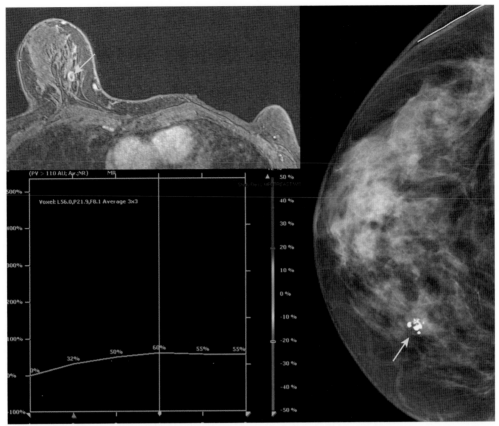

FIGURE 13-10 **Mass on MRI That Is Stable by Mammography.** There is an apparent rim enhancing mass (*arrow*) on this screening MRI in a 58-year-old woman who had a prior left mastectomy. The mass has persistent enhancement, which is uncommon for rim enhancing masses. On the mammogram, this mass corresponds to a degenerating fibroadenoma (*arrow*) that had been stable for many years. The lack of enhancement in the center of the fibroadenoma is due to signal dropout from the calcifications.

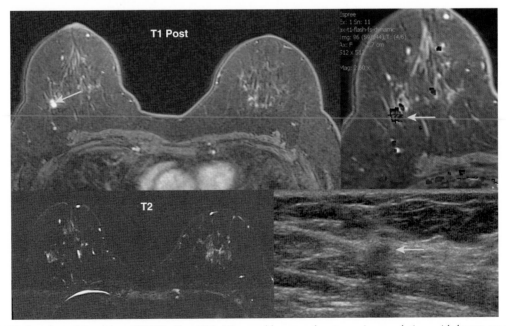

FIGURE 13-11 **US Correlate of Suspicious MRI Finding.** This 59-year-old woman has two primary relatives with breast cancer. Her screening MRI shows an oval well-defined mass with rapid initial and washout delayed enhancement (*arrows*). There is a suggestion of a nonenhancing septation, but this is a very nonspecific finding. It is not T2 hyperintense. This is BI-RADS 4. US performed for biopsy planning shows a correlative subtle hypoechoic mass (*arrow*) with posterior acoustic shadowing. Biopsy revealed IDC, grade I.

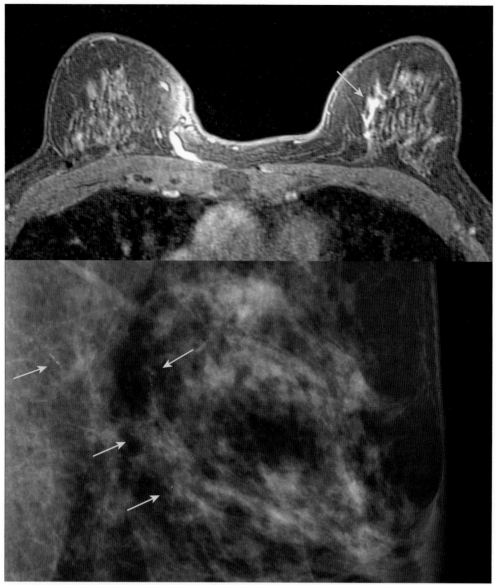

FIGURE 13-12 **Suspicious Calcifications in an Area of NME.** Segmental NME in the left medial breast (*arrow*) on this high-risk screening MRI correlates with new segmental fine pleomorphic calcifications on mammography (*arrows*). The patient's prior mammogram 6 months earlier had only a few calcifications in this area. Stereotactic biopsy showed DCIS, high-grade.

frequent on the first (prevalent) examination compared with subsequent (incident) MRI screens.

False-negative findings can also occur with screening MRI (Fig. 13-13). Most of the same rules from screening mammography apply to screening MRI. A new mass is suspicious unless you can prove that it is a definitely benign, such as a lymph node, no matter what the modality. Use the same tools that we use for screening mammography (remember Chapter 3?): know where cancers live and where we miss them, and audit the performance of each radiologist and of your group practice.

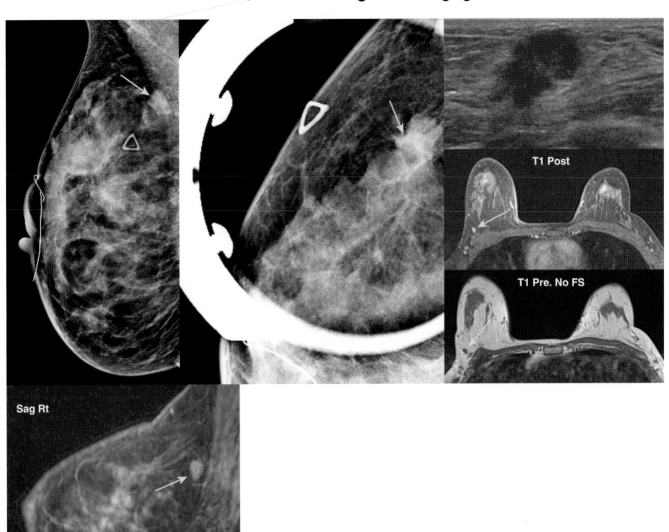

FIGURE 13-13 **False-Negative MRI.** This 39-year-old woman of Ashkenazi Jewish ancestry and a primary relative with breast cancer presented with a palpable lump in the right breast at 11 o'clock. On mammography, the palpable lump corresponded to an irregular mass with spiculated margins (*arrows*). This was also highly suspicious on US, BI-RADS 5. Biopsy showed IDC, grade III. In retrospect, the mass was present on her screening MRI 10 months earlier (*arrows*). The reader likely assumed that the mass represented a lymph node due to the location and shape.

KEY POINTS

- Breast cancer risk factors can be divided into three categories: personal, breast-related, and genetic. Carriers of certain genetic mutations (e.g., *BRCA1* and *BRCA2*) are at high lifetime risk.
- Breast cancer risk models are used to estimate risk given a combination of factors. All underestimate lifetime risk and do not yet include breast density.
- Risk reduction strategies include prevention (e.g., tamoxifen, prophylactic mastectomy) and intensive screening. Breast MRI is recommended for women with a lifetime risk of greater than 20% to 25% using a family history model (i.e., not the Gail model).
- Screening US detects additional mammographically occult cancers in moderate-risk women. However, the false-positive rate is high (a biopsy will be recommended for 7%-8% of women having screening US), and the PPV is less than 10%.
- Many skills used for interpretation of screening mammography also apply to screening MRI such as comparison with prior studies, management of developing lesions, assessment of mass margins, and management of multiple masses.
- Foci are generally benign but may be suspicious when a new or a sole finding, or if they display suspicious kinetics.
- Kinetic analysis of enhancement is most helpful in the evaluation of masses with benign features. It is not as helpful in the evaluation of NME.

References

Abe H, Schmidt RA, Shah RN, et al. MR-directed ("second-look") ultrasound examination for breast lesions detected initially on MRI: MR and sonographic findings. Am J Roentgenol 2010;194: 370-377.

Baltzer PAT, Benndorf M, Dietzel M, et al. False-positive findings at contrast-enhanced breast MRI: A BI-RADS descriptor study. Am J Roentgenol 2010;194:1658-1663.

Barlow WE, White E, Ballard-Barbash R, et al. Prospective breast cancer risk prediction model for women undergoing screening mammography. J Natl Cancer Inst 2006;98:1204-1214.

Berg WA. Tailored supplemental screening for breast cancer: What now and what next? Am J Roentgenol 2009;192:390-399.

Berg WA, Blume JD, Cormack JB, et al. Combined screening with ultrasound and mammography vs. mammography alone in women at elevated risk of breast cancer. JAMA 2008;299:2151-2163.

Berg WA, Zhang Z, Lehrer D, et al. Detection of breast cancer with addition of annual screening ultrasound or a single screening MRI to mammography in women with elevated breast cancer risk. JAMA 2012;307:1394-1404.

Bigenwald RZ, Warner E, Gunasekara A, et al. Is mammography adequate for screening women with inherited BRCA mutations and low breast density? Cancer Epidemiol Biomarkers Prev 2008;17: 706-711.

Chen J, Pee D, Ayyagari R, et al. Projecting absolute invasive breast cancer risk in white women with a model that includes mammographic density. J Natl Cancer Inst 2006;98:1215-1226.

Clemons M, Loijens L, Goss P. Breast cancer risk following irradiation for Hodgkin's disease. Cancer Treat Rev 2000;26:291-302.

DeMartini WB, Eby PR, Peacock S, Lehman CD. Utility of targeted sonography for breast lesions that were suspicious on MRI. Am J Roentgenol 2009;192:1128-1134.

Goss PE, Sierra A. Current perspectives on radiation-induced breast cancer. J Clin Oncol 1998;16(1):338-347.

Haas JS, Kaplan CP, DesJarlais G, et al. Perceived risk of breast cancer among women at average and increased risk J Womens Health 2005;14:845-851.

Hooley RJ, Greenberg KL, Stackhouse RM, et al. Screening US in patients with mammographically dense breasts: Initial experience with Connecticut Public Act 09-41. Radiology 2012;265:159-169.

Liberman L, Mason G, Morris EA, Dershaw DD. Does size matter? Positive predictive value of MRI-detected breast lesions as a function of lesion size. Am J Roentgenol 2006;186:426-430.

Mahoney MC, Gatsonis C, Hanna L, et al. Positive predictive value of BI-RADS MR imaging. Radiology 2012;264(1):51-58.

McTiernan A, Gralow J, Talbott L. Breast Fitness: An Optimal Exercise and Health Plan for Reducing Your Risk of Breast Cancer. New York, Macmillan, 2001.

Million Women Study Collaborators. Breast cancer and hormone-replacement therapy in the Million Women Study. Lancet 2003;362: 419-427.

Saslow D, Boetes C, Burke W, et al. American Cancer Society guidelines for breast screening with MRI as an adjunct to mammography. CA Cancer J Clin 2007;57(2):75-89.

Weigert J, Steenbergen S. The Connecticut experiment: The role of ultrasound in the screening of women with dense breasts. Breast J 2012;18:517-522.

CASE QUESTIONS

CASE 13-1. A 58-year-old woman has a family history of breast and ovarian cancer. What are your BI-RADS assessment and recommendation based on her high-risk screening MRI?

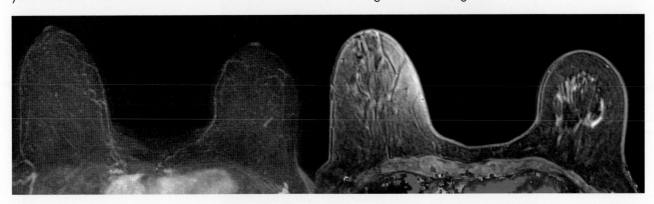

CASE 13-2. This 58-year-old woman was recalled from screening for left breast calcifications (*box*). Stereotactic and subsequent excisional biopsy showed ADH. Her mother had breast cancer at age 76. Is she considered at high risk for breast cancer? Would you suggest screening MRI?

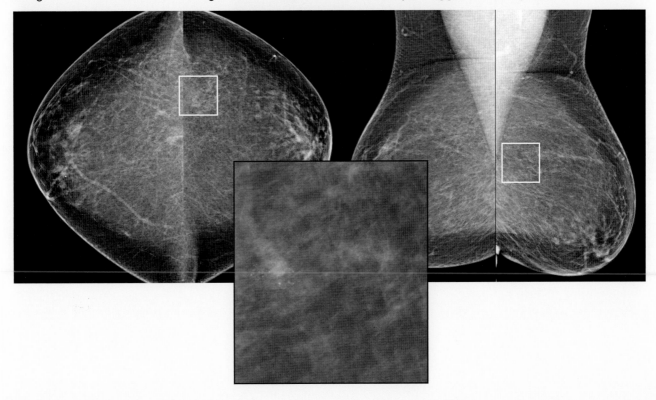

CASE 13-3. A 50-year-old woman undergoes her first screening MRI due to lifetime risk for breast cancer of 52%. Selected images are provided here. What are your assessment and recommendation?

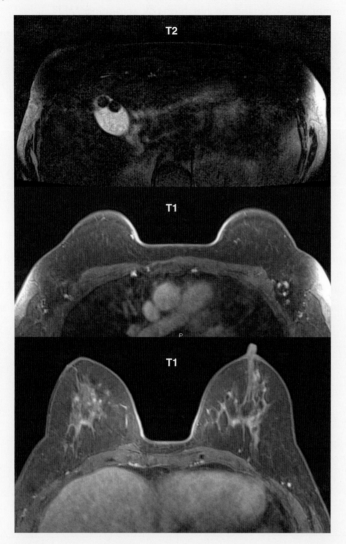

CASE 13-4. A 56-year-old woman undergoes screening MRI due to prior biopsy showing LCIS and dense breast tissue. No family history of breast cancer. What do you think of her screening MRI?

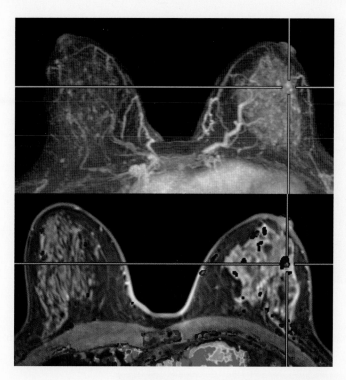

CASE 13-5. A 33-year-old woman undergoes her first screening MRI. She has a strong family history of breast cancer. Her lifetime risk of breast cancer is 42%. How would you manage the enhancing mass in her right breast?

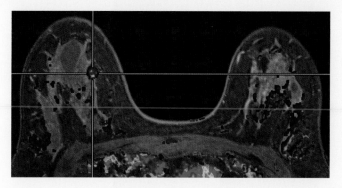

CASE 13-6. A 53-year-old high-risk woman underwent screening MRI. A 1-minute subtraction image is shown. Should the enhancing finding in the right breast (*arrow*) be considered a mass or a focus? What would you recommend?

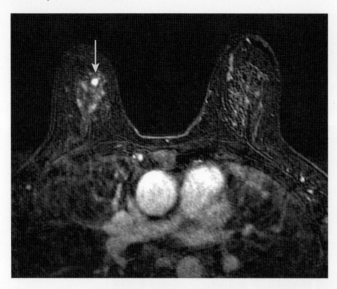

CASE 13-7. This 64-year-old woman had a right breast biopsy 5 years ago showing LCIS and has dense breast tissue. What do you think of her MRI?

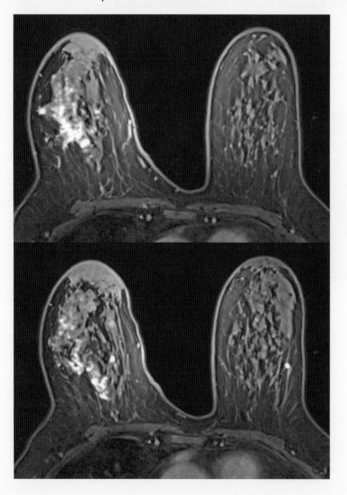

CASE 13-8. A 55-year-old woman has a screening MRI. She has had prior left breast cancer. Her mother was diagnosed with breast cancer at age 61. What is the finding (*arrow*)? What are your BI-RADS assessment category and recommendation? Her MRI was otherwise negative.

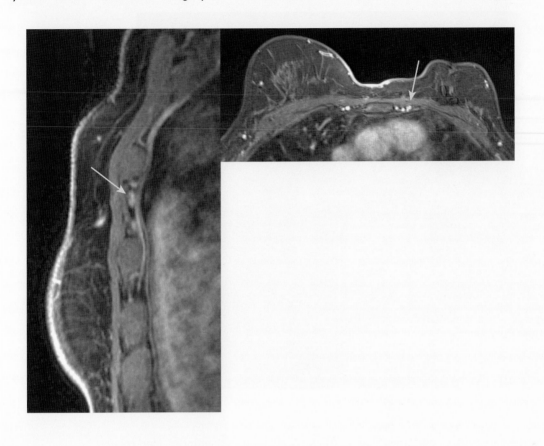

CASE 13-9. A 59-year-old woman with a mother, maternal grandmother, and maternal aunt with breast cancer presents for high-risk screening MRI. The curve represents the enhancing area in the right breast. What are your BI-RADS assessment and recommendation for this patient?

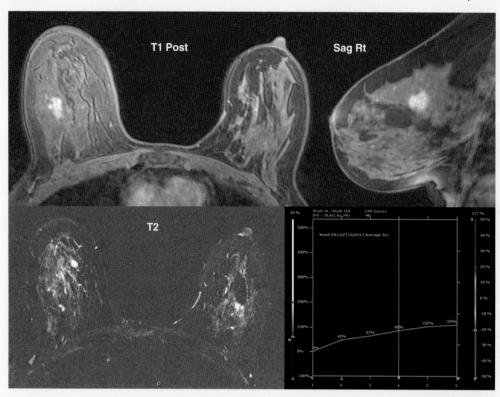

CASE 13-10. A screening MRI is performed on a 60-year-old high-risk woman. Her recent mammogram was negative. How would you describe the findings? What are your BI-RADS assessment and recommendation?

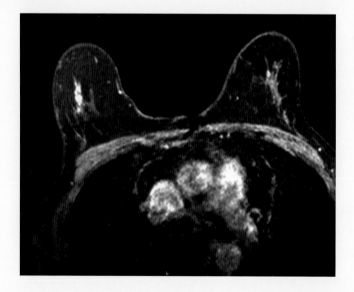

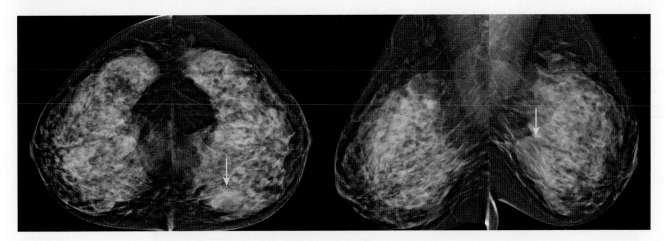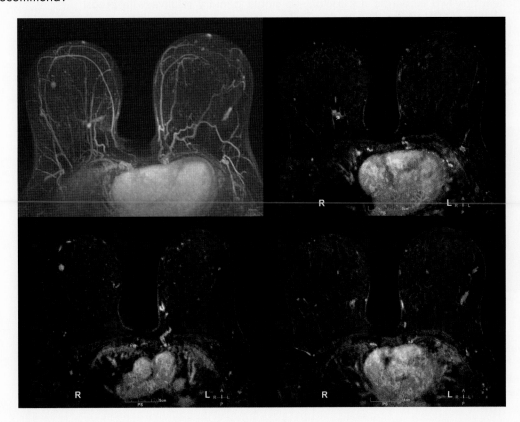

CASE 13-11. A 51-year-old average-risk woman with extremely dense tissue is recalled from screening for evaluation of a new mass in her medial left breast (*arrows*). Because the mass is likely a cyst, diagnostic mammography was not performed and the patient was evaluated by US. Should scanning be performed of the new mass only, or should the examination be expanded to include the entire breast or even both breasts?

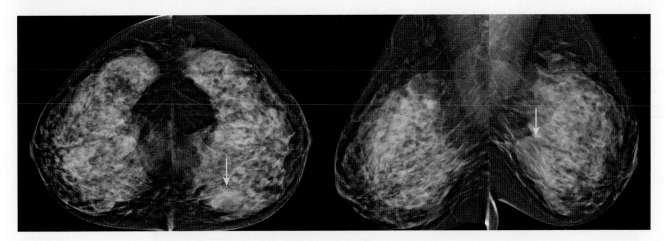

CASE 13-12. A 53-year-old woman had a less than 1 cm mass in her medial right breast detected on screening mammography. IDC was diagnosed by stereotactic biopsy, and she is referred for preoperative MRI. How would you describe the findings? What do you recommend?

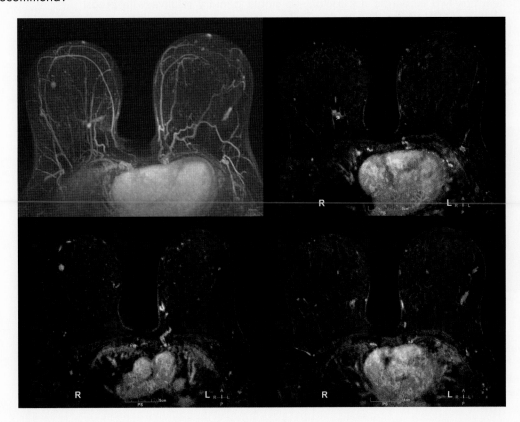

CASE ANSWERS

CASE 13-1. There is an 11-mm linear area of NME in the lateral left breast (*arrows*). It does not matter that the NME does not show color. This is BI-RADS 4. Her screening mammogram last month was negative. Small areas of NME such as this are not commonly identified on US, which was not performed. MRI-guided biopsy showed DCIS, intermediate-grade.

There is also a small focus of enhancement in the right breast at 6 o'clock (*arrow*). Despite benign features, this focus is the sole finding in the right breast. BI-RADS 3. This area underwent MRI-guided biopsy as well, which showed fibrocystic changes.

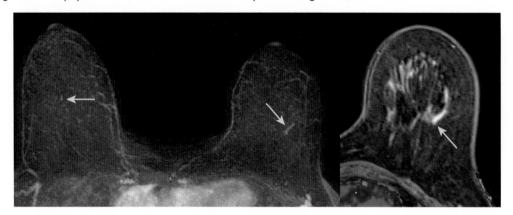

CASE 13-2. This patient has two moderate risk factors—a single primary relative with breast cancer and a biopsy showing ADH. According to the Gail model, she has a 29% lifetime risk for breast cancer, which is higher than the 20% risk for which MRI screening is recommended. It does not matter that her breast tissue is fatty-replaced. Her MRI is shown here.

Her screening MRI performed only 4 months after her screening mammogram shows clumped NME in the right breast at 6 o'clock (*arrows*) with rapid enhancement with delayed washout (*red*). Biopsy of an US correlate showed invasive lobular carcinoma.

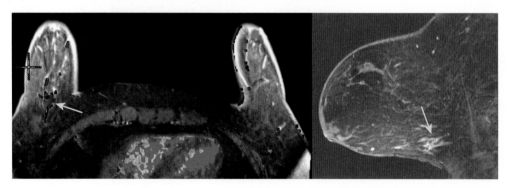

CASE 13-3. Remember to look outside the breasts. A good strategy to reading screening breast MRI is to look at the MIPs (the big picture), the T1 precontrast without fat-saturation, T2, and then go to the T1 postcontrast and sagittal sequences. This patient has gallstones that she didn't know about. She has some foci scattered in both breasts, but nothing is dominant or concerning.

CASE 13-4. There is marked asymmetry in parenchymal enhancement in the left breast. There is a focus of enhancement in the left breast at 3 o'clock that shows washout (*crosshairs*). This is BI-RADS 4. MRI-guided biopsy and subsequent surgical excision showed extensive LCIS.

LCIS is typically occult on mammography, but can result in marked enhancement on MRI. This patient will need close monitoring with imaging and has been counseled regarding other risk reduction strategies.
P.S. Enhancement of the sternum is a normal variant.

CASE 13-5. There is a 10-mm round mass with smooth margins in the medial right breast that has persistent enhancement (*blue* on color map). This has benign features, but if it is new, then biopsy may be indicated. This is her first screening MRI, but she has had prior mammograms, so let's take a look at those. Her right mammogram from 2 years earlier shows the mass (*arrow*), so it is stable: BI-RADS 2. It is likely a fibroadenoma.

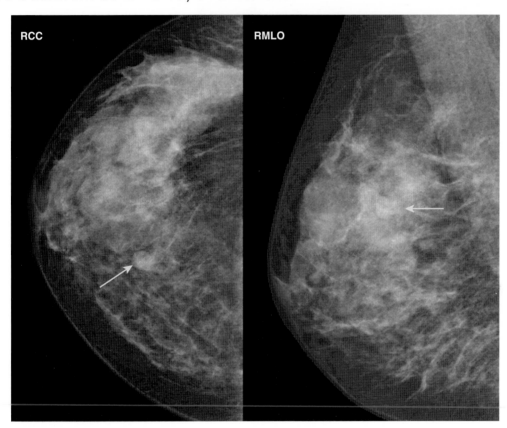

CASE 13-6. The round area of enhancement measures 7 mm and is therefore consistent with a mass rather than a focus. Furthermore, it shows intense enhancement on the 1-minute sequence, which is suspicious. This is a BI-RADS 4 lesion. A corresponding solid mass with indistinct margins was identified on US. Ultrasound-guided core biopsy revealed IDC with DCIS.

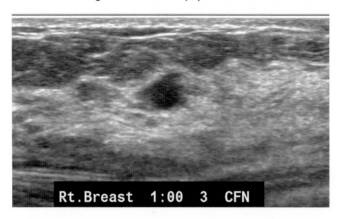

CASE 13-7. This is similar to Case 13-6. There is asymmetric enhancement in the right breast. This NME is segmental and associated with subtle distortion. Biopsy showed ILC. Did you also notice the focus in the left breast? This was the only enhancing finding in the left breast: MRI-guided biopsy also showed ILC.

CASE 13-8. A small internal mammary lymph node is present. On the sagittal view, a fatty hilum is suggested. This is uncommon but normal on MRI and is BI-RADS 2. Recommend routine high-risk screening.

CASE 13-9. There is an oval mass with ill-defined margins in the right breast at 11 o'clock that has persistent enhancement and is not T2 hyperintense. The enhancement pattern is benign, but morphologic appearance always trumps the curve. This is BI-RADS 4. MRI-guided biopsy showed DCIS, high grade, with a 3-mm focus of IDC.

CASE 13-10. There is clumped NME in a linear distribution in the lateral right breast. This is BI-RADS 4. Targeted US revealed no abnormalities. MRI-guided biopsy showed intermediate-grade DCIS.

CASE 13-11. This is a controversial topic, and there is no right or wrong answer. Certainly, by broadening our search, we may generate false-positive findings for which follow-up or biopsy will be recommended.

In our practices, we often view this type of scenario as an opportunity to informally screen dense tissue, knowing that the sensitivity of mammography is reduced in these women. In doing so, we are looking for findings suspicious for invasive cancer, not complicated cysts or other masses with benign features. In this patient, the mass seen on mammography was a simple cyst (**A**). Screening of that breast was also performed, identifying a highly suspicious mass nearby (**B**) that was IDC with DCIS on core biopsy. This lesion was occult on mammography, even in retrospect.

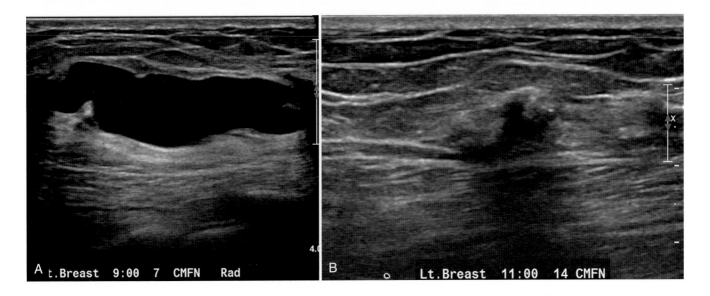

CASE 13-12. The biopsy-proven carcinoma is seen in the medial right breast (*arrow*). A slowly enhancing mass without color assignment (*arrow*) is seen in the anterior lateral right breast. Although this is of low suspicion, core biopsy was performed due to the ipsilateral malignancy and revealed fibroadenoma.

More concerning is linear NME in the lateral left breast (*arrow*). This shows persistent enhancement; however, morphologic appearance is suspicious. MRI-guided biopsy revealed DCIS. So what's this case doing in a chapter about screening? After breast cancer is diagnosed, preoperative MRI screens the contralateral breast, and detects unsuspected contralateral malignancy in 3% to 4% of patients.

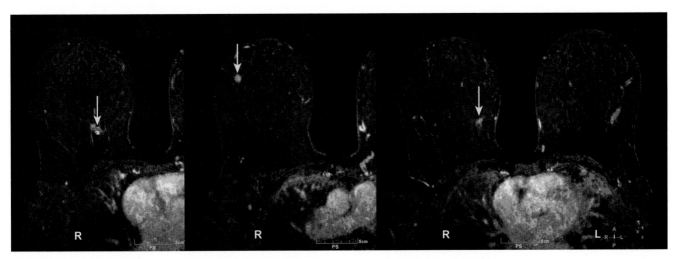

DIAGNOSTIC EXAMINATIONS AND MANAGEMENT

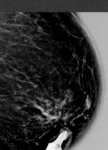

CHAPTER **14**

The Painful and the Palpable

Four o'clock and you are winding down the day. The mammography technologist brings you a mammogram of a 41-year-old woman with a breast lump. It looks negative. You ask the ultrasound technologist to scan the area, or how about scanning both breasts just to be safe. She returns a bit later with 24 images from each radian of both breasts. Looks okay.

Are you done? Wait. Don't let her leave. Go talk with her. Examine the lump and put the ultrasound transducer directly over it and really look. It will only take a few minutes and could save her life and your neck! Yes, your technologists can be trained to do this well too, though it takes dedication and feedback from the radiologist.

Radiologists have few opportunities to actually see patients, with the exception of breast imaging and interventional radiology. A busy breast-imaging practice may seem more like a clinic than a typical reading room. The radiologist covering diagnostics may spend more time out of the reading room talking with and examining patients than reading mammograms. Interacting with patients can seem intimidating at first, but hey, we all went to medical school. Obtaining a history and doing a focused clinical breast examination are extremely helpful in directing you to a significant finding.

Clinical Signs and Symptoms

Breast pain (mastalgia) is a common complaint. About 60% of women will seek medical attention at some point in their life for evaluation of breast pain. Fortunately, pain is rarely the sole presenting complaint for breast cancer. On the other hand, a palpable breast finding that is painful can definitely be cancer.

Breast pain can be classified as cyclic or noncyclic. Breast pain that is worst just before the menstrual cycle (luteal phase) is due to swelling resulting from elevated progesterone levels. Reassurance is all that is needed in most cases. For severe mastalgia, treatment with androgens or antiestrogens may be recommended.

However, very commonly when you ask a woman to point to the area of tenderness, she points to a costochondral junction or rib. In fact, noncyclic breast pain is often not due to pain in the breasts at all, but to costochondritis. Most women are just really worried that they have breast cancer; they are usually very happy to find out that their symptoms are not even related to their breasts.

In a study of 916 women presenting to a breast clinic with the primary symptom of breast pain, six women were diagnosed with breast cancer. All of these women either had a palpable lump in the symptomatic region or cancers unrelated to the symptomatic region that were detected mammographically. In addition, this study found that rather than providing reassurance to these women, immediate imaging evaluation for breast pain increased subsequent unnecessary utilization of medical services.

Bilateral or cyclic breast pain does not require diagnostic evaluation. For women with focal noncyclic breast pain and a normal clinical examination, diagnostic evaluation may be performed but is not mandatory. If a patient with mastalgia has negative mammography and the breasts are fatty replaced, it is unlikely that ultrasonography (US) will add useful information. Additional imaging may serve to reassure the patient, but our experience and the preceding study show that the likelihood of finding a cancer is exceedingly low.

If the patient with mastalgia has an abnormal clinical examination, diagnostic evaluation should be performed and management based on evaluation of the palpable abnormality. For women age 40 or older, a mammogram is a good place to start. US is usually performed as well, and when a dominant cyst is found, aspiration may provide some relief (Fig. 14-1). Cysts that are more round and distended are more likely to cause tenderness than those that are more flaccid.

Skin dimpling, focal skin thickening, or nipple retraction. Retraction or dimpling of either the skin or nipple may be due to an underlying invasive carcinoma. Focal skin thickening may be due to invasion of the dermis by carcinoma. Spot compression or tangential views and US

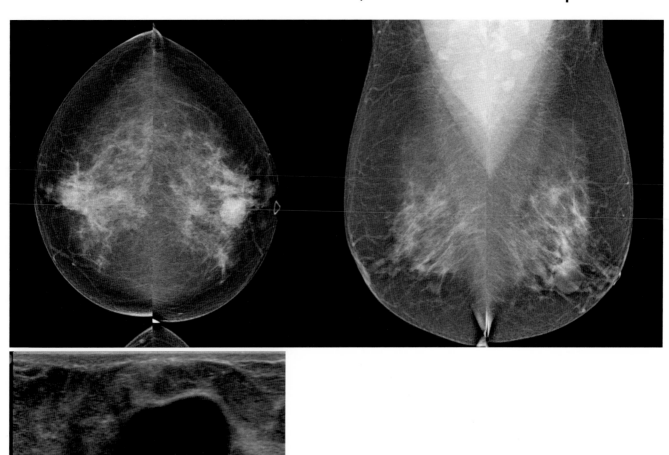

FIGURE 14-1 **Painful Breast Cyst.** A 46-year-old woman with a painful palpable mass in the left breast. Mammogram shows a round circumscribed equal density mass that corresponds to the palpable lump (*triangle marker*). On US, there is an oval simple cyst that corresponds to the painful lump. Aspiration was performed at the request of the patient for pain relief: 3 mL of yellow fluid were obtained; 2 cm³ of room air were then injected to reduce the likelihood of cyst recurrence.

of the underlying area will identify most malignancies causing these findings (Fig. 14-2). If the clinical finding is suspicious and the imaging is negative, patients in our practices are often referred for surgical evaluation. When the clinical findings are of high suspicion, an MRI may also be performed and may reveal a malignancy that is not apparent on either mammography or US.

Paget disease (nipple eczema) presents as excoriation of the skin of the nipple (Fig. 14-3) and is often diagnosed by a dermatologist. Most women with this presentation have cancer cells—most commonly high-grade ductal carcinoma in situ (DCIS)—involving the cutaneous tissues of the nipple. An invasive ductal component is often present and may be distant from the nipple. The diagnosis can be made by punch biopsy of the nipple skin by a surgeon or dermatologist. The punch biopsy will show

cancer cells percolating up to the dermis. If an invasive cancer is identified, there will virtually always be DCIS extending between the invasive carcinoma and the nipple. Paget disease is rarely associated with invasive lobular carcinoma (ILC).

Excoriation of the nipple can also occur with discharge due to an intraductal papilloma, though this is a much less common cause. In these cases, the nipple punch biopsy will be negative.

Breast edema is often due to benign causes such as fluid overload, congestive heart failure, or renal failure. This usually results in bilateral symmetric edema, though it is sometimes asymmetric due to sleeping habits or prior surgery or radiation. Unilateral breast edema is more concerning, but is also frequently benign as long as there is no erythema. On mammography, edema produces skin

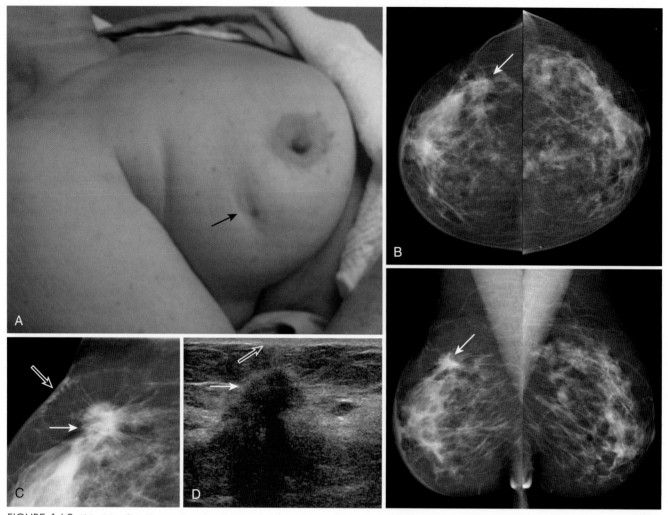

FIGURE 14-2 **Skin Dimpling Due to Invasive Cancer. A,** This 53-year-old woman presents with skin dimpling (*arrow*). **B,** On the mammogram, an irregular mass (*arrows*) with spiculated margins is present just beneath the area of dimpling. **C** and **D,** The spot compression view and US demonstrate focal skin thickening (*open arrows*) adjacent to the mass. More diffuse skin thickening is also seen in the anterior breast.

and trabecular thickening (Fig. 14-4). The findings are usually diffuse and may be more pronounced in the dependent portions of the breasts.

Breast inflammation presents as a warm red breast and is concerning for either mastitis or inflammatory breast cancer (Fig. 14-5). Mammography will show breast edema. If a suspicious mass is identified on imaging, biopsy should be performed. If mastitis is suspected, the patient can be given a trial of antibiotics for 10 to 14 days. With mastitis, the symptoms should resolve. Women with inflammatory breast cancer often have mild associated cellulitis and can show some improvement in symptoms with antibiotic treatment. If the inflammatory signs and symptoms do not clear completely, a dermal punch biopsy is necessary to exclude inflammatory breast cancer. The punch biopsy will show invasion of dermal lymphatics by tumor cells.

Focal pain associated with warmth and redness may indicate an underlying abscess. Breast abscesses are more common in women who smoke, and unfortunately, tend to be recurrent and difficult to treat with antibiotics alone. Mammography may show focal skin thickening

but is usually not specific and often painful. US can be helpful in identifying the presence, location, and size of an abscess (Fig. 14-6). In some cases, smaller abscesses can be successfully treated by ultrasound-guided aspiration and antibiotic therapy. Surgical drainage is often necessary, especially for larger collections. Abscesses can also be relatively cold in the breast, presenting with minimal or no symptoms, and can even mimic breast cancer.

Palpable breast lumps are common. Most palpable lumps are discovered by the patient, and most are benign (Box 14-1). Those in postmenopausal women have a higher chance of malignancy. Malignant palpable lumps often produce nonspecific clinical findings that cannot be distinguished from benign lesions (Fig. 14-7). In one study, about 6% of women ages 40 to 69 in a large HMO (health maintenance organization) presented for evaluation of a breast lump over a 10-year period. Of those women, about 10% were subsequently diagnosed with breast cancer.

Palpable breast thickening is defined as firmness of the breast tissue that is less discrete than a palpable lump.

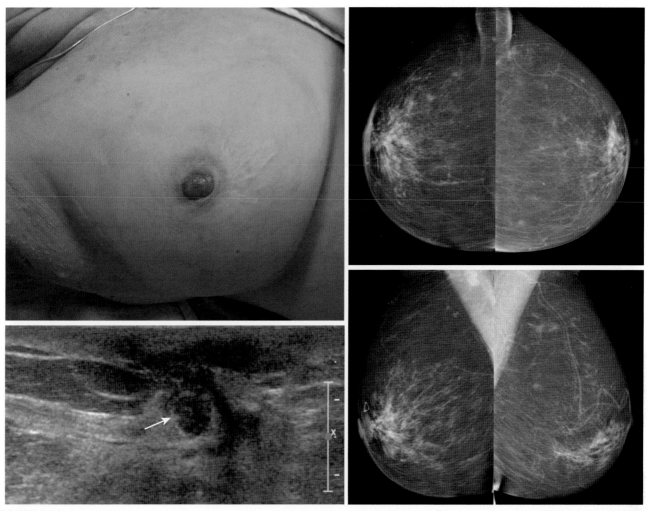

FIGURE 14-3 **Paget Disease.** A 70-year-old woman with a complaint of skin changes and retraction of her right nipple. On examination, there is erosion of the skin of the right nipple with mild retraction. The mammogram shows thickening and retraction of the right nipple with underlying architectural distortion. US of the subareolar region shows a hypoechoic mass (*arrow*). Histologic evaluation showed invasive ductal carcinoma (IDC), grade III.

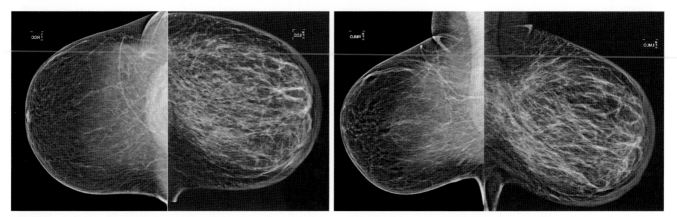

FIGURE 14-4 **Unilateral Edema Due to Mastitis.** A 42-year-old woman presented with a swollen left breast. She had mild erythema. Her symptoms resolved following a 10-day course of cephalexin.

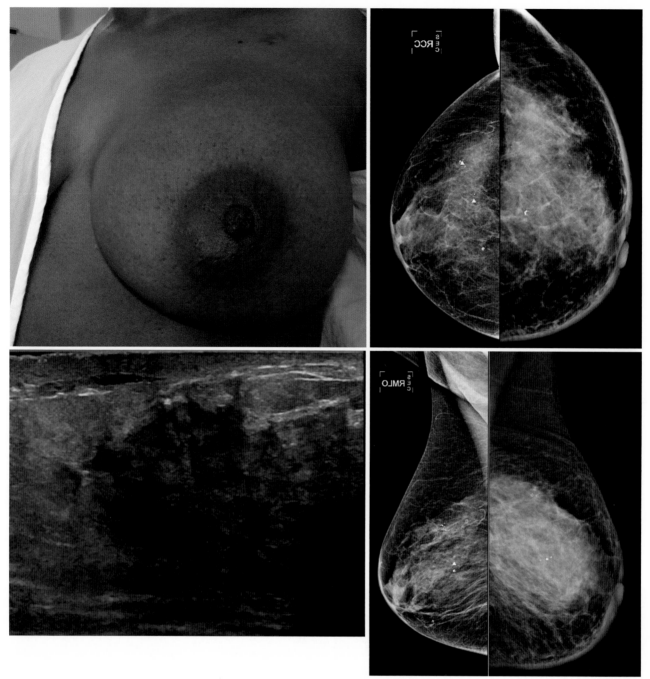

FIGURE 14-5 **Inflammatory Breast Cancer.** This 56-year-old woman presented with a warm red left breast. On mammography, there is unilateral skin thickening with increased density in the left breast. US revealed diffuse hypoechogenicity with distortion and shadowing. Histologic diagnosis: IDC.

We evaluate palpable thickening in the same manner as palpable lumps, with routine and spot compression mammographic views and US. Comparing the potentially abnormal area with the palpable texture of the rest of that breast or the opposite breast on clinical examination is very helpful in gauging the level of suspicion. Thickening is often normal, although about 5% of women with this symptom may have breast cancer. ILC and DCIS may present with palpable thickening (Fig. 14-8).

Neglected breast cancer manifests clinically as a shrunken very hard breast, often with associated erythema (Fig. 14-9). This is sometimes referred to as a "mummified" breast. Palpable ipsilateral axillary adenopathy is common. Skin nodules or erosion due to dermal metastasis may also be present. Mammography is quite difficult and may not be helpful in management. Imaging for evaluation of regional and distant disease may be helpful in staging and management. The most frequent histologic finding associated with this presentation is invasive ductal carcinoma–not otherwise specified (IDC-NOS). This appearance should not be confused with the mammographic finding of the "shrinking

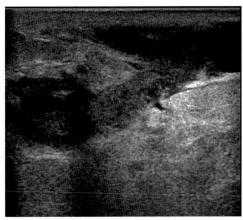

FIGURE 14-6 **Breast Abscess.** A 32-year-old woman presents with a very tender right breast with focal erythema in the upper outer quadrant. US shows a complex fluid collection under the areola that extends into the upper outer quadrant.

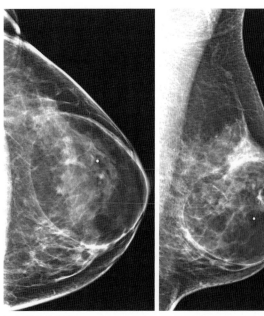

FIGURE 14-7 **Palpable Lipoma.** A 32-year-old woman presents with a palpable lump in her left breast. Mammography shows a large lipoma corresponding to the palpable finding. BI-RADS 2.

BOX 14-1 Causes of Palpable Breast Lumps

- Normal tissue
  - Ridge of tissue
  - Lactiferous sinus
  - Lymph node
  - Montgomery gland cyst
- Skin lesions (sebaceous cyst, epidermal inclusion cyst)
- Benign lesions
  - Cyst or fibrocystic change
  - Lipoma
  - Oil cyst
  - Hamartoma
  - Galactocele
  - Fibroadenoma
  - Papilloma
  - Scar
- Cancer (IDC > ILC > DCIS)

BOX 14-2 Questions to Ask a Patient with a Breast Lump

- Who found the lump and when?
- If your doctor found it, has this doctor examined you before?
- Do you perform breast self-examination on a regular basis?
- Has the finding changed? Have you had a menstrual cycle since it was found?
- Are there multiple lumps or one dominant lump?
- Have you had surgery to that region?
- Have you had recent trauma to that region?
- Have you had any signs or symptoms of infection?

breast" of ILC, which is associated with minimal clinical symptoms.

Evaluation of the Symptomatic Patient

Clinical history is helpful in assessing the relative importance of the clinical finding (Box 14-2). The easiest way to start is to simply ask the patient, "Can you tell me about the lump?" as you are washing your hands. (P.S. *Always* do this in front of the patient. Love, Mom and Dad) This will usually provide you with all of the information that you need. In our experience, a history of, "Well, it was here last week, but now it has moved over to this spot. It moves around a lot," has a negative predictive value of nearly 100%.

Clinical breast examination is usually performed in conjunction with US and can be limited to the area of concern (Fig. 14-10). If the patient can only find the palpable abnormality when in a certain position (e.g., sitting up), the examination should take place in that position. If the area is firm and different in texture compared with the rest of the breast, the level of suspicion should be high.

If the patient cannot identify the area of concern, clinical examination prior to mammography can be helpful in accurately placing a marker over the suspicious area. Ask the patient if she can show you the general region where it is located. The finding may then become obvious on your examination. If the location is still unclear, a quick call to the referring provider will often provide the specific location. We ask our providers to describe the

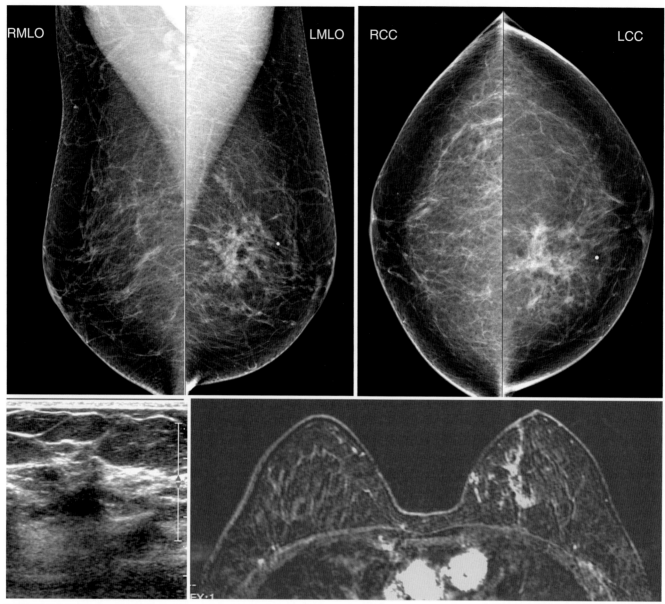

FIGURE 14-8 Palpable Thickening Due to Malignancy. A 48-year-old woman with palpable thickening in the medial left breast. Mammography shows a corresponding focal asymmetry with architectural distortion. US reveals abnormal echotexture with several hypoechoic subcentimeter ill-defined masses. Subtracted postcontrast MRI shows extensive nonmass enhancement in the region of thickening. Diagnosis: IDC and DCIS.

palpable finding and to specify its precise location on their requests by noting the clock position and distance from the nipple.

Mammography and Ultrasonography

We perform diagnostic evaluation of women presenting with palpable lumps, thickening, suspicious skin or nipple changes, focal persistent noncyclic pain, or suspicious nipple discharge (reviewed in Chapter 15). For women age 40 and older, a radiopaque marker should be placed over the clinical finding. The marker can be a metallic BB or a radiopaque triangle. A diagnostic mammogram is then performed, including spot compression views of the area of concern. If the patient has had a recent negative

mammogram (within 3 to 4 months) spot compression views of the finding may suffice. US is nearly always indicated following the mammogram though there are some exceptions, as we will discuss next.

For younger women—those under 30 or 40 in most practices—referred for evaluation of a palpable finding, US is typically used for the initial evaluation. In these women, there should be a low threshold for performing mammography, especially when the palpable finding is clinically suspicious or when the patient is at elevated risk for breast cancer. If US shows a cyst or normal tissues that account for the clinical finding, then no further evaluation may be necessary (Fig. 14-11). However, if the US findings are suspicious, confusing, or equivocal, mammography should be performed. For example, if echogenic foci suggestive of calcifications or

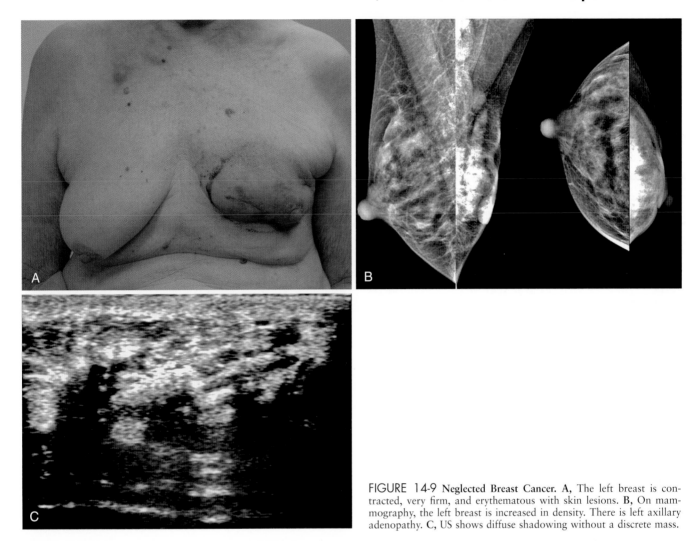

FIGURE 14-9 **Neglected Breast Cancer. A,** The left breast is contracted, very firm, and erythematous with skin lesions. **B,** On mammography, the left breast is increased in density. There is left axillary adenopathy. **C,** US shows diffuse shadowing without a discrete mass.

FIGURE 14-10 **Focused Clinical Examination with Targeted US for Evaluating a Palpable Finding. A,** Breast palpation is performed using the three middle fingers with the pads placed flat on the breast. Using small concentric circles light, medium, and then deep pressure is applied. **B,** An ink mark over the lump can be helpful as palpation may become more difficult after the application of US gel. **C,** The US probe is placed directly over the palpable finding in order to best determine its cause. *(From Harvey JA. Sonography of palpable breast masses. Semin Ultrasound CT MR 2006;27(4):284-297.)*

FIGURE 14-11 **Normal US in a Young Woman.** A 32-year-old woman with a palpable ridge of breast tissue. US demonstrates hyperechoic breast tissue *(arrows)* surrounded by fat on both sides. BI-RADS 1 or 2. *(From Harvey JA. Sonography of palpable breast masses. Semin Ultrasound CT MR 2006;27(4):284-297.)*

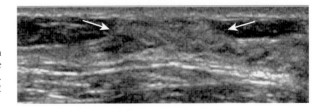

a suspicious mass are seen, mammography should be performed.

Ultrasound should be focused as precisely as possible on the palpable finding. This gives us the best chance to identify and determine the cause of the clinical finding. If necessary, the palpable finding can be pinned between two fingers and the transducer placed between them. A standoff pad can be helpful for correlating the US and clinical findings (Fig. 14-12). US of the quadrant of tissue surrounding the clinical finding can also be performed but is not mandatory.

When we are scanning, we find that women can often tell precisely when the transducer passes over a palpable finding. This provides confirmation that the area of concern was specifically evaluated, even if no imaging abnormalities are detected. Occasionally, as you are scanning, a patient will inform you of another area that is of concern to her on self-examination. We generally scan those regions as well, even if they were not considered suspicious on the clinical examination performed by the health care provider.

Magnetic resonance imaging (MRI) may occasionally be useful if the clinical examination is very suspicious but the imaging is negative (Fig. 14-13).

Imaging Management Scenarios

Mammogram shows a definitely benign mass, such as a lipoma, oil cyst, or coarsely calcified fibroadenoma (Fig. 14-14): No further evaluation is needed. US can be skipped if it is clear that the benign mass represents the palpable finding. This is BI-RADS 2. If it is not clear, then US can be helpful to confirm that the clinical and mammographic findings are the same.

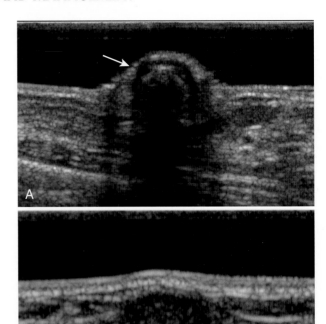

FIGURE 14-12 US Correlation of a Palpable Finding. **A,** A finger (*arrow*) is placed on top of the palpable lump between a stand-off pad and the breast. **B,** The finger is slid out of the way. The palpable mass is then seen indenting the gel pad (*arrows*). *(From Harvey JA. Sonography of palpable breast masses. Semin Ultrasound CT MR 2006;27(4):284-297.)*

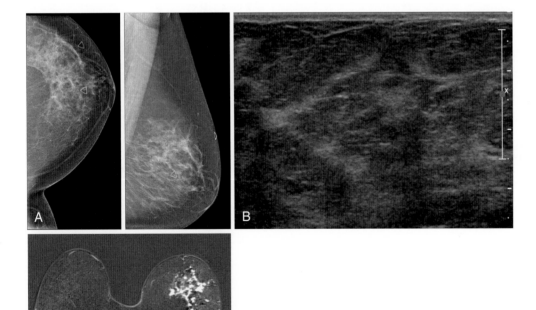

FIGURE 14-13 Diagnostic MRI to Evaluate a Palpable Finding. **A,** Left mammogram suggests subtle architectural distortion, but no definable abnormality. **B,** US did not show any abnormalities in the region of the palpable finding. **C,** Subtraction image from contrast-enhanced MRI shows extensive nonmass enhancement in the left breast. Pathologic findings showed ILC.

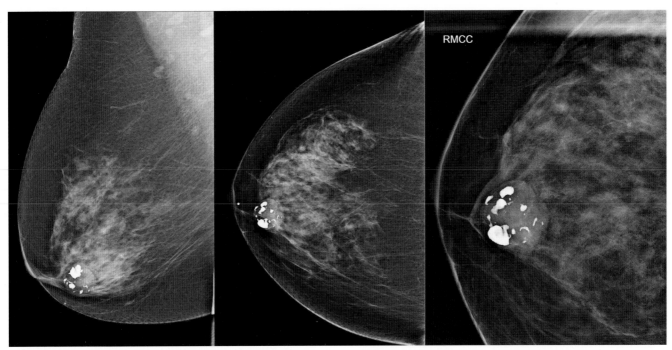

FIGURE 14-14 **Palpable Fibroadenoma.** A 65-year-old woman with no prior mammograms presents with a palpable mass in her right breast (marked with a *BB* on the craniocaudal (CC) and mediolateral oblique (MLO) views). There is a circumscribed mass with coarse calcifications corresponding to the palpable finding. These features are characteristic of a hyalinized fibroadenoma. BI-RADS 2.

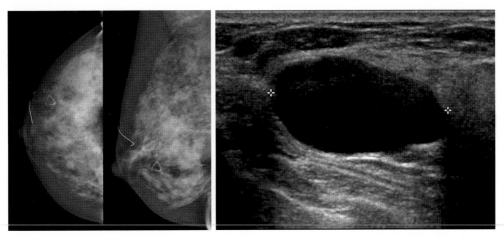

FIGURE 14-15 **Negative Mammogram with Palpable Benign Cyst.** BI-RADS 2. Aspiration is needed only if desired by the patient for symptomatic relief.

Mammogram is negative and US shows a definitely benign mass, such as a lymph node or simple cyst (Fig. 14-15): No further evaluation is needed. BI-RADS 2.

Mammogram shows only fatty tissue in the area of the palpable finding: You must ask yourself if the palpable finding was definitely on the mammogram. If it could be back by the chest wall, then US will help ensure that a mass was not missed.

Performing US on these patients can also help identify a definitive benign cause for a palpable lump (Fig. 14-16). By your demonstrating a benign mass such as an area of fat necrosis or a lipoma, the patient will be reassured and may be less likely to seek unnecessary intervention.

Mammography or US shows a normal structure. Normal structures that can present as a palpable finding include the inframammary ridge, lymph nodes, ribs, costochondral joints, lactiferous sinuses, and Montgomery glands (Fig. 14-17). Normal fibroglandular tissue may also present as a palpable lump, ridge, or thickening. Careful correlation of the palpable finding with US can ensure that the clinical finding is benign.

Mammogram and US show a nonspecific mass with benign features. On the mammogram, this includes round or oval circumscribed masses. On US benign features include homogeneously hypoechoic solid masses with parallel orientation, abrupt well-defined margins, and no shadowing. The scenario is similar whether the mammogram is negative and the US shows a mass with benign features or the mammogram shows a mass with benign features and the US is negative. The situation is not the

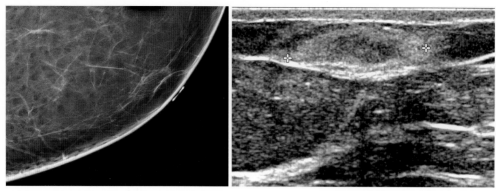

FIGURE 14-16 **Palpable Lump with a Fatty Mammogram.** Spot compression view of a palpable lump (marked by a *triangle*) shows only fatty tissue. On US, the palpable lump corresponded to a superficial oval hyperechoic mass with central hypoechogenicity. The findings are consistent with fat necrosis. BI-RADS 2. On clinical examination, the lump was soft, but easily palpable. Without a specific diagnostic finding on US, this patient may have sought an unnecessary surgical intervention.

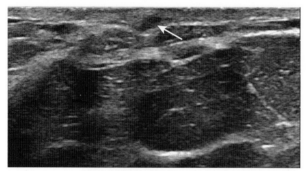

FIGURE 14-17 **Palpable Montgomery Gland Cyst.** This young woman palpated a superficial BB-sized round mass in the areola. US shows a small cyst (*arrow*) in the dermis of the areola consistent with a Montgomery gland cyst.

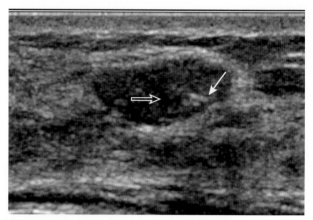

FIGURE 14-18 **Palpable Probable Fibroadenoma.** The mass is oval, parallel in orientation, homogeneously hypoechoic, with a very well-defined abrupt margin. There is a suggestion of a septation (*arrow*) and a small cyst centrally (*open arrow*). Short-term follow-up was performed, and the mass has been stable for over 2 years.

same if either mammography or US shows a suspicious mass and the other modality shows a mass with benign features. The mass should be managed based on the most suspicious features.

The vast majority of these masses represent fibroadenomas (Fig. 14-18). If this is a baseline mammogram and the lesion is palpable, then either short-term follow-up (BI-RADS 3) or biopsy (BI-RADS 4A) can be used (Box 14-3). If follow-up is recommended, then the lesion should have all of the characteristics of a fibroadenoma: oval shape, well-defined margins, parallel orientation, and homogeneous echo texture. If the mass is visible on mammography as a new or enlarging finding, then biopsy should be considered (BI-RADS 4).

Mammogram and US show a mass with suspicious features. These masses must undergo biopsy (BI-RADS 4 or 5) unless definitively shown to be benign by another modality (Fig. 14-19). For example, an apparently suspicious mass on US may be shown to represent a benign oil cyst on mammography, eliminating the need for biopsy (BI-RADS 2).

Mammogram and US show a highly suspicious mass. Excellent! You made the finding for this patient. However, don't stop looking; our job is not yet done. The role of imaging for these patients shifts from detection and diagnosis to evaluating the extent of disease and staging. This

> ### BOX 14-3 Can I Use BI-RADS 3 for a Palpable Finding?
>
> Series including at least 1000 women with palpable masses that have benign features on US have been published in the literature. The cancer incidence in these series ranges from 0% to 0.8%, which is lower than the incidence in the series of nonpalpable masses with benign imaging features. Given these results, short-interval follow-up of palpable solid masses is a reasonable alternative to biopsy if there are only benign features.

includes looking for additional abnormal calcifications or masses and using US to evaluate axillary lymph node morphologic appearance (Fig. 14-20).

Mammogram and US are both negative. When malignancies are large enough to detect on clinical breast examination, they almost always produce suspicious findings on mammography or US focused on the palpable

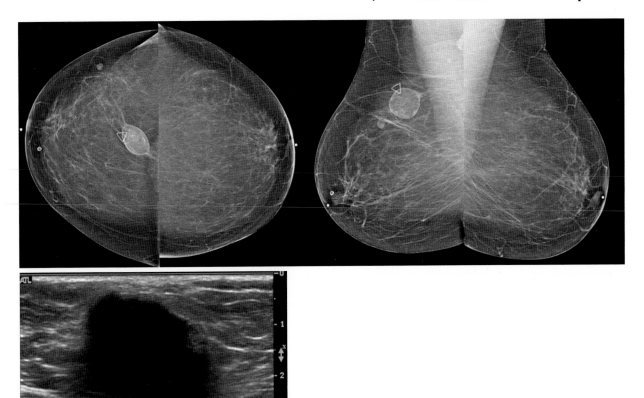

FIGURE 14-19 **Suspicious US, but Specific Benign Mammogram.** A 68-year-old woman presents with a palpable lump in the right breast. Mammogram shows a round, circumscribed, fat-containing mass with rim calcifications that corresponds to the palpable mass (*triangle*). It would be appropriate to stop at this point because the mammogram has a specific benign finding. US shows a complex mass with posterior acoustic shadowing. The US findings are suspicious, but fortunately the mammogram shows a clearly benign mass. BI-RADS 2.

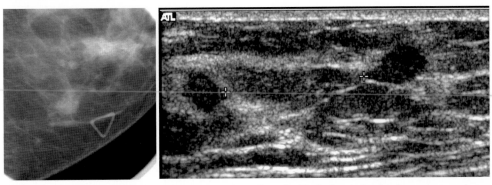

FIGURE 14-20 **Multifocal Invasive Carcinoma.** Spot compression view of a palpable finding (*triangle*) shows an irregular mass. Corresponding US shows a highly suspicious mass with ill-defined margins and an echogenic halo. A second mass was identified on US between the palpable lump and the nipple. Both masses represented IDC on core biopsy. *(From Harvey JA. Sonography of palpable breast masses. Semin Ultrasound CT MR 2006;27(4):284-297.)*

area. The negative predictive value of mammography and US in the setting of a palpable finding ranges from 97% to 100% in the literature. For the vast majority of women, all that is needed after negative imaging is reassurance.

However, some symptomatic malignancies—particularly noncalcified DCIS or ILC—may be occult on routine imaging, and this possibility should be conveyed to the patient (Fig. 14-21). If the clinical findings are very suspicious, surgical consultation should be considered without delay, even when mammography and US are negative or equivocal. MRI may also be useful in this setting (see Fig. 14-13).

When the clinical examination seems fine and imaging is negative, the patient needs reassurance. However, a very small number of these women will have breast cancer in that region, so a good approach is to reassure but emphasize that the palpable finding should be monitored. It is important not to dismiss the clinical finding. Let her know that everything looks fine and that you don't see anything concerning. Then close the conversation by saying, "However, this is not a perfect test. Keep an eye on that area. Continue to examine yourself regularly, and if you notice any concerning changes, give your provider a call to get it rechecked, even if it's next week. If you or your provider are worried, we are also happy to see you back for imaging if your provider requests it."

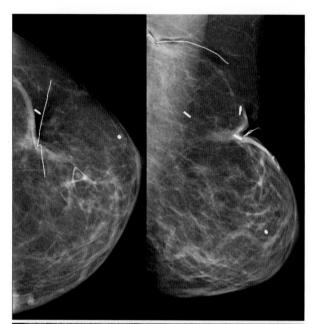

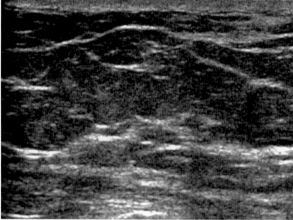

FIGURE 14-21 **Suspicious Clinical Examination with Negative Mammogram and US.** The patient had a firm palpable area in the left breast at 12 o'clock (*triangle*) inferior to a prior lumpectomy site. The mammogram and US are normal. MRI was also normal. Core biopsy of the palpable area was performed using manual guidance showing DCIS, intermediate grade. Extensive DCIS was found in that region on mastectomy.

If the clinical examination is very concerning, radiologists who are experienced and comfortable performing clinical examinations can help facilitate referral of these patients for prompt surgical consultation. Consider how the palpable finding feels on clinical examination. Is it simply a lumpy area in the background of a lumpy breast or something more suspicious? The clinical examination is very concerning when the finding is firm and distinct from the rest of the breast tissue. If your practice does not manage patient referrals or you're not experienced deciding the level of suspicion of a clinical finding, then patients should be advised to follow-up with their referring providers, who will direct the patient's management.

If you lack confidence in your clinical skills because you haven't done a breast examination in a long time, breast imaging provides an excellent opportunity to learn. This is a skill that you can develop over time. Because we have the advantage of immediate feedback about our examination from US, radiologists can become very good at discerning what is likely to be normal or not, even before we start scanning. You do not need to examine both breasts or even the entire breast. An examination focused to the area of concern is typically adequate. Give it a try!

Palpable unilateral axillary adenopathy. You must be highly suspicious of ipsilateral invasive breast carcinoma (Fig. 14-22). Biopsy of an axillary lymph node is a good place to start to obtain a diagnosis of metastatic breast carcinoma, although sometimes the biopsy will show lymphoma or a nonbreast metastasis such as melanoma. A core biopsy will yield enough tissue for the pathologist to perform receptor assays and special stains if needed. When a diagnosis of metastatic breast cancer is established, identification of the primary breast lesion is helpful in management. If the mammogram is negative, US can be useful to screen the breast. If both are negative, then MRI will detect the primary carcinoma in about 90% of women. Occasionally, the primary breast lesion is never identified.

Final Comments

It seems counterintuitive that radiologists, the specialists most worried about lawsuits, may be satisfied with having a technologist do a nontargeted US of the entire breast to evaluate a woman with a palpable lump. To take full advantage of the high sensitivity of mammography and US in evaluating palpable findings, the examination should be focused on the clinical finding. Performing a *targeted* clinical examination and correlating the findings with US can save you and your patient!

P.S. Seeing patients is also very rewarding. They are so grateful for your care. You will get hugs, cupcakes, and excellent survey responses in return.

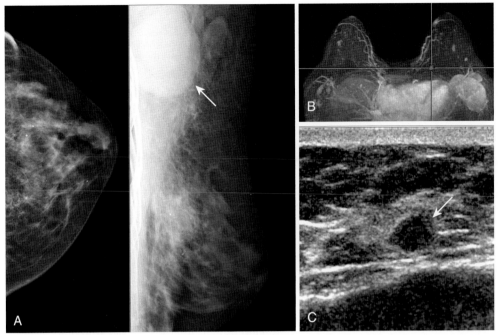

FIGURE 14-22 **Palpable Unilateral Axillary Adenopathy Due to Invasive Breast Carcinoma. A,** There is a large left axillary lymph node on the mammogram (*arrow*). The remainder of the mammogram and whole breast US were negative. **B** and **C,** MRI identified a 10-mm mass in the left breast at 7 o'clock (*crosshairs*) that was identified by second-look US (*arrow*). Histologic diagnosis: IDC, grade III.

KEY POINTS

- For the symptomatic patient to benefit from the full capabilities of mammography and US, it is important for the imaging evaluation to be as focused as possible on the clinical finding.
- History and limited clinical examination complement the imaging and permit direct correlation of the imaging and clinical findings.
- Breast cancer rarely presents with pain as the sole complaint. However, focal pain associated with a palpable abnormality may be due to breast cancer and warrants diagnostic evaluation.
- In women 40 years of age and older, suspicious palpable lumps, thickening, or skin or nipple changes are evaluated by routine and spot compression mammographic views, and US. In younger women, US is used as the initial study.
- The negative predictive value of mammography and US in evaluating a palpable abnormality is over 95%. These patients can be reassured that the finding is very unlikely to be malignant but should be monitored with clinical examination. If the clinical findings are highly suspicious and routine imaging is negative, MRI may be of value.
- Inflammatory changes involving the breast may be due to mastitis or inflammatory carcinoma. If the signs and symptoms persist after antibiotic treatment, punch biopsy of the skin should be performed.

References

Dennis MA, Parker SH, Klaus AJ, et al. Breast biopsy avoidance: The value of normal mammograms and normal sonograms in the setting of a palpable lump. Radiology 2001;219:186-191.

Harvey JA, Nicholson BT, LoRusso AP, et al. Short-term follow-up of palpable breast lesions with benign imaging features: evaluation of 375 lesions in 320 women. Am J Roentgenol 2009;193:1723-1730.

Hook GW, Ikeda DM. Treatment of breast abscesses with US-guided percutaneous needle drainage without indwelling catheter placement. Radiology 1999;213:579-582.

Howard MB, Battaglia T, Prout M, Freund K. The effect of imaging on the clinical management of breast pain. J Gen Intern Med 2012;27(7):817-824.

Smith RL, Pruthi S, Fitzpatrick LA. Evaluation and management of breast pain. Mayo Clin Proc 2004;79:353-372.

Soo MS, Rosen EL, Baker JA, et al. Negative predictive value of sonography with mammography in patients with palpable breast lesions. Am J Roentgenol 2001;177:1167-1170.

CASE QUESTIONS

CASE 14-1. A 64-year-old woman has erosion of the skin on her right nipple. Here is her mammogram. What would you do next?

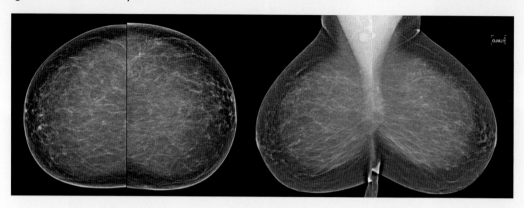

CASE 14-2. A 48-year-old woman with a palpable lump behind the right nipple with mild associated nipple retraction. What is your differential diagnosis? Your BI-RADS assessment and recommendation?

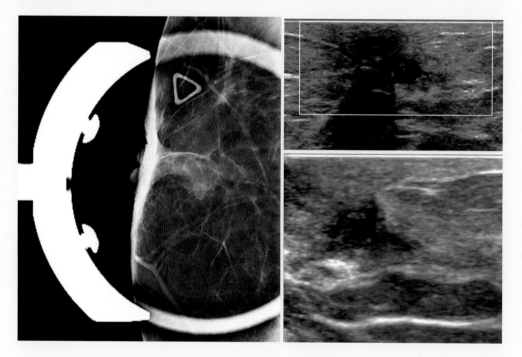

CASE 14-3. A 52-year-old woman has a palpable lump in the left breast (*triangle*). She had a normal screening mammogram 3 months ago. Your technologist brings these images. What would you do?

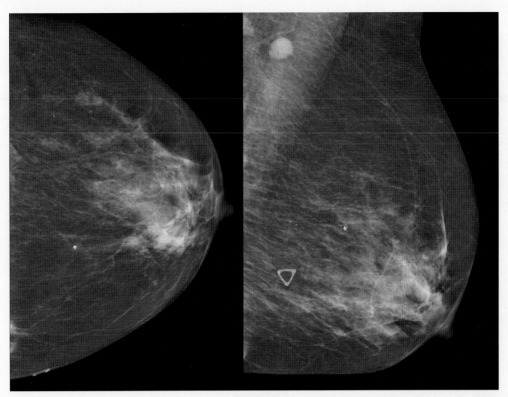

CASE 14-4. A 45-year-old woman presents with a palpable mass in her lateral left breast (marked with a *BB*). What are the findings? What do you recommend?

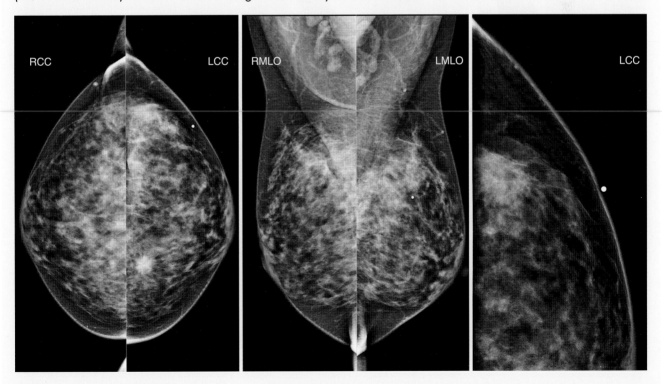

CASE 14-5. A 62-year-old woman with a history of benign surgical biopsy of the left breast 10 years ago presents with a small palpable lump she detected near the scar marked with a *BB*. Diagnostic mammography and US are performed. The sonographer tells you she can only feel scar tissue and brings you these images. What do you recommend?

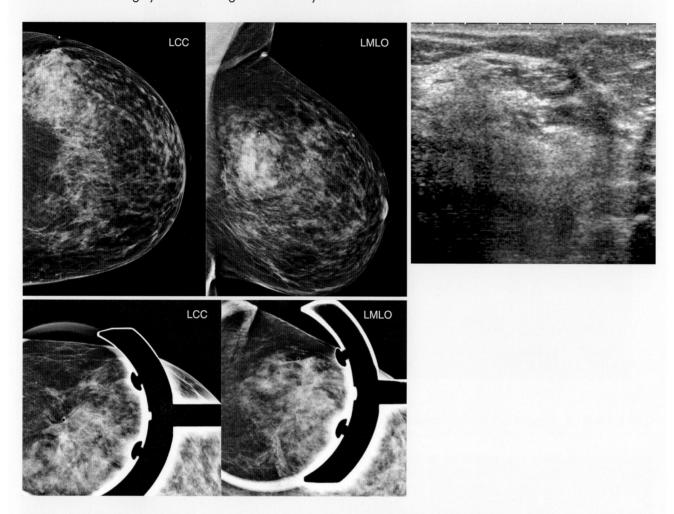

CASE 14-6. A 64-year-old woman who had a normal mammogram 3 months earlier presents with a new palpable lump in her upper right breast. She had a motor vehicle accident 1 month ago. US is shown here. What do you recommend?

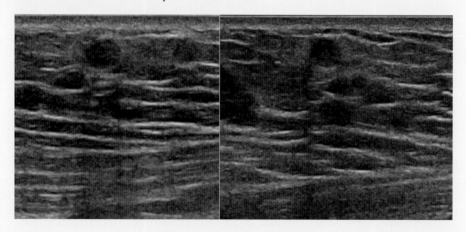

CASE 14-7. A 51-year-old woman has a history of pain and swelling of the left breast and axilla. Mastitis was suspected. She completed a course of antibiotics with slight improvement. Mammography was performed, although she could not tolerate optimal compression. US of the breast and axilla was also performed. How would you describe the findings? What are your management recommendations?

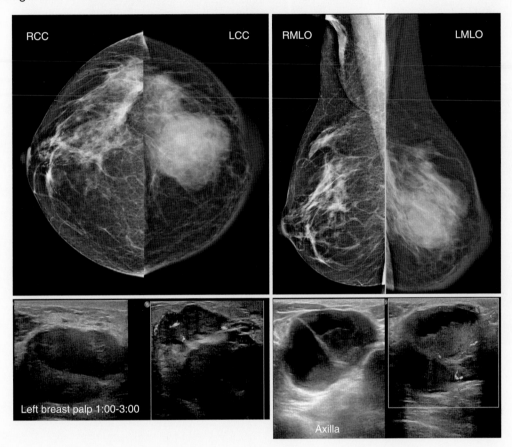

CASE 14-8. An 85-year-old woman presents with new retraction of the left nipple. What are the mammographic findings? What do you recommend?

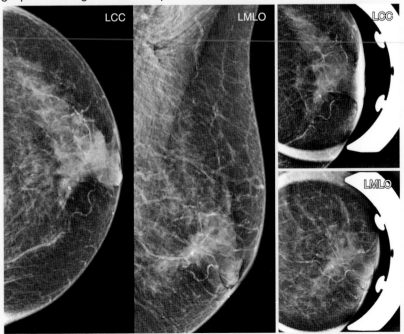

CASE 14-9. A 52-year-old woman presents with a palpable left breast mass. Mammography and US were performed. She has two clips in the left breast from previous benign biopsies. The sonographer found one dominant cyst accounting for the palpable mass as well as two small masses in the same region. What do you recommend?

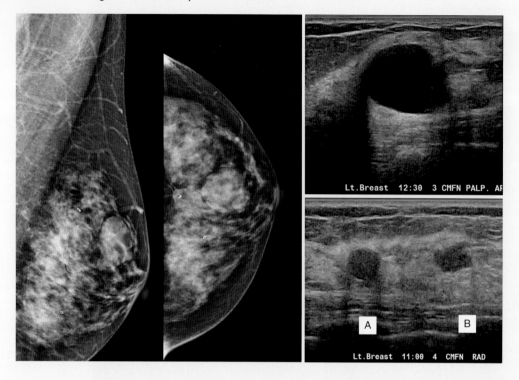

CASE 14-10. A 60-year-old woman presents with a palpable mass in her left breast marked with *BB*. Diagnostic mammography was performed. What are the findings? What do you recommend?

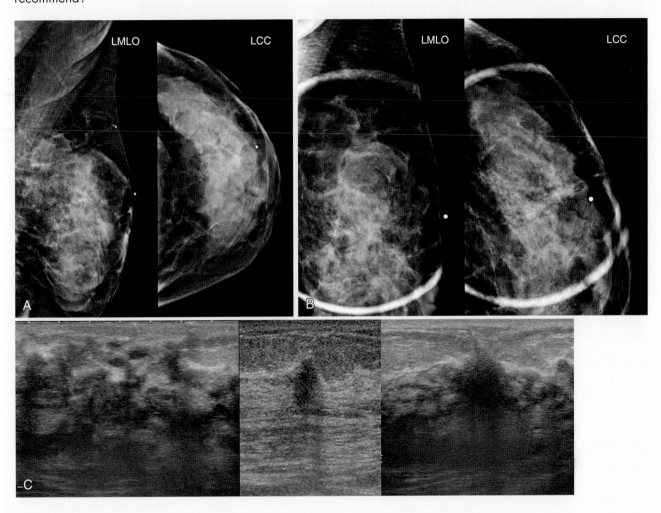

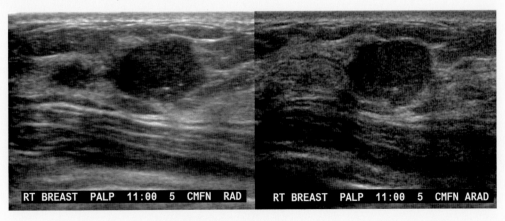

CASE 14-11. A 27-year-old woman presents with a palpable right breast mass. US images are shown here. What do you recommend?

CASE 14-12. A 54-year-old woman with a tender, palpable cordlike area in her right axilla (*arrow*). What do you think is the most likely cause?

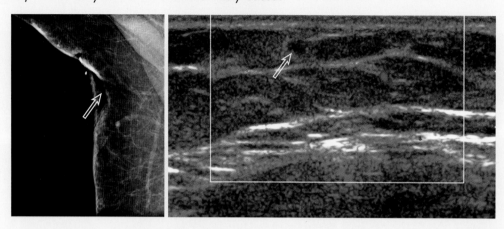

CASE ANSWERS

CASE 14-1. Her mammogram is negative. US was also negative. Her dermatologist performed a punch biopsy of the right nipple that shows adenocarcinoma. This patient's symptoms are concerning for Paget disease, and the skin punch biopsy confirms the diagnosis. An MRI was performed to evaluate the extent of disease. **A** and **B,** Subtraction contrast-enhanced MRI shows asymmetric enhancement of the right nipple (*arrow*) compared with the left (*open arrow*). **C,** There is nonmass enhancement in the right breast at 11 o'clock (*arrow*). Histologic evaluation showed high-grade DCIS. (Skin enhancement in the left medial breast is due to an inflamed sebaceous cyst.)

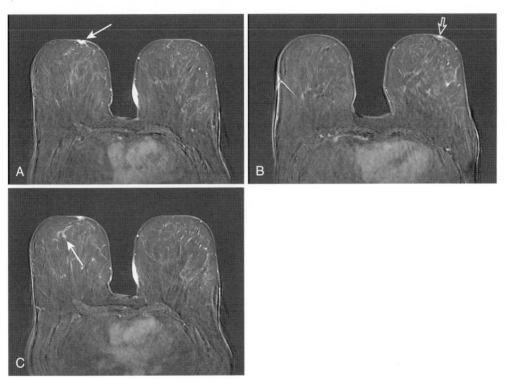

CASE 14-2. There is a low-density mass in the subareolar region of the right breast. The US is very suspicious, showing a hypoechoic irregular mass with increased vascularity. BI-RADS 4. Recommend ultrasound-guided core biopsy. Histologic findings showed abscess! Hey, it happens. She noted only minimal tenderness, was afebrile, and there was no erythema. Good news for her!

CASE 14-3. Spot compression views were obtained showing a portion of an irregular mass in the posterior breast on the CC view. Her US shows a malignant-appearing solid mass. Ultrasound-guided core biopsy showed IDC. This is not a sternalis muscle, which is visualized on the CC view only and is never palpable.

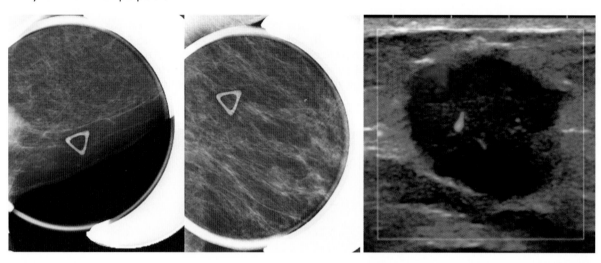

CASE 14-4. A mass is seen in the region of the palpable finding. Did you also notice the spiculated lesion in the medial left breast? US shows multiple irregular masses (three are shown). Core biopsy of lesions in the 2 o'clock and 7 o'clock positions revealed infiltrating carcinoma with ductal and lobular features. Due to multicentric disease, mastectomy was performed. In this case, mammography and US determined disease extent to be much greater than suspected clinically.

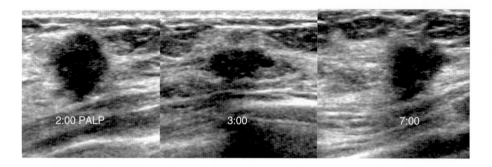

CASE 14-5. The tissue is dense. There is mild architectural distortion at the previous biopsy site. The next step is to examine and scan the patient yourself! When asked, the patient was able to put one finger precisely on the newly palpable finding that was anterior to the scar. Repeat US of this region (image shown here) shows a shadowing mass with ill-defined margins separate from the scar. Core biopsy revealed ILC.

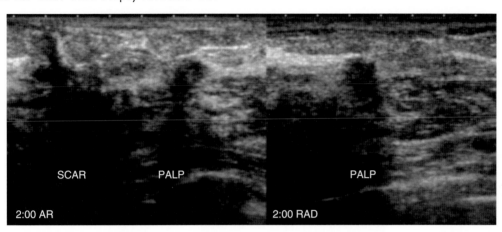

CASE 14-6. There are several hypoechoic masses corresponding to the palpable finding. These have a nonspecific US appearance. Although the patient has had a recent mammogram, a repeat limited mammogram should be performed. An MLO view with a *BB* over the lump shows fat necrosis with oil cysts. Now we know with certainty that the lump is benign. BI-RADS 2.

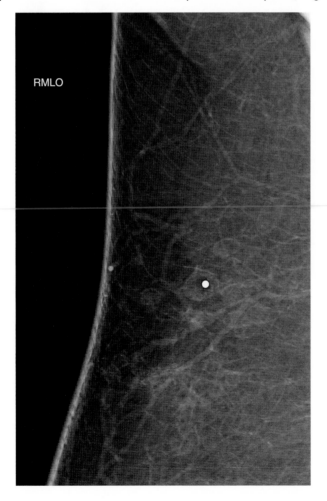

CASE 14-7. Mammography shows a large mass in the central left breast and marked left skin thickening. US shows complex masses with flow on color Doppler in the central left breast and axilla. The differential diagnosis includes abscess and necrotic tumor.

Purulent material was aspirated from the breast mass. Core biopsy of the residual mass revealed IDC. The axillary mass was aspirated, yielding bloody fluid. Cytologic examination was positive for ductal carcinoma. Secondary infection of a cancer is very uncommon. Diagnosis: necrotic IDC, grade III, complicated by abscess formation. Necrotic axillary adenopathy.

CASE 14-8. There is a spiculated mass in the retroareolar region that accounts for the nipple retraction (*arrows*). US shows an irregular hypoechoic mass in the 12 o'clock position. BI-RADS 5. Recommend ultrasound-guided core biopsy. Diagnosis: ILC.

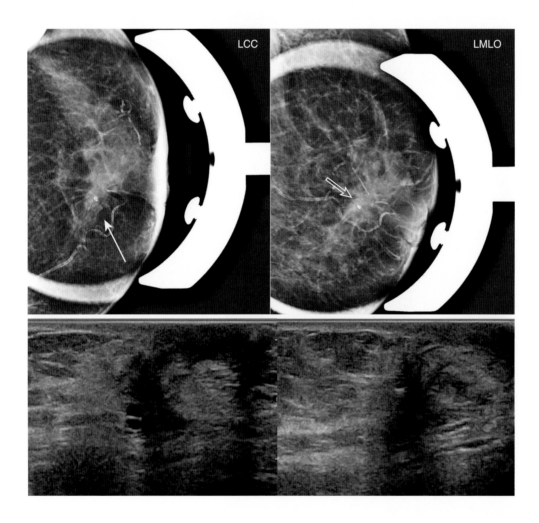

CASE 14-9. The palpable mass is visible on mammography and is a benign simple cyst by US. The two smaller masses (A and B) do not represent simple cysts. Mass A is round with well-defined margins; however, mass B is irregular in shape with angular margins. Lesion A was aspirated and represented a complicated cyst. Core biopsy of lesion B revealed IDC.

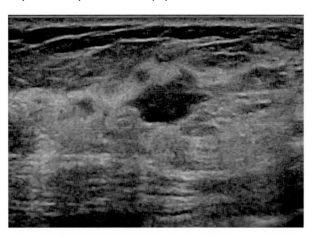

CASE 14-10. The tissue is extremely dense. There is subtle architectural distortion in the upper outer breast. This is best seen at the lateral border of the fibroglandular tissue (*arrows*). Note the focal areas of skin thickening (*open arrows*).

US revealed diffusely abnormal echotexture throughout the upper outer breast (first image). Multiple hypoechoic masses were also seen in this quadrant. BI-RADS 5. Diagnosis: Multicentric ILC.

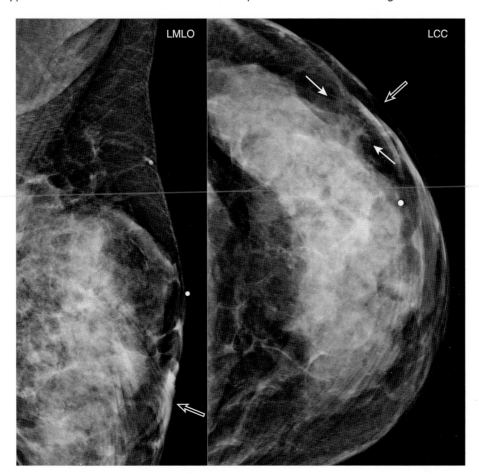

CASE 14-11. US shows two solid masses, the smaller (*arrow*) with microlobulated margins and the larger with angular margins. There are echogenic foci in the posterior aspect of the larger mass (*open arrow*) suggesting calcifications. Because of these suspicious features mammography was performed, showing a mass with associated fine pleomorphic calcifications. Biopsy revealed IDC with high-grade DCIS.

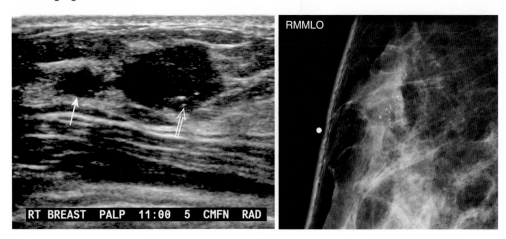

CASE 14-12. There is a tubular density on the mammogram in the region of the palpable finding. On US, this is hypoechoic without flow. Diagnosis: clotted superficial vein (Mondor disease). This may be treated conservatively. Anticoagulation is not necessary.

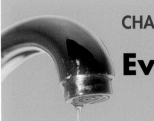

CHAPTER 15

Evaluation of Nipple Discharge

She's a little embarrassed. And she's more than a little nervous. She saw a spot of blood in her bra. Does she have cancer? Her mammogram last month was normal, so everything must be fine.

Don't let this make you nervous. Figuring out who has concerning versus benign discharge is actually pretty straightforward. One of the most helpful things you can do now is go talk with her and examine her. Ask her to show you the discharge. With a few questions, you can usually tell whether she needs reassurance or imaging. (P.S. The mammogram is almost always normal.)

In a typical history for worrisome discharge a woman notices a spot of blood in her bra or a wet spot on her nightgown upon awakening. Worrisome discharge is usually unilateral, but can occur in women with preexisting bilateral benign nipple discharge. It may occur only once or a few times and seem to resolve. A typical history for benign nipple discharge is discharge that is expressed or occurs during mammographic compression and can be any color except bloody. A warm bath or shower relaxes the smooth muscle in the nipple, so discharge that only appears following bathing is not considered spontaneous and is usually benign.

Discharge that is bloody is concerning, but so is serous discharge. If the discharge is yellow or clear, the fluid can be checked for the presence of blood using a urine dipstick. A dipstick that turns green within the first 30 seconds indicates blood products and should be considered a true positive. If you look at the dipstick later, it will eventually turn green due to the lactoferrin that is normally secreted in breast fluid, which is a false positive (Table 15-1).

Etiology of Nipple Discharge

Milky discharge (galactorrhea) is not concerning for breast cancer but may be due to a brain tumor—specifically a pituitary prolactinoma. Women with thyroid disorders can also have milky discharge because thyroid-stimulating hormone (TSH) can cross-talk with prolactin. Serum prolactin and TSH should be checked in women with milky discharge. Some medications can also result in milky discharge, including psychotropic medications, such as antidepressants, neuroleptics, and metoclopramide. These medications are dopamine antagonists, which stimulate prolactin production.

Benign nipple discharge (not milky) (Fig. 15-1) in premenopausal women is most commonly due to fibrocystic change in which cysts communicate with the ducts (Fig. 15-2). In postmenopausal women, duct ectasia is the most common cause. With duct ectasia, the ducts are dilated in the subareolar region and become attenuated more posteriorly (Fig. 15-3).

Worrisome discharge (Fig. 15-4) is due to an intraductal papilloma 90% of the time (Fig. 15-5), but is due to ductal carcinoma in situ (DCIS) about 8% of the time (Fig. 15-6). A single intraductal mass near the nipple is most likely to represent a papilloma; however, the imaging appearance is not definitive, and a tissue diagnosis is needed. Multiple intraductal masses (see Fig. 15-6) are concerning for DCIS but may be due to papillomatosis or even debris. Trauma (e.g., injury due to a motor vehicle collision), core or surgical biopsy, and cyst aspiration are rare causes of bloody discharge. Occasionally, a cause is not identified.

Evaluating Nipple Discharge

Clinical history and examination are important in order to triage who needs blood work (milky), reassurance (benign), or workup (worrisome). The first question to ask is how the patient noticed the discharge. This will tell you if it is spontaneous or expressible. You will also want to know the color and duration of the discharge, and whether it is unilateral or bilateral. Women should also be asked about medications that could explain milky discharge and whether there is any recent history of trauma.

Mammography may reveal suspicious calcifications indicating DCIS as the cause, but is nearly always negative. Sometimes a solitary dilated duct will correlate with the offending duct. This finding is not very specific, although it becomes more suspicious if it is new or increasing, associated with concerning calcifications, or in a non-subareolar location. Don't bother with spot compression or magnification views behind the nipple unless an abnormality is suspected on the routine views.

Ultrasound can be very useful for evaluating ductal pathology (Fig. 15-7). The location of the discharging orifice on the nipple can be helpful in guiding the ultrasonography (US) examination. For example, if the orifice is on the lateral aspect of the nipple, it is likely that the abnormal duct system will also be in the lateral breast. If

TABLE 15-1	Distinguishing Worrisome from Benign Nipple Discharge	
POTENTIALLY CANCEROUS	**PROBABLY BENIGN**	
Unilateral	Often bilateral	
Bloody or serous	Yellow, green, black, milky	
From a single orifice	From multiple orifices	
Spontaneous	Expressible	

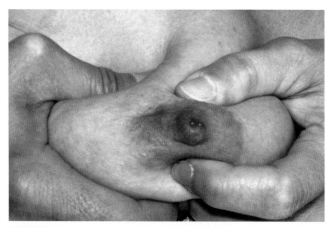

FIGURE 15-1 **Benign Nipple Discharge.** Multiduct green discharge. The discharge was bilateral and not spontaneous.

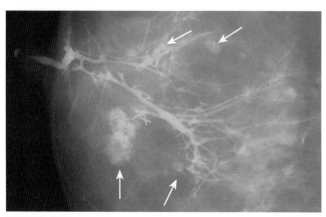

FIGURE 15-2 **Fibrocystic Changes on Galactogram.** One large and several small cysts are filling (*arrows*). This patient had serous, heme-negative nipple discharge.

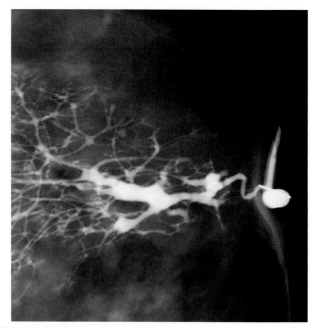

FIGURE 15-3 **Duct Ectasia on Galactogram.** The patient had a few spontaneous episodes of minimal serous discharge. Only duct ectasia is seen on galactography. No further evaluation is necessary.

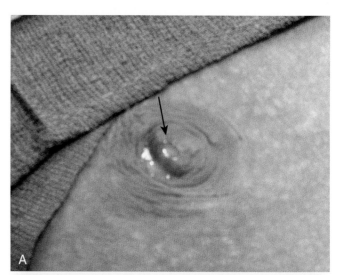

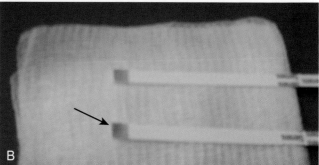

FIGURE 15-4 **Worrisome Nipple Discharge. A,** Serous, single-duct discharge that is heme-positive. **B,** The green color indicates blood in the fluid on these urine dipsticks.

there is a known trigger point—a specific site that elicits discharge on palpation—it can also be used to localize the abnormal duct system. If an intraductal mass is identified on a galactogram, US can be performed to see if the mass is amenable to wire localization using ultrasound guidance. However, US is poor in identifying peripheral intraductal masses (Fig. 15-8), so if the US is negative, additional evaluation will be necessary.

Galactography involves cannulation of the offending duct and injection of contrast material. Central and peripheral intraductal masses are equally well identified.

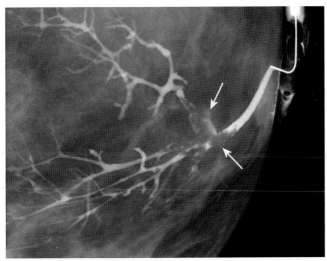

FIGURE 15-5 **Large Single Intraductal Mass.** The mass is centrally located on galactography (*arrows*). Diagnosis: intraductal papilloma.

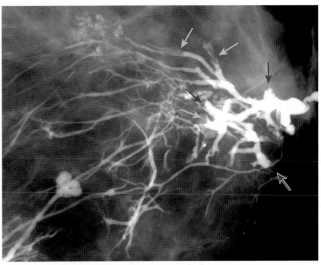

FIGURE 15-6 **Multiple Intraductal Masses.** Multiple intraductal masses (*yellow arrows*) are present as well as abrupt duct termination (*blue arrows*) on the galactogram. Incidental fibrocystic change is present with filling of some benign cysts. Diagnosis: DCIS, high grade.

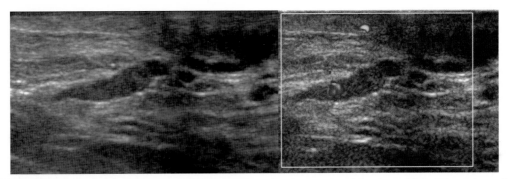

FIGURE 15-7 **Intraductal Mass on US.** Doppler flow confirms that the mass is solid and not debris. Diagnosis: papilloma.

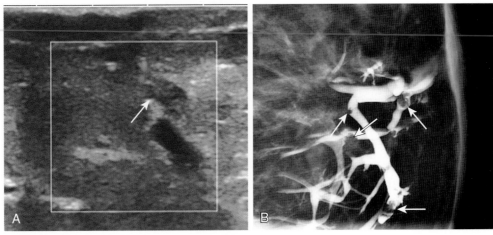

FIGURE 15-8 **Multiple Intraductal Masses Not Seen on US. A,** US shows a single proximal intraductal mass (*arrow*). **B,** Galactogram shows multiple intraductal masses (*arrows*). Central duct excision showed papillomatosis.

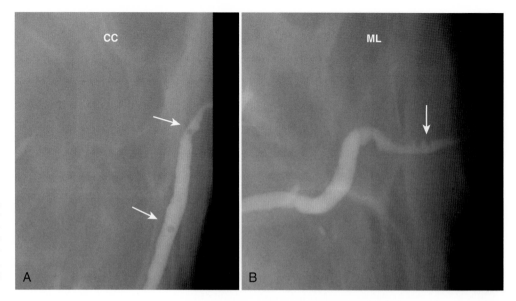

FIGURE 15-9 **Air Introduced During Galactogram.** On the craniocaudal (CC) view (**A**), two small round intraductal lesions are identified (*arrows*). On the mediolateral view (**B**), they both shift in position to the nondependent duct wall (*arrow*).

Also known as ductography, galactography is our procedure of choice for evaluating nipple discharge. An abnormal galactogram may show abrupt duct termination, a single filling defect (intraductal mass), multiple filling defects, or irregular narrowing of the duct lumen.

Air can be introduced into the duct inadvertently through the galactography catheter (Fig. 15-9). Although DCIS can present as tiny, round, intraductal masses, the masses will not shift in position like air bubbles. Debris can mimic intraductal masses as well.

Contrast-enhanced magnetic resonance imaging (MRI) may be helpful in identifying papillomas and DCIS in women with nipple discharge. The abnormal duct can sometimes appear hyperintense on the T2-weighted sequences (Fig. 15-10). Postcontrast sequences reveal the lesion causing the discharge in about 90% of cases. Although more expensive, MRI is a useful alternative if the duct cannot be cannulated for galactography and US is negative. Ductoscopy is a less common procedure that is performed at a few institutions with reasonable success.

Managing the Abnormal Galactogram or US

Nice job! You found an intraductal mass 3 cm behind the nipple. It will need to be excised for definitive diagnosis. Now how will the surgeon excise the correct area? Here are the options:

In ***central duct excision*** the lactiferous sinuses and major ducts are removed from the subareolar region. This includes the ductal structures within 1 to 2 cm from the nipple. This therapeutic procedure will resolve the patient's symptom of nipple discharge but may or may not be diagnostic, depending upon the location of the causative lesion (Fig. 15-11). If the patient has an

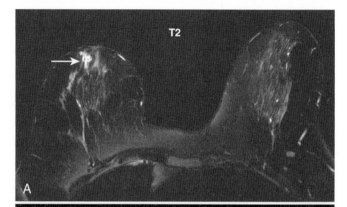
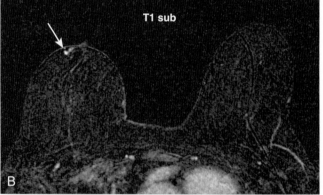
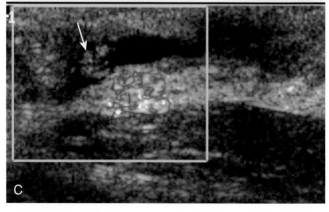

FIGURE 15-10 **MRI Evaluation of Nipple Discharge.** In this patient, there is high T2 signal in the duct (**A**) with a corresponding enhancing intraductal mass on T1 (**B**, *arrow*). US identified a correlative mass (**C**, *arrow*). Histologic examination showed intraductal papilloma.

intraductal mass identified by US or galactography that is within 1 to 2 cm from the nipple, then central duct excision is a good procedure. However, if our patient has an intraductal mass that is 3 cm from the nipple, there is a good chance that it will not be removed during central duct excision.

Clip placement after galactogram using mammographic guidance (Fig. 15-12) allows wire localization and surgical excision when the timing is convenient without repeating the galactogram. This is our typical strategy for intraductal masses identified on galactography that are more than 1 to 2 cm behind the nipple.

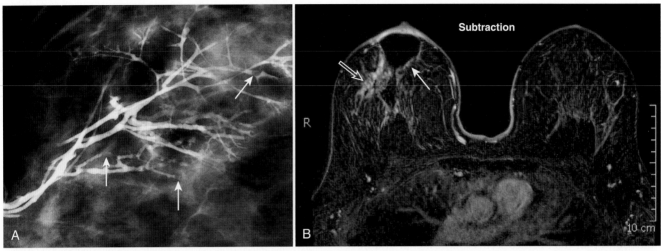

FIGURE 15-11 **False Negative Central Duct Excision. A,** Galactogram shows multiple intraductal masses. Central duct excision showed a single minute papilloma. Her subsequent MRI (**B**) shows segmental nonmass enhancement (*open arrow*) directly posterior to the central duct cavity (*arrow*). Re-excision showed extensive DCIS, high grade.

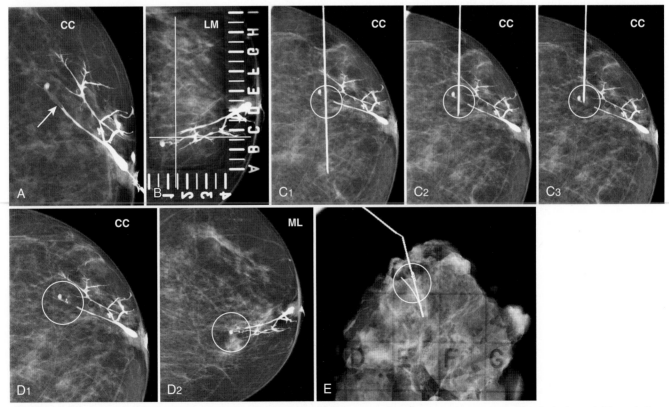

FIGURE 15-12 **Clip Placement After Galactogram. A,** Galactogram shows an intraductal mass 5 cm posterior to the nipple (*arrow*). The technique is similar to wire localization. **B,** The breast is placed in an alphanumeric grid. A lateromedial approach was used in this case. The intraductal mass is at 1.4 and B.7. The clip device is placed perpendicular to the skin. **C,** The breast is released from compression, and an orthogonal view is obtained (a CC view in this case). The tip of the needle is pulled back to the location of the intraductal mass (*arrow*). **D,** The clip is placed. On the day of surgery (several weeks later in this case), the clip is localized with a wire. **E,** Specimen radiograph documents removal of the clip. Histologic examination showed intraductal papilloma.

Ultrasound-guided wire localization is a useful alternative to mammographic wire localization if an intraductal mass is visible by US.

Core biopsy using either stereotactic guidance after a galactogram or with ultrasound guidance will yield a definitive diagnosis in most women with an intraductal mass, but will often not provide relief of the patient's symptoms. Excision is both diagnostic and therapeutic.

Immediate excision may be performed following galactography with wire localization of the intraductal mass and injection of dye into the offending duct. With this approach, galactography has to be performed only once. The downside is that time in the operating room may be held unnecessarily if the galactogram is negative or unsuccessful.

Repeat galactogram on the day of surgery with localization and injection of dye into the offending duct allows more flexible scheduling of operating room time. However, it is sometimes difficult to repeat cannulation of the same duct.

If the Attempt at Galactography Fails

Sometimes that duct orifice seems to know that you have a meeting at noon and will not relax. Warm compresses and distracting conversation about family or other personal interests may help the patient relax. If you still cannot cannulate the duct, another attempt can be made in a week or two. Imaging with other modalities such as US and MRI can be used as well. However, do *not* let the patient disappear. Just because the discharge goes away does not mean that she does not have breast cancer. At a minimum, we see our patients back for a unilateral ipsilateral mammogram in 6 months.

KEY POINTS

- Nipple discharge is caused by benign processes in over 90% of cases but may be a presenting sign of malignancy.
- The most suspicious presentation is spontaneous bloody discharge. Serous discharge may also be caused by malignancy. Galactography evaluates the entire duct system and is useful in identifying the location of ductal lesions and in guiding surgical management.
- US is useful for identifying and localizing lesions of the central ducts.
- MRI can be used to evaluate nipple discharge when galactography is unsuccessful and US is negative or inconclusive.

References

Baker KS, Davey DD, Stelling CB. Ductal abnormalities detected with galactography: Frequency of adequate excisional biopsy. Am J Roentgenol 1994;162:821-824.

Cardenosa G, Doudna C, Eklund G. Ductography of the breast: Techniques and findings. Am J Roentgenol 1994;162:1081-1087.

Gomez A, Mata JM, Donoso L, Rams A. Galactocele: Three distinctive radiographic appearances. Radiology 1986;158(1):43-44.

Hou MF, Huang TJ, Liu GC. The diagnostic value of galactography in patients with nipple discharge. J Clin Imaging 2001;25:75-81.

Nicholson BT, Harvey JA, Cohen MA. Nipple-areolar complex: Normal anatomy and benign and malignant processes. Radiographics 2009;29(2):509-523.

Tabar L, Dean PB, Pentek Z. Galactography: The diagnostic procedure of choice for nipple discharge. Radiology 1983;149:31-38.

CASE QUESTIONS

CASE 15-1. A lovely 84-year-old woman is waiting for you to perform her galactogram. When you walk in the room, she is rubbing her temples. You ask her to tell you about her discharge and she says, "I feel like I'm going to have a baby." She has copious bilateral milky discharge. Her mammogram is shown here. What is the most likely cause of her discharge? Does she need a galactogram?

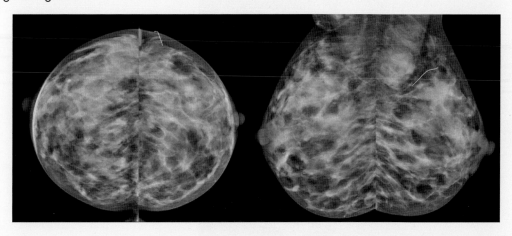

CASE 15-2. A 45-year-old woman has had several episodes of bloody discharge over the last few months. What do think of her galactogram? How would you manage her?

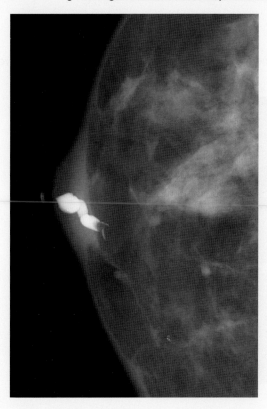

CASE 15-3. This 64-year-old woman has noticed spots of blood on her bra. Her mammogram is normal. She had a benign stereotactic biopsy 5 years ago. Here is her galactogram. What is the most likely diagnosis? What is your recommendation?

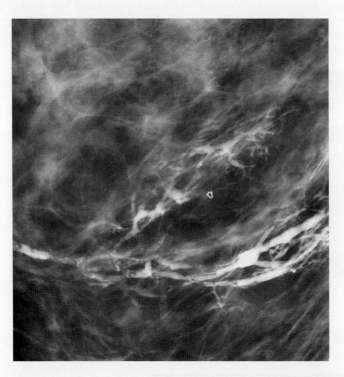

CASE 15-4. A 55-year-old woman has heme-positive serous nipple discharge. How would you interpret her galactogram?

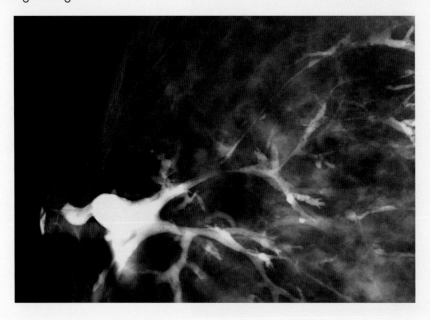

CASE 15-5. A 32-year-old woman presents with right nipple discharge and a palpable lump (*triangle*). What is the most likely diagnosis? What are your BI-RADS assessment and recommendation?

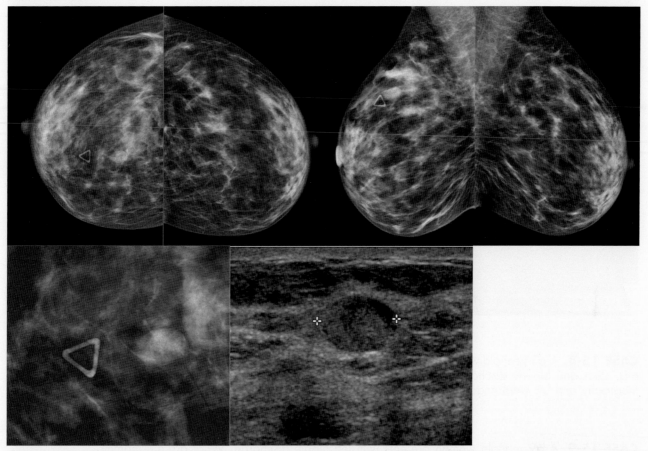

CASE 15-6. A 69-year-old woman has noticed occasional damp spots on her nightgown over the right breast. On examination, she has serous discharge from a single duct on the right nipple. It tests heme-positive. Her mammogram is normal. A galactogram is attempted, but no discharge could be expressed on the day that she presented for the test. What do you suggest?

This is a good story for pathologic discharge in a postmenopausal woman. Discharge severity can wax and wane, so we must continue to pursue the cause even if there is currently no discharge. If galactography cannot be performed, consider performing an MRI. She underwent central duct excision showing atypical ductal hyperplasia (ADH). What do you think of her postoperative MRI?

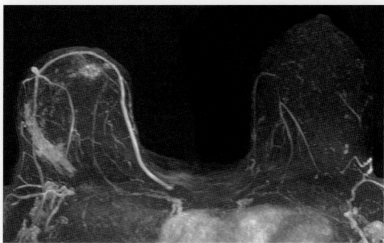

CASE 15-7. A 46-year-old woman is referred for evaluation of bloody discharge from the left nipple. Magnification views of the left breast were obtained. How would you describe the findings? What do you recommend? Galactography was performed. What are the findings?

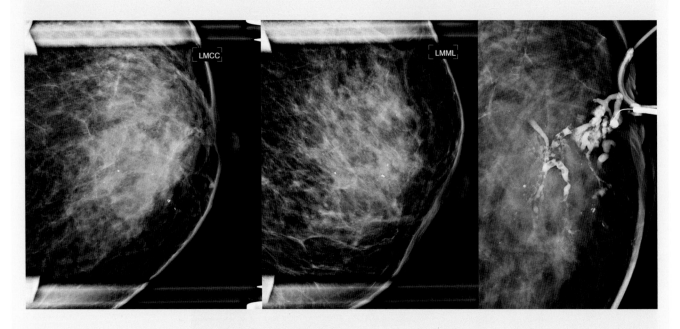

CASE 15-8. A 63-year-old woman with a history of left mastectomy presents with new, spontaneous, clear and bloody discharge from the right nipple. Galactography was unsuccessful. Mammography and US were negative. What do you recommend?

CASE 15-9. A 69-year-old woman presents with left nipple discharge. What are the mammographic findings?

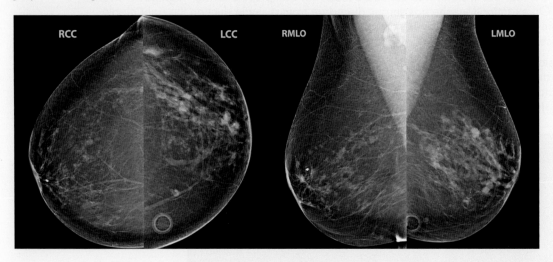

CASE 15-10. A 49-year-old woman with history of benign ultrasound-guided core biopsy of a complicated cyst in the left breast 9 months ago, now presents with a 5-month history of intermittent left nipple bloody discharge. What do you think about her galactogram? What is the most likely cause of her discharge?

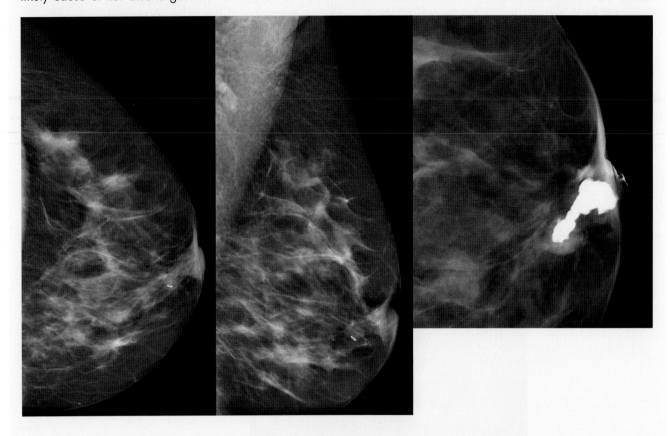

CASE ANSWERS

CASE 15-1. Her mammogram is normal other than being very dense for her age. Her discharge is almost certainly due to a pituitary prolactinoma given her symptoms of breast engorgement and headache. She does not need a galactogram. She may, however, need a brain surgeon.

CASE 15-2. There is abrupt duct termination just beneath the nipple. Because this is so close to the nipple, there is no reason to place a clip. This lesion should be easily removed by central duct excision. If you are not sure whether the lesion would be excised during a central duct excision, see whether one of your surgical colleagues can review the case with you before the patient leaves. The surgeon can let you know whether he or she would like a clip placed. Diagnosis: papilloma.

CASE 15-3. There are multiple filling defects in the ductal system that are highly concerning for DCIS. An irregularly narrowed duct segment is seen anteriorly (arrow in image). A clip can be placed at the time of galactography to aid in localization. Diagnostic core biopsy can also be performed. Diagnosis: DCIS.

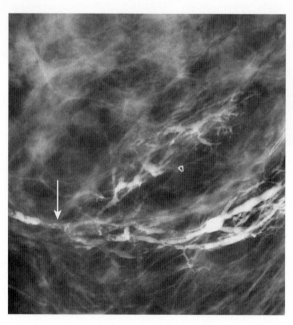

CASE 15-4. There are multiple intraductal masses. The tiny defects in some areas should not be confused with air bubbles (*arrows*). She had extensive DCIS.

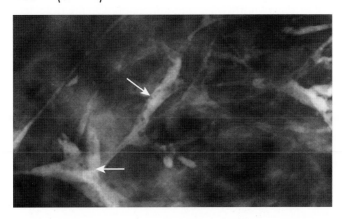

CASE 15-5. There is an oval, circumscribed mass in the right breast that correlates with the palpable finding. On US, this corresponds to an intraductal mass. Given the history of nipple discharge and the young age, papilloma is a likely diagnosis. Tissue diagnosis is needed, however. BI-RADS 4: Suspicious finding. Ultrasound-guided wire-localization was performed showing intraductal papilloma. Excision is not only diagnostic but also therapeutic, resulting in elimination of the discharge.

CASE 15-6. There is segmental nonmass enhancement in the right lateral breast. The subareolar rim enhancing "lesion" is due to the seroma from her recent central duct excision. Histologic finding: extensive DCIS, intermediate grade.

CASE 15-7. There are coarse, heterogeneous calcifications with segmental distribution in the medial breast. These are suspicious, especially given the history of bloody discharge. There are multiple intraductal filling defects as well as ductal narrowing and truncation. On the galactogram the abnormal duct system corresponds to the location of the calcifications. There is also suspicion of an irregular mass medially (*arrow*). US showed an abnormal duct segment in the medial breast, and ultrasound-guided core biopsy revealed invasive ductal carcinoma.

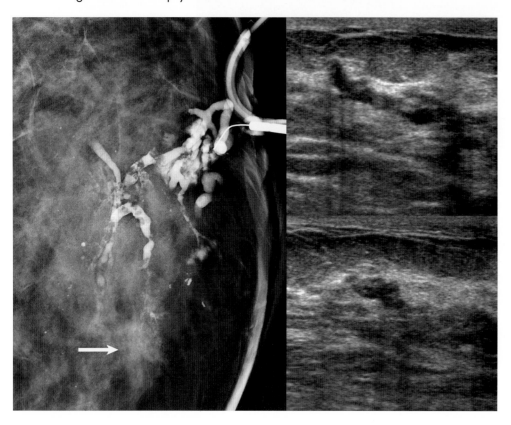

CASE 15-8. MRI can frequently identify the cause of suspicious nipple discharge when galactography is unsuccessful. In this case, there was segmental nonmass enhancement in the central lateral breast, as shown on the postcontrast T1 fat-saturation images below. Diagnosis: high-grade DCIS.

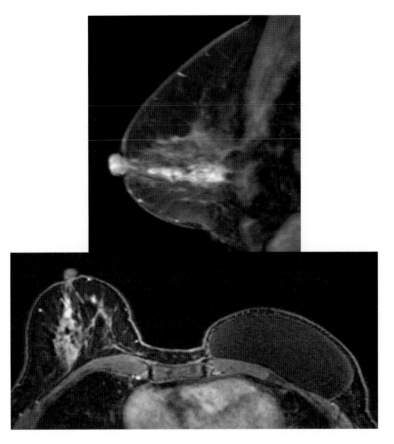

CASE 15-9. There is ductal dilatation in the lateral left breast. This is a nonspecific finding that is usually insignificant but may be caused by papilloma(s) or DCIS. US images of the 1 o'clock position of the left breast 5 cm from the nipple is shown below. How can you aid surgical management?

A small intraductal lesion was identified on US that is most likely a papilloma. Because US may miss more peripheral lesions, galactography can also be performed prior to surgery to determine whether other lesions are present. Excision will be facilitated by preoperative wire localization using ultrasound guidance. Diagnosis: papilloma.

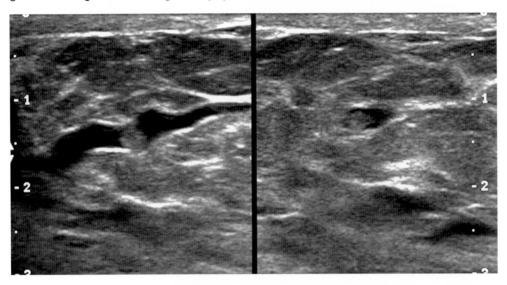

CASE 15-10. On the galactogram, contrast is filling the duct and center of the cystic lesion that underwent biopsy. Although very uncommon, bloody discharge can be due to prior surgery, core biopsy, trauma, or even cyst aspiration.

CHAPTER 16

The Male Breast

*A sheepish older guy with a breast lump is in your depart-
ment. Without even seeing him, you know that the most
likely diagnosis is gynecomastia. But let's make sure that
it's not more serious. At diagnosis, breast cancer in men
tends to be more advanced than in women and will nearly
always be invasive. The distinction between gynecomastia and cancer is important—a delay in diagnosis may
change the stage of the disease.*

Men are pretty easy in the world of breast imaging.
Lesions other than gynecomastia and invasive ductal carcinoma (IDC) are really uncommon. Fortunately, male
breast cancer is much less common than gynecomastia
and distinguishing between the two is usually very straightforward. Sometimes gynecomastia is mass-like in appearance, and the features on ultrasonography (US) can be
suspicious. In this chapter, we'll focus on how to tell gynecomastia and cancer apart and review a few uncommon
male breast lesions that you might see in your practice.

Male Breast Tissue Composition

Until puberty, male and female breasts are the same.
During puberty, female breasts experience ductal elongation and branching followed by lobular proliferation, but
male breasts do not. Normal male breasts therefore only
have atrectic ducts and few lobules. The normal male
breast consists primarily of fat with a small amount of
ductal tissue in the subareolar regions. Intramammary
and axillary lymph nodes are commonly seen (Fig. 16-1).
Lesions of lobular origin, such as fibroadenomas, cysts,
and lobular carcinoma, are uncommon.

Gynecomastia

Gynecomastia is non-neoplastic enlargement of the male
breast due to hyperplasia of epithelial and stromal elements. Gynecomastia develops as a result of an imbalance
between estrogen and androgen actions within the breast
tissue. *Physiologic gynecomastia* presents at times when
there is a normal change in the balance between these
hormones. It occurs in over half of adolescent boys and
usually regresses within 6 months of diagnosis. Gynecomastia is also present in about half of older men—usually
over 65—in whom it is often asymptomatic.

Between these age peaks, gynecomastia is usually pathologic. It may be caused by one of a variety of different

diseases, syndromes, medications, or other substances
that increase estrogen or decrease testosterone (Box 16-1).
The clinical history can give clues to the cause. Is he an
awkward teenager? A bartender with a red nose? An older
guy being treated for prostate cancer? Gynecomastia is
often idiopathic, so the cause is not always apparent.
Confirming a diagnosis of gynecomastia is important
because it often allows the patient to be successfully
treated if the cause is identified, and provides reassurance
to the patient that the findings are not malignant.

Breast enlargement can also be caused by *pseudogynecomastia*, which is an increase in adipose tissue rather
than enlargement of the fibroglandular tissue. Gynecomastia can usually be differentiated from pseudogynecomastia on clinical examination. In gynecomastia, a mound
of tissue concentric to the nipple is generally appreciated.
However, this finding is absent in pseudogynecomastia.
Because there is no suspicious palpable mass and the
enlargement is due to fat, the diagnosis is usually apparent on clinical examination and mammography (Fig.
16-2).

Mammographic Patterns of Gynecomastia

There are three patterns of gynecomastia based on the
mammographic appearance: nodular, dendritic, and
diffuse fibroglandular. In one series, among 61 cases of
biopsy-proven gynecomastia, 47 (77%) were nodular, 12
(20%) dendritic, and 2 (3%) were diffuse fibroglandular.
An awareness of these patterns aids in the recognition of
gynecomastia, and helps differentiate it from potentially
malignant findings.

With the nodular type, there is typically a flame-shaped
density (also described as triangular or fan-shaped), centered behind the nipple, that radiates posteriorly and
blends into fat (Figs. 16-3 and 16-4). This type occurs
during the acute florid phase and usually lasts for less
than 1 year. The breast is often tender. If US is performed,
prominent hypoechoic ducts and edematous adjacent
tissues are often visualized, and increased blood flow is
common on Doppler examination (Fig. 16-5). The main
histologic findings in this phase are ductal proliferation
with loose, cellular stroma and edema.

If gynecomastia persists, the findings may progress to
the dendritic pattern. This is a chronic, fibrotic phase that
can develop when gynecomastia has been present for
at least 1 year. The term "dendritic" originates from
the Greek language and refers to a tree branching.

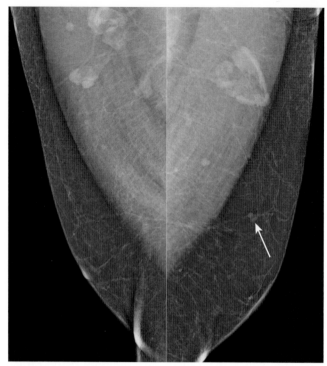

FIGURE 16-1 **Normal Male Mammogram.** There is only fatty tissue present with a normal intramammary lymph node in the upper left breast (*arrow*).

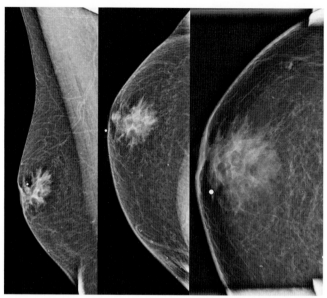

FIGURE 16-3 **Nodular Gynecomastia.** The retroareolar density is concentric to the nipple and radiates posteriorly, gradually blending into the fat. It is compressible and interspersed with fat, characteristics that are best seen on the magnification view.

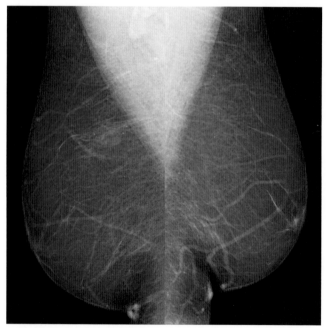

FIGURE 16-2 **Pseudogynecomastia.** Male patient referred for evaluation of bilateral breast enlargement shows fatty breast tissue with no evidence of mass or gynecomastia.

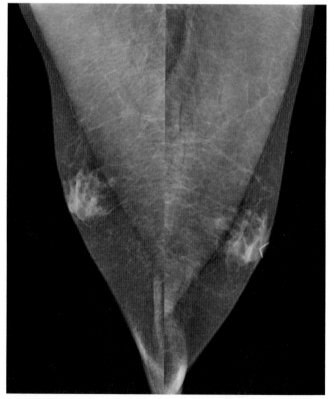

FIGURE 16-4 **Bilateral Symmetric Nodular Gynecomastia.** Bilateral retroareolar density typical for gynecomastia.

BOX 16-1   Causes of Gynecomastia

- Physiologic
- Idiopathic
- Increased body mass index
- Medications
  - Chemotherapeutic agents
  - Cimetidine
  - Diazepam
  - Digitoxin
  - Estrogen
  - Metoclopramide
  - Phenytoin
  - Prostate cancer therapy (antiandrogens, estrogen)
  - Spironolactone
  - Steroid hormones
  - Thiazides
  - Tricyclic antidepressants
- Drug use
  - Anabolic steroids
  - Alcohol
  - Marijuana
  - Opioids
- Hyperthyroidism
- Cirrhosis
- Chronic renal failure
- Neoplasms
  - Hepatocellular carcinoma
  - Adrenal carcinoma
  - Testicular tumors
- Klinefelter syndrome

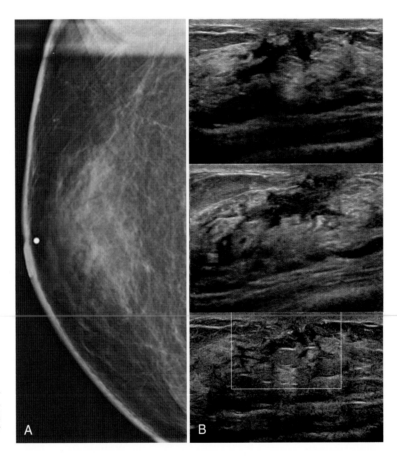

FIGURE 16-5 **Medication-Induced Early Nodular Gynecomastia. A,** Magnified craniocaudal (CC) view showed retroareolar density typical for gynecomastia. **B,** US revealed edematous ducts. Flow was demonstrated on color Doppler examination.

Mammography shows retroareolar breast tissue that radiates posteriorly in a fairly typical pattern, resembling tree branches (Figs. 16-6 and 16-7). At this stage, symptoms have usually abated and the gynecomastia is unlikely to regress either spontaneously or with treatment. If US is performed, the appearance will be similar to female breast tissue with mostly hyperechoic fibrous tissue and small ducts. Edema and increased blood flow have resolved. The histologic findings at this stage are dominated by periductal fibrosis and hyalinization of the stroma.

Diffuse fibroglandular gynecomastia is another pattern that occurs in men receiving estrogen treatment. The breasts are enlarged with a diffuse increase in density, producing an appearance similar to that of a mammogram of a female patient with dense tissue (Fig. 16-8). With this pattern, both nodular and dendritic features may be present.

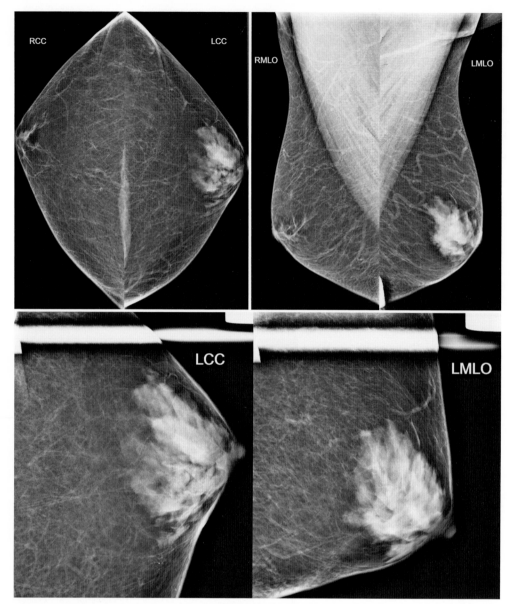

FIGURE 16-6 **Dendritic Gynecomastia.** Posterior soft tissue density extensions from the left subareolar region produce the typical appearance of dendritic gynecomastia. There is minimal gynecomastia on the right.

Male Breast Cancer

Breast cancer is uncommon in men, accounting for about 0.5% of all breast cancers and less than 1% of all malignancies diagnosed in men. Incidence increases with age and plateaus at about 80 years of age; the median age of diagnosis is 67 years. Breast cancer is very uncommon in younger men.

Family cancer history is important for men and women. About 25% of men diagnosed with breast cancer are *BRCA* gene carriers, more commonly *BRCA2*. Men with a *BRCA2* mutation have a 7% risk of being diagnosed with breast cancer by age 70 years. Diagnosis of breast cancer in a man is much more likely to be associated with a *BRCA* mutation than diagnosis of breast cancer in a woman, and a man's family is therefore at higher risk for a genetic mutation as well. Men with breast cancer

and women with a first-degree male relative with breast cancer are typically referred for genetic counseling.

Risk factors for male breast cancer other than family history include Klinefelter syndrome, androgen deficiency (undescended testes, orchitis, testicular trauma or torsion), cirrhosis, and chronic alcoholism. Some of the risk factors for male breast cancer involve chronic elevation of the ratio of estrogen to androgen, which is interestingly the same hormonal imbalance that underlies the development of gynecomastia. Although it has been difficult to establish gynecomastia as a risk factor for breast cancer, the two often occur together; this is not surprising given the overlapping risk factors and high prevalence of gynecomastia. In one study, 22 out of 55 (40%) male breast cancers occurred in patients with gynecomastia.

Most male breast cancers arise from ducts in the subareolar region, and the most common clinical presentation is a palpable mass that is eccentric but near the nipple. Palpable axillary adenopathy is common at the time of presentation. However, axillary adenopathy is rarely the sole presenting finding. Nipple discharge is an uncommon presentation.

The large majority of male breast cancers are infiltrating ductal carcinomas, not otherwise specified. Ductal carcinoma in situ (DCIS) may also occur, usually in association with IDC. Pure DCIS is uncommon. Other subtypes of ductal carcinoma are much less common; however, all subtypes that occur in women have also been reported in men. Infiltrating lobular carcinoma is rare. In a large series, 93.7% of male breast tumors were either ductal or unclassified carcinomas, 2.6% were papillary carcinomas, and only 1.5% were lobular carcinomas (Box 16-2).

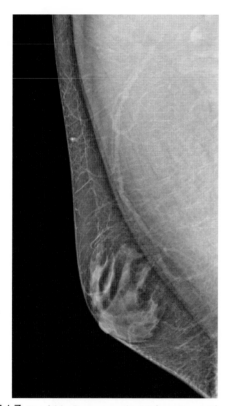

FIGURE 16-7 **Dendritic Gynecomastia.** Male patient with a history of right breast enlargement for over 2 years.

BOX 16-2 Do Men Need Screening Mammograms?

- In the United States, the screening threshold is set as the risk of breast cancer equal to or greater than that of a 40-year-old woman, which is 120/100,000 per year. To screen any other population with mammography, the risk should be equal to or greater than this risk level.
- Overall, the risk of breast cancer for men is 1.2/100,000, which is well below the threshold for screening in the United States.
- Men who are known or suspected *BRCA* carriers may benefit from screening mammography. These men are at substantially increased risk compared with the general male population. Their risk approaches that of women in their 40s.
- Of male patients with gynecomastia, only those with Klinefelter syndrome approach the screening range. Screening of these men remains controversial. Men with gynecomastia due to gender reassignment with hormone therapy are not at high risk for breast cancer. Routine screening mammography is not indicated.

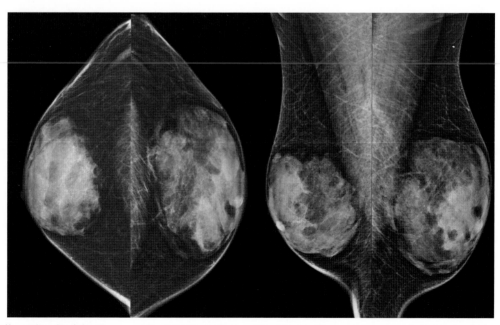

FIGURE 16-8 **Diffuse Fibroglandular Gynecomastia.** Middle-aged man with a history of long-term estrogen treatment producing diffuse symmetric gynecomastia.

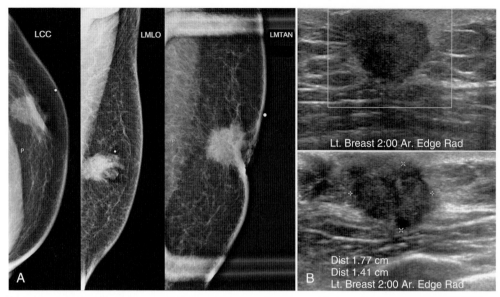

FIGURE 16-9 **Infiltrating Carcinoma.** An 83-year-old man presents with palpable mass in the 1 o'clock position of the left breast near the nipple. **A,** Mammography shows an irregular mass with spiculated margins. The nipple is retracted. **B,** US shows a mass with indistinct margins. Diagnosis: infiltrating carcinoma with ductal and lobular features. *(Case courtesy of Cheri Nguyen, MD.)*

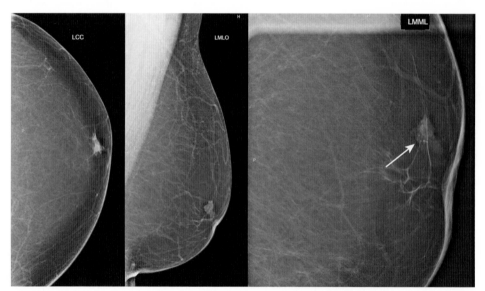

FIGURE 16-10 **Ductal Carcinoma in Situ (DCIS).** A 56-year-old man presents with bloody discharge from the left nipple. Mammography shows an eccentric subareolar mass containing a few coarse calcifications *(arrow).* Diagnosis: DCIS. *(Case courtesy of Cheri Nguyen, MD.)*

Mammographic Findings

Male patients with clinically suspicious palpable findings should first be evaluated by bilateral mammography. At our centers, we perform routine CC and mediolateral oblique (MLO) projections of the ipsilateral breast. An MLO with or without a CC view is obtained of the contralateral breast. Spot compression or magnification views may also be performed to provide a more detailed evaluation of the palpable finding. Some men have very large pectoralis muscles, so spot compression views may be more helpful than full views.

The mammographic appearance of male breast cancer is most commonly a mass with suspicious features similar to malignant masses found in women (Fig. 16-9). DCIS is much less common in men presumably because the ducts are atretic. Calcifications can occur with DCIS, and tend to be more coarse and less numerous than those seen in women with DCIS (Fig. 16-10). Microcalcifications alone are an uncommon finding in male breast cancer.

Sonographic Findings

US of malignant masses in the male patient has a similar appearance to that of malignant masses in women (see Fig. 16-9). Cysts and fibroadenomas, which are common in women, are rare in male patients. Because benign masses are very uncommon in men, biopsy should be considered for essentially any solid or complex mass in a man.

In men with nipple discharge, US of the ducts in the subareolar region may identify an intraductal papilloma or carcinoma. Galactography may also be useful in the evaluation of male patients with discharge.

Is It Cancer or Gynecomastia?

This is usually the primary question when evaluating a male patient with a breast lump. As a breast imager, your most important role in evaluating the male patient is to diagnose malignant lesions without delay. However, your most frequent role—by a wide margin—will be to confirm the diagnosis of benign gynecomastia. Remember that over 90% of male patients will be referred for signs and symptoms caused by benign lesions.

Age and Incidence of Disease

The patient's age is an important key to accurate diagnosis. Most young adult and middle-aged men presenting for imaging will have gynecomastia rather than breast cancer; various medications and drug use are common causes in this age group. One caveat: a young man with no obvious cause for his gynecomastia may have testicular carcinoma, which is the most common cancer in young men. A simple physical examination by the health care provider can exclude this possibility in most patients.

Family History

If there is a family history of breast cancer, the patient may be at genetic risk for breast cancer as well. The *BRCA* genes are carried by both men and women.

Clinical Presentation

How long has the patient been symptomatic? Does the patient take any medications known to cause gynecomastia? Is he living in his parents' basement with red eyes and a ravenous appetite? Is he a little too buff for gym time alone? Is the palpable finding soft and tender or hard and painless? Subareolar or eccentric from the nipple? Is there any adenopathy? Answers to these questions should be considered in your interpretation of the imaging findings.

Mammographic Findings

Mammography is very sensitive and specific in differentiating benign from malignant disease in men. Mammography is the examination of choice in evaluating symptomatic men.

The easiest approach is to think of your male patient as a female presenting for a screening mammogram. Would you pass the study as a negative screening in a female patient? Then the diagnosis is gynecomastia. Is there a mammographic finding that would prompt you to recall her from screening? If so, then cancer is more likely.

Findings in a man that should raise the level of suspicion include eccentric location of a mass, defined margins, and increased density. A mass that is not centered behind the nipple-areolar complex has a high chance of malignancy and generally warrants biopsy. Malignant masses in men tend to have discrete margins. Malignant masses are typically noncompressible, are more dense centrally, and do not contain fat.

Gynecomastia is bilateral and asymmetric about 80% of the time. Gynecomastia will be unilateral in about 15% of men. Bilateral findings are therefore more likely to represent gynecomastia. But be careful. Cancers can develop in men with gynecomastia and may be obscured by dense tissue in these cases. In patients with gynecomastia and a palpable mass, the mammogram needs to be read just like in a woman with a palpable lump. Is there a discrete mass or asymmetric tissue that is separate from the confluent dense tissue of gynecomastia? Always search for calcifications and secondary signs of malignancy (skin/nipple retraction, skin thickening, axillary or intramammary adenopathy) as well.

Problem Solving and Pitfalls of Ultrasonography

Many radiologists are reluctant to perform US in a man. There is no question that US of patients with nodular gynecomastia can lead to false-positive findings because prominent hypoechoic ducts in the subareolar region may simulate a shadowing mass (Fig. 16-11). When the clinical and mammographic findings are typical for gynecomastia, US rarely contributes additional useful information and may result in an unnecessary biopsy.

However, when the clinical and mammographic findings are unclear, US may be quite helpful. *Don't be afraid to scan a male patient if you need more information!* The convex borders of nodular gynecomastia can occasionally mimic a mass with ill-defined margins on mammography. US may be helpful when mammography cannot differentiate between a mass and gynecomastia. It also allows direct correlation with the physical findings. If US demonstrates a discrete mass, biopsy is indicated.

Here is a practical tip for performing US in men. Shadowing from the nipple may be minimized by scanning from the side of the areola while compressing the opposite side of the breast against the transducer with the nonscanning hand (see Fig. 16-11).

A summary of features that may be helpful in distinguishing gynecomastia from male breast cancer is shown in Table 16-1. Occasionally, the findings of gynecomastia cannot be confidently differentiated from malignancy by mammography or US and biopsy is needed (Box 16-3).

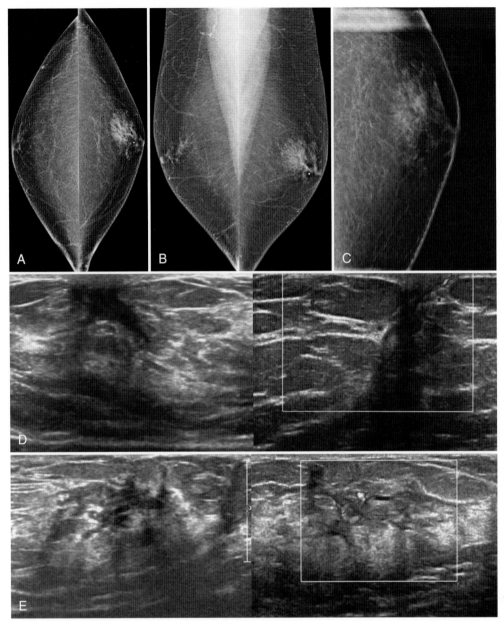

FIGURE 16-11 **Nodular Gynecomastia. A** to **C,** The subareolar density is concentric to the nipple, blends into adjacent fat, is compressible, and is bilateral and asymmetric. There is fat interspersed within the tissue. **D,** US was performed, and initially, an irregular, hypoechoic, shadowing lesion was questioned. **E,** Additional scanning with greater compression revealed only ducts and no evidence of mass.

BOX 16-3 Indications for Breast Ultrasonography in the Male Patient

- A breast mass that is eccentric to the nipple
- A mammographic mass with suspicious features (margin, shape, density)
- A mammogram that is not definitive for gynecomastia
- Nipple discharge
- Guidance for biopsy

Other Breast Lesions in Male Patients

After gynecomastia, lipomas are the most common palpable lesions for which male patients are referred for breast imaging (Fig. 16-12). Fat necrosis (Fig. 16-13), sebaceous cysts, epidermal inclusion cysts, pseudoangiomatous stromal hyperplasia (PASH), diabetic mastopathy, hematomas, abscesses, cysts (Fig. 16-14), and intraductal papillomas are also seen in men. Unilateral axillary adenopathy may be caused by malignant lesions, such as metastatic tumor from breast, lung, or melanoma, or from lymphoma or leukemia. Adenopathy may also be reactive or due to infection or granulomatous disease.

TABLE 16-1 Distinguishing Features of Gynecomastia Versus Cancer

FEATURE	GYNECOMASTIA	CANCER
Clinical		
Palpable findings	Usually soft or rubbery and mobile	Firm or hard; may be fixed
Tenderness	Common in early phase	Uncommon
Nipple bleeding or discharge	Uncommon	May occur
Skin/nipple retraction or ulceration	Not seen	May occur
Axillary adenopathy	Not seen	Common: seen in about half of all cases
Mammographic/Ultrasound		
Location	Concentric to nipple	Frequently eccentric to nipple
Calcifications	Not seen	Seen in about a third of cases
Increased trabecular markings	Not seen	May be present
Skin thickening	Not seen	May be present
Unilateral/bilateral	Bilateral in about 85% of cases	Usually unilateral; may develop with gynecomastia
Discrete complex or solid mass	Rare	Common
Abnormal axillary lymph nodes	Not seen	Common

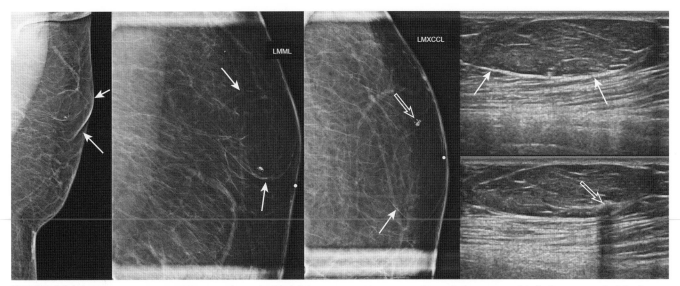

FIGURE 16-12 **Lipoma.** A 51-year-old man with a palpable left breast mass. Mammographic and ultrasonographic findings are typical for lipoma (*arrows*), which contains coarse calcifications due to fat necrosis (*open arrows*).

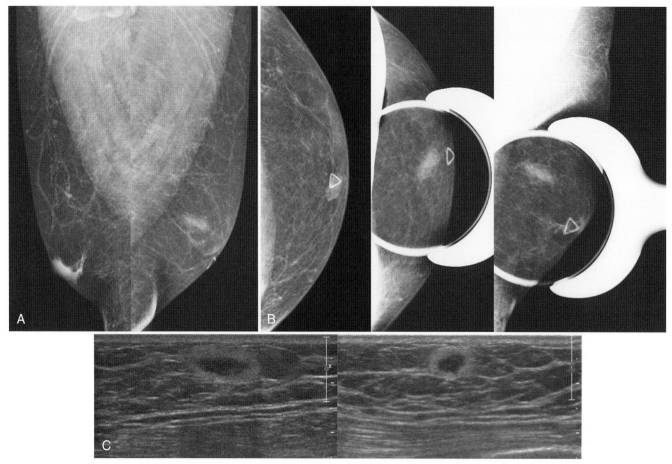

FIGURE 16-13 **Fat Necrosis.** A male patient who developed a palpable mass following trauma to the breast. **A** and **B,** Mammography showed an oval mass with ill-defined margins. **C,** US revealed a hypoechoic mass with an echogenic halo.

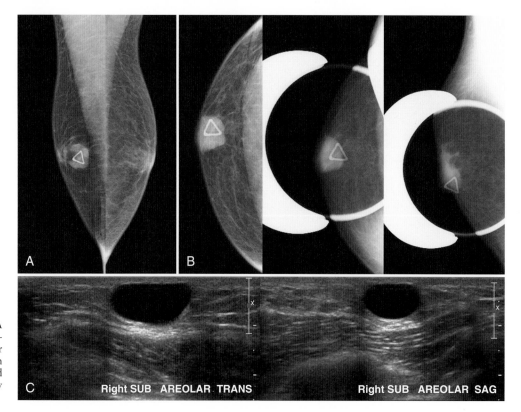

FIGURE 16-14 **Simple Cyst.** A male patient presented with a palpable mass in the right subareolar region. The mass had smooth margins on mammography (**A** and **B**) and represented a simple cyst by US (**C**).

KEY POINTS

- Over 90% of men referred for breast-related complaints will have benign lesions, most commonly gynecomastia.
- There are three mammographic patterns of gynecomastia: nodular, which is an early phase; dendritic, which is a chronic phase; and diffuse fibroglandular, which occurs in men receiving estrogen treatment. Gynecomastia is typically concentric to the nipple, blends into adjacent fat, and is compressible and interspersed with fat. It is most commonly bilateral and asymmetric.
- Mammography can differentiate male breast cancer from gynecomastia and other benign lesions with a high degree of accuracy. US is helpful in select cases.
- Indeterminate discrete masses usually warrant biopsy.

References

Appelbaum AH, Evans GFF, Levy KR, et al. Mammographic appearance of male breast disease. RadioGraphics 1999;19:559-568.

Braunstein GD. Gynecomastia. N Engl J Med 2007;357:1229-1237.

Chantra PK, So GJ, Wollman JS, Bassett LW. Mammography of the male breast. AJR 1995;164:853-858.

Chen L, Chantra PK, Larsen LH, et al. Imaging characteristics of malignant lesions of the male breast. RadioGraphics 2006;26:993-1006.

Dershaw DD. Male mammography. AJR 1985;146:127-131.

Evans GF, Anthony T, Appelbaum AH, et al. The diagnostic accuracy of mammography in the evaluation of male breast disease. Am J Surg 2001;181:96-100. [Erratum, Am J Surg 2001;181:579.]

Giordano SH, Cohen DS, Buzdar AU, et al. Breast carcinoma in men: A population-based study. Cancer 2004;101:51-57.

Goss PE, Reid C, Pintilie M, et al. Male breast cancer: A review of 220 patients who presented to the Prince Margaret Hospital during 40 years: 1955-1996. Cancer 1999;85:629-639.

Mathew J, Perkins GH, Stephens T, et al. Primary breast cancer in men: Clinical, imaging, and pathologic findings in 57 patients. AJR 2008; 191:1631-1639.

Michels LG, Gold RH, Arndt RD. Radiology of gynecomastia and other disorders of the male breast. Radiology 1977;122:117-122.

Narula HS, Carlson HE. Gynecomastia. Endocrinol Metab Clin North Am 2007;36(2):497-519.

Risch HA, McLaughlin JR, Cole DE, et al. Population BRCA1 and BRCA2 mutation frequencies and cancer penetrances: A kin-cohort study in Ontario, Canada. J Natl Cancer Inst 2006;98(23): 1694-1706.

Sandler B, Carman C, Perry RR. Cancer of the male breast. Am Surg 1994;60:816-820.

Stavros AT. Breast ultrasound. Philadelphia, Lippincott Williams & Wilkins, 2004, pp 712-741.

CASE QUESTIONS

CASE 16-1. This 48-year-old man was referred for evaluation of bilateral breast enlargement. What is your impression and recommendation?

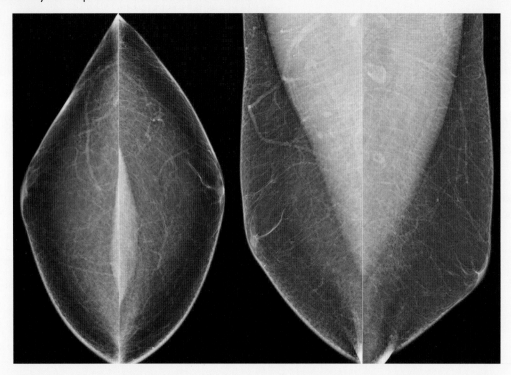

CASE 16-2. Male patient presents with a palpable mass in the left breast (*BB* marker). What is the cause of the palpable finding?

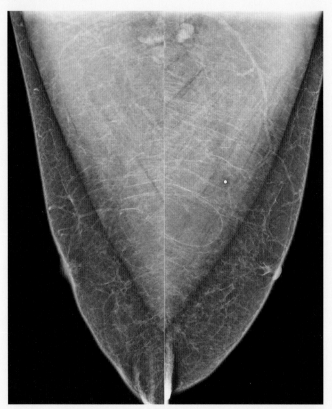

CASE 16-3. You are just starting a diagnostic session and the technologist presents you with the first case: "He's a 23-year-old guy who's really built. His right breast is enlarged and tender." What is your diagnosis?

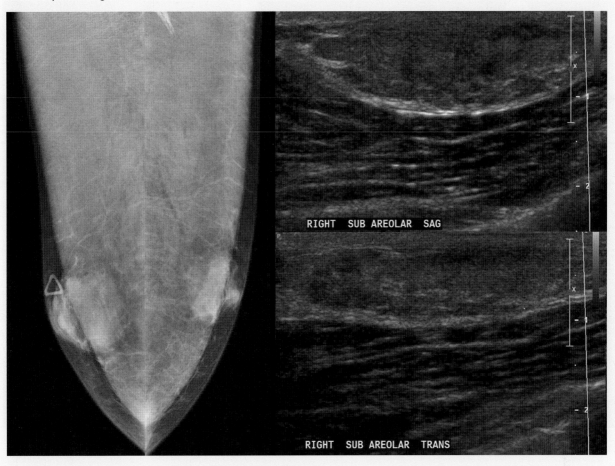

CASE 16-4. A 38-year-old man with right breast enlargement. If this were a screening mammogram on a woman, how would you read it? What is the most likely diagnosis? Are the findings more likely to be of recent onset or chronic?

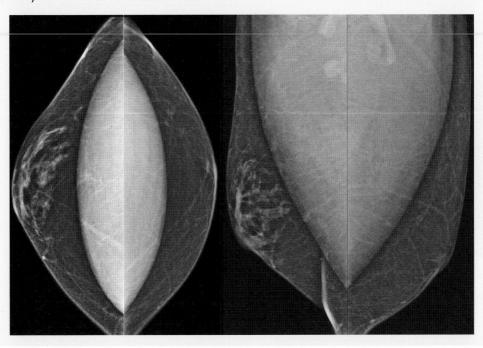

CASE 16-5. An 89-year-old man presents with a palpable mass in his right breast. If this were a screening mammogram on a woman, how would you read it? What are the findings?

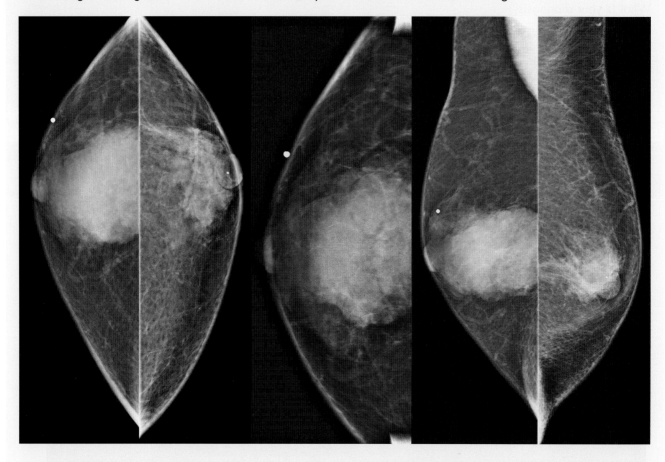

CASE 16-6. A 42-year-old gender-reassigned genotypic male who has been taking estradiol for 10 years is referred for screening mammography. There are no breast complaints and no family history of breast cancer. What is your recommendation?

CASE 16-7. A 78-year-old man is referred for US of a palpable mass in the left subareolar region. Based on these images, what do you recommend?

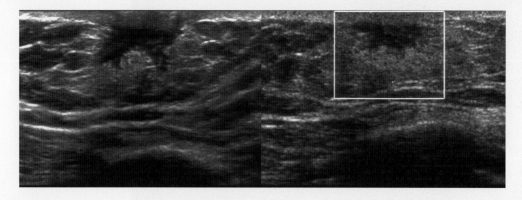

CASE 16-8. A 77-year-old man presents with a palpable abnormality in his right breast. If this were a mammogram of a woman, how would you read it? What are the findings? What are your assessment and recommendation?

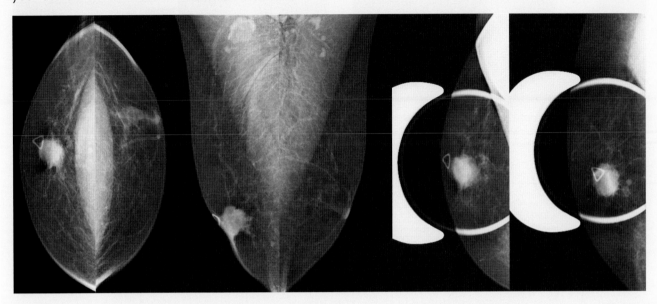

CASE 16-9. A 77-year-old man presents with a palpable mass in his right breast. What are the findings? What are your assessment and recommendation?

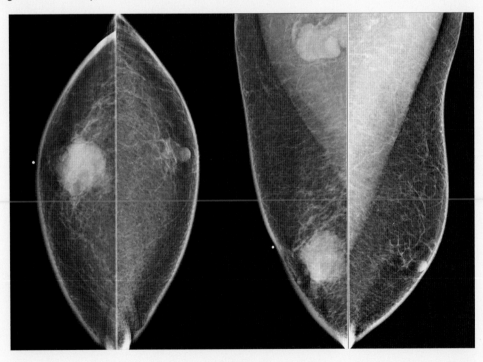

CASE 16-10. This male patient was referred for evaluation of a palpable mass in the left subareolar region. What are your assessment and recommendation?

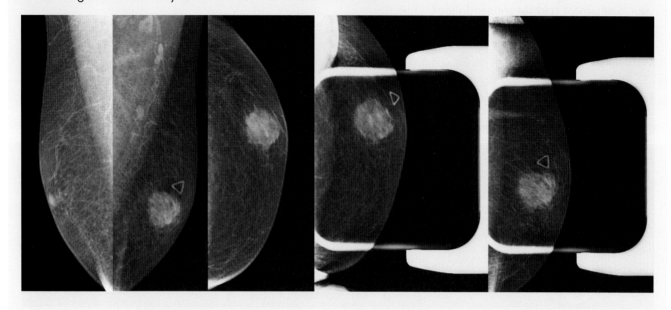

CASE ANSWERS

CASE 16-1. The tissue consists almost entirely of fat. There is no evidence of mass or gynecomastia. The findings are due to pseudogynecomastia producing symmetric breast enlargement. No additional evaluation is needed. BI-RADS 2.

CASE 16-2. There is a fat-containing mass near the marker, overlying the pectoralis muscle, consistent with lipoma. This is a benign finding and requires no additional evaluation. There is no evidence of malignancy or gynecomastia. BI-RADS 2.

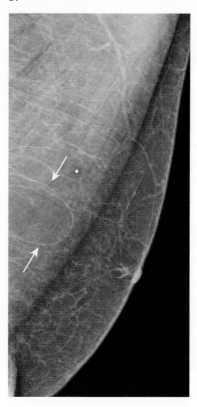

CASE 16-3. Mammography shows bilateral asymmetric dense tissue in the subareolar regions, right larger than left, that is concentric to the nipples. US of the right breast shows hypoechoic edematous tissue. The chance of malignancy in a 23-year-old man is remote. Diagnosis: bilateral nodular gynecomastia, more pronounced on the right. Upon questioning he confessed to some use of exogenous steroids.

CASE 16-4. If this were a screening mammogram in a woman, the category would be BI-RADS 1 or 2. Recall would not be indicated. The appearance is typical for gynecomastia, specifically the dendritic type on the right, which is a chronic finding. In this patient, the clinical findings had been present for several years. There are no findings to suggest malignancy.

CASE 16-5. If this were a screening mammogram in a woman, the asymmetry would catch your attention. On the right, the tissue is mass-like and dense, with a discrete margin and without interspersed fat. On the left, the subareolar tissue is lower in density, centered behind the nipple, and blends into adjacent fat. The left mammogram looks like normal breast tissue in a woman—and therefore gynecomastia in a man. US of both breasts reveals a solid mass on the right breast for which biopsy is indicated (*upper image*). There are no visible abnormalities on the left and no further evaluation of the left breast is needed (*lower image*). Diagnosis: IDC and DCIS in the right breast and bilateral gynecomastia.

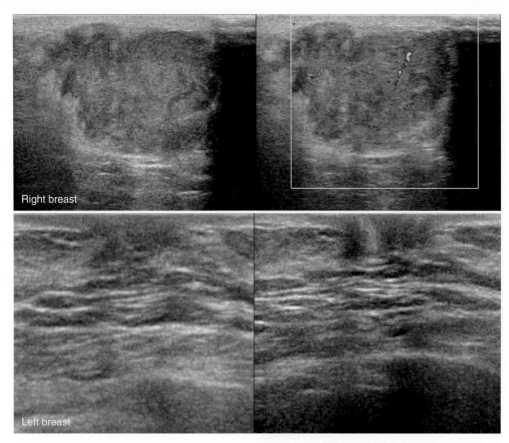

CASE 16-6. This patient does not need screening mammography. In genotypic women, estradiol alone does not significantly elevate breast cancer risk, though combined estrogen-progesterone therapy does increase risk. Even if the use of estradiol *doubled* the breast cancer risk in this male patient, the absolute risk (2.4/100,000) would be equivalent to that for a genotypic woman in her 20s. The low prevalence of breast cancer in this population therefore does not justify the use of routine screening mammography.

CASE 16-7. US shows an irregular area of decreased echogenicity behind the left nipple. The sonographic findings are indeterminate. This could represent either nodular gynecomastia or invasive cancer. Recommend mammographic evaluation.

Mammography reveals retroareolar density with a pattern typical for nodular gynecomastia. The US finding represents prominent ducts. Remember that mammography is more helpful than US in diagnosing gynecomastia and that the sonographic findings may be misleading.

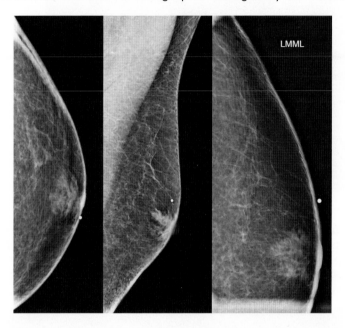

CASE 16-8. If this were a mammogram performed on a woman, you would be very worried about the dense mass with spiculated margins in the subareolar region. This lesion should not be confused with gynecomastia. Note skin thickening and nipple retraction on the MLO view. The mass does not blend into the adjacent fat, is more dense than gynecomastia, and is not compressible on spot views. BI-RADS 5. Diagnosis: IDC.

CASE 16-9. There is a dense mass with ill-defined margins in right subareolar region. This is not gynecomastia. The mass corresponds to the palpable finding. Did you also see the right axillary adenopathy? That definitely bumps up the level of suspicion. US was performed and shows a solid mass with microlobulated discrete margins. The US findings do not resemble gynecomastia. BI-RADS 5. Diagnosis: IDC with axillary lymph node metastasis. *(Case courtesy of Cheri Nguyen, MD.)*

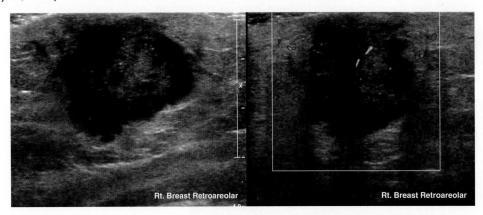

CASE 16-10. There is a mass-like area in the left retroareolar region. The mammographic features are more mass-like than is typical for gynecomastia. The outward convex margins are concerning. US shows a discrete hypoechoic area in the subareolar region. This could be either nodular gynecomastia or invasive cancer. BI-RADS 4. Core biopsy was performed, revealing nodular gynecomastia and no evidence of malignancy.

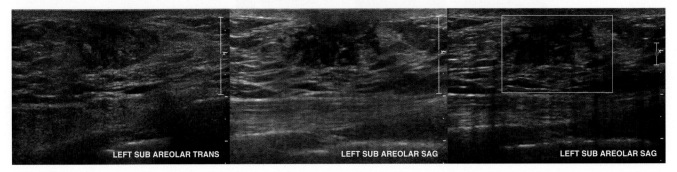

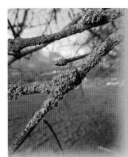

CHAPTER 17

Imaging the Patient with Breast Cancer

Do you have trees in your yard? If you see a diseased area on a branch of a dogwood tree, you will likely also look up and down that branch to see the extent of the process. Then you are probably going to look at the other branches to see if there are other areas involved. And because whatever is in the ground or air that resulted in the disease could also affect your other dogwood trees, you'll probably look around the yard to see if they might also be having a problem.

YES! You found a highly suspicious lesion on mammography. Nice work! But wait—there's more. Our work is not done here. After identifying a lesion on imaging that is very suggestive of breast cancer, our job shifts from detection to evaluating the extent of disease and the staging of the cancer. Let's thoroughly evaluate the patient so that we make the surgeon's job easier. Oh, and don't forget about that other breast!

For women with a very suspicious (BI-RADS 4C) or highly suspicious (BI-RADS 5) finding on mammography or ultrasonography (US), evaluation of the extent of disease and the staging can occur at the initial diagnostic appointment. If biopsy of a less suspicious lesion results in a cancer diagnosis, then imaging evaluation of the extent of disease and the staging should be performed prior to surgical intervention. In women with recently diagnosed breast cancer, the incidence of contralateral cancer is 0.1% to 2% on mammography and 3% to 5% by magnetic resonance imaging (MRI), so careful review of the mammogram and consideration of breast MRI are important.

Imaging contributes to patient care by guiding surgical management and providing information about staging. Surgical management of the breast is determined by accurate assessment of the size and location of the cancer, and identification of multifocal or multicentric disease. Imaging affects staging by identifying invasive tumor for women with ductal carcinoma in situ (DCIS), accurately measuring tumor size, evaluating regional lymph nodes, and identifying skin or chest wall involvement. Imaging to identify systemic disease is also important in staging, but will not be reviewed here.

Size and Extent of the Primary Tumor

Invasive Tumor Size

In the TNM system for staging breast cancer, the T is based on the size of the largest invasive component. Although measurement of the tumor in three dimensions

is helpful for monitoring change for women undergoing neoadjuvant chemotherapy, only the longest dimension is used in staging. When there is more than one invasive focus, only the largest is considered in staging. Tumors are classified as Tis (in situ), T1 (≤20 mm), T2 (21-50 mm), or T3 (>50 mm). T1mi refers to microscopic invasion of less than 1 mm.

Tumor size is measured at histologic examination. However, there are times when the size on imaging may be used, such as when the tumor is very small and mostly removed at core biopsy or in the setting of neoadjuvant chemotherapy. For invasive carcinoma, US size that includes the echogenic rim correlates best with histologic size (Fig. 17-1). Measurements of invasive carcinoma on MRI correlate best with size at histologic evaluation. This is especially true for invasive lobular carcinoma (ILC) (Fig. 17-2).

Associated Ductal Carcinoma in Situ

Now that you have identified a mass that is suspicious for invasive carcinoma, let's look to see whether there is also associated DCIS. Mammography is a good place to start. Breast cancer typically affects a single ductal system. If we recall the tree branch analogy from Chapter 5, Breast Anatomy and Physiology, we will want to focus our attention on the ductal system where the mass is located. We will especially want to look for calcifications between the mass and the nipple, as well as between the mass and the chest wall (Fig. 17-3). Recall that one ductal system can extend over a wide area in the breast, so even calcifications that are not immediately adjacent to an invasive carcinoma may represent DCIS.

MRI can also be very helpful in assessing the extent of DCIS associated with a primary invasive cancer. The associated DCIS will usually present as nonmass enhancement in the same ductal distribution (Fig. 17-4).

Extent of Ductal Carcinoma in Situ

The extent of calcifications on mammography typically correlates well with DCIS that is high grade, but low-grade DCIS often has more extensive noncalcified disease.

When the primary lesion presents as suspicious calcifications, other calcifications that are morphologically similar are likely to represent additional disease (Fig. 17-5). Calcifications of differing morphologic appearance may also need to undergo sampling if they are also

437

suspicious based on morphologic appearance, distribution, or change over time (Fig. 17-6).

This does not mean that you must biopsy every cluster of calcifications in the breast! If the calcifications are of similar morphologic appearance, do a biopsy of the most suspicious finding first (see Fig. 17-5). If the biopsy shows cancer and the patient desires mastectomy, doing a second biopsy will not alter her management. On the other hand, if the patient desires breast-conserving therapy, an additional biopsy may be needed to establish the extent of disease. In our practice, a second biopsy of the ipsilateral breast is not typically performed until the results of the biopsy showing cancer have been discussed with the patient and she has seen a breast surgeon to discuss surgical options.

DCIS with Associated Invasive Disease

When the primary lesion is malignant-appearing calcifications and you are suspecting DCIS, finding an invasive component changes the stage from 0 to I. Providing the patient and surgeon with the higher stage of disease is helpful because the patient may then need a sentinel lymph node biopsy. An invasive component may be

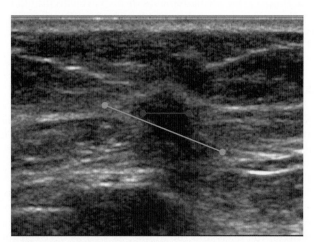

FIGURE 17-1 **Ultrasound Measurement of Tumor Size.** The longest dimension that includes the echogenic margin (*green line*) correlates better with the size at histologic examination than does just the hypoechoic mass (*red line*). The measurement does not need to be parallel to the face of the transducer.

suspected when there is density that looks like a puff of smoke overlying the calcifications (Fig. 17-7). US is useful in evaluating these patients. An invasive focus will appear as a hypoechoic mass, whereas DCIS will appear as an expanded duct with calcifications (see Fig. 17-7). US is also useful when malignant calcifications are present in dense breast tissue that could be masking an invasive carcinoma (Fig. 17-8). US does *not* need to be performed for every patient with suspicious or malignant calcifications. If an associated mass is not definitely identified by US, stereotactic biopsy is preferred over ultrasound-guided biopsy because it is less likely to show only atypical ductal hyperplasia because of undersampling.

Multifocal Invasive Carcinoma

Small masses or asymmetries in the same ductal distribution as the primary lesion should be viewed with suspicion. When additional invasive disease is separated by less than 4 cm, the cancer is considered to be multifocal (Fig. 17-9). Although different criteria are used to determine whether carcinomas should be classified as multifocal (vs. multi*centric*), the less-than-4-cm measurement correlates well with a lower chance of local recurrence when compared with more extensive lesions (Box 17-1).

US is very useful to identify multifocal invasive carcinoma. Remember our tree? With the transducer oriented in the radial plane, sweep the area between the cancer and the nipple and then the cancer and the periphery of the breast to identify additional lesions within the branches of the involved ductal system (see Fig. 17-9).

MRI is very sensitive for detecting additional invasive breast carcinoma (Fig. 17-10).

Multicentric Carcinoma

Additional ipsilateral cancer that is more than 4 cm from the primary lesion is considered multicentric. This may or may not be identified in a different quadrant. Satisfaction of search is difficult to overcome. Ignore that really concerning finding and *really* look at the rest of that breast (see Fig. 17-6). Diagnosis of multicentric carcinoma is generally a contraindication for breast-conserving therapy, though it is not an absolute contraindication.

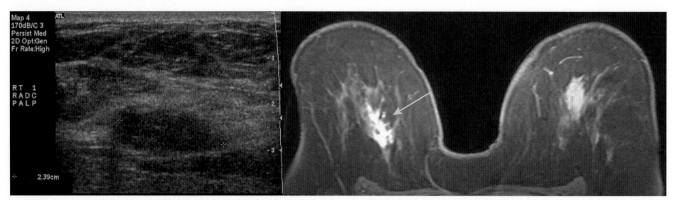

FIGURE 17-2 **Size of ILC on MRI.** On mammography and US, this palpable ILC measures 2.4 cm. On MRI, however, the mass was considerably larger, measuring 4.5 cm. At histologic examination, the mass measured 5 cm. The enhancement in the left breast is due to a contralateral MRI-detected invasive ductal carcinoma (IDC).

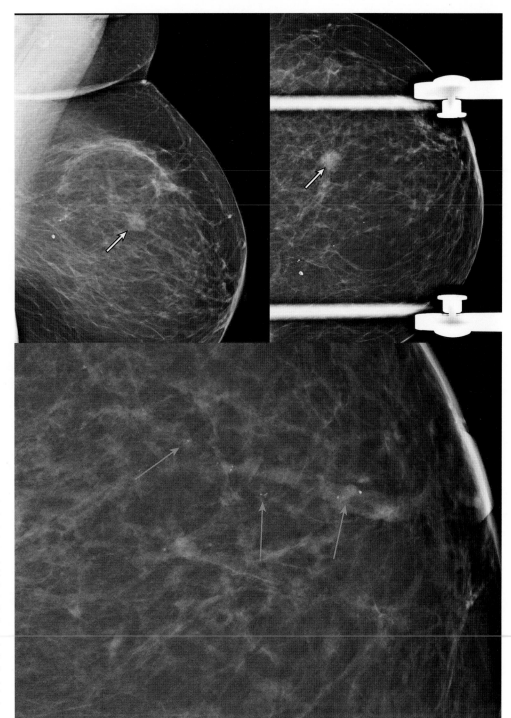

FIGURE 17-3 **IDC with Associated DCIS.** A 48-year-old woman with a screening detected mass in her left breast (*arrows*). On a magnification view, round and punctuate calcifications in a segmental distribution are seen extending between the mass and the nipple (*blue arrows*). Mild ductal dilatation is also seen. Although the morphologic appearance of the calcifications is of low suspicion, their segmental distribution is suspicious especially because they lie in the same ductal system as the mass. Biopsy of the mass revealed IDC with DCIS; the retroareolar calcifications represented additional DCIS.

Skin or Chest Wall Involvement

Remember the T classification earlier? We only gave you T0 to T3, but there is also a T4 category that is defined by involvement of the skin or chest wall with tumor. Skin involvement is defined as skin nodules or ulceration (Fig. 17-11), not just dermal invasion. Chest wall involvement is invasion into the intercostal muscles or ribs. Invasion of the pectoral muscles may influence surgical or medical management, but is not considered chest wall invasion. Inflammatory cancer is also considered T4.

If you are a "lumper," then skip this paragraph. If you are a "splitter," then you'll want to know the T4 subcategories. T4a is invasion of the chest wall. T4b is tumor associated with skin ulceration, ipsilateral skin nodules, or skin edema that does not meet criteria for inflammatory breast carcinoma. T4c is findings of both T4a and T4b. T4d is inflammatory carcinoma.

Inflammatory carcinoma is most commonly associated with invasive ductal carcinoma—not otherwise specified (IDC-NOS). It is not associated with DCIS alone. The diagnosis of inflammatory carcinoma may be clinical (red, swollen breast in a patient with invasive carcinoma)

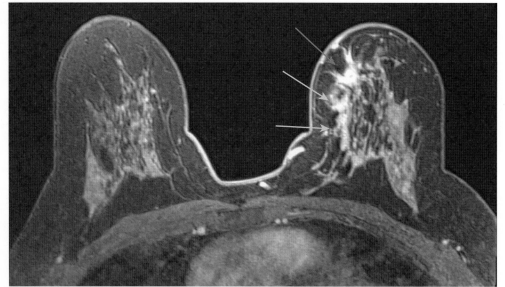

FIGURE 17-4 **MRI-Detected DCIS in Patient with IDC.** This patient presented with a palpable lump in the left breast that corresponded to a suspicious mass on US. Her mammogram was negative. Biopsy showed IDC. MRI performed to evaluate extent of disease shows the mass (*blue arrow*) with associated segmental nonmass enhancement (*yellow arrows*) that represented extensive DCIS.

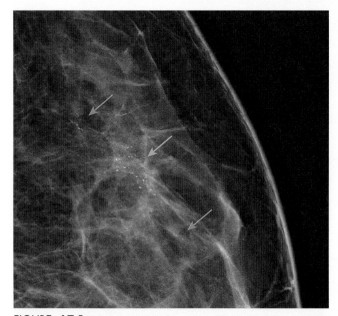

FIGURE 17-5 **Suspicious Calcifications with Similar Morphologic Appearance.** Biopsy of the most suspicious area (*yellow arrow*) showed DCIS. If the patient desires breast-conserving therapy, then biopsy of the posterior and anterior groups (*green arrows*) can help determine extent of disease.

BOX 17-1 Managing Multiple Suspicious Findings

- If there is a BI-RADS 5 lesion present, start with a biopsy there first to establish a diagnosis.
- If there are two different BI-RADS 4 lesions, biopsy of each may be indicated because one might be cancer and the other benign.
- Once a cancer diagnosis is made, give the patient a chance to digest the news and think about her surgical options.
- If the biopsy shows invasive carcinoma and the patient desires mastectomy, no further breast biopsies are needed.
- For women desiring breast-conserving therapy
  - If a second area is present but within a centimeter or so from the primary carcinoma, the surgeon can likely remove the finding during the primary resection. Review the case with your surgeon.
  - If the associated disease is more extensive, choose an area for biopsy that is as far away from the known cancer that is likely to yield a cancer diagnosis.

or histologic (punch biopsy of the skin showing invasion of the dermal lymphatics).

Paget Disease Is Not T4

Although Paget disease is tumor ulceration of the skin of the nipple, it is not considered T4 disease. If Paget disease is only associated with DCIS, then it is stage Tis. If a woman with Paget disease has an associated invasive carcinoma, then the T status is based on the size of the invasive carcinoma.

Contralateral Breast Cancer

The incidence of synchronous contralateral breast cancer is 0.1% to 2% by mammography and 3% to 5% by MRI (Fig. 17-12). Ignore the ipsilateral breast for a moment and really focus on the other breast. Bilateral breast cancer diagnosed at the same time is considered synchronous, whereas diagnosis that occurs at least 6 months apart is considered metachronous.

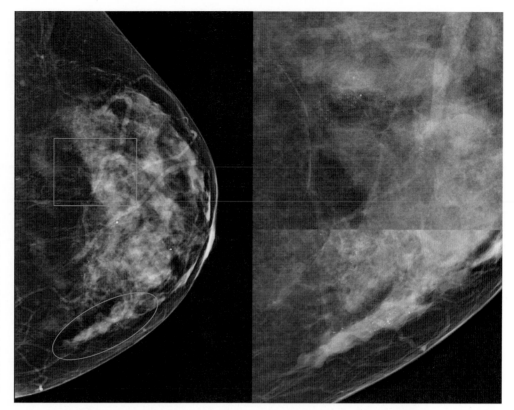

FIGURE 17-6 Suspicious Calcifications of Differing Morphologic Appearance. *Green marks* denote two areas of calcifications on the screening craniocaudal (CC) view. Calcifications in the lateral breast are fine pleomorphic, whereas those in the medial breast are coarse heterogeneous. Biopsy of either cluster could be benign or malignant and acted upon independently. Therefore, biopsy of both should be performed. Histologic diagnoses: DCIS, low-grade lateral breast; DCIS, high-grade medial breast.

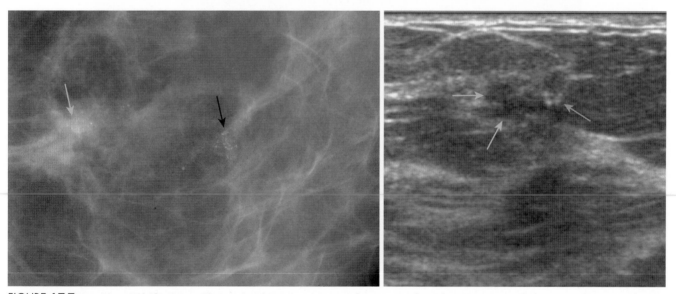

FIGURE 17-7 Suspicious Calcifications with Associated Density. CC magnification view from this screening recall shows two adjacent suspicious groups of calcifications with similar morphologic appearances in the same ductal distribution. The posterior group (*yellow arrow*) has an associated density that corresponds to a hypoechoic mass (*yellow arrows*) with calcifications (*green arrow*) on US. Histologic diagnosis: multifocal DCIS with IDC at the posterior site.

Evaluating Regional Lymph Nodes

Lymph from the breast drains mostly to the axillary lymph nodes, though some drains to the internal mammary lymph nodes. About one third of breast cancers will have metastasized to the regional lymph nodes or other surrounding tissues at the time of diagnosis.

Axillary lymph nodes are divided into levels with relationship to the pectoralis minor muscle. Lymph nodes that are lateral, posterior, or medial to the pectoralis minor muscle are level I, II, and III, respectively. Lymph nodes located in the space between the pectoralis major and minor are interpectoral (Rotter) nodes and are managed as level II lymph nodes.

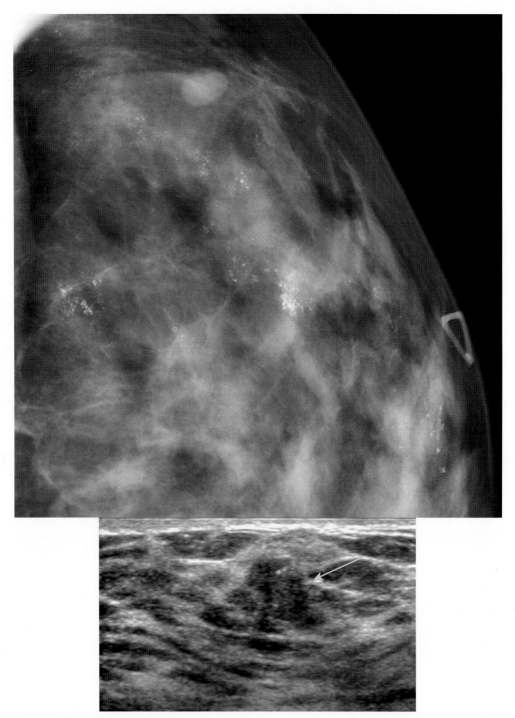

FIGURE 17-8 **Malignant Calcifications with Suspicious Mass on US.** CC magnification view shows malignant coarse heterogeneous and fine pleomorphic calcifications in a segmental distribution that are highly suspicious for DCIS (BI-RADS 5). US is useful to identify an invasive component in the setting of malignant calcifications in dense breast tissue. US shows a hypoechoic solid mass (*arrow*) with calcifications. Ultrasound-guided core needle biopsy showed IDC, grade III. You may have noticed a small round mass at the top of the CC magnification view. This was a metastatic intramammary lymph node. These are generally managed as though they were another focus of invasive cancer.

Level I axillary lymph nodes are seen on mammography, US, and breast MRI (see Fig. 17-9). Level II and III axillary and supraclavicular lymph nodes are seen to varying degrees on US and breast MRI. Internal mammary lymph nodes are most commonly found in the second or third intercostal spaces and can be identified on US or MRI (Fig. 17-13). Small normal internal mammary

lymph nodes may occasionally be seen on MRI. If seen on US, an internal mammary lymph node is usually abnormal.

Lymph fluid enters the node on the outside cortical surface and exits via the hilum. Metastatic deposits are often first seen beneath the lymph node capsule. These can result in cortical thickening, which can be focal or

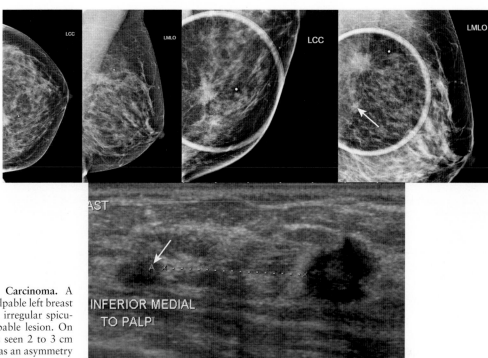

FIGURE 17-9 **Multifocal Invasive Carcinoma.** A 51-year-old woman presents with a palpable left breast mass marked with a *BB*. There is an irregular spiculated mass corresponding to the palpable lesion. On US a second, smaller mass (*arrow*) is seen 2 to 3 cm from the palpable mass. This appears as an asymmetry (*arrow*) on the mediolateral oblique (MLO) spot compression view. The palpable mass was IDC and the nonpalpable lesion IDC with DCIS.

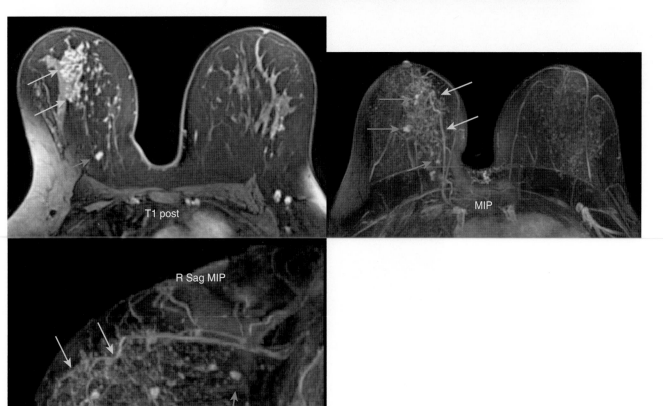

FIGURE 17-10 **DCIS with Multifocal Invasive Carcinoma on MRI.** This patient had a stereotactic core biopsy for a group of calcifications in the right breast showing DCIS. Axial T1 postcontrast image, axial maximum intensity projection (MIP), and sagittal right breast MIP show nonmass enhancement (*yellow arrows*) with several enhancing masses (*blue arrows*) in the same ductal distribution. Histologic examination showed DCIS with multifocal IDC.

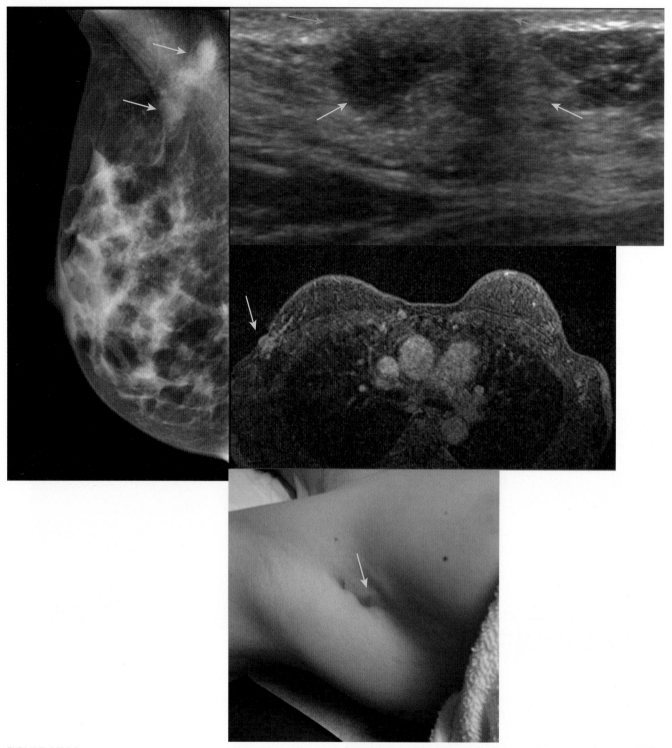

FIGURE 17-11 **Skin Involvement, Stage IIIB.** RMLO shows an irregular mass in the low axilla (*arrows*). US shows a heterogeneous mass (*yellow arrows*) involving the dermis (*green arrows*). MRI shows an enhancing mass in the tail of the breast with enhancement of the skin (*arrow*). On clinical examination, the patient has a skin nodule. Histologic diagnosis: ILC.

diffuse (Fig. 17-14). The definition of abnormal cortical thickness is variable and ranges from 2.3 to 4 mm. This is not a very specific finding because normal bulges can mimic focal thickening. The most specific sign of metastasis is loss of the fatty hilum, though this is not very common. Infiltration of the fat surrounding an axillary node is suggestive of extranodal extension of tumor.

Occasionally, malignant calcifications can develop within lymph nodes involved by metastatic disease.

As for staging, this isn't actually that hard because current staging considers level I and II lymph nodes together, and level III and supraclavicular lymph nodes together. So if you are scanning the axilla in a patient with breast cancer and see suspicious axillary lymph

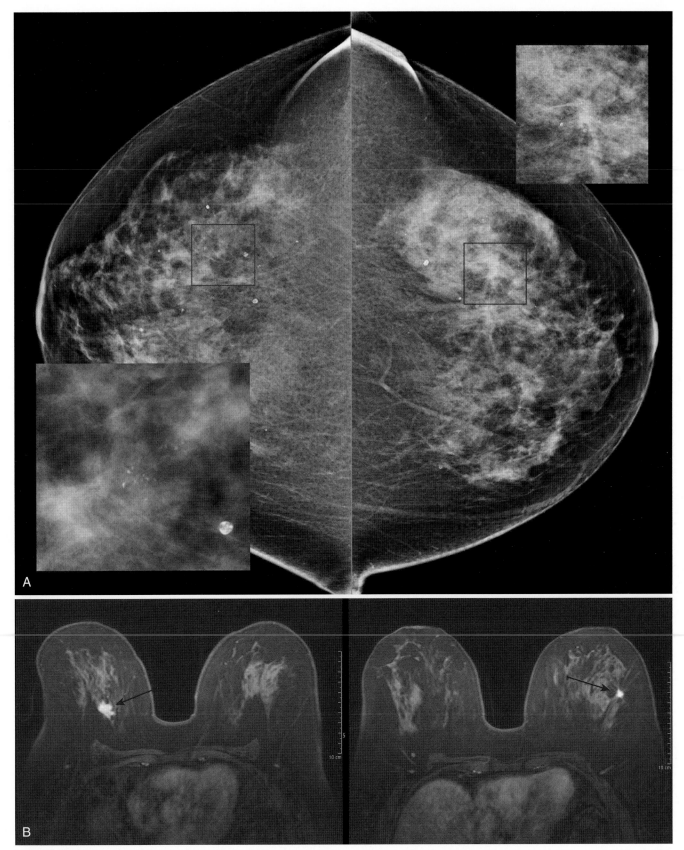

FIGURE 17-12 **Contralateral Synchronous Breast Cancer in Two Patients.** This may be diagnosed on mammography (**A**) or MRI (**B**). **A,** This patient had right calcifications that were DCIS and a left mass that was a tubular carcinoma. **B,** MRI on a different patient who had a known right ILC with a left IDC detected on MRI.

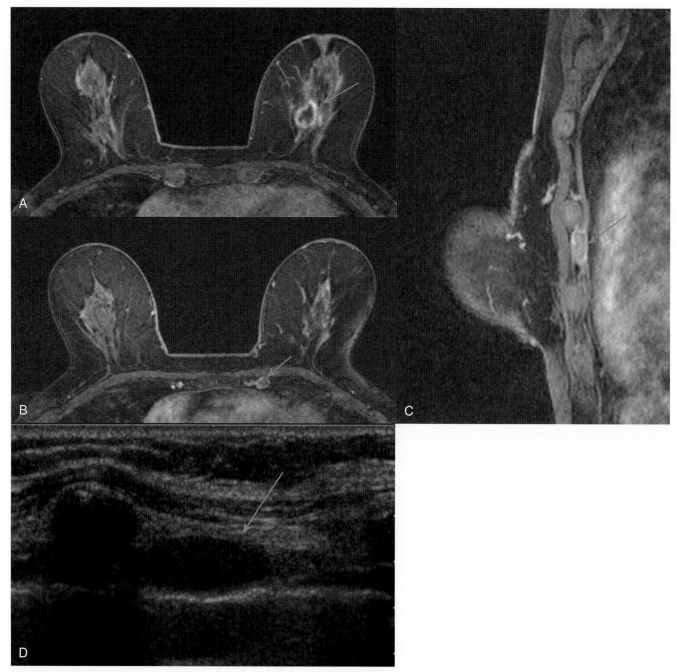

FIGURE 17-13 **Internal Mammary Lymph Node Metastasis. A,** Rim enhancing IDC in the left breast (*arrow*). **B,** Axial postcontrast T1 image shows an enlarged internal mammary lymph node (*arrow*). **C,** Same lymph node in the sagittal plane (*arrow*). **D,** US in the sagittal plane shows the same lymph node between ribs (*arrow*).

nodes, slide the transducer medially under the clavicle (level III) and also above the clavicle. Internal mammary lymph nodes that appear abnormal by imaging are also taken into consideration at staging (Table 17-1).

Why do we care about any of this? Doesn't the surgeon sort all of this stuff out? Well, yes, but imaging can help. The surgical approach to management of the axilla has become less aggressive over time. Complete axillary dissection was the standard of care for decades, to be replaced by sentinel lymph node biopsy for women without evidence of axillary disease by clinical

examination. If image-guided biopsy diagnosed axillary metastasis in these women, axillary dissection was performed instead of sentinel lymph node biopsy.

Management of the axilla is now becoming even less aggressive as studies are showing that axillary surgery may not affect morbidity or mortality rates in women with early stage disease. Systemic and radiation therapy to the axilla probably provide adequate control for the vast majority of these women. The Z11 trial showed that for women meeting certain criteria (including early stage [T1 or T2] breast cancer and 1 or 2 sentinel lymph nodes

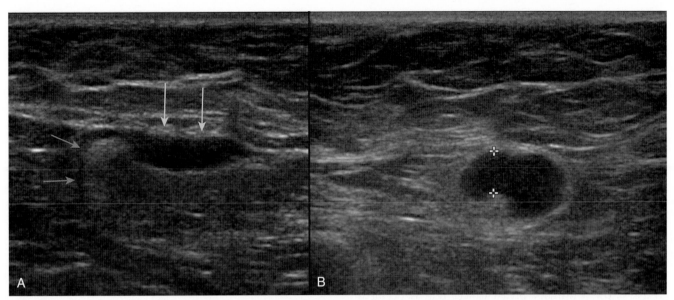

FIGURE 17-14 **Metastatic Axillary Lymph Nodes. A,** The cortex is focally thickened (*yellow arrows*) compared with the normal thin cortex of the remainder of the node (*blue arrows*). **B,** Diffuse cortical thickening

TABLE 17-1 Breast Cancer Staging

Stage 0	DCIS with no axillary or distant metastasis
Stage I	Invasive tumor, 2 cm or smaller without distant metastasis IA: No axillary LN metastasis IB: Micrometastasis in 1 to 3 axillary LNs
Stage IIA	Invasive tumor, 2 cm or smaller with metastasis in 1 to 3 axillary LNs, tiny metastasis in internal mammary LNs on sentinel LN biopsy, or both, OR invasive tumor >2 cm but <5 cm with no axillary or distant metastasis
Stage IIB	Invasive tumor >2 cm but <5 cm with metastasis in 1 to 3 axillary LNs and/or tiny metastasis in internal mammary LNs on sentinel LN biopsy but no distant disease OR invasive tumor >5 cm without chest wall or skin involvement and no axillary metastasis
Stage IIIA	Tumor <5 cm with axillary metastasis in 4 to 9 LNs or to internal mammary LNs but no distant disease OR tumor >5 cm without chest wall or skin involvement and metastasis in up to 9 axillary LNs or enlarged internal mammary LNs
Stage IIIB	Invasive tumor of any size that has grown into the skin or chest wall and metastasis in 0 to 9 axillary LNs or any internal mammary LNs and no distant disease Includes inflammatory breast cancer without distant disease
Stage IIIC	Invasive tumor of any size with metastasis in 10 or more axillary LNs, level III LNs, supraclavicular LNs, any axillary LNs with enlarged internal mammary LNs, or more than 3 axillary LNs with micrometastasis in internal mammary LNs No distant disease
Stage IV	Tumor of any size or nodal status with evidence of distant metastasis

The American Joint Committee on Cancer (AJCC) tumor-node-metastasis (TNM) system is used to stage breast carcinoma. Staging is based on the TNM characteristics of the lesion.
From Edge SB, Byrd DR, Compton CC, et al (eds). AJCC Cancer Staging Manual, 7th ed. New York, Springer, 2009.

containing metastatic tumor), there was no significant difference in mortality rates or recurrence rates whether or not axillary dissection was performed. With median patient follow-up of 6.3 years, the findings suggest that the morbidity and potential complications of axillary node dissection can be avoided in these patients. On the other hand, women undergoing mastectomy or with larger invasive tumors may still undergo axillary lymph node dissection. The Z11 trial was not large, but management of the axilla is likely to change over the next 5 to 10 years. Good communication with your surgical colleagues will be key to a well–thought-out approach.

Imaging of potentially abnormal axillary lymph nodes may not change management for some women, but this doesn't mean that we don't look! Documentation of the number and location of abnormal regional lymph nodes is often helpful for many women. For example, a woman with a 1-cm invasive ductal carcinoma who has ipsilateral metastatic axillary and supraclavicular adenopathy is stage IIIC with a poorer prognosis than if she did not have adenopathy and may undergo neoadjuvant chemotherapy (Table 17-2).

Occasionally, breast carcinoma will present as metastatic axillary adenopathy due to an invasive carcinoma that is occult on mammography (Fig. 17-15). MRI will detect the invasive carcinoma in about 90% of women.

A last note about lymph nodes: Metastatic tumor can completely replace a lymph node so that the normal nodal architecture is obliterated both on imaging and even histologic examination. The differentiation between a metastatic intramammary or low axillary lymph node versus a primary invasive breast cancer can be difficult (Fig. 17-16). If there is DCIS associated with the mass at histologic examination, then it is a primary breast cancer. Without the presence of DCIS, an MRI may be needed to assess for a primary breast cancer that is occult on mammography.

TABLE 17-2	Breast Cancer Stage and Survival Rates
STAGE	**5-YEAR SURVIVAL RATE**
0	93%
IA	88%
IB	88%
IIA	81%
IIB	74%
IIIA	67%
IIIB	41%
IIIC	49%
IV	15%

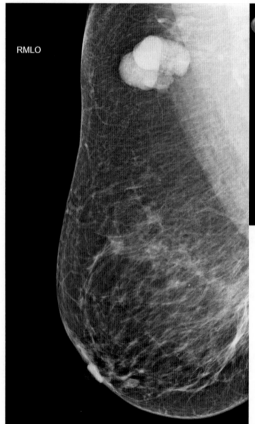

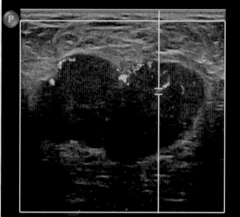

FIGURE 17-15 **Breast Cancer Presenting as Metastatic Axillary Adenopathy.** A 68-year-old woman presents with palpable fullness in her lower right axillary region. Mammography and US show a solid mass with well-defined margins. No other mammographic abnormalities are seen. The differential diagnosis includes both primary and metastatic breast cancer. Core biopsy revealed metastatic adenocarcinoma consistent with breast primary. No primary lesion was identified in this patient on mammography or MRI.

FIGURE 17-16 **Low Axillary Mass.** This 63-year-old woman presented with a palpable lump in her right breast at 10 o'clock at the periphery of the breast, which corresponded to a round mass on mammography (*triangle*) and a very hypoechoic round mass with well-defined margins and internal blood flow on US. US of the axilla was also performed and shows a similar very hypoechoic mass suspicious for a metastatic lymph node. So is the palpable mass a primary breast cancer or a metastatic low axillary lymph node? MRI was performed to exclude a mammographically occult breast cancer. On MRI, the palpable mass is a round rim-enhancing mass (*arrow*). Although no other suspicious findings were identified in the right breast, an irregular enhancing mass was detected in the left breast (*arrow*). Diagnosis: IDC, grade III in the right breast (palpable lump) with a metastatic lymph node and IDC, grade II in the left breast.

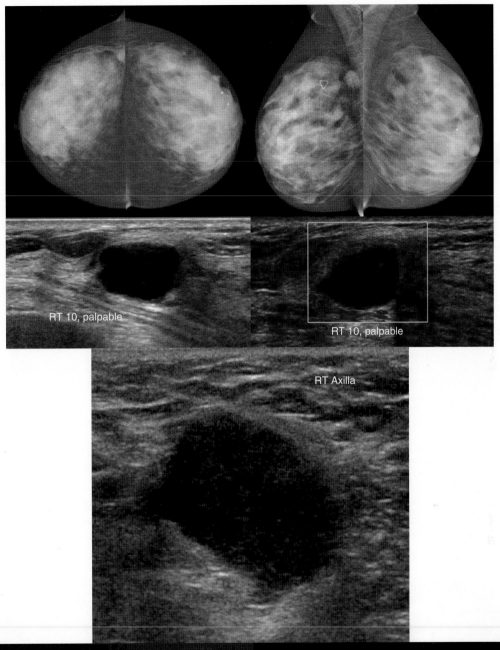

RT 10, palpable

RT 10, palpable

RT Axilla

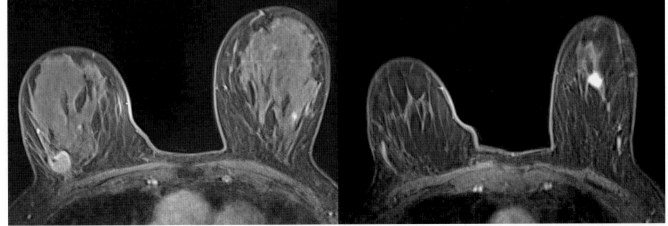

MRI and Women with Recently Diagnosed Cancer

MRI has been used since the mid-1990s to evaluate women with a recent diagnosis of breast cancer. More than 50 studies have been published describing the outcome for women undergoing MRI in this setting. MRI detects additional ipsilateral breast cancer not detected on conventional imaging in 10% to 25% of women (Fig. 17-17). However, the risk of local recurrence is about 6% for women undergoing breast-conserving therapy. This indicates that many of these additional foci of disease

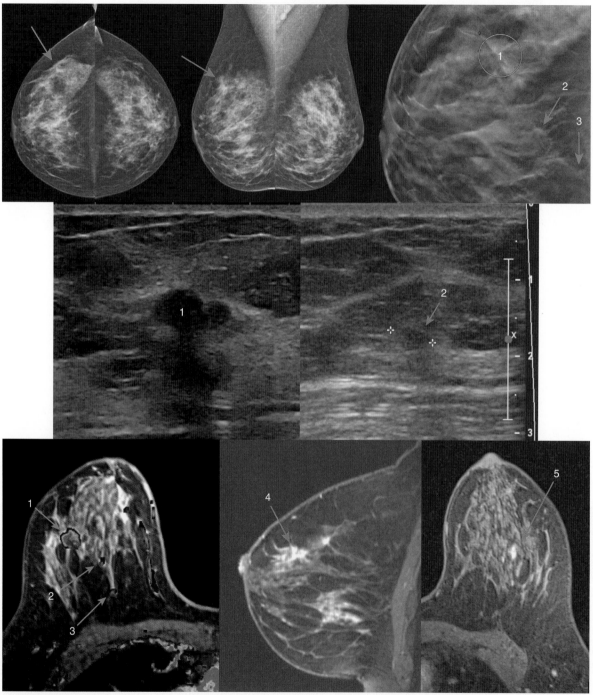

FIGURE 17-17 **Extent of Disease on Several Modalities.** This 49-year-old woman was recalled from screening to evaluate a focal asymmetry in the right breast at 10 o'clock (*arrows*). The asymmetry was highly suspicious on diagnostic imaging. On tomosynthesis, the primary lesion (*1*) is well seen as well as two additional irregular masses (*2* and *3*) that represent multifocal IDC. On US, lesions *1* and *2* were seen but not lesion *3*. On MRI, these three foci of IDC were seen as well as another irregular mass (*4*) in the right breast that was ILC on biopsy. A small linear area of nonmass enhancement was detected in the left breast only on MRI (*5*) that was benign stromal fibrosis on MRI-guided biopsy.

would have been adequately treated with radiation or systemic therapies. Many women having preoperative MRI may undergo more extensive excision or mastectomy unnecessarily.

A meta-analysis of 50 studies was published in 2012 (Plana and associates) that included over 10,000 women. Additional ipsilateral breast disease was identified in 20% of women undergoing preoperative MRI. Of these, 9.1% of women underwent more extensive surgical resection; about half of these (4.6%) were due to false-positive MRI findings. About 10% of women underwent mastectomy due to MRI findings; 8.7% were due to true-positive MRI findings, but 1.7% were due to false-positive findings. Contralateral breast cancer was identified on MRI in 5.5% of women.

Two prospective randomized trials have evaluated preoperative MRI:
- The COMICE (Comparative Effectiveness of MRI in Breast Cancer) Trial randomized 1623 women scheduled for breast-conserving surgery to either receive or not receive preoperative MRI. Seven percent of these patients underwent initial mastectomy compared with 1% of those not having a preoperative MRI. There was no difference in the percentage of women undergoing re-excision after initial lumpectomy. The total mastectomy rate was 13% for women undergoing MRI compared with 9% of women not undergoing MRI.
- The MONET (Mammography of Nonpalpable Breast Tumors) Trial randomized 418 women with nonpalpable, screen-detected BI-RADS 3, 4, or 5 lesions to receive or not receive MRI. Of these patients, 148 were diagnosed with breast cancer. In this smaller study, the initial and final mastectomy rates were similar between groups. Surprisingly, the re-excision rate was significantly higher for the women who had undergone MRI (34% compared with 12%).

Critics of the COMICE trial point out that many centers that participated in the trial had little experience with breast MRI and some did not have the ability to perform MRI-guided biopsies, which may have led to the higher mastectomy rate.

A meta-analysis of 22 studies evaluated the incidence of contralateral breast cancer detected on preoperative breast MRI. A total of 131 contralateral breast cancers were detected in 3253 women (4.1%). Of these, 35% were DCIS and 65% were invasive. Of 114 cancers for which staging information was provided, all but two were invasive and larger than 2 cm. Because these are nearly all small early cancers, the authors suggest that detection by MRI may not provide a significant life-saving advantage over later detection with mammography.

MRI may be more effective in particular subsets of women with a recent cancer diagnosis. This is an evolving area of research. In 2010, the European Society of Breast Cancer Specialists (EUSOMA) published guidelines for recommending breast MRI. In addition, the EUSOMA work group suggested additional study to evaluate the role of preoperative MRI for women with dense tissue; young age; ER/PR (estrogen receptor/

> **BOX 17-2 EUSOMA Work Group Recommendations for MRI in Women with Recently Diagnosed Breast Cancer**
>
> - Invasive lobular carcinoma
> - High risk for breast cancer due to genetic mutation or family history
> - Age < 60 years with a discrepancy in size of the lesion of more than 1 cm between mammography and US with a potential impact on treatment decision
> - Partial breast irradiation candidate

progesterone receptor) negative tumors; close or positive margins; multifocal, multicentric, or bilateral cancers; DCIS to evaluate for invasion; and Paget disease (Box 17-2).

Situations Where Imaging Helps with Staging

So let's put all of our knowledge to work now. Let's think through when imaging can help our surgical and medical colleagues with staging or management.
- **Identifying an invasive component in woman with DCIS.** This changes her from stage 0 to at least stage I.
- **Identifying metastatic axillary adenopathy.** This is at least stage II disease.
- **Identifying extensive axillary adenopathy.** If there are four or more metastatic axillary lymph nodes, the stage is at least IIIA.
- **Identifying abnormal internal mammary lymph nodes.** If metastasis to the internal mammary lymph nodes is identified, the stage is at least IIIA.
- **Identifying skin or chest wall involvement with tumor.** The stage is at least IIIB. Chest wall invasion is different from pectoral muscle invasion. Invasion of the pectoral muscle can be documented by enhancement of the muscle on breast MRI. However, chest wall invasion is tumor invading the ribs or intercostal muscles. Likewise, skin nodularity or erosion must be present, not just dermal invasion.
- **Identifying abnormal level III axillary or supraclavicular lymph nodes.** The stage is at least IIIC.
- **Identifying systemic disease.** If you are reading a breast MRI for a woman with a history of breast cancer, look carefully at structures other than the breast. Findings that may make you worry about metastasis include mass(es) in the lung, liver, or bones. Small pleural effusions are common and normal as long as they are less than 7 mm on the right and 5 mm on the left. Enhancement of the sternum is also common and need not be cause for alarm.

KEY POINTS

- When a breast cancer is suspected or known, our attention turns to evaluating the size and extent of the tumor, detecting multifocal or multicentric disease, and staging the regional lymph nodes.

- Look between the primary lesion and the nipple, as well as between the primary lesion and the chest wall, for calcifications and small masses that may represent additional DCIS or invasive cancer.

- In the setting of calcifications, US may be helpful to detect invasive cancer if there is an associated mass or density or if overlying breast tissue may obscure a mass.

- In the setting of multiple ipsilateral findings, the initial goal is to establish a diagnosis of breast cancer, whereas the later goal is to establish extent of disease for women desiring breast-conserving surgery.

- Remember to look at the contralateral breast because synchronous breast cancer occurs in 1% to 2% of patients as detected by mammography and 3% to 4% as detected by MRI.

- For women with recently diagnosed breast cancer, the use of MRI in the preoperative setting may or may not benefit the patient. However, MRI may be more helpful in some subsets of women, including those with a lifetime risk greater than 20%, ILC, and discrepant size in women younger than age 60.

References

American Cancer Society Breast Cancer Facts & Figures. 2011-2012. Atlanta, GA, American Cancer Society, Inc.

Brennan ME, Houssami N, Lord S, et al. Magnetic resonance imaging screening of the contralateral breast in women with newly diagnosed breast cancer: Systemic review and meta-analysis of incremental cancer detection and impact on surgical management. J Clin Oncol 2009;27:5640-5649.

Deurloo EE, Tanis PJ, Gilhuijs KGA, et al. Reduction in the number of sentinel lymph node procedures by preoperative ultrasonography of the axilla in breast cancer. Eur J Cancer 2003;39:1068-1073.

Edge SB, Byrd DR, Compton CC, et al. (eds). AJCC Cancer Staging Manual, 7th ed. New York, Springer, 2010.

Fischer U, Zachariae O, Baum F, et al. The influence of preoperative MRI of the breasts on recurrence rate in patients with breast cancer. Eur Radiol 2004;14:1725-1731.

Giuliano AE, Hunt KK, Ballman KV, et al. Axillary dissection or no axillary dissection in women with invasive breast cancer and sentinel node metastasis. A randomized clinical trial. JAMA 2011; 305(6):569-575.

Godinez J, Gombos EC, Chikarmane SA, et al. Breast MRI in the evaluation of eligibility for accelerated partial breast irradiation. AJR Am J Roentgenol 2008;191:272-277.

Houssami N, Ciatto S, Macaskill P, et al. Accuracy and surgical impact of magnetic resonance imaging in breast cancer staging: Systematic review and meta-analysis in detection of multifocal and multicentric cancer. J Clin Oncol 2008;26:3248-3258.

Hwang N, Schiller D, Crystal P, et al. Magnetic resonance imaging in the planning of initial lumpectomy for invasive breast carcinoma: Its effect on ipsilateral breast tumor recurrence after breast-conservation therapy. Ann Surg Oncol 2009;16:3000-3009.

Kropcho LC, Steen ST, Chung AP, et al. Preoperative breast MRI in the surgical treatment of ductal carcinoma in situ. Breast J 2011;18:151-156.

Kuhr M, Wolfgarten M, Stolzle M, et al. Potential impact of preoperative magnetic resonance imaging of the breast on patient selection for accelerated partial breast irradiation. Int J Radiat Oncol Biol Phys 2011; 81:e541-e546.

Lindquist D, Hellberg D, Tot T. Disease extent ≥4 cm is a prognostic marker of local recurrence in T1-2 breast cancer. Pathology Research International 2011; Article ID 860584, 6 pages, doi:10.4061/2011/860584.

Mann RM, Loo CE, Wobbes T, et al. The impact of preoperative breast MRI on the re-excision rate in invasive lobular carcinoma of the breast. Br Cancer Res Treat 2010;119:415-422.

McGhan L, Wasif N, Gray R, et al. Use of preoperative magnetic resonance imaging for invasive lobular cancer: Good, better, but maybe not the best? Ann Surg Oncol 2010;17:255-262.

Morrow M, Waters J, Morris E. MRI for breast cancer screening, diagnosis, and treatment. Lancet 2011;378:1804-1811.

Nguyen J, Nicholson BT, Patrie JT, Harvey JA. Incidental pleural effusions on screening breast MRI. AJR Am J Roentgenol 2012; 199(1):W142-145.

Peters NHGM, van Esser S, van den Bosch MAAJ, et al. Preoperative MRI and surgical management in patients with nonpalpable breast cancer: The MONET—Randomised controlled trial. Eur J Cancer 2011;47:879-886.

Plana MA, Carreira C, Muriel A, et al. Magnetic resonance imaging in the preoperative assessment of patients with primary breast cancer: Systematic review of diagnostic accuracy and meta-analysis. Eur Radiol 2012;22:26-38.

Sardanelli F, Boetes C, Borish B, et al. Magnetic resonance imaging of the breast: Recommendations from the EUSOMA working group. Eur J Cancer 2010;46:1296-1316.

Turnbull TL, Brown S, Harvey I, et al. Comparitive effectiveness of MRI in breast cancer (COMICE) trial: A randomized controlled trial. Lancet 2010;375:563-571.

CASE QUESTIONS

CASE 17-1. A 48-year-old woman presents with a palpable mass (*triangle*) in the left breast. US of her left axilla was also performed. Are you done? What else might you look at?

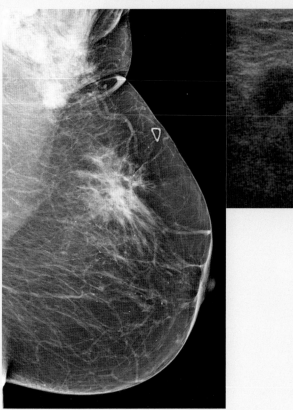

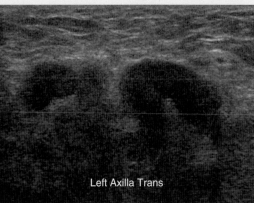

Left Axilla Trans

CASE 17-2. A 52-year-old woman presents with a palpable mass in the left breast (*triangle*), shown by core biopsy to represent IDC. The axillary lymph nodes were normal by US. Based on the imaging below, what stage is her cancer?

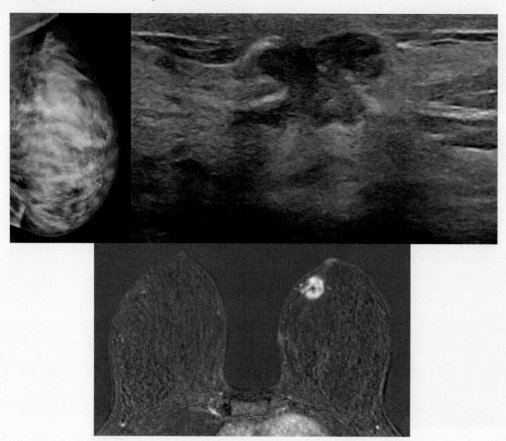

CASE 17-3. This patient had a left mastectomy 2 years ago with five positive axillary lymph nodes. She has a strong family history of breast cancer but cannot undergo MRI due to an expander implant reconstruction on the left. Her right mammogram is negative, but she has dense tissue. Breast-specific gamma imaging was performed to screen the right breast. What do you think of her images?

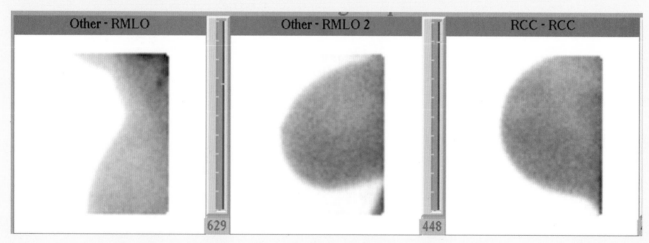

CASE 17-4. A 76-year-old woman with a mass (*arrow*) detected on her screening mammogram. US showed a solid mass. Ultrasound-guided core needle biopsy showed IDC. The patient desires breast-conserving therapy. You are reviewing the images with her breast surgeon. What are the findings? What would you recommend?

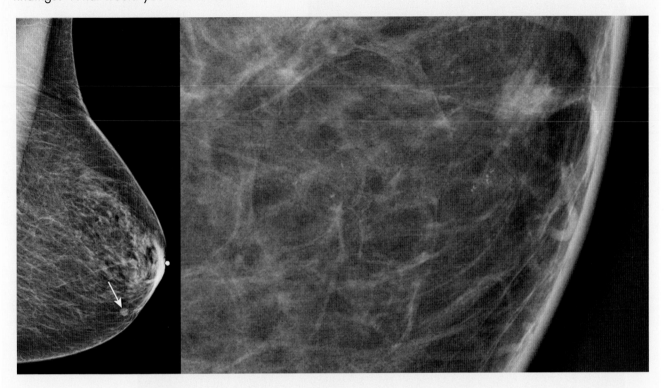

CASE 17-5. Postcontrast MRI of a woman with newly diagnosed IDC of the left breast. What is the cause of the enhancing mass (*arrows*)? What is her stage?

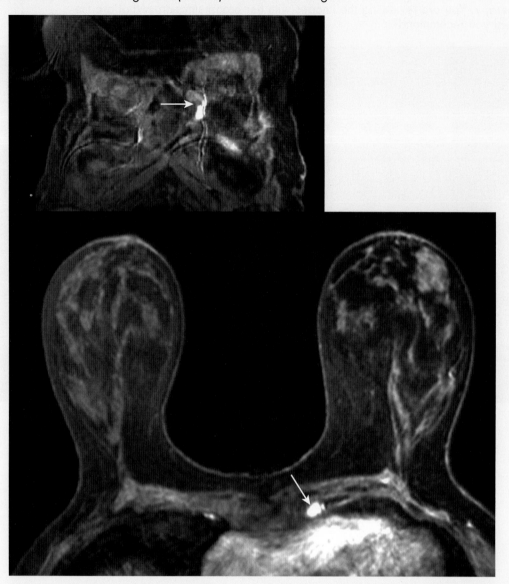

CASE 17-6. A 67-year-old woman with a history of left mastectomy for carcinoma presents with a palpable concern in the medial right breast. Mammography and US of the medial breast are negative. The sonographer also scanned the right axilla and brings you the image shown here. How can you explain the US findings? What are your BI-RADS category and recommendation?

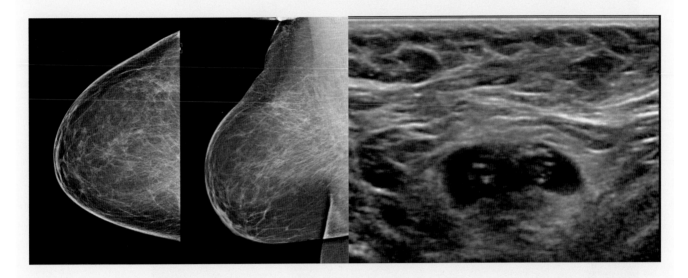

CASE 17-7. A 60-year-old woman presents with thickening and erythema of the right breast. T1-weighted, postcontrast subtraction, and maximum intensity projection images are shown. How would you describe the findings? What is the most likely histologic finding?

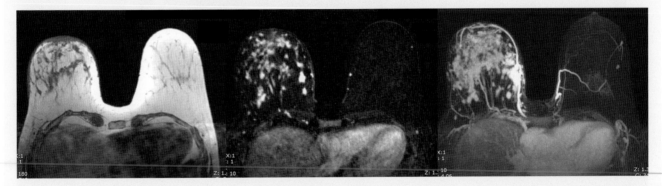

CASE 17-8. A 58-year-old woman presents with a palpable mass (marked with a *BB*) in her right breast. The mammogram and US of the palpable finding are shown here. Where else would you look with US?

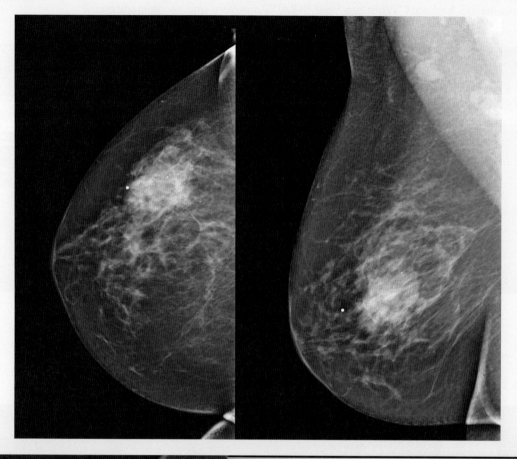

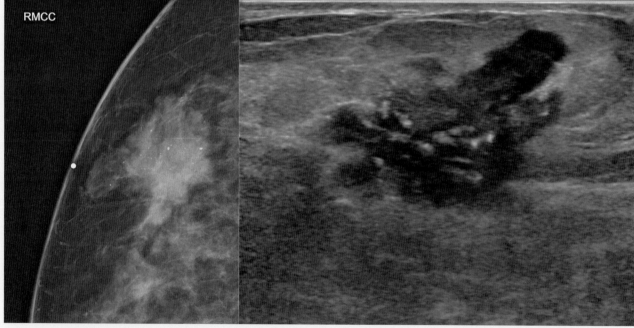

RMCC

CASE 17-9. A 55-year-old woman presents with a palpable mass in her upper outer left breast. Core biopsy revealed IDC. Fine-needle aspiration biopsy of an enlarged axillary node adjacent to the palpable tumor showed metastatic disease. Subtraction and T1-weighted images are shown here. What is her stage?

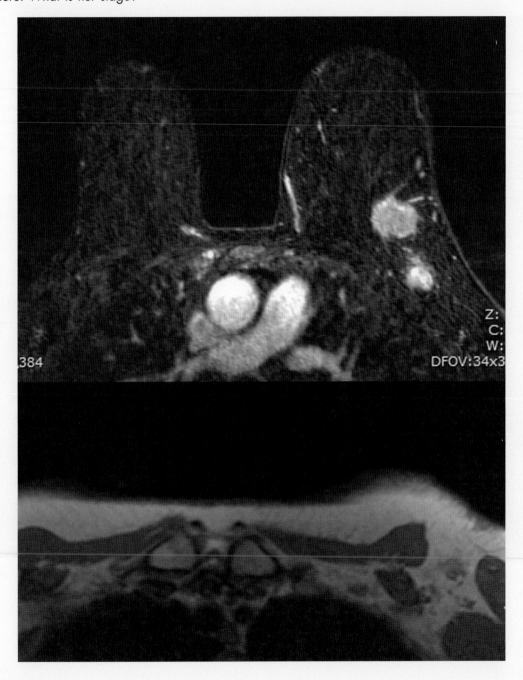

CASE 17-10. A 65-year-old woman has a focal asymmetry with associated fine pleomorphic calcifications in her right breast (*boxes*) detected on screening mammography. Stereotactic biopsy of the calcifications revealed pleomorphic ILC and pleomorphic LCIS. What do you recommend?

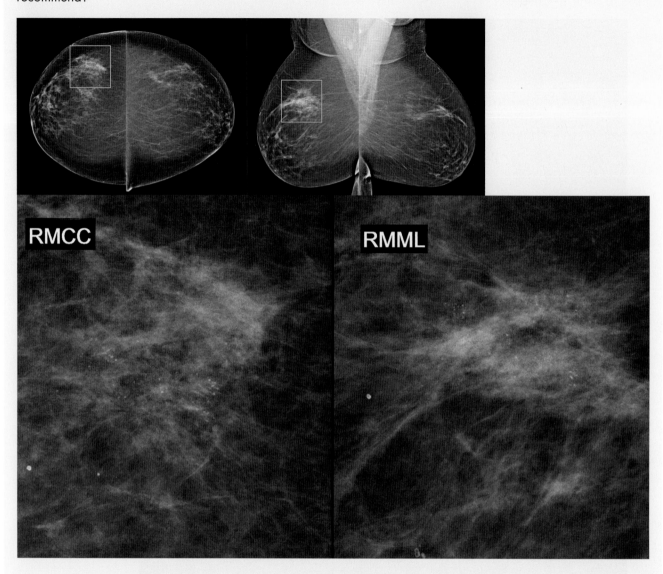

CASE 17-11. A 51-year-old woman is recalled from screening because of a new cluster of fine pleomorphic calcifications. Stereotactic biopsy showed DCIS, high grade. Her mother, maternal aunt, and maternal grandmother all have a history of breast cancer. Because of her strong family history, she had a preoperative MRI. What are the findings? What are your BI-RADS category and recommendation?

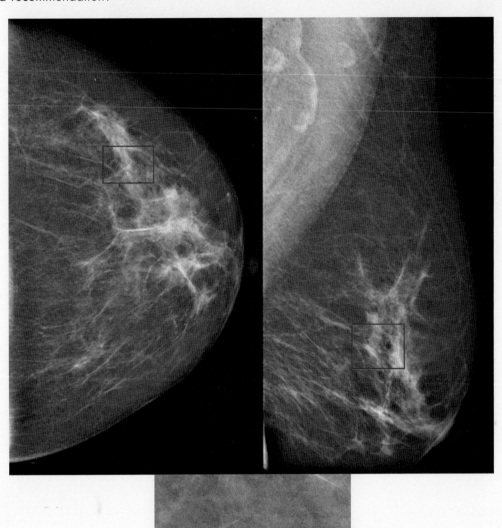

Figure continued on next page.

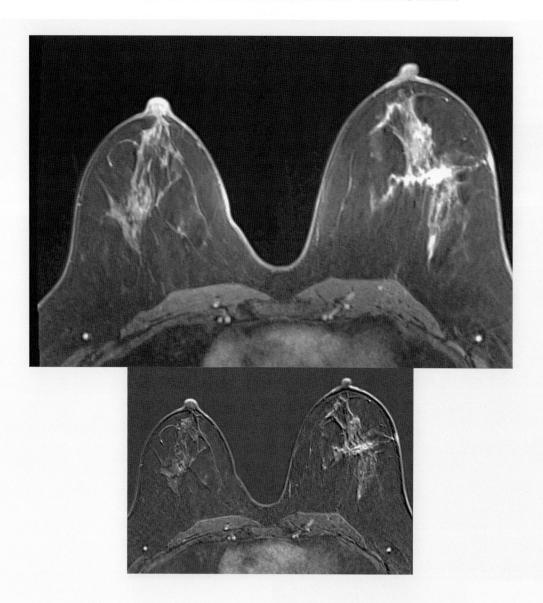

CASE 17-12. This 49-year-old woman was recalled from screening due to calcifications in her right breast at 10 o'clock, posterior third. Biopsy showed DCIS, high grade. Given the appearance of her mammogram and biopsy results, what would you recommend for her?

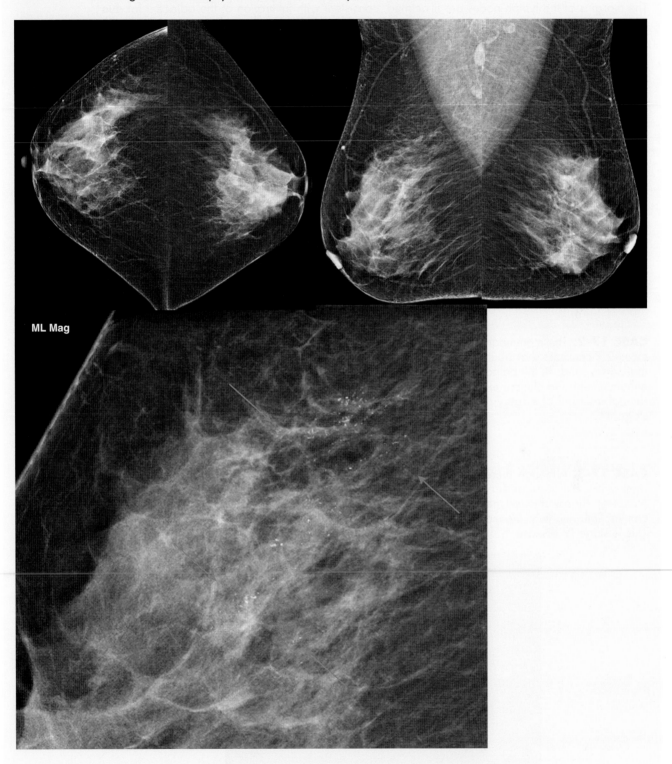

ML Mag

CASE ANSWERS

CASE 17-1. There is clearly left axillary adenopathy present, highly suspicious for metastases. The margins of the lymph nodes are ill-defined, consistent with infiltration of the adjacent fat due to extranodal extension of tumor. Great observation, but don't stop there. Keep going up. Look for level III and supraclavicular lymph nodes. Below is an image of her supraclavicular fossa that shows a very abnormal lymph node. It is amenable to image-guided, fine-needle aspiration, which was positive, making this patient at least stage IIIC.

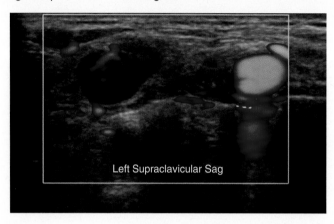

Left Supraclavicular Sag

CASE 17-2. The mammogram is normal, but with dense tissue. On US, there is a highly suspicious 2.8-cm mass that abuts the skin. On MRI, there is a round, well-defined, enhancing mass that corresponds to the palpable finding. Although the mass is close to the skin, there is no dermal enhancement. On clinical examination, there were no skin changes. Even if there is microscopic dermal invasion at surgery, this patient is not stage IIIB. If her lymph nodes are negative, she is stage IIA.

CASE 17-3. Although there is no activity in the right breast, there is abnormal uptake in the right axilla. Her right axillary US (below) shows a lymph node with abnormal cortical thickening (*calipers*). Biopsy showed metastatic invasive breast carcinoma that resembled her prior left breast cancer. Unfortunately, the metastasis to the right axilla is due to her contralateral left breast cancer. This is stage IV disease.

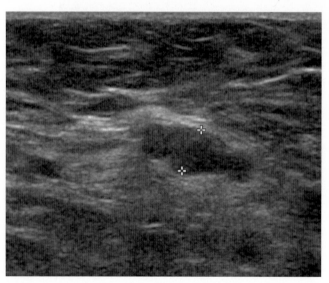

CASE 17-4. Fine pleomorphic calcifications posterior to the mass are concerning for associated DCIS. Unfortunately, this was not recognized. The patient had one wire placed for excision. At excision, the mass was on the edge of the specimen image (*arrow*). There were also calcifications at the margin (*open arrow*), and DCIS was present at the margin. Residual calcifications were present on the postexcision mammogram, and the patient required re-excision. If the calcifications had been recognized in advance, two wires could have been placed—at the anterior and posterior aspects of the mass/calcifications—to aid in complete excision.

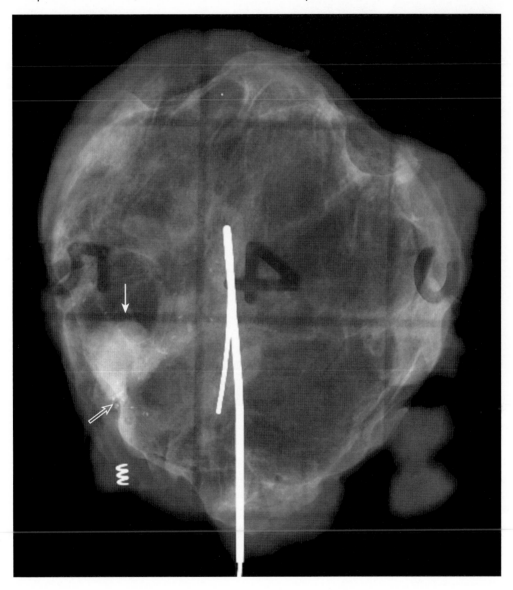

CASE 17-5. Enhancing internal mammary adenopathy is present on the left. The cancer is therefore at least stage III.

CASE 17-6. Mammography reveals no abnormalities. The US image shows an axillary node with cortical thickening and echogenic foci suspicious for calcifications, confirmed on the axillary tail view here. This is concerning for metastatic disease due to mammographically occult ipsilateral breast cancer or metastasis due to her prior left breast cancer. BI-RADS 4: Suspicious. Biopsy revealed metastatic axillary metastasis identical to the patient's contralateral left breast carcinoma, indicating stage IV disease.

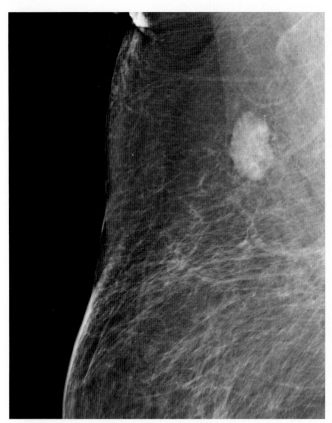

CASE 17-7. There is skin thickening of the right breast. On postcontrast images, numerous enhancing masses are seen throughout the breast with intervening areas of nonmass enhancement. The findings are consistent with inflammatory carcinoma. This is usually caused by IDC; in this case, however, biopsy revealed ILC. The stage is at least IIIB.

CASE 17-8. There is a BI-RADS 5 irregular mass with fine pleomorphic and coarse heterogeneous calcifications corresponding to the palpable lesion. Prominent right axillary nodes are seen on mammography. Once you have finished scanning the palpable mass, look for other foci of invasion by scanning between the mass and the periphery of the breast and between the mass and the nipple. Then evaluate the axilla.

The palpable mass is located at 10 o'clock, 4 to 5 cm from the nipple. A second 4-mm mass is seen at the 10 o'clock position, 9 cm from the nipple. In the low axilla, a round mass without an echogenic hilum is seen, suspicious for metastatic adenopathy. Core biopsy of the palpable mass revealed IDC, grade III. Core biopsy of the 10 o'clock lesion showed metastasis to an intramammary lymph node. Fine-needle aspiration biopsy of the axillary mass confirmed lymph node metastasis.

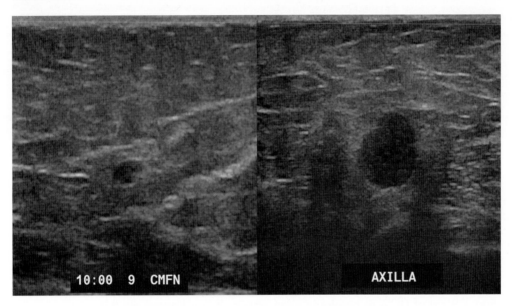

CASE 17-9. The primary tumor and adjacent metastatic axillary lymph node are seen on the subtracted image. On the T1-weighted image, a level III node is seen (*arrow*), medial to the pectoralis minor muscle (*pm*). This finding is suspicious for metastatic involvement, consistent with at least stage IIIC.

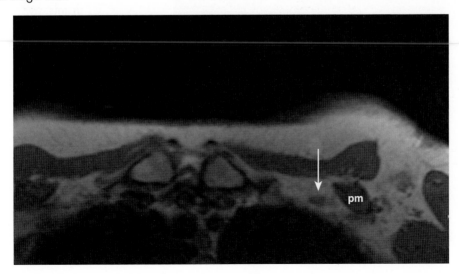

CASE 17-10. The pleomorphic subtype of ILC is more aggressive and carries a worse prognosis than the classic type. The extent of ILC is frequently underestimated on mammography, and the focal asymmetry in this patient is suspicious for additional tumor.

MRI for preoperative evaluation of ILC is one of the EUSOMA Work Group Recommendations discussed previously and was performed on this patient. Postcontrast maximum intensity projection and subtracted images reveal extensive nonmass enhancement in the anterior and middle thirds of the breast. Mastectomy showed extensive ILC and pleomorphic LCIS.

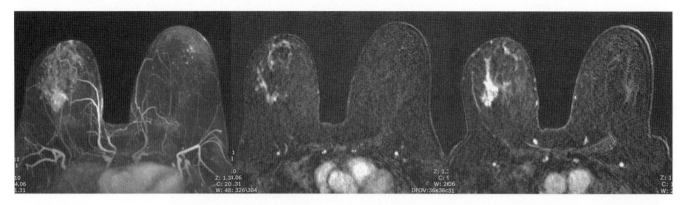

CASE 17-11. On the mammogram, there is a single small cluster of calcifications. The extent of high-grade DCIS usually corresponds pretty well to the extent of calcifications. On MRI, there is linear nonmass enhancement in the left breast at 3 o'clock, middle third (*blue arrows*). Did you notice how it is oriented in the transverse plane rather than in a segmental distribution? Did you also notice that there is no enhancement in the center (best seen on the subtraction image)? That's because it represents the enhancing biopsy track from her recent stereotactic biopsy, not DCIS. You can even make out the skin nick (*yellow arrow*). Because of her family history, she opted for bilateral mastectomy and had 1.8 cm of DCIS at histologic examination. If you figured out this one, great job!

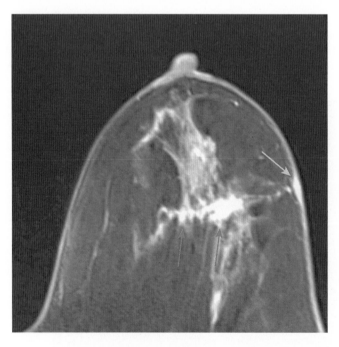

CASE 17-12. Did you notice that there is a mildly enlarged lymph node in the right axilla? If so, then nice job! The enlargement proved real and was due to metastatic disease. Let's try to find the invasive carcinoma because DCIS alone would not result in metastasis (though a microscopic focus of invasion may never be identified). Here is her MRI. On the subtraction image, there is segmental nonmass enhancement (*arrows*) in the right breast at 10 o'clock consistent with extensive DCIS. On the sagittal image, there is an enhancing mass (*yellow arrow*) just inferior to the biopsy clip (*blue arrow*). Ultrasound-guided biopsy showed IDC.

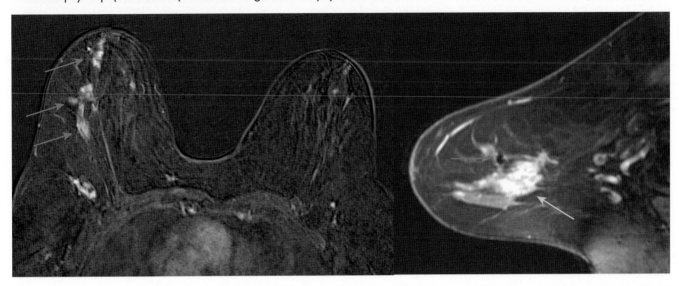

POSTOPERATIVE STUDIES

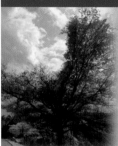

CHAPTER 18

The Postoperative Breast

Do you see the branch that has been cut out on the left side of the tree in the picture? If the branch had been removed due to disease, where would you look to see if the disease had resurfaced? You would look really carefully at the remainder of that branch. You would also probably check the rest of the tree to be sure there was no new sign of disease in any other branches.

When imaging the patient with known or suspected breast cancer (Chapter 17), we focused our attention on the affected ductal system to evaluate extent of disease. Likewise, when looking for recurrent cancer in women who have undergone breast-conserving therapy (BCT), we will focus on the ductal system where the cancer developed. We will start by looking at the lumpectomy scar and then within that ductal system.

In this chapter, we will review benign surgical changes and then turn our attention to detection of residual and recurrent breast cancer. We will give you our best tips for differentiating benign postoperative changes from those that may represent cancer.

Reduction Mammoplasty and Mastopexy

Reduction mammoplasty, mastopexy, and breast augmentation are typically performed by plastic surgeons rather than breast surgeons. Breast augmentation is discussed in Chapter 19.

Reduction mammoplasty is performed to reduce the overall size of the breasts. It is often performed for women with back or shoulder problems due to the weight of large breasts. After mastectomy with reconstruction, the contralateral breast may be reduced to improve symmetry of breast size. Mastopexy, or a "breast lift," is similar in surgical approach, but breast tissue is not removed. This is performed for women with ptotic breasts wishing to reverse the effects of living on a gravitational planet.

For both reduction mammoplasty and mastopexy, a keyhole incision is made (Fig. 18-1). The scars of

reduction mammoplasty are therefore seen primarily on the inferior breasts.

The breast tissue has a "swirled" appearance in the inferior aspect of the mediolateral oblique (MLO) views—the ducts are heading toward the prior location of the nipple, which has been moved up to a perkier location (Fig. 18-2). Isolated islands of breast tissue may be seen and are the result of separation of the tissue during surgery (Fig. 18-3). Dermal calcifications are very common in the scar tissue (Fig. 18-4). Oil cysts are also very common after both reduction and mastopexy (Fig. 18-5).

Benign Surgical Biopsy

Surgical Biopsy Terminology

"Lumpectomy" literally means removal of a palpable lump. However, by convention, "lumpectomy" is used to describe the surgical removal of a cancer, regardless of whether or not it is palpable. "Excisional biopsy" refers to the surgical removal of an entire breast lesion. For example, a palpable fibroadenoma may undergo surgical excision. "Incisional biopsy" indicates a surgical biopsy in which only a portion of a lesion is removed. This type of biopsy may be performed when a core biopsy shows a high-risk lesion or was benign discordant. The goal of incisional biopsy is to obtain tissue for diagnosis rather than to completely remove a palpable finding or known carcinoma.

Changes of Surgical Biopsy

In the immediate postoperative period, small hematomas and seromas are common. Large fluid collections necessitating drainage are very uncommon. Fluid collections in the biopsy cavity decrease in size and have typically resolved by the time imaging is next performed. Imaging after a benign surgical biopsy may be helpful to confirm

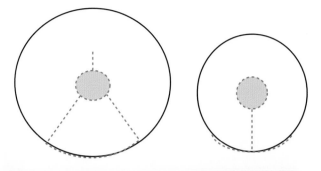

FIGURE 18-1 **Keyhole Incision.** This incision is used for reduction mammoplasty and mastopexy. Incisions are made around the areola, at 4 and 8 o'clock, and along the inframammary fold (*blue lines*). For reduction, the fatty tissue and skin are removed from the inferior breast. For mastopexy, the skin is removed but not the underlying breast tissue. The skin is then pulled together leaving scars at 6 o'clock and along the inframammary fold. If the surgery stopped here, the nipple would now be under the breast mound because that tissue and skin have been removed. The plastic surgeon therefore makes a small incision at 12 o'clock, and the areola is moved cephalad.

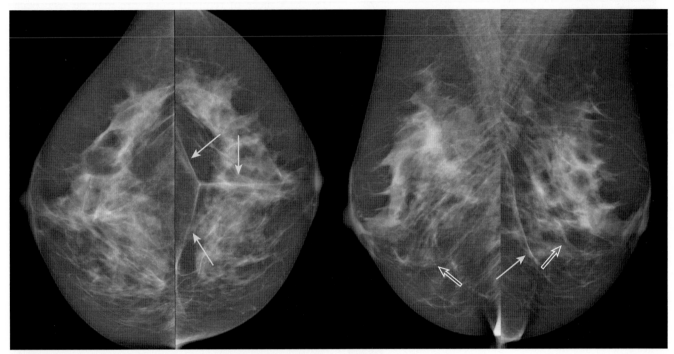

FIGURE 18-2 **Typical Changes of Reduction Mammoplasty.** Scars are present in the inferior breast (*arrows*), and the breast tissue has a swirled appearance on the MLO views (*open arrows*).

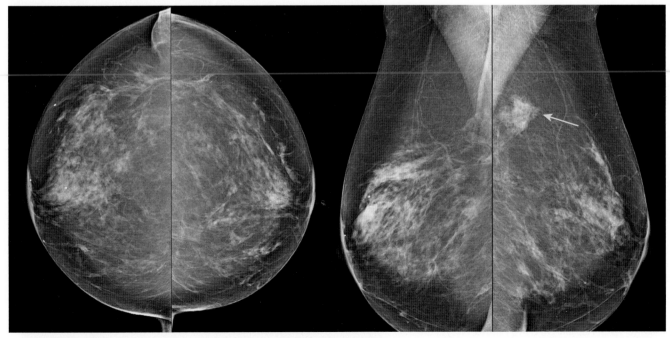

FIGURE 18-3 **Isolated Islands of Breast Tissue.** Isolated islands of breast tissue (*arrow*) are common after reduction mammoplasty.

that the targeted lesion has been sampled or removed, but it is not required.

The first postoperative mammogram is often obtained 6 to 12 months after biopsy. Distortion from scarring will be worst on this earliest mammogram. The size and density of the scar will improve with time. Scars are

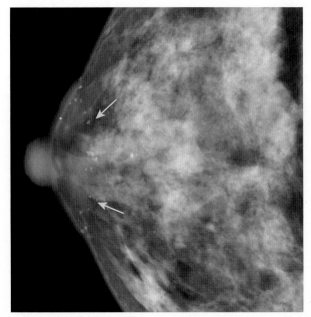

FIGURE 18-4 **Dermal Calcifications in Reduction Scars.** Dermal calcifications in reduction scars (*arrows*) are present in the circumareolar area.

planar (Fig. 18-6). After about 5 years, distortion after benign biopsy becomes difficult to identify in most women. Significant architectural distortion more than 10 years after a benign biopsy is uncommon and should be viewed with suspicion. Don't assume that the architectural distortion you see is due to a fibroadenoma that was removed in 1995! Comparison with older mammograms or diagnostic evaluation may be indicated.

Fat necrosis and benign dystrophic calcifications may evolve over the first year or two. The detritus of surgery may also be seen. Sutural calcifications may develop (Fig. 18-7). A piece of retained hookwire may be seen occasionally (Fig. 18-8).

Surgery for Breast Cancer

Lumpectomy for Carcinoma

Imaging of women undergoing BCT is important for detecting residual disease in the early postoperative period (prior to radiation therapy [RT]), for identifying recurrent breast cancer after therapy, and for diagnosing metachronous breast cancer (Box 18-1).

Residual Disease

There are several opportunities to identify residual disease in women undergoing BCT. These include positive or close margins of the excised specimen at pathologic examination, a specimen radiograph showing the lesion near the radiographic margin, and the pre-RT mammogram.

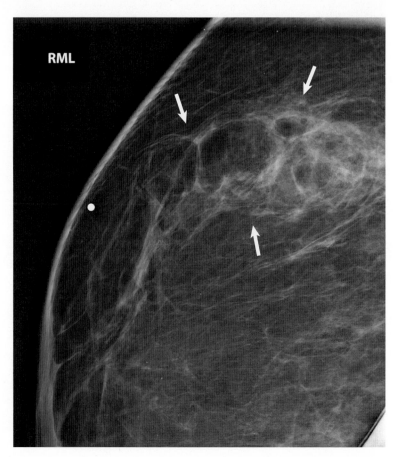

FIGURE 18-5 **Palpable Oil Cysts.** Palpable oil cysts are seen following reduction mammoplasty (*arrows*).

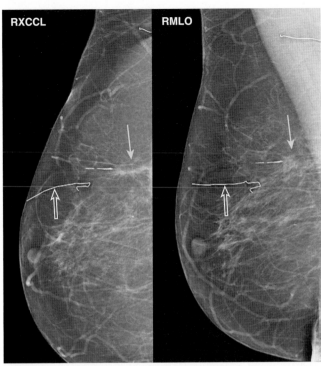

FIGURE 18-6 **Normal Benign Biopsy Scar.** The scar is planar, like a piece of paper. It appears linear on the exaggerated craniocaudal view (*arrow*) but is less dense and more diffuse on the MLO view (*arrow*). A wire (*open arrows*) has been placed on the skin to mark the scar in these and other images throughout this chapter.

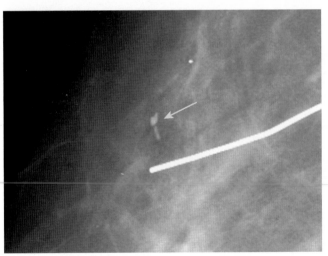

FIGURE 18-7 **Sutural Calcification** (*arrow*).

A pathology report of *positive or close margins* is associated with a high likelihood of cancer remaining in the breast. If the patient had calcifications associated with the cancer, magnification views of the operative region prior to re-excision may demonstrate concerning residual calcifications that can be localized as part of the re-excision surgery (Fig. 18-9). These calcifications may be difficult to visualize because of the postoperative changes, so look back at the preoperative magnification views for comparison.

Magnetic resonance imaging (MRI) is also very useful in assessing the amount of residual disease to assist decision making about whether another excision is likely to

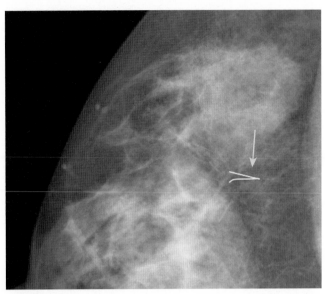

FIGURE 18-8 **Retained Hookwire.** Retained hookwire (*arrow*) after a wire-localized benign biopsy.

BOX 18-1 Typical Post-BCT Imaging Protocol

- Ipsilateral pre-RT mammogram (all calcification cases, others on a case-by-case basis)
- Ipsilateral mammogram every 6 months for 2 to 3 years
- Contralateral mammogram every year
- Magnification views of the lumpectomy bed with each mammogram for 5 years

be successful (Fig. 18-10). It can also detect additional previously occult lesions distant from the site of known tumor. When the MRI is abnormal (Fig. 18-11), additional disease should be confirmed by biopsy before mastectomy is recommended. False-positive and false-negative MRI findings are fairly common; the sensitivity and specificity of MRI in identifying residual cancer in women with positive or close margins are 61.2% and 69.7%, respectively. A negative MRI does not indicate that the patient can forgo re-excision. Microscopic or nonenhancing carcinoma may still be present.

A pathology report of negative margins does not ensure that there is no residual disease present. Pathologic assessment of margins is an imperfect science; four to five small samples of tissue are taken from the areas that appear most suspicious for cancer on the surface of the lumpectomy tissue by gross inspection. Pathologists estimate that around 16% of the surface of a lumpectomy specimen is sampled for microscopic examination.

Radiologists have an opportunity to help; the *specimen radiograph* not only confirms whether the lesion was removed or not, but also where the lesion was located within the specimen (Fig. 18-12). If the lesion is at or near an edge, the chance of incomplete excision is 79% to 98%. In these cases, communication with the surgeon in

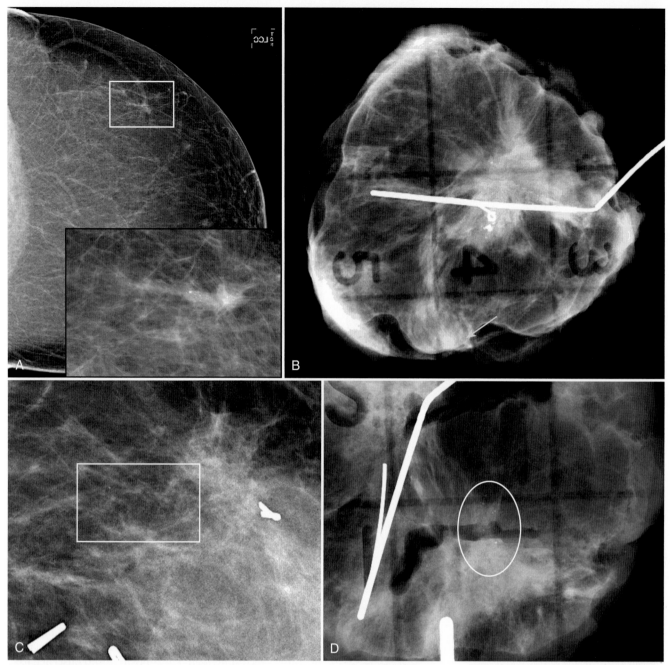

FIGURE 18-9 **Positive Margin with Residual Calcifications. A,** Screening recall for a mass with associated calcifications. Core biopsy showed invasive ductal carcinoma (IDC) with ductal carcinoma in situ (DCIS). **B,** Specimen radiograph shows excision of the mass, though the posterior extent including calcifications may not be completely excised (*arrow*). DCIS was present at the margin. **C,** Magnification view after lumpectomy shows residual calcifications (*box*). These were wire localized to aid re-excision. **D,** Radiograph of the re-excision specimen documents removal (*circle*). Residual DCIS was present with negative margins.

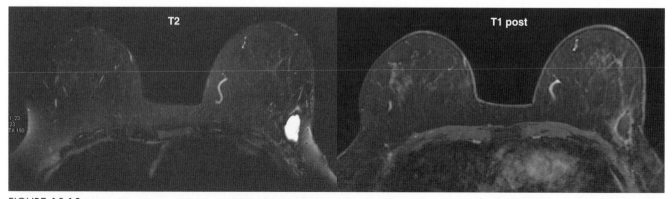

FIGURE 18-10 **Normal Lumpectomy Cavity on MRI.** This patient had a close margin at lumpectomy. She desired breast conserving therapy. The T2 (*left*) shows the location of the seroma. The T1 postcontrast sequence (*right*) shows a thin rim of enhancement around the seroma. There is no imaging evidence of residual disease. She had successful BCT with low-volume re-excision.

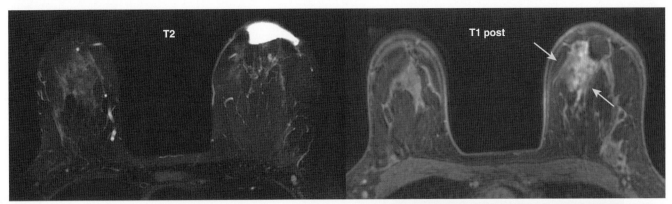

FIGURE 18-11 **Extensive Residual Disease on MRI.** This patient had a wire-localized removal of a small cluster of microcalcifications that were DCIS on core biopsy. Surgical margins were positive. The T2 sequence shows the left subareolar seroma. Postcontrast T1 sequence shows extensive nonmass enhancement in the medial left breast that represented residual noncalcified DCIS (*arrows*).

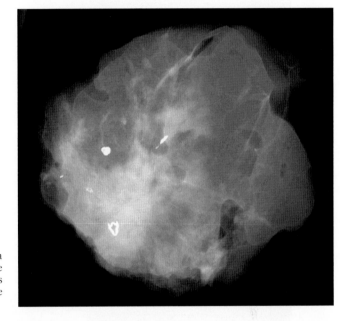

FIGURE 18-12 **Mass at Edge of the Specimen.** Yes, the mass that is a biopsy-proven IDC has been removed, but it is located at the edge of the specimen. It is highly likely that the margin will be positive unless this situation is communicated to the surgeon so that additional tissue can be removed.

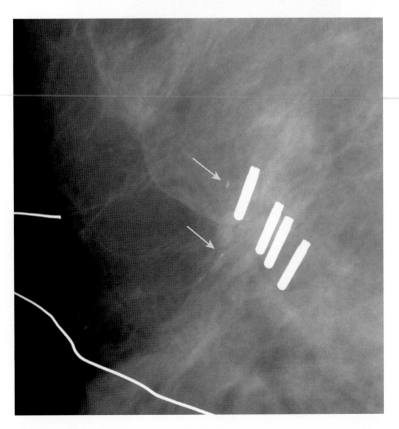

FIGURE 18-13 **Abnormal Pre-RT Mammogram.** Residual calcfications are seen in the lumpectomy bed (*arrows*). Surgical margins were negative at the time of resection. Re-excision showed residual DCIS. The patient then proceeded to have successful BCT with RT.

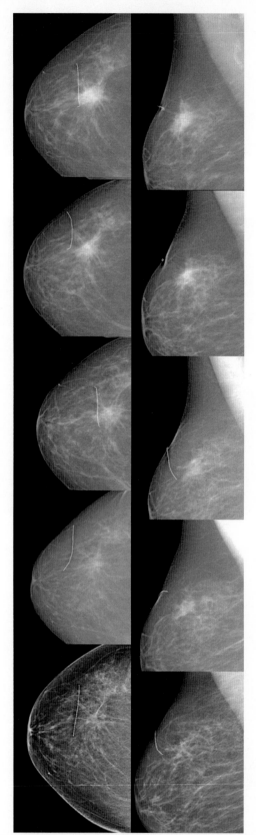

FIGURE 18-14 Evolution of a Normal Lumpectomy Scar. The scar is largest and most dense on the first postoperative mammogram (*top*) and decreases in size and density over the next 10 years.

the operating room may guide immediate resection of the suspect margin. This can result in a negative margin, eliminating the need for additional surgery.

Radiologists have one more opportunity to identify residual disease: the *pre-RT mammogram*. In the early BCT trials, women with residual calcifications in or near the lumpectomy bed had a local recurrence rate of 60% compared with a 6% recurrence rate of women overall. That's a huge difference, so we have a job to do! For women with breast cancer presenting as calcifications with or without an associated mass, an ipsilateral mammogram with magnification views prior to RT may identify residual calcifications in or near the lumpectomy bed (Fig. 18-13). If a pre-RT mammogram is not obtained and residual carcinoma is identified after RT is administered, the patient must undergo mastectomy.

Normal Lumpectomy Changes

Scars are tricky. Has the distortion increased? Is it denser? We struggle with this almost daily in mammography.

Just as with a benign biopsy scar, the appearance should be worst on the first mammogram after surgery. After this the breast is healing, so the scar should decrease in size and density over time (Fig. 18-14). If the scar is increasing in size, density, or amount of distortion, then local recurrence may be present.

Scars are typically thin and linear on ultrasonography (US) (Fig. 18-15). Focal mass-like areas of thickening in the scar on US are suspicious for local recurrence. US can also be confusing, however, because of suspicious masses related to fat necrosis or shadowing from scar tissue or benign calcifications.

Radiation Therapy Changes

RT results in some edema acutely that often leads to fibrosis. On mammography, this appears as skin and trabecular thickening (thickening of the Cooper ligaments) (Fig. 18-16). These changes will peak on the first post-RT mammogram. If the patient has chemotherapy, the post-RT mammogram is often about 1 year after diagnosis. If skin and trabecular thickening improve and then become worse, the patient may have inflammatory breast cancer (Fig. 18-17).

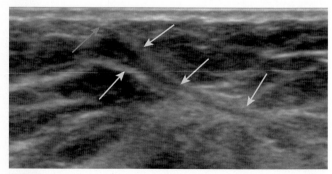

FIGURE 18-15 US of a Normal Lumpectomy Scar. The skin is a little thicker at the site of surgical incision (*blue arrow*). The scar is thin and linear as it extends down into the breast (*yellow arrows*).

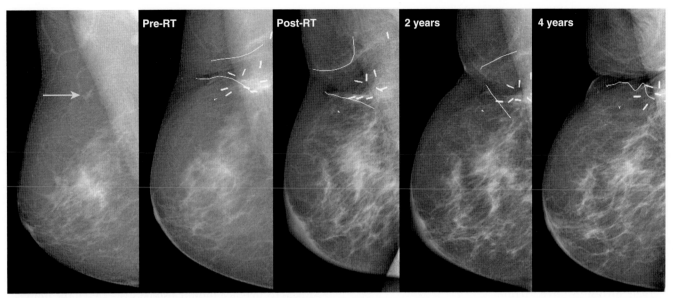

FIGURE 18-16 **Radiation Therapy Changes.** The asymmetry in the superior right breast (*arrow*) was an 8-mm IDC. The lumpectomy bed is densest on the first postsurgical (pre-RT) mammogram. The skin and trabecular thickening peak on the first mammogram after treatment (post-RT).

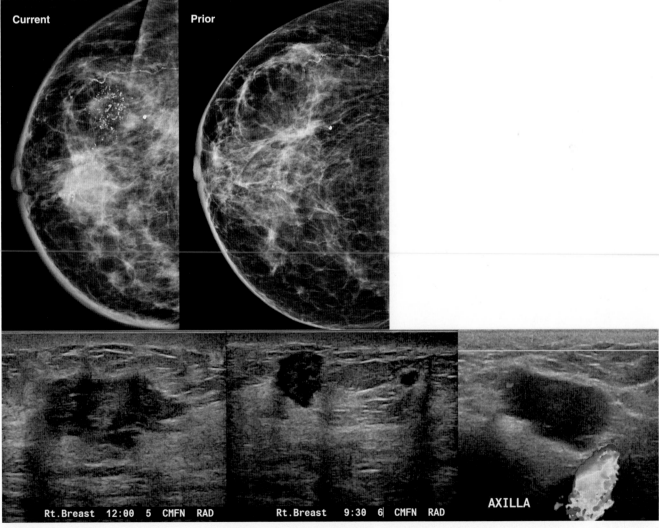

FIGURE 18-17 **Recurrent Carcinoma.** A 71-year-old woman who had lumpectomy and RT for right breast carcinoma 4 years earlier. Compared with the prior study, mammography shows increased skin thickening, new coarse heterogeneous calcifications, and a developing asymmetry in the central breast. US revealed multiple irregular masses and axillary adenopathy.

Mastectomy Without Reconstruction or Implant Reconstruction

These women do not need routine imaging. The risk of local recurrence is small, and typically presents as a small palpable mass. Imaging, usually with US, is helpful in evaluating a palpable finding.

Mastectomy with Autologous (Tissue Flap) Reconstruction

This is a common procedure with good aesthetic outcome. Women typically have a skin-sparing mastectomy with removal of the nipple-areolar complex. The tissue flap can originate from the abdomen (transverse rectus abdominis myocutaneous [TRAM] or deep inferior epigastric perforator [DIEP]), shoulder (latissimus dorsi), or buttocks. A tissue flap can be attached to a vascular pedicle or not (a "free" flap).

On imaging, fatty tissue replaces the breast mound with scars in the subcutaneous regions (Fig. 18-18). The muscular pedicle is often seen. Fat necrosis and oil cysts are common.

Detecting Recurrent Disease

Local recurrence affects 6% to 8% of women undergoing BCT. Most local recurrence will occur between years 1 and 7 after lumpectomy, with the peak at year 4. Recurrence within the first 2 years after treatment is fortunately uncommon; by the time most cancers recur, the findings caused by lumpectomy and RT have usually stabilized. Without RT, local recurrence is much more common,

affecting 30% to 40% of women. Be very suspicious when reviewing the mammograms of women who decline RT.

Local recurrence typically occurs in the same ductal system (segment) as the original cancer. Therefore, after we look at the scar itself, we must pay special attention to the region between the scar and the nipple, and the scar and the chest wall (Fig. 18-19). A developing asymmetry, mass, or even a few calcifications in these regions are suspect.

Among patients initially treated for DCIS, 75% with local recurrence will present with calcifications. Benign calcifications tend to develop earlier than calcifications of recurrent disease (median time 2 versus 4 years) (Fig. 18-20). Of women initially diagnosed with DCIS who have a local recurrence, about half will have an invasive component (Fig. 18-21). Mastectomy is usually indicated for treatment of local recurrence after RT because the patient will have already received the maximum allowable radiation dose to the breast.

Local recurrence should also be suspected if the lumpectomy scar is becoming thicker or denser over time. A focal lesion may be identified on US in some cases (Fig. 18-22). Diffuse thickening of the scar is less specific and may be due to fat necrosis. If there is not a clear focal finding on mammography or US, then MRI may be helpful (Fig. 18-23).

Most scars more than a couple of years old do not show suspicious enhancement on MRI. A small amount of linear enhancement of a scar or residual seroma is not uncommon, however, even many years after surgery. Mass or nonmass enhancement in or near the lumpectomy bed is concerning for local recurrence (Fig. 18-24).

Fat necrosis is a big mimicker of cancer on any modality. The most common appearance is a lipid-containing

Text continued on p. 483

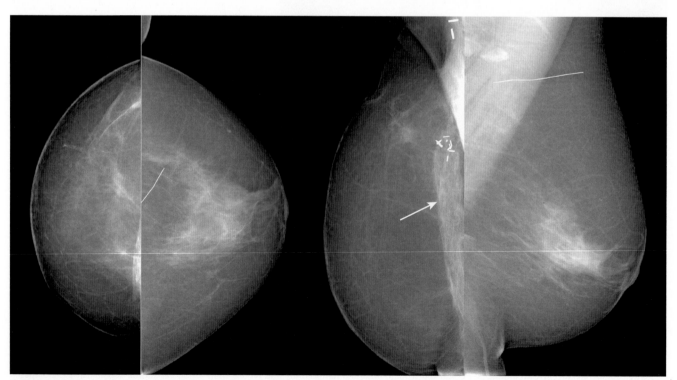

FIGURE 18-18 **TRAM Reconstruction.** This patient has had a right mastectomy with TRAM reconstruction. The muscular pedicle (*arrow*) is seen posteriorly.

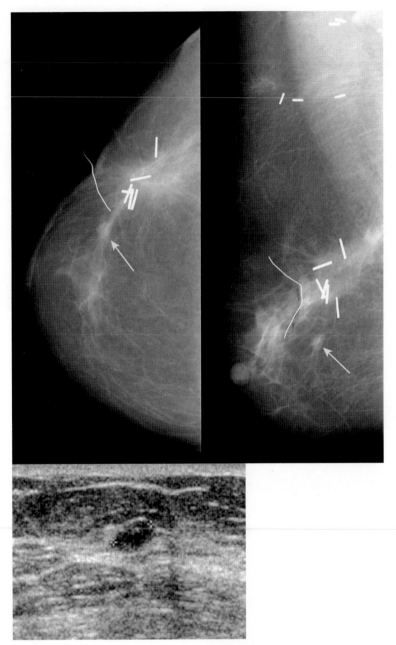

FIGURE 18-19 **Local Recurrence in the Same Ductal System.** The patient is 5 years after BCT. Right mammogram shows a small mass between the lumpectomy bed and the nipple (*arrow*). On US, there is a corresponding hypoechoic solid mass. Histologic examination showed IDC. The patient underwent mastectomy.

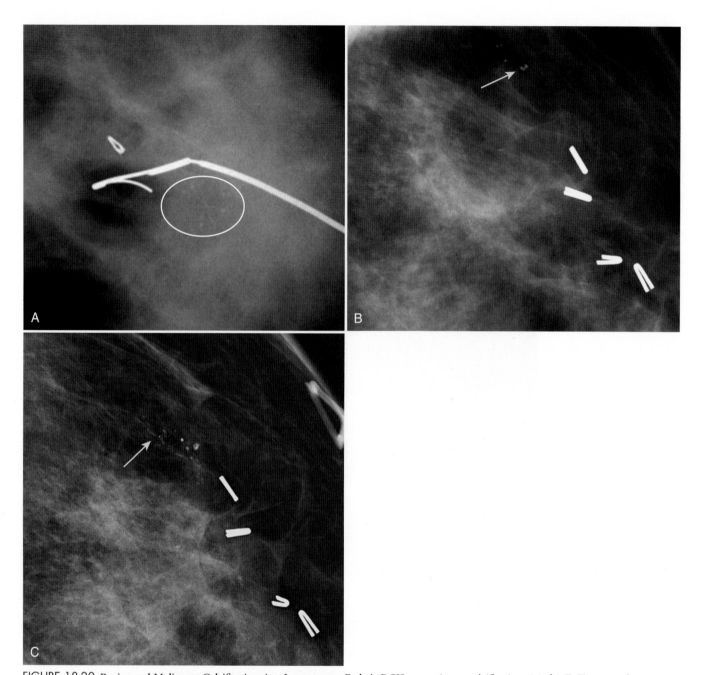

FIGURE 18-20 **Benign and Malignant Calcifications in a Lumpectomy Bed. A,** DCIS presenting as calcifications (*circle*). **B,** Two years later, coarse calcifications developed that are benign (*arrow*). **C,** Four years later, fine pleomorphic calcifications similar to the original DCIS appeared in the lumpectomy bed (*arrow*). Stereotactic biopsy showed recurrent DCIS.

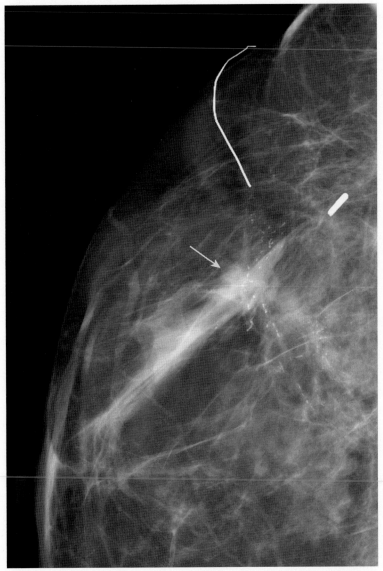

FIGURE 18-21 **Recurrent DCIS with IDC.** This patient had lumpectomy and RT for treatment of DCIS 5 years earlier. Pleomorphic calcifications associated with a small mass (*arrow*) between the lumpectomy site and the nipple represent recurrent DCIS with IDC.

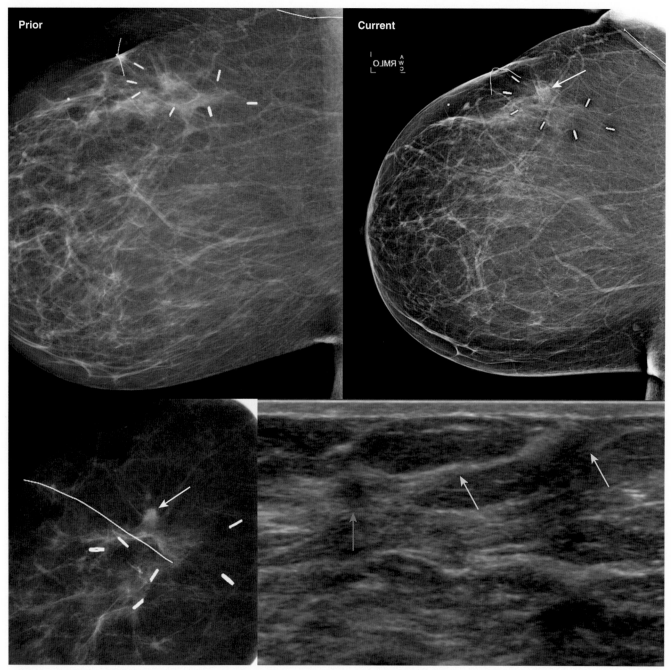

FIGURE 18-22 **Increased Density in Lumpectomy Bed Due to Recurrence.** Four years after lumpectomy, the scar is increasing in density (*arrow*) compared with 2 years prior. The spot compression view shows a small mass (*arrow*). US confirms a small hypoechoic mass (*blue arrow*) adjacent to the scar (*yellow arrows*).

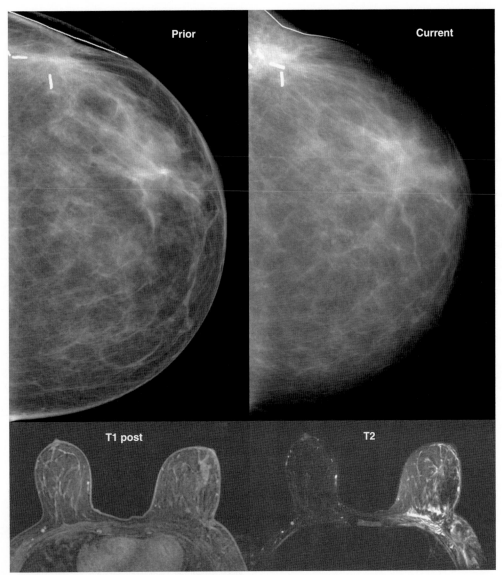

FIGURE 18-23 **Interval Increase in Density of a Scar.** There is an interval increase in density at the scar compared with 1 year prior. MRI shows no enhancement of the scar on the T1 postcontrast sequence. There is increased signal on the T2-weighted sequence. The findings are consistent with fat necrosis.

mass. On MRI, check the T1 without fat saturation. Unfortunately, fat necrosis can also appear as an irregular mass on MRI, and the enhancement pattern is variable. A small handful of women tend to have progressive fat necrosis after BCT (Fig. 18-25). If you are doing MRI on women with BCT, you will biopsy fat necrosis at some point.

Local recurrence can also occur in the dermis, usually in or near the scar (Fig. 18-26). This can mimic a sebaceous cyst, so don't be fooled! If a dermal lesion is near a lumpectomy scar, consider fine-needle aspiration (FNA).

Sentinel Lymph Node Failure

Sentinel lymph node biopsy (SLNB) is about 95% accurate. It's unfortunate that 95% is not 100%. Some women

with axillary metastasis have a negative SLNB, and may present later with an abnormal axillary lymph node (Fig. 18-27).

Local Occurrence in a Tissue Flap

Local recurrence in a tissue flap occurs in the residual breast tissue, not the relocated abdominal fat. Because many women now have skin-sparing mastectomy, local recurrence typically occurs along the subcutaneous scar line (Fig. 18-28). This may present as a palpable mass or be detected by screening. Routine screening of tissue flap reconstructed breasts is controversial. Mammographic screening of 106 women with a history of mastectomy and TRAM flap reconstruction detected two recurrent cancers in one series. However, a later similar series found no cancers in 265 women.

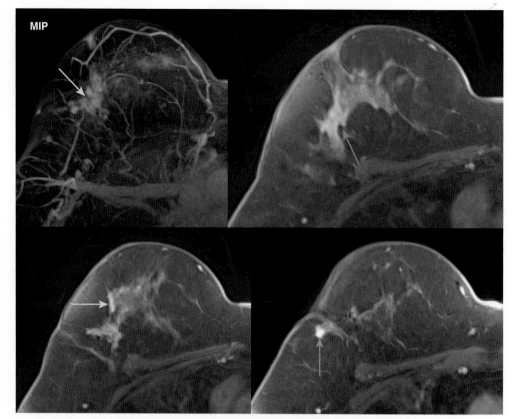

FIGURE 18-24 **Local Recurrence on MRI.** The maximum intensity projection (MIP) shows both mass and nonmass enhancement at the lumpectomy site (*arrow*). T1 post-contrast images show nonmass enhancement at the lumpectomy scar (*blue arrow*), linear nonmass enhancement anterior to the scar (*yellow arrow*), and a round enhancing mass lateral to the scar (*green arrow*). Ultrasound-guided biopsy of the mass confirmed local recurrence. Mastectomy showed DCIS and IDC.

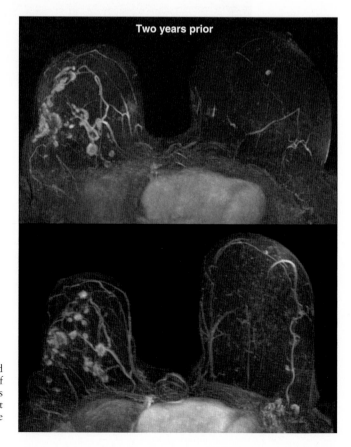

FIGURE 18-25 **Progressive Fat Necrosis After BCT.** This 71-year-old woman had lumpectomy with RT for treatment of a small area of intermediate-grade DCIS with negative margins 10 years ago. She has had three prior biopsies showing fat necrosis. Some areas in the right breast have regressed, although other focal areas have become more prominent.

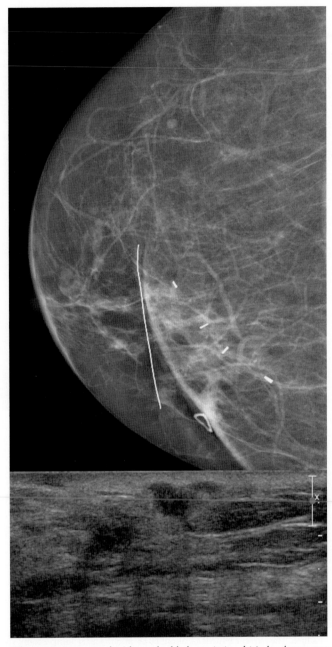

FIGURE 18-26 **Dermal Recurrence.** This patient presented with a palpable lump (*triangle*) in her lumpectomy scar. On US, there is a corresponding irregular hypoechoic mass. Fine-needle aspiration showed recurrent IDC.

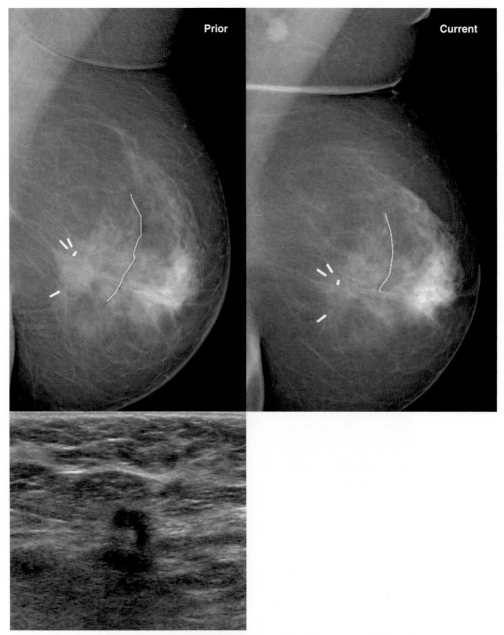

FIGURE 18-27 **Sentinel Lymph Node Failure.** The current left MLO obtained 18 months after lumpectomy shows an increase in size of an axillary lymph node compared with the mammogram from 1 year prior. US shows an irregular cortical margin of the lymph node. Biopsy showed lymph node metastasis with extracapsular extension.

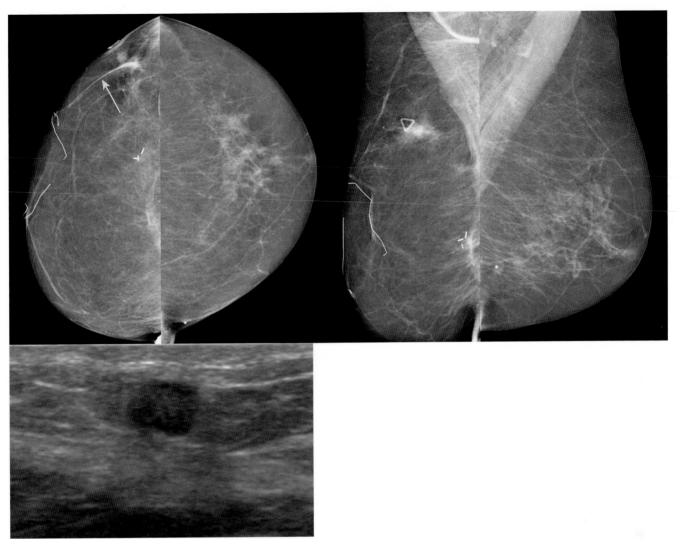

FIGURE 18-28 **Local Recurrence in a TRAM Reconstruction.** This patient had a right skin-sparing mastectomy with TRAM reconstruction 4 years ago. There is a mass on mammography corresponding to a palpable lump (*triangle*). Note that the mass is just superficial to the scar from the skin-sparing mastectomy (*arrow*). US shows an oval solid well-circumscribed mass in the subcutaneous tissue. Biopsy showed IDC.

KEY POINTS

- Reduction mammoplasty and mastopexy often result in fat necrosis, dermal calcifications in scar tissue, and a swirled appearance to the fibroglandular tissue in the inferior breast.

- Distortion and density of a postsurgical scar are most pronounced on the first postoperative study, whether due to benign biopsy or lumpectomy for cancer. Skin and trabecular thickening due to RT are greatest on the first mammogram after RT.

- Identification of calcifications in or near the lumpectomy bed on mammographic magnification views prior to RT allows excision of residual disease and reduces the local recurrence rate. Residual calcifications are associated with a 60% local recurrence rate.

- View small masses or calcifications in the same ductal system as the original cancer (between the scar and the nipple and the scar and the chest wall) with suspicion. Be even more suspicious for women who declined RT—their risk of local recurrence is 30% to 40%.

- The key to detecting recurrent breast cancer on mammography is change over time based on comparison with previous mammograms. After stabilization of the post-therapeutic changes, any new or more prominent findings should be viewed with suspicion.

References

Graham RA, Homer MJ, Sigler CJ, et al. The efficacy of specimen radiography in evaluating the surgical margins of impalpable breast carcinoma. Am J Roentgenol 1994;162:33-36.

Krishnamurthy R, Whitman GJ, Stelling CB, Kushwaha AC. Mammographic findings after breast conservation therapy. RadioGraphics 1999;19:S53-S62.

Lee CH, Carter D. Detecting residual tumor after excisional biopsy of impalpable breast carcinoma: Efficacy of comparing preoperative mammograms with radiographs of the biopsy specimen. Am J Roentgenol 1995;164:81-86.

Lee JM, Georgian-Smith D, Gazelle GS, et al. Detecting nonpalpable recurrent breast cancer: The role of routine mammographic screening of transverse rectus abdominis myocutaneous flap reconstructions 1. Radiology 2008;248:398-405.

Lee JM, Orel SG, Czerniecki BJ, et al. MRI before reexcision surgery in patients with breast cancer. Am J Roentgenol 2004;182:473-480.

Mark A, Helvie MA, Bailey JE, et al. Mammographic screening of TRAM flap breast reconstructions for detection of nonpalpable recurrent cancer. Radiology 2002;224:211-216.

Mendelson EB. Evaluation of the postoperative breast. Radiol Clin North Am 1992;30:107-138.

Philpotts LE, Lee CH, Haffty BG, et al. Mammographic findings of recurrent breast cancer after lumpectomy and radiation therapy: Comparison with the primary tumor. Radiology 1996;201:767-771.

CASE 18-1. Screening mammogram on a 43-year-old woman. What are the findings? What are your BI-RADS assessment and recommendation?

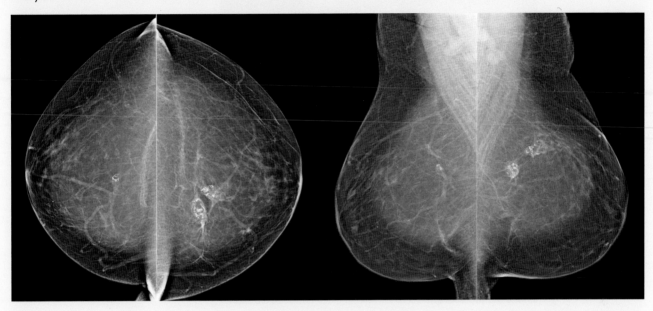

CASE 18-2. Sagittal T1 image after contrast. What type of surgery has this patient had? What is the artifact?

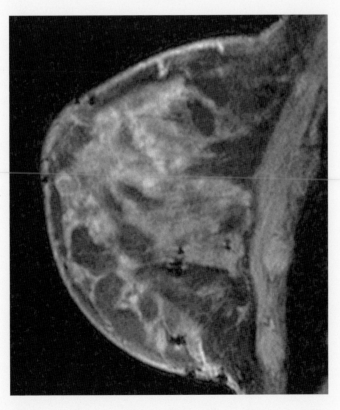

CASE 18-3. This is a 45-year-old woman with prior left breast cancer treated with skin-sparing mastectomy with TRAM reconstruction. Her mother and maternal aunt have also had breast cancer. Here is her screening MRI. What are your BI-RADS assessment category and recommendation?

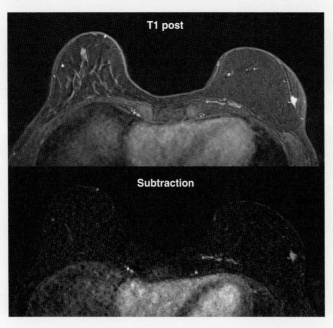

CASE 18-4. This is a screening MRI on a patient with personal (right mastectomy with implant reconstruction) and family history of breast cancer. What are your BI-RADS assessment category and recommendation?

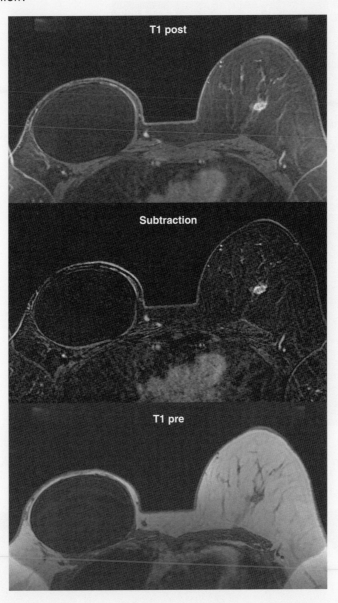

CASE 18-5. Screening mammogram on a 71-year-old woman with a history of lumpectomy and RT for left breast carcinoma over 20 years ago. What do you recommend?

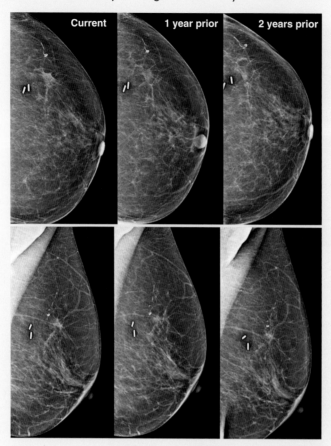

CASE 18-6. A 41-year-old woman with a history of right mastectomy for carcinoma with TRAM flap reconstruction has a screening MRI performed. How do you explain the enhancement in the posterior aspect of the reconstructed breast (*arrow*)?

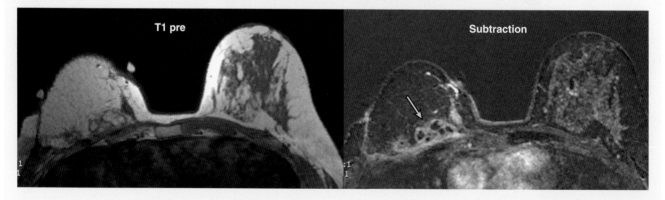

CASE 18-7. Earlier this morning, you did a wire localization for calcifications that were DCIS on stereotactic biopsy. A technologist brings you this specimen radiograph. The surgeon is on the phone and wants to know if the specimen looks good. What will you say?

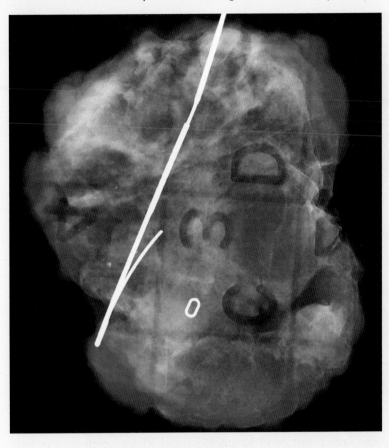

CASE 18-8. A 60-year-old woman with a history of BCT for left breast cancer is recalled for evaluation of an axillary lymph node that is normal in size but has become more dense since her previous mammogram. How would you describe the findings? What do you recommend?

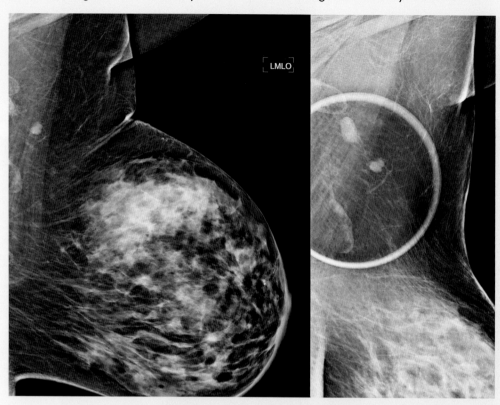

CASE 18-9. A 78-year-old woman with a history of lumpectomy and RT for carcinoma in her lateral left breast. What change has occurred at the lumpectomy site?

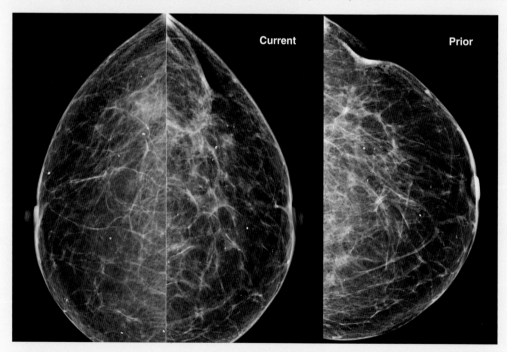

CASE 18-10. This 60-year-old woman had lumpectomy and RT for treatment of prior invasive lobular carcinoma (ILC) in the right breast at 1 o'clock (*arrows*) 8 years ago. Are there findings suspicious for recurrent breast cancer?

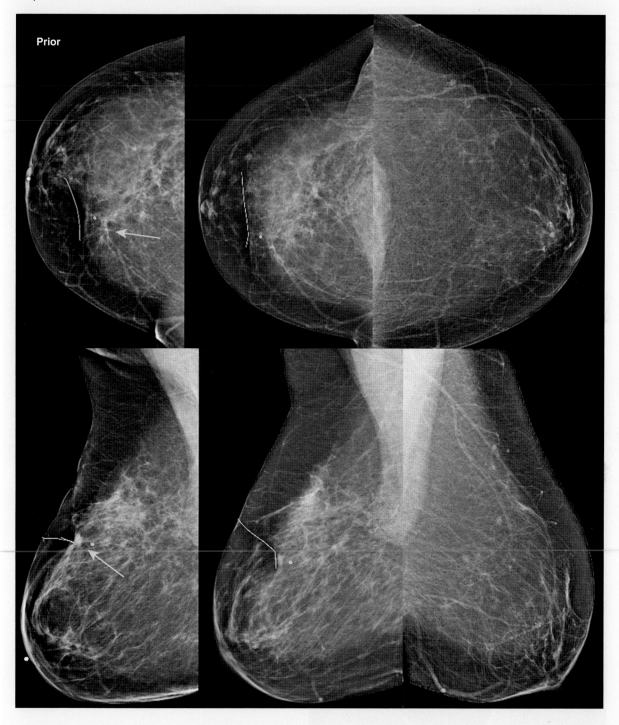

CASE 18-11. This 56-year-old woman had a lumpectomy 4 years ago. She had an MRI due to a personal and strong family history of breast cancer. What are your BI-RADS assessment and recommendation?

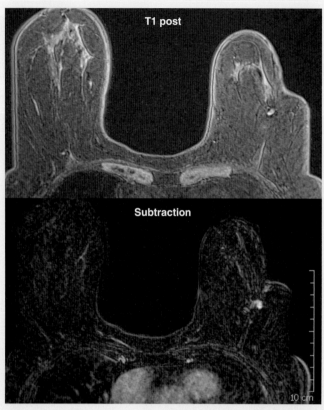

CASE 18-12. This 59-year-old woman had prior lumpectomy and RT for left breast ILC 5 years ago. What do you think of her MRI? What are your BI-RADS assessment and recommendation?

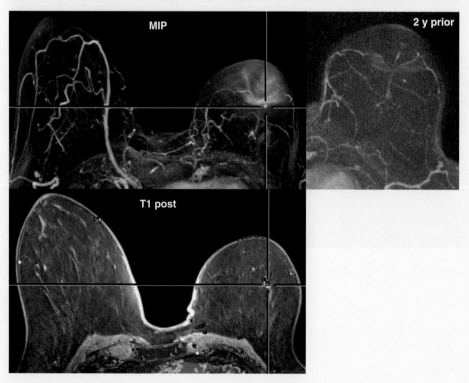

CASE ANSWERS

CASE 18-1. There are bilateral inferior scars with a distribution typical for reduction mammoplasty. Calcified oil cysts are present bilaterally. BI-RADS 2. Recommend annual mammographic screening.

CASE 18-2. This patient has had mastopexy. The scars in the inferior breast and areolar region are identified by the signal dropout artifact from metallic fragments that occur during the surgical procedure, often associated with use of the electrocautery device.

CASE 18-3. There is an enhancing mass in the subcutaneous tissue of the lateral left TRAM flap. This is suspicious for a local recurrence. BI-RADS 5. Ultrasound-guided biopsy was performed. Diagnosis: IDC.

CASE 18-4. There is an oval, circumscribed, rim-enhancing mass in the 12 o'clock region of the left breast. Did you notice that the mass contains fat on the T1 precontrast image without fat saturation? This is consistent with a small oil cyst. She had reduction mammoplasty on the left at the time of her mastectomy for symmetry. Here is the mammogram that confirms the finding (*arrow*).

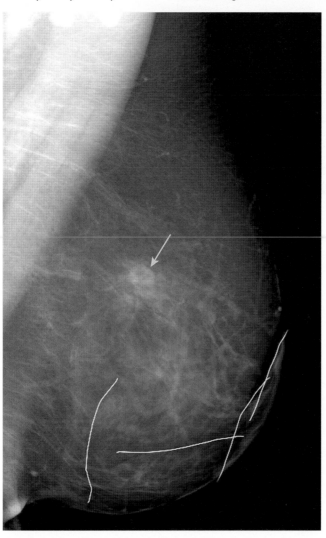

CASE 18-5. There is increasing density at the lumpectomy site that is inconsistent with the normal evolution of post-treatment changes. This finding persists on spot compression views. US shows an echogenic mass. Although echogenic lesions are usually benign, the change on mammography is suspicious and warrants biopsy. Ultrasound-guided core biopsy revealed ILC.

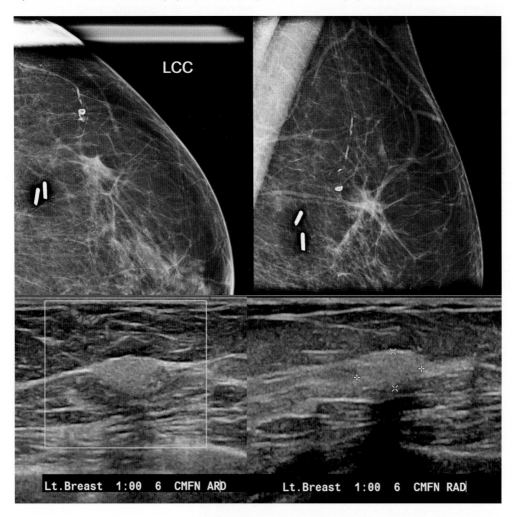

CASE 18-6. There are multiple rim-enhancing masses in the posterior right breast with high signal on T1 indicative of fat. The findings are therefore consistent with fat necrosis, which is common following TRAM flap reconstruction. BI-RADS 2.

CASE 18-7. The specimen contains the biopsy marker and some calcifications. However, the calcifications are near the edge of the specimen (*arrows*). It would be prudent for the surgeon to remove a little more tissue at the deep end of the surgical bed (where the tip of the wire is located). The pathologist did find a positive margin on the original lumpectomy sample, but the margins of the additional tissue taken by the surgeon were negative.

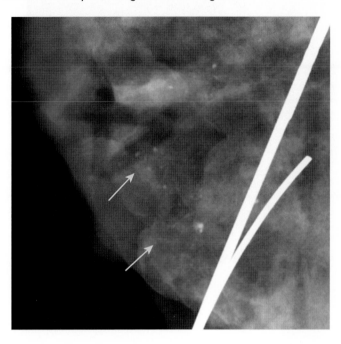

CASE 18-8. On the spot compression view two dense nodes without fatty hila are seen. The larger node has indistinct margins. On US, both shadow and have indistinct margins. Core biopsy showed metastatic IDC in both nodes.

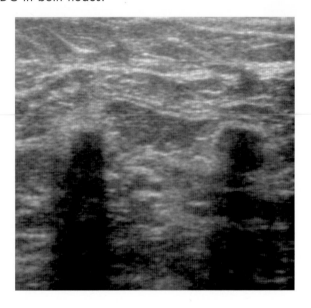

CASE 18-9. There is a new asymmetry anterior to the lumpectomy scar (*arrow*). US revealed a hypoechoic shadowing mass with indistinct margins. Core biopsy revealed recurrent IDC.

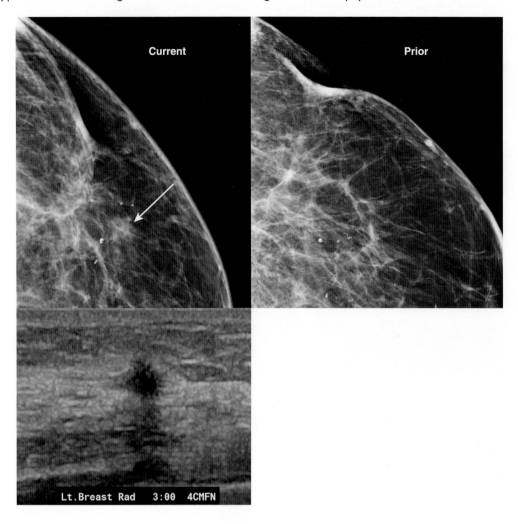

CASE 18-10. There is a new one-view asymmetry in the lateral right breast (*blue arrow*). This was localized to the 9 o'clock position on her diagnostic mammogram. US showed a small hypoechoic solid mass. Her lumpectomy scar is located in a different quadrant (*yellow arrow*), so this is more likely to be a second primary carcinoma rather than local recurrence. Ultrasound-guided core biopsy showed IDC.

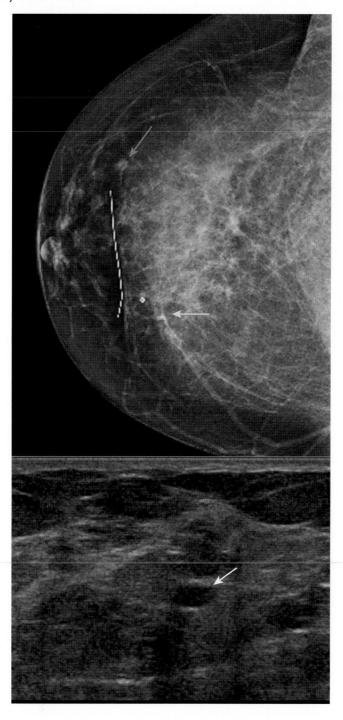

CASE 18-11. There is increased signal intensity with signal dropout at the edges located at the lumpectomy site on the T1 postcontrast sequence (*arrow*). This could be due to signal flare from a clip in the lumpectomy bed or local recurrence. There is increased signal in this area on the subtraction image, which can only be due to an enhancing mass and not signal flare. BI-RADS 4. Ultrasound-guided biopsy showed recurrent IDC.

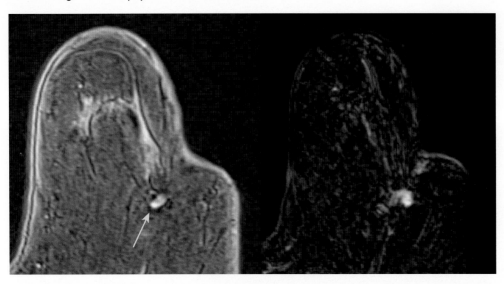

CASE 18-12. There is an enhancing focus in the left breast. Although small and with persistent enhancement, the size has increased compared with the prior MRI. Ultrasound-guided biopsy showed recurrent ILC. Great job if you figured this one out!

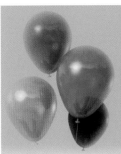

CHAPTER 19

Evaluating Women with Implants

She had breast implants years ago and now she's nervous: I wonder if that lump that my doctor feels is related to my implant or if it's something more serious. What if it's cancer? Should I take their advice and get a mammogram? What if my implants rupture?

The primary goal of mammography in patients with implants remains the detection of potentially malignant lesions. Cancer detection in the augmented breast can pose unique challenges. Mammography may be hindered by limitations in positioning and compression of the tissue. Women referred because of clinical findings must be evaluated with a wider differential diagnosis in mind: implants and their complications can produce false-positive findings for malignancies, and conversely, breast cancer may be mistaken for implant-related complications.

Breast augmentation is common—11/1000 in one large series. The first sealed breast implant was a silicone gel-filled prosthesis developed and introduced in the early 1960s. Since that time, breast augmentation has become the most commonly performed cosmetic surgery in the United States, and over 389,000 breast augmentation and reconstruction procedures were performed in 2010. About 20% of implant surgeries were performed in breast cancer patients, most commonly for reconstruction following mastectomy.

Mammography, ultrasonography (US), and magnetic resonance imaging (MRI) can be used to differentiate findings of concern for malignancy from those related to implants, their complications, or their sequelae after rupture or explantation. It is therefore important to be familiar with the terminology and imaging findings related to implants and their complications.

Implant Terminology

Since their introduction, over 240 styles of breast implants and tissue expanders have been introduced by American manufacturers alone. The major differences among implant types relate to the number of lumens, the substances that fill them, and the location of the implant.

Implant Shell

The implant shell (synonyms: elastomer shell, envelope, or membrane) used for both saline- and silicone-containing implants is an elastic, semipermeable membrane made of a solid silicone polymer (Fig. 19-1). The outer surface of shell is textured in some implants to reduce the incidence of implant rotation and capsular contracture. Texturing may cause the outer edge of the implant to appear indistinct on mammography.

Implant Lumens and Contents

Implants almost always have one or two lumens—triple-lumen implants have been manufactured but are rarely seen in practice. Single-lumen implants outnumber the multilumen varieties by a large margin. Implants are filled with either saline or silicone gel (Fig. 19-2). Of breast implants placed in 2010, 60% contained silicone gel and the remainder saline. Double-lumen models usually have an inner lumen filled with silicone and an outer lumen filled with saline. However, the opposite configuration (reverse double lumen) with inner saline and outer silicone as well as silicone-within-silicone implants may also be seen but are very uncommon.

Saline implants have a valve or diaphragm through which fluid can be instilled or removed. An expander implant has a metal valve through which saline can be added over time. These implants are usually placed after mastectomy and exchanged for permanent saline or silicone implants after full expansion. Because of the metallic valve, expander implants are not safe for MRI.

On mammography, silicone is radiopaque but saline is much more radiolucent. The two types can be distinguished on routine mammography and dual-lumen implants may be appreciated if the outer lumen is saline and the inner silicone (see Fig. 19-2). On US, saline and silicone implants are normally anechoic. Silicone implants may have strong reverberation artifact even when intact. MRI evaluation of implants is not necessary for saline implant integrity. "Silicone" sequences are typically heavily T2-weighted, often with both fat and water suppression. Silicone will be bright white on these sequences (Fig. 19-3).

Patients who have had direct injection of silicone, paraffin, polyacrylamide gel, or other substances into the breast for augmentation may occasionally be encountered. Silicone injections produce dense masses on mammography, some with peripheral calcifications, and areas of fat necrosis (Fig. 19-4). Paraffin injections can appear initially as masses representing fluid collections and later as masses representing paraffinomas with calcifications

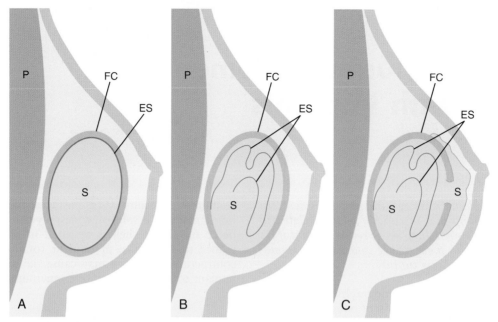

FIGURE 19-1 **Silicone Implant Rupture. A,** Normal subglandular implant. **B,** Intracapsular rupture. **C,** Extracapsular rupture. *ES,* elastomer shell; *FC,* fibrous capsule; *P,* pectoralis major; *S,* silicone.

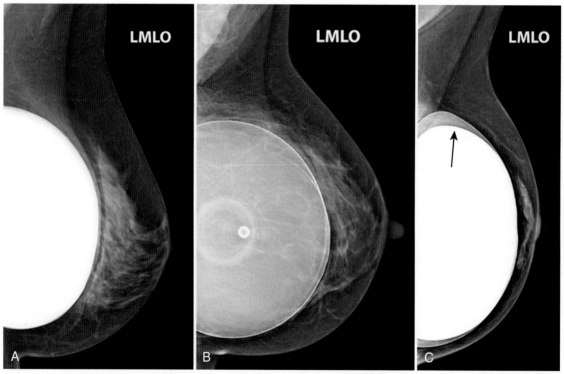

FIGURE 19-2 **Normal Implants. A,** Subpectoral silicone implant. **B,** Subpectoral saline implant. The valve is apparent. **C,** Subglandular inner-silicone outer-saline dual-lumen implant. The edge of the silicone-filled implant is visible within the saline component (*arrow*).

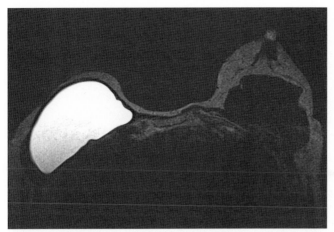

FIGURE 19-3 **Silicone and Saline Implants on MRI.** The right implant contains silicone, which is bright white. The left saline implant is dark due to water suppression on this T2-weighted image.

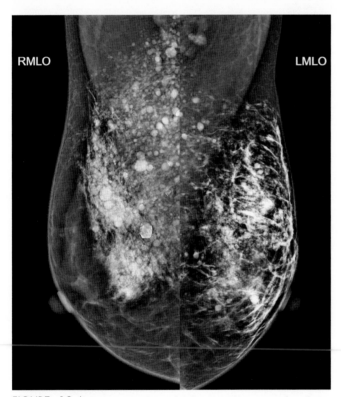

FIGURE 19-4 **Direct Injection of Silicone.** Mammography shows multiple high-density round masses, some of which have rim calcifications.

and architectural distortion. Direct injection of these substances markedly limits clinical and mammographic evaluation.

Implant Location

Most implants are placed either behind the glandular tissue and anterior to the pectoralis major muscle (subglandular, retroglandular, prepectoral), or between the pectoralis major and minor muscles (subpectoral,

BOX 19-1 Complications of Breast Implants

- Intracapsular rupture
- Extracapsular rupture
- Silicone granuloma
- Distant migration of silicone
- Silicone adenopathy
- Capsular contracture
- Bulge in contour
- Herniation through fibrous capsule
- Infection
- Hemorrhage
- Implant migration

submuscular). The terms *subglandular* and *subpectoral* will be used in this chapter (see Fig. 19-2).

Fibrous Capsule

When an implant is placed, it incites an inflammatory reaction in the surrounding tissues leading to the formation of a fibrous capsule. This may be visible on the mammogram as a thin band of soft tissue immediately adjacent to the implant shell. The fibrous capsule has a smooth inner surface that is closely apposed to the outer surface of the implant shell, creating a potential space between the two. Calcifications often develop within the fibrous capsule typically years after placement of the implant.

Implant Complications (Box 19-1)

Mammography, US, and MRI have different strengths and limitations in detecting and characterizing implant complications. Mammographic screening of women with implants will detect some complications in the asymptomatic patient. In one study of 350 women with implants, 16 (5%) had evidence of rupture on screening mammography, including two with bilateral rupture. The decision to evaluate implants with US is usually based on clinical or mammographic findings. MRI is the most accurate imaging modality for determining implant status. The gold standard for determining whether an implant is intact is examination after surgical removal.

Capsular Contracture

Capsular contracture is the most common complication of implants and is due to contraction of the fibrous capsule around the implant. It can occur with either silicone or saline implants but is most common with silicone implants in a subglandular location. This is a clinical diagnosis in which fibrous tissue displaces or changes the shape of the implant or limits its movement. In its most

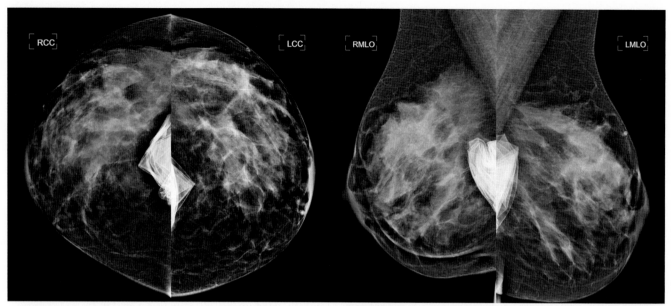

FIGURE 19-5 **Saline Implant Rupture.** Collapsed bilateral subglandular saline implants are present at the posterior aspect of both breasts.

severe form, the breast becomes hard and there is distortion of the implant. The mammography technologist may not be able to displace the implant, limiting evaluation of the breast parenchyma. On mammography, rounding or distortion of the implant may be seen. Comparison with several previous mammograms may reveal progressive rounding of the implant coinciding with progressive loss of the technologists' ability to displace it.

Capsular contracture was previously treated by closed capsulotomy. In this procedure, the surgeon manually disrupted the fibrous bands without surgical incision while the patient was under anesthesia. In some women, this converted the problem from a firm, intact implant to a softer, ruptured one. Because of the risk of rupture, this procedure is no longer commonly performed.

Gel Bleed

Many toys are made out of silicone, like the bag of eyeballs at the science museum. They're really fun to squeeze and play with, but have you ever noticed that your hands are kind of sticky afterward? Just as with those kids' toys, silicone molecules can pass through the semipermeable implant shell even when the implant is not ruptured. Now you will understand silicone gel bleed. In this process, silicone gel can coat the exterior surface of the shell. This gel can travel, and silicone may appear in axillary lymph nodes even without rupture.

Rupture

The main predisposing factor for rupture is the age of the implant. Rupture may occur spontaneously or be caused by a specific event, including trauma, closed capsulotomy, and complications of surgical or needle biopsy or other interventional procedures. The implant shell can

withstand a compression force much greater than is typically used for mammography; rupture during mammography is rare.

Saline Implant Rupture

Rupture of saline implants is usually obvious clinically and on mammography. The extraluminal saline is resorbed, and on mammography the implant shell is partially or wholly collapsed (Fig. 19-5), which looks like someone took your wadded-up plastic sandwich bag and stuck it in the back of the breast. You don't need US or MRI to make this diagnosis!

Silicone Implant Rupture

Diagnosis of silicone implant rupture can be more challenging both clinically and by imaging. There are two types or stages of silicone implant rupture—intracapsular and extracapsular (see Fig. 19-1). With intracapsular rupture, the implant shell is disrupted but the silicone is still contained by the fibrous capsule. These patients are typically asymptomatic. With extracapsular rupture, both the implant shell and fibrous capsule are disrupted. These patients may complain of pain or tenderness, palpable nodules, or decreased implant size, but they may also be asymptomatic.

Intracapsular rupture is often not apparent on clinical examination or mammography because the contour of silicone contained by the fibrous capsule is similar or identical to that produced by the intact shell.

US is not very sensitive or specific in the evaluation of intracapsular rupture, limiting its value in this role. One finding suggestive of rupture are multiple parallel echogenic lines within the sonolucent silicone, creating an appearance known as the "stepladder sign" (Fig. 19-6). Another US finding suggestive but not diagnostic of intracapsular rupture is that of low-level echoes internally, within the silicone gel, which is typically more sonolucent when the implant is intact.

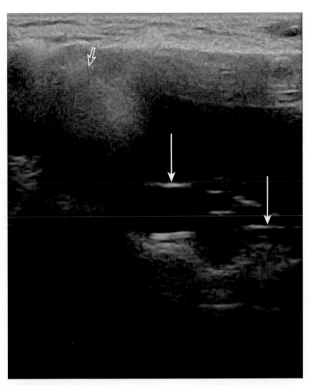

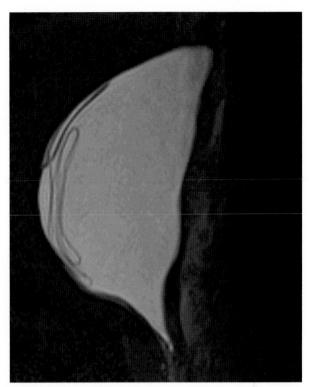

FIGURE 19-6 **Intracapsular Rupture on US.** Multiple echogenic lines within silicone (*long arrows*), producing the stepladder sign. This is akin to the "linguine" sign on MRI. Echogenic extracapsular silicone is also apparent (*short arrow*).

FIGURE 19-7 **Intracapsular Rupture on MRI.** Sagittal image shows curvilinear signal in the implant: the "linguine" sign.

MRI is the most sensitive and specific imaging modality for evaluating implant rupture. In one series, sensitivity and specificity for gross rupture were 98% and 91%, respectively. With intracapsular rupture, MRI shows curvilinear low-intensity signal within the implant, an appearance known as the linguine sign (Fig. 19-7). This appearance can be caused by the elastomer shell floating in the silicone, contained by the fibrous capsule. However, in some cases, the linear signal is not actually the shell but is caused by water mixing with the silicone. This is a moot point because the imaging finding suggests intracapsular rupture whether those linear signals are due to the elastomer shell or water mixing with silicone.

The sensitivity of MRI is lower when only a small amount of silicone has leaked outside the shell but the shell has not collapsed. The subcapsular line sign reveals silicone adjacent to both surfaces of the ruptured shell. The inverted teardrop (also known as the keyhole or noose sign) is another appearance of silicone leakage within a fold in the shell (Fig. 19-8). Rupture of the inner silicone lumen of a double-lumen implant results in mixture of silicone and saline, producing an appearance known as the "salad oil" sign.

Extracapsular rupture is usually a relatively easy diagnosis on any modality. Mammography is quite effective in demonstrating extracapsular silicone because its density is higher than that of breast parenchyma (Figs. 19-9 to 19-11). When interpreting the mammogram, trace the edge of the implant to see if it is smooth. Look for any contour abnormalities and for globules or linear tracking

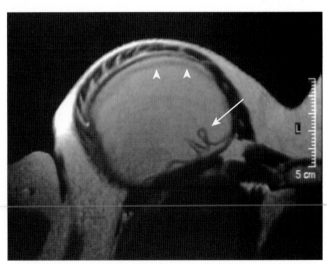

FIGURE 19-8 **Intracapsular Rupture.** Axial MRI (T2-weighted image) shows a subpectoral implant with the subcapsular line (*arrowheads*) and inverted teardrop signs (*arrow*).

of silicone outside the fibrous capsule. Silicone within breast tissue may form silicone granulomas, and occasionally, silicone may be seen extending into ducts. It may also be visible within axillary lymph nodes (Fig. 19-12) and migrate to more distant sites.

US is also quite helpful in diagnosing extracapsular rupture. Globules of silicone in the breast tissue usually produce a unique highly echogenic finding with loss of posterior detail forming a pattern known as the "snowstorm" appearance (Figs. 19-10 and 19-13). Usually, the

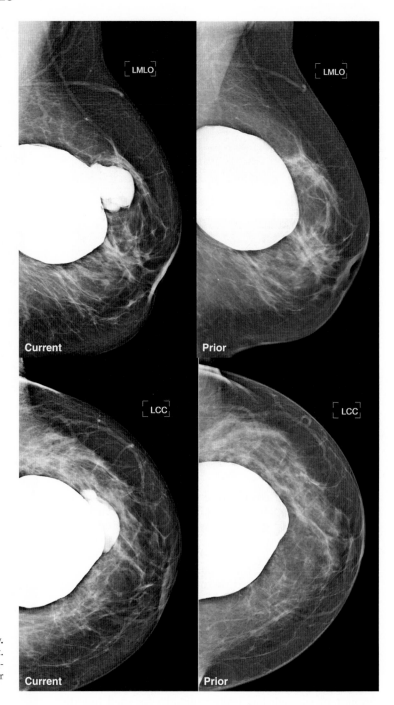

FIGURE 19-9 **Extracapsular Rupture on Mammography.** Screening mammogram shows a subglandular silicone implant. Extracapsular rupture has occurred since the previous mammogram with free silicone collecting within the tissue anterior to the implant.

echogenic noise extends deep to the silicone. This appearance is also seen within lymph nodes containing silicone, which can help differentiate silicone-containing lymph nodes from adenopathy due to other causes. The snowstorm pattern is also seen in silicone that has migrated to other sites. Extracapsular silicone does not always have this characteristic US appearance. It may also contain hypoechoic regions, have a complex cystic appearance, or appear as a shadowing lesion.

On MRI, extracapsular silicone usually has very low signal on fat-suppressed T1-weighted images and high signal on water-suppressed T2-weighted images (Fig. 19-14).

Radial Folds Versus Intracapsular Rupture

In order to be soft and supple, implants are not tightly expanded. The shell can fold into the implant. These radial folds are common and normal but can be mistaken for intracapsular rupture on US or MRI. On US, these appear as continuous echogenic lines radiating to the edges of the implant. On MRI, radial folds can be linear or curvilinear but should be contiguous with the shell. Careful evaluation of sequential slices and in multiple planes can usually distinguish radial folds from rupture (Fig. 19-15). Another clue is that the lines of a radial fold are thicker than those of a collapsed shell because they represent a double layer of shell.

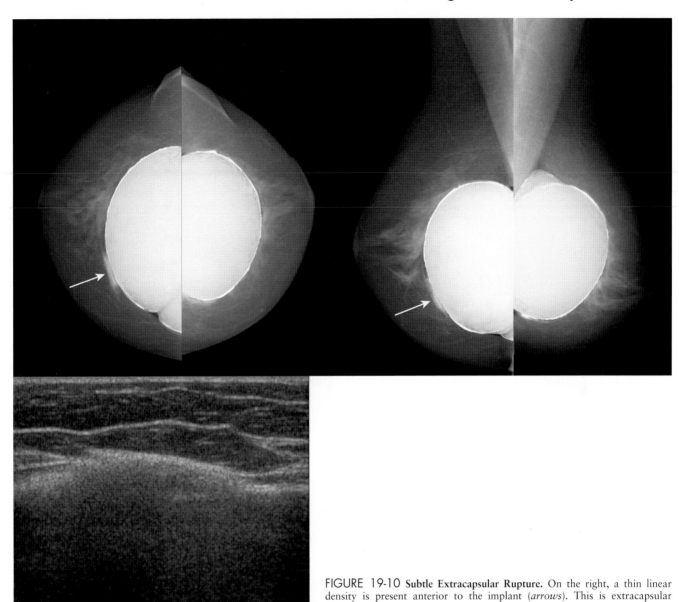

FIGURE 19-10 **Subtle Extracapsular Rupture.** On the right, a thin linear density is present anterior to the implant (*arrows*). This is extracapsular rupture. US confirms extracapsular rupture producing the highly echogenic snowstorm appearance anterior to the implant. Also note contour deformity of the superior implant on the left and capsular calcifications bilaterally.

Contour Irregularities

About half of women with implants have contour deformities. A focal outpouching of the contour—typically forming an obtuse angle with the adjacent implant—can represent a bulge or herniation. Bulge refers to a focal protrusion of the implant within an intact fibrous capsule. With herniation, a portion of the implant extends through a defect in the fibrous capsule. This is the opposite of intracapsular rupture—the implant is intact, but the fibrous capsule is disrupted. Implant herniation may present as a palpable mass. Contour deformities may also be associated with or progress to rupture. Mammography alone often cannot differentiate between bulge and herniation and cannot exclude the presence of rupture (Fig. 19-16).

Screening Women with Implants

Mammography

The sensitivity of mammography is reduced in women with breast implants. In one series the sensitivity of mammography was only 45% for women with augmentation compared to 66% for those without. Although the quality of mammography may be compromised in some women with implants, it remains the primary screening modality in this population. Screening mammography for women with implants routinely includes four views of each breast. For these patients, craniocaudal (CC) and mediolateral oblique (MLO) views are obtained, including as much breast tissue as possible with the implant in the field of view. For these views, the technologist should

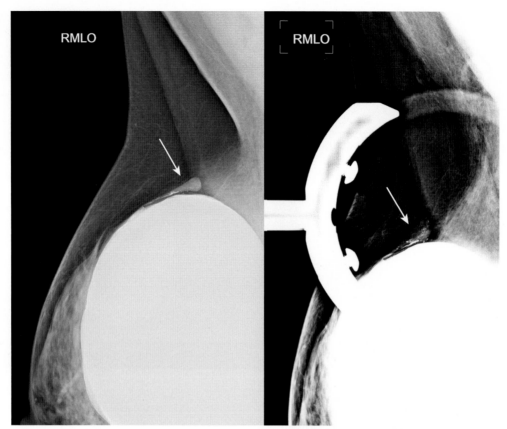

FIGURE 19-11 **Extracapsular Rupture.** Ruptured subglandular silicone implant with a small amount of extracapsular silicone (*arrows*).

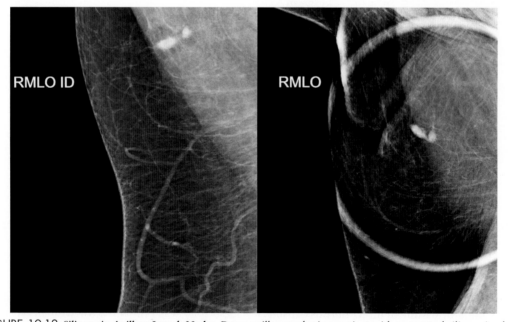

FIGURE 19-12 **Silicone in Axillary Lymph Nodes.** Dense axillary nodes in a patient with a ruptured silicone implant.

compress only enough to immobilize the implant. These views evaluate the more posterior breast and axillary region, which may not be included on implant-displaced (ID) views, and also evaluate the implant itself.

ID views are modified compression views also obtained in the CC and MLO projections. The implant is displaced posteriorly while the breast tissue is pulled forward. This technique, described by Eklund and associates (1988), improves both the amount of tissue evaluated and the adequacy of tissue compression, and it poses little risk of damaging the implant (Fig. 19-17).

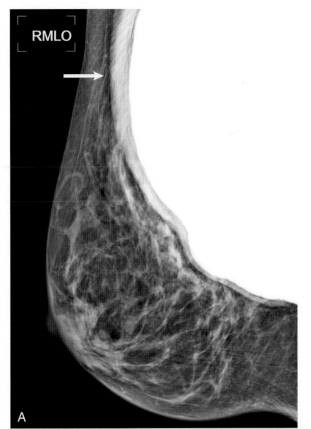

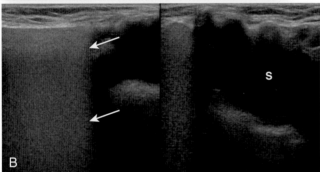

FIGURE 19-13 **Subpectoral Silicone Implant with Extracapsular Rupture. A,** Mammography shows a subpectoral silicone implant with an irregular contour and increased density overlying the pectoralis muscle (*arrow*). **B,** US shows the snowstorm appearance of extracapsular silicone (*arrows*) and irregularly shaped residual silicone (*S*) within the fibrous capsule.

The amount of tissue that can be included on the ID views is influenced by the location of the implant and the ability to displace the implant away from the tissue. Subpectoral implants are the easiest to displace. In one series, among 252 women with implants undergoing screening mammography, 94% of those with subpectoral implants had ID views rated as excellent or good, compared with only 47% of women with subglandular implants.

When the implant cannot be fully displaced, some tissue can still usually be compressed by carefully excluding the implant, and can add to the diagnostic value of the study. In this case, mediolateral views may also be taken to provide additional visualization of tissue above and below the implant.

Nonmammographic Screening

In some women with implants, mammography may be limited due to suboptimal tissue inclusion and compression that limits cancer detection. Evaluation of patients who have had direct injection of silicone or other substances is also severely limited. When our ability to evaluate the breast is significantly compromised by implants, US or MRI screening can be considered.

Diagnostic Evaluation of Women with Implants or Their Sequelae: Implant-Related Versus Breast Pathology

Women with implants or their sequelae may be recommended for diagnostic evaluation because of findings detected on screening mammography, because of palpable findings, or for other clinical signs or symptoms that may either be implant-related or due to breast pathology.

Mammographic Findings

Silicone Granulomas

Free silicone or silicone granulomas within the breast tissue are usually easily recognized owing to their high density. They may have circumscribed or indistinct margins (Fig. 19-18). Silicone granulomas occasionally

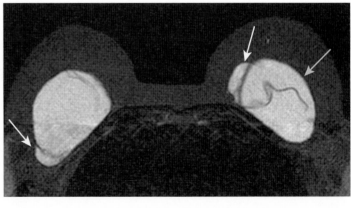

FIGURE 19-14 **Intracapsular and Extracapsular Rupture on MRI.** Curvilinear signal is seen in both implants consistent with intracapsular rupture. The fibrous capsule is a dark band around the implant (*yellow arrow*). There is high signal outside the fibrous capsule (*white arrows*) indicating bilateral extracapsular rupture as well.

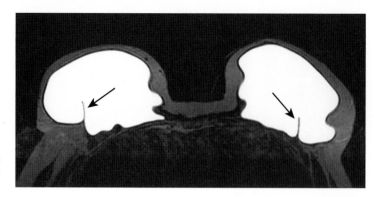

FIGURE 19-15 **Intact Implants with Radial Folds.** The folds (*arrows*) extend into the implant. Note how the line of the fold is always contiguous with the implant shell.

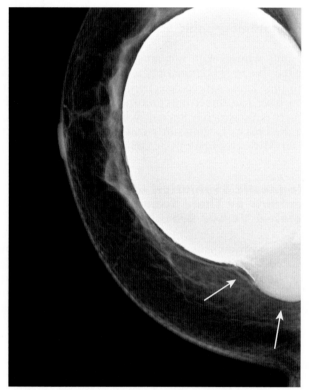

FIGURE 19-16 **Contour Deformity.** CC view shows medial bulge with apparent herniation of the implant through the calcified fibrous capsule (*arrows*). This appearance can also be due to rupture.

appear suspicious for malignancy on mammography, particularly when they are not dense enough for a definite diagnosis.

Explantation

Following removal of an implant (explantation), scarring and fat necrosis may produce a mass-like appearance (Fig. 19-19). Comparison with previous studies is most helpful in these patients. If a soft tissue density mass is new, enlarging, or of uncertain stability, additional mammographic views and US are often indicated, and biopsy may be needed.

The fibrous capsule, which commonly contains calcifications, is usually but not always removed with the implant during explantation. Residual capsular calcifications have the potential to raise concern for malignancy

on subsequent mammography, but their ovoid distribution and location together with history of implant removal are clues to their benign nature (Fig. 19-20). Larger dystrophic calcifications and calcified oil cysts may also be seen.

Dystrophic Calcifications

When calcifications have a distribution that is defined by the implant or the fibrous capsule, rather than the segmental anatomy of the breast, they are rarely suspicious for malignancy (Fig. 19-21). Also realize that calcifications adjacent to implants in the subpectoral region are outside the breast parenchyma and therefore, not suspicious for breast cancer. If calcifications are morphologically indeterminate and appear unrelated to the implant, they should be evaluated and managed based on the criteria for morphology and distribution discussed in Chapter 6.

Postoperative Scarring

Architectural distortion in patients with implants or who have had implants removed should be correlated with the location of scars on the skin. If needed, additional mammographic views taken after marking the scars with a wire will usually determine whether the distortion and scar correspond. Identification of associated oil cysts or dystrophic calcifications may also provide a clue to their benign character. Comparison with previous mammograms is very important in these cases. Architectural distortion that has developed or enlarged since a previous postoperative mammogram is not a normal postsurgical change and should be considered suspicious. In this case, US may be helpful in defining an associated mass and guiding biopsy. MRI can be useful in a problem-solving role to help differentiate scarring from a potentially malignant finding.

Clinical Findings

The etiology and significance of clinical findings in women with implants are often unclear and the differential diagnosis needs to be expanded to include implant-related as well as nonimplant-related explanations. Mammography and US are frequently used to evaluate these patients. MRI may be helpful in cases that remain unclear after routine evaluation.

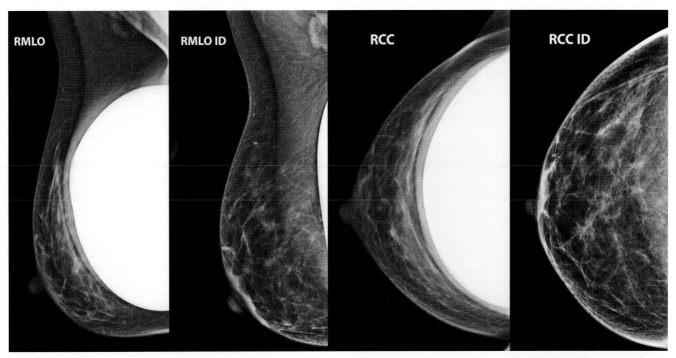

FIGURE 19-17 **Implant-Displaced Views.** Posterior displacement of the subpectoral implant allows for improved compression of the breast tissue.

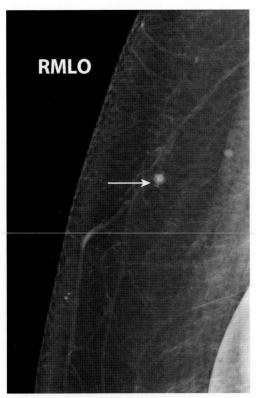

FIGURE 19-18 **Silicone Granuloma.** Dense silicone granuloma with indistinct margins (*arrow*) in a patient with a history of ruptured silicone implant. This finding was not suspicious due to its very high density and stability.

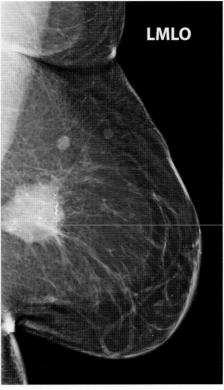

FIGURE 19-19 **Postoperative Fibrosis.** A 36-year-old woman with a history of removal of silicone implants. There is residual mass-like fibrosis in the posterior breast with associated coarse calcifications. This finding was stable on mammography.

Focal Palpable Finding

In women with a focal palpable finding, mammography and US may provide a specific diagnosis that the clinical finding is related to the implant and therefore not suspicious for malignancy (Box 19-2).

When a palpable lump corresponds to high-density silicone within the breast parenchyma, the diagnosis is straightforward. Silicone granulomas are usually high-density masses but may not be as dense as free silicone. If a mass is not dense enough on mammography to definitely represent silicone or is obscured by dense tissue or the implant, US may be helpful. When US shows the snowstorm appearance, the diagnosis of free silicone or silicone granuloma can be made with confidence. However, some silicone granulomas have a mammographic and US appearance indistinguishable from malignancy, and biopsy may be indicated (Fig. 19-22).

A palpable finding may also be due to a prominent implant fold, valve, bulge, or herniation of the implant through a defect in the fibrous capsule. The cause of these findings will usually be apparent on mammography or US.

When mammography and US do not reveal a specific implant-related explanation for a clinical finding, all of the pathologic findings encountered in women without

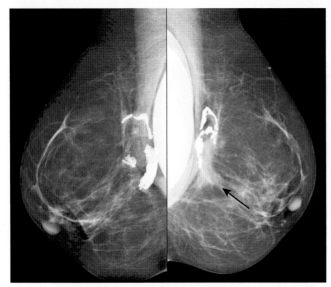

FIGURE 19-20 **Residual Calcified Fibrous Capsule After Explantation.** This patient previously had subglandular silicone implants that were removed with new dual-lumen subpectoral implants placed. There are large coarse calcifications in the posterior breast that represent the retained calcified fibrous capsule. The soft tissue density on the left (*arrow*), which was stable on the mammogram, is also part of the remaining fibrous capsule.

BOX 19-2 Typically Benign Palpable Finding Related to Implant or Surgery

- Implant fold
- Implant valve
- Implant bulge or herniation
- Dense free silicone
- Dense silicone granuloma
- Dense silicone-containing lymph node
- Oil cysts
- Characteristically benign calcification (dystrophic, lucent-centered)

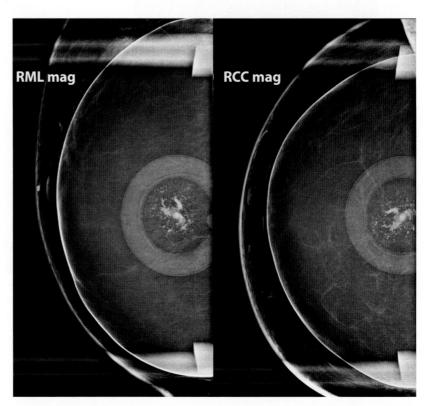

FIGURE 19-21 **Dystrophic Calcifications or Other Opaque Substance Related to the Implant.** In this case, there is high-density material associated with the diaphragm fill value of a saline implant.

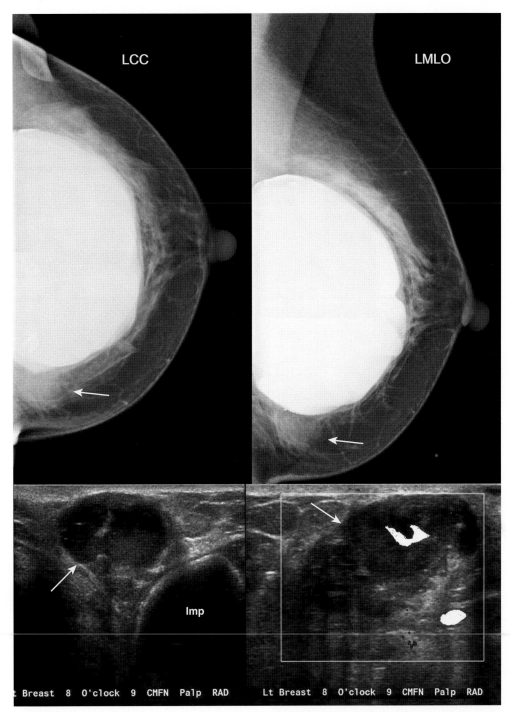

FIGURE 19-22 **Palpable Silicone Granuloma.** Mass in a patient with known implant rupture that is not dense enough on mammography (*arrows*) to characterize as free silicone or a silicone granuloma. US (*bottom*) shows a solid mass (*arrows*) with flow on Doppler adjacent to the implant (*Imp*). Core biopsy revealed findings consistent with silicone granuloma.

implants must be considered in the differential diagnosis. Keep in mind that the large majority of palpable malignancies will produce suspicious findings on diagnostic mammography, US, or both (Fig. 19-23).

Swelling or Enlargement of the Breast
Enlargement of the breast with recently placed implants may be due to hematoma, seroma, mastitis, or abscess (Fig. 19-24). Even when implant placement was not recent, a small amount of fluid adjacent to the implant is considered normal. Larger or increasing amounts of fluid may be caused by implant rupture, infection, localized or generalized edema, or inflammatory carcinoma. Hemorrhage may also increase breast size. Fluid surrounding an implant may resemble a double-lumen implant on US and MRI. Correlation of the imaging findings with the patient's history and type of implant is important in these cases (Box 19-3).

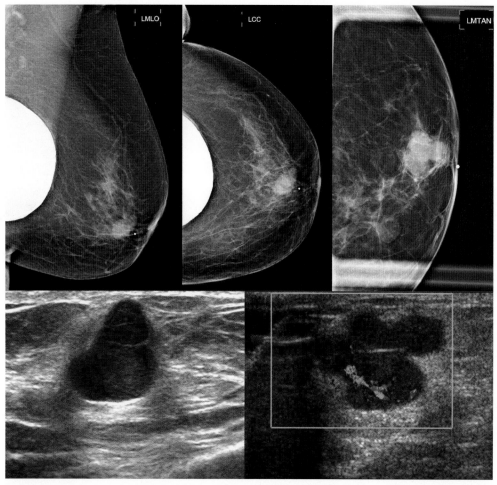

FIGURE 19-23 **Carcinoma in a Patient with Implants.** A 64-year-old woman with subpectoral silicone implants presents with a palpable mass in her left breast. Mammography shows an irregular mass that is solid by US. The mass is unrelated to the implant. Biopsy revealed invasive ductal carcinoma (IDC).

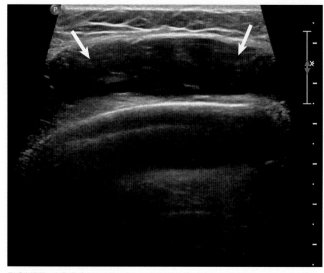

FIGURE 19-24 **Peri-implant Fluid.** A 53-year-old woman with a history of recent mastectomy and implant reconstruction is referred because of swelling. US reveals a fluid collection (*arrows*) surrounding the implant. The US and clinical findings were most consistent with seroma. Abscess or hemorrhage may also have this appearance.

BOX 19-3 Differential Diagnosis of Peri-implant Fluid

- Small amount may be normal
- Implant rupture
- Infection
- Seroma
- Hematoma
- Neoplasm

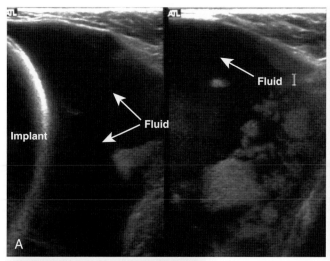

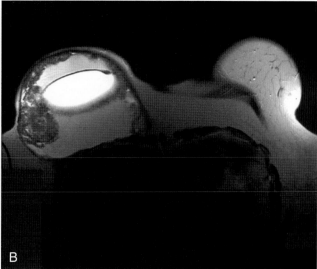

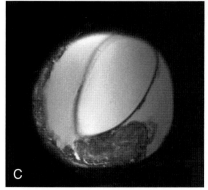

FIGURE 19-25 **Large Cell Lymphoma Associated with an Implant.** This patient had right mastectomy with implant reconstruction and presented with swelling. **A,** US shows fluid surrounding the implant with solid projections from the fibrous capsule into the fluid. **B,** Axial and, **C,** coronal magnetic resonance images show an intact implant with a large amount of peri-implant fluid and multiple masses. The differential diagnosis (DDx) includes recurrent breast cancer, lymphoma, or hemorrhage. Biopsy revealed anaplastic large-cell lymphoma.

The possibility of breast cancer should be considered as a cause of an apparent increase in breast size. Breast implants have not been shown to be associated with increased risk for breast cancer; however, in January 2011, the U.S. Food and Drug Administration (FDA) published a Medical Device Safety Communication (www.FDA.gov) describing a possible association between anaplastic large-cell lymphoma and breast implants (Fig. 19-25).

Palpable Axillary Mass

Axillary masses may be shown by mammography to have the typical high-density appearance of silicone uptake by a lymph node. US may be helpful in showing the snowstorm appearance within a lymph node, confirming silicone adenopathy. Lymph node enlargement without high-density silicone or the snowstorm appearance on US should raise concern for other causes of adenopathy, particularly metastatic disease from a breast or nonbreast cancer or lymphoma. Just as in women without implants, axillary masses such as lipoma or even primary breast cancer can present as a palpable finding.

KEY POINTS

- The primary focus when interpreting mammograms of women with implants is to detect breast cancer. ID views are required in addition to routine mammographic views for breast cancer screening. If mammography is limited, screening US or MRI can be considered, especially for women who are at high risk for breast cancer.
- Extracapsular rupture may be diagnosed by mammography, US, or MRI.
- MRI is the most sensitive modality for detecting intracapsular implant rupture. US can be used but has lower sensitivity and specificity.
- Diagnostic evaluation of women with implants using mammography and US can identify most findings suspicious for malignancy and in need of biopsy. When the findings remain unclear, MRI may be of value.

References

ACR Practice Guidelines for the Performance of Contrast-Enhanced Magnetic Resonance Imaging (MRI) of the Breast. Rev. ed. 2008 (Resolution 25). Accessed at www.acr.org.

American Cancer Society. Cancer Facts & Figures – 2011. American Cancer Society, Atlanta, Georgia, 2011. Accessed at http://www.cancer.org.

American Society of Plastic Surgeons. Report of the 2010 Plastic Surgery Statistics. Accessed at www.plasticsurgery.org.

Berg WA, Caskey CI, Hampter UM, et al. Single- and double-lumen silicone breast implant integrity: Prospective evaluation of MR and US criteria. Radiology 1995;197:45-52.

Cronin TD, Gerow F. Augmentation mammoplasty: A new "natural feel" prosthesis. In Transactions of the Third International Congress on Plastic Surgery. Amsterdam, Excerpta Medica, 1964, pp 41-49.

Destouet JM, Monsees BS, Oser RF, et al. Screening mammography in 350 women with breast implants: Prevalence and findings of implant complications. AJR 1992;159:973-978.

Eklund GW, Busby RC, Miller SH, Job JS. Improved imaging of the augmented breast. AJR 1988;151:469-473.

Erguvan-Dogan B, Yang WT. Direct injection of paraffin into the breast: Mammographic, sonographic, and MRI features of early complications. AJR 2006;186:888-894.

Everson LI, Parantainen H, Detile T, et al. Diagnosis of breast implant rupture: Imaging findings and relative efficacies of imaging techniques. AJR 1994;163:57-60.

Handel N, Silverstein MJ, Gamagami P, et al. Factors affecting mammographic visualization of the breast after augmentation mammoplasty. JAMA 1992;268:1913-1917.

Middleton MS. Breast implant classification. In Gorczyca DP, Brenner RJ (eds). The Augmented Breast. Radiologic and Clinical Perspectives. New York, Thieme, 1997, Chap. 4, p 28.

Miglioretti DL, Rutter CM, Geller BM, et al. Effect of breast augmentation on the accuracy of mammography and cancer characteristics. JAMA 2004;291:442-450.

Phillips JW, de Camara DL, Lockwood MD, Grebner WC. Strength of silicone breast implants. Plast Reconstr Surg 1996;97:1215-1225.

Silverstein MJ, Gierson ED, Gamagami P, et al. Breast cancer diagnosis and prognosis in women with augmented silicone gel-filled implants. Cancer 1990;66:97-101.

Soo MS, Kornguth PJ, Walsh R, et al. Complex radial folds versus subtle signs of intracapsular rupture of breast implants: MR findings with surgical correlation. AJR 1996;166:1421-1427.

CASE QUESTIONS

CASE 19-1. Screening MLO views of a 54-year-old woman who had ruptured implants removed 10 years ago. What is the abnormal finding and its significance? What are your BI-RADS assessment and recommendation?

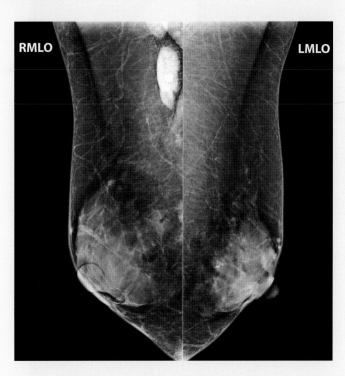

CASE 19-2. Diagnostic evaluation of a 44-year-old high-risk woman with a palpable left breast mass (indicated by the metallic marker). What are the findings? What do you recommend?

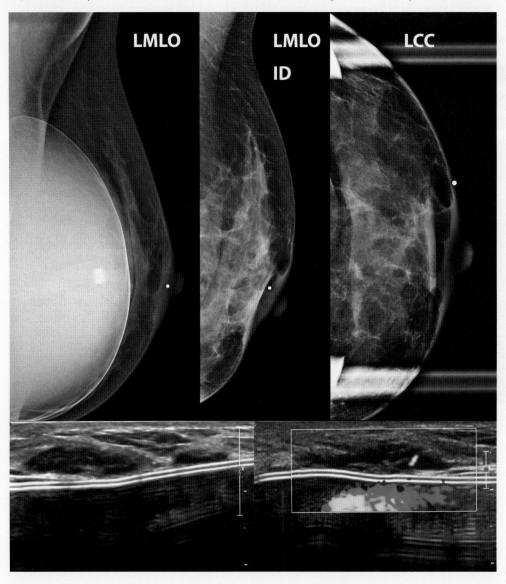

CASE 19-3. Screening mammogram on a 67-year-old who had implants placed 25 years ago. The technologist was unable to displace the left implant. US images are of the left implant (**A, B**) and axilla (**C**). What are the mammographic and US findings?

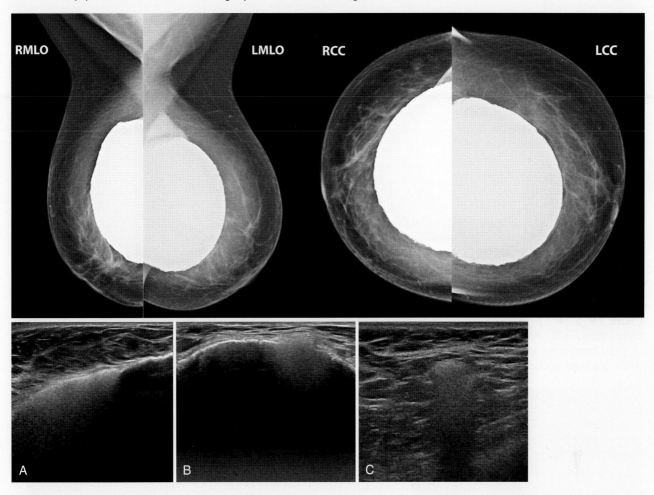

CASE 19-4. Screening mammogram of a 55-year-old woman who had implants placed 30 years ago. The technologist could not displace the left implant. What are your findings and recommendations?

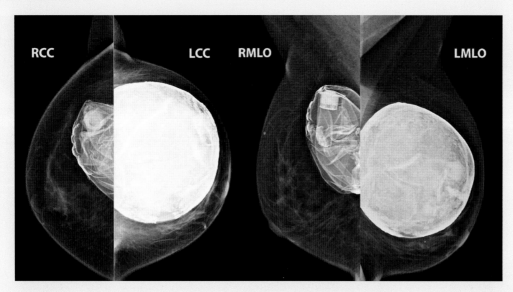

CASE 19-5. A 56-year-old woman with prior right mastectomy with transverse rectus abdominus myocutaneous (TRAM) flap reconstruction. An implant was placed on the left side for symmetry of size. Here are her screening views. What is the finding? What is your BI-RADS category and what are your recommendations?

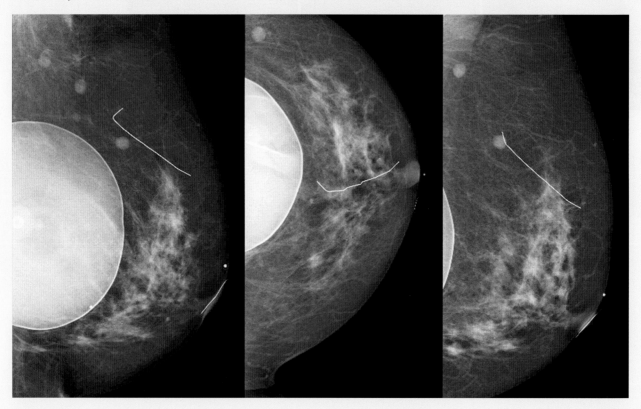

CASE 19-6. A 62-year-old woman presents for screening mammography. What are your BI-RADS category and recommendation?

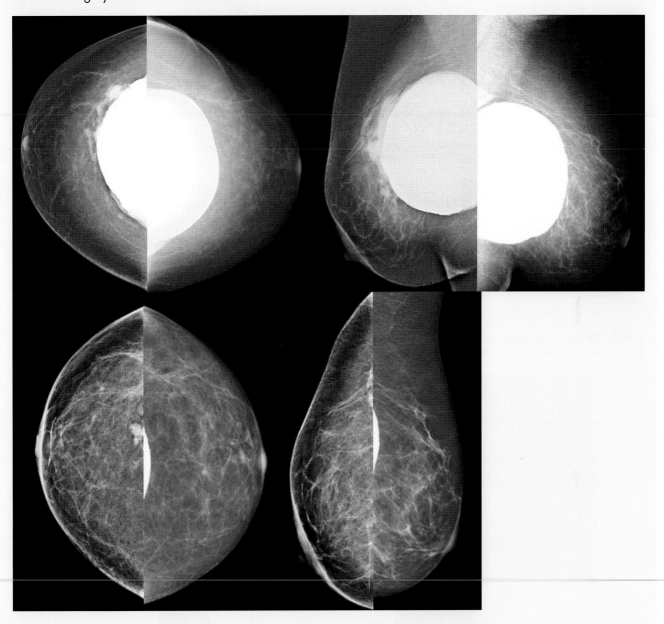

CASE 19-7. A 57-year-old woman with subglandular silicone implants presents with a history of left breast enlargement over an 8-month period. T2-weighted axial and coronal unenhanced magnetic resonance images are shown. What are the findings and DDx?

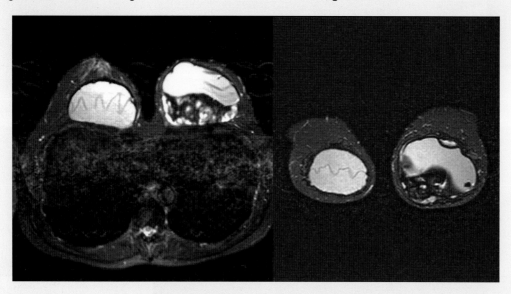

CASE 19-8. A 55-year-old woman presents with a palpable left breast mass, marked with a *BB*. Describe the findings. What is your recommendation?

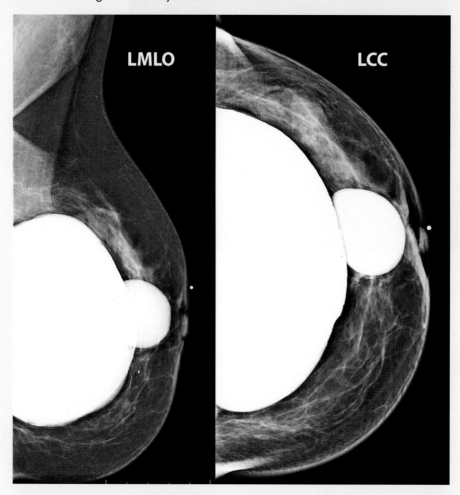

CASE 19-9. Screening mammogram on a patient who had silicone implants removed 3 years ago because of rupture on the right. What are the findings?

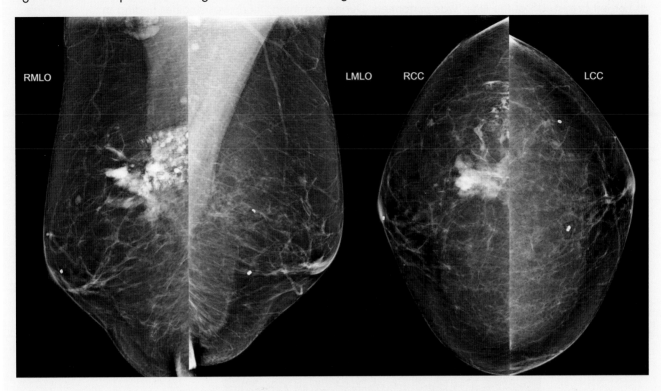

CASE 19-10. A 47-year-old woman with a history of left breast cancer who underwent bilateral mastectomy and implant reconstruction presents with multiple palpable masses in the subcutaneous tissues overlying the left implant. Mammography and US were performed. What is your DDx for the findings?

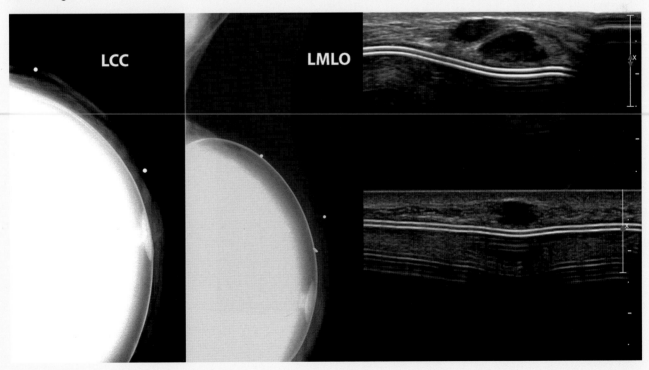

CASE 19-11. A 47-year-old woman with saline implants had minor trauma to the left breast. She then felt her implant decrease in size and noticed a palpable lump in the 3 o'clock position of her left breast. US of the lump was performed. During scanning, there was another finding in the 9 o'clock position of the left breast. Are the US findings suspicious for malignancy?

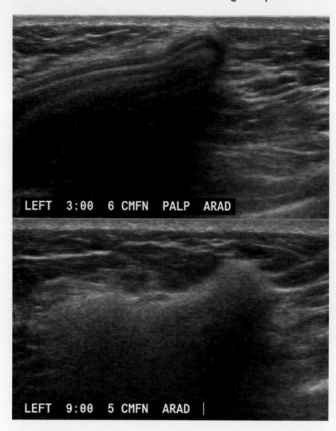

CASE 19-12. This 42-year-old woman complains of a palpable mass in the left axilla. She reports that she had saline implants when she was younger but had them removed a few years ago. Here are her mammogram and US of her axilla. What would you tell her is the cause of her palpable lump?

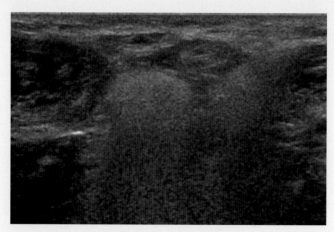

CASE ANSWERS

CASE 19-1. There is a prominent dense lymph node within the right axilla. The appearance is consistent with silicone uptake after implant rupture. There are no suspicious findings. BI-RADS 2. Recommend annual mammographic screening.

CASE 19-2. The tissue is heterogeneously dense. A saline implant is present. Mammography shows no implant-related or breast findings in the region of the palpable mass. US reveals two hypoechoic solid masses adjacent to the implant. Flow is seen within one mass on Doppler examination. The findings are suspicious, and biopsy is recommended (BI-RADS 4). Diagnosis: ductal carcinoma in situ, low and intermediate grade, associated with a fibroadenoma.

CASE 19-3. There are no findings suspicious for malignancy. A triangular collection of silicone is seen adjacent to the upper left implant representing extracapsular rupture. The left implant is rounded, suggesting capsular contracture. There is extensive calcification of the fibrous capsule bilaterally, causing the edges of the implants to appear irregular.

US image **A** shows the snowstorm pattern corresponding to the extracapsular silicone seen on mammography. Image **B** shows another focus of extracapsular silicone near the anterior implant. Note the different appearance of the snowstorm pattern compared with the echogenic calcified fibrous capsule. Image **C** reveals the snowstorm appearance within the axilla consistent with nodal uptake of silicone.

CASE 19-4. There are bilateral subglandular saline implants. The right implant is ruptured and collapsed with adjacent capsular calcifications. There are extensive capsular calcifications on the left with rounding of the implant, consistent with capsular contracture. There are no findings suspicious for malignancy. Recommend annual mammographic screening.

CASE 19-5. There is an intact saline implant. There is a possible small mass in the medial left breast that is denser than the rest of the tissue (*arrow*). It may be located in the inferior breast on the MLO ID view. BI-RADS 0. CC and lateral medial spot compression views and US were performed. The diagnostic examination confirms a small, solid, round mass in the left breast at 8 o'clock. BI-RADS 4. US-guided core biopsy revealed IDC.

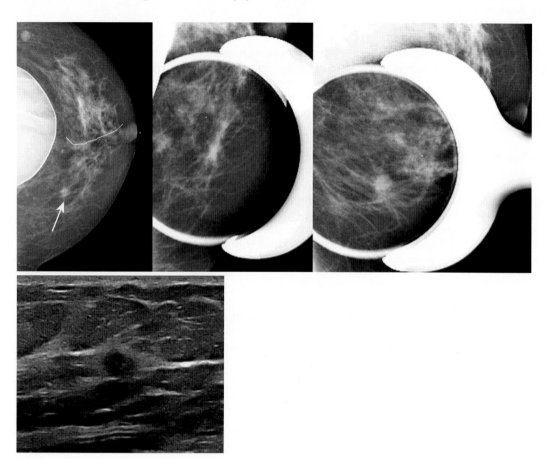

CASE 19-6. There is silicone outside the implant on the right consistent with extracapsular rupture. This is Bi-RADS 2 because it is not suspicious for breast carcinoma. However, she may wish to see a plastic surgeon for evaluation and management of her rupture.

CASE 19-7. There is a mixed signal mass within the fibrous capsule posterior to the left implant. The implant is displaced anteriorly. The DDx included lymphoma, primary breast cancer, metastatic disease, and hemorrhage. The patient had a known coagulopathy. Diagnosis on explantation: chronic hemorrhage with organized blood clots on the left and bilateral intracapsular ruptures.

CASE 19-8. The palpable finding corresponds to extracapsular silicone. Note how the silicone forms an acute angle with the rest of the implant, indicating extracapsular silicone rather than bulge or herniation. There is no evidence of malignancy. No additional imaging is needed.

This palpable finding developed shortly after core biopsy guided by palpation. Although this complication is uncommon with imaging-guided core biopsy, patients with implants should be informed about the risk of implant rupture when informed consent is obtained.

CASE 19-9. There is dense residual silicone in the posterior right breast with bilateral scarring. No additional evaluation is needed. BI-RADS 2.

CASE 19-10. In a case such as this, the hope is that mammography will reveal typically benign findings such as oil cysts or rim calcifications due to fat necrosis. However, the palpable masses could not be visualized mammographically. US did not show the palpable findings to be related to implant folds or the valve. There were multiple solid masses, less than 1 cm, in the subcutaneous tissues adjacent to the implant. Core biopsy of two masses revealed recurrent IDC.

CASE 19-11. US of the palpable finding (3 o'clock) reveals the collapsed elastomer shell. There are no suspicious findings. The snowstorm appearance is seen in the medial breast (9 o'clock). The patient had prior ruptured silicone implants that were exchanged about 10 years ago. Mammography confirms the sonographic findings: a collapsed saline implant and residual free silicone.

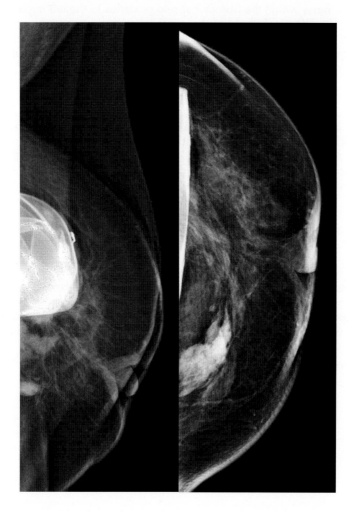

CASE 19-12. The snowstorm pattern is visualized. The palpable lump in her left axilla is therefore due to silicone adenopathy. Her implants were NOT saline!

INTERVENTIONS

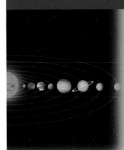

CHAPTER **20**

Breast Needle Biopsy: Tips for Challenging Cases

Aha! You've identified a suspicious lesion at diagnostic evaluation and now it needs a biopsy. You're pretty sure you can see it on ultrasonography (US), so maybe you'll do the biopsy that way. It's so much quicker, although sometimes it's a struggle to see the needle and get all of those angles right. And then sometimes the clip is close to but not in the lesion. If the pathologic finding is benign, will I be sure that the biopsy was of the correct area?

When we are performing breast biopsy with imaging guidance, our goal is to obtain enough material for diagnosis using an approach that is safe and well tolerated by the patient. We need to consider how to target the lesion accurately while minimizing the invasiveness of the procedure. We also need to consider how the procedure fits into the care of the patient from a larger perspective—specifically, how the biopsy approach and results will impact future management.

Adhering to a specific routine works well for some aspects of breast imaging. When interpreting screening mammograms or breast magnetic resonance imaging (MRI), using a systematic approach will improve the consistency and efficiency of our interpretations. However, with breast interventions, it helps to keep a more flexible mindset. Keeping an open mind about using a different approach or a different modality for guidance can improve the chance of a successful outcome.

We will assume that you have at least basic proficiency in breast biopsy procedures, including an understanding of the indications, points to review while obtaining informed consent, and the use of sterile technique. We also assume a basic understanding of how lesions are targeted for biopsy and familiarity with the operation of the biopsy equipment. This foundation will allow us to focus on more challenging cases.

In this chapter, we will give you our best tips on breast biopsy that we hope will help make these interventions safer and more comfortable for you and your patients. For US biopsy, we'll help you find that needle and adapt your technique for biopsy of small, deep, and vanishing lesions with confidence. We'll give you some ideas for

identifying and targeting posterior lesions on stereotactic biopsy, and what to do with thin breasts and superficial lesions. Finally, we'll move to MRI and review how to biopsy posterior and multiple lesions, and how to manage those lesions that you really can't get to with a biopsy needle.

Choosing Biopsy Guidance and Device

Ultrasound-guided biopsy has many advantages over stereotactic or MRI-guided biopsy, including patient comfort, low cost, flexibility of approach, shorter procedure time, sampling with real-time visualization, and the ability to access virtually any lesion. We therefore almost always use ultrasound guidance for biopsy of suspicious lesions that are well seen by this modality.

However, not every lesion that is seen on US is best sampled using ultrasound guidance. If you are struggling to identify the lesion that your partner saw on US when it is obvious on mammography, then by all means switch her to a stereotactic biopsy (Fig. 20-1). Likewise, a lesion that is easily seen on MRI with a questionable correlate on US would be best sampled using MRI guidance (Fig. 20-2). Keeping an open mind about guidance can keep you out of some difficult situations. More on this later.

Masses generally require less tissue removal for accurate diagnosis than calcifications. Therefore, for most ultrasound-guided biopsies, a 14-gauge automated spring-loaded device provides adequate sampling and is very cost effective. Vacuum-assisted devices offer larger tissue samples, single insertion, and directional capability. These devices are preferred for stereotactic biopsy for calcifications as they are less likely to yield a result of atypical ductal hyperplasia (ADH) in the setting of ductal carcinoma in situ (DCIS). For US biopsy, vacuum biopsy is usually overkill, but it can be really helpful for certain lesions, such as small or complex masses, or lesions with calcifications. A coaxial guide can shorten procedure time for US biopsies (especially when teaching residents) and makes it easier to place the biopsy needle into a good

FIGURE 20-1 **Stereotactic Biopsy Was a Better Choice. A,** This patient presented for ultrasound-guided biopsy of a mass detected on mammography (*arrow*). **B,** The US correlate is somewhat vague (*arrow*), and the post-US biopsy image (C) shows that the ribbon marker (*arrow*) is not located within the mammographic mass. **D,** The patient underwent immediate stereotactic biopsy, and the ring marker (*yellow arrow*) is within the mass. Histologic diagnosis from the ultrasound-guided biopsy showed mild hyperplasia, although the stereotactic biopsy showed invasive ductal carcinoma (IDC). If an US correlate of a mammographic finding is questionable, perform a stereotactic biopsy instead.

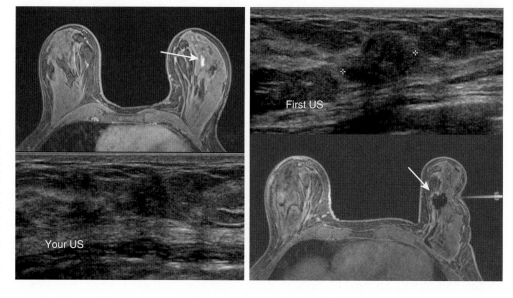

FIGURE 20-2 **Unclear US Correlate of an MRI Finding.** This patient had a small, suspicious, enhancing mass on screening MRI (*arrow*). Your colleague (who is now at lunch) identified an US correlate (*calipers*) that you cannot reproduce. This patient was therefore rescheduled for an MRI-guided biopsy. Targeting was confident with the lesion removed (*arrow*). Histologic examination showed stromal fibrosis.

pre-fire position before each pass. However, the use of a guide may also result in the introduction of more air into the biopsy site.

Ultrasound-Guided Biopsy

The operator dependence of US is well known, and this dependence rises to an even higher level with ultrasound-guided biopsy. It takes practice to develop the skills needed for these procedures. Performing your initial patient procedures under the supervision of a more experienced radiologist is extremely helpful. If you are just learning these techniques or modifying your current ones, try practicing on phantoms first. A raw turkey breast with olives between the pectoralis major and minor muscles makes a very good and inexpensive phantom. This can be really fun even if you are very experienced at US biopsy and just want to practice some of the more advanced moves we describe later on.

The Basic Ultrasound-Guided Biopsy: Warning—Geometry in Use

Do you remember your high school geometry teacher? The one who kept promising that someday you would find a practical use for the subject and thank them for teaching you? That day has arrived! Don't worry, we won't ask you the cosine of a scalene triangle. However, understanding the basic geometry of an ultrasound-guided breast biopsy—how the lesion, transducer, skin nick, and biopsy needle can be kept in alignment—will help us confidently biopsy lesions using a safe angle of approach. Later, we'll modify these angles when we discuss sampling of more challenging lesions.

Positioning
First we do all of the obvious things—review the images, set up the biopsy tray, and obtain consent. Next we position the patient. Yes, we want to ensure that the patient is comfortable and can remain still during the procedure, but this is also our first chance to use geometry in our favor. Positioning can be used to thin out the tissue in the region of the lesion. As a result, the lesion will not be as deep and the approach will be easier. For example, if a lateral right breast lesion is being biopsied and the patient rolls about halfway onto her left side, the lateral tissue will be thinner. Likewise, lowering the patient's head so that she is lying flat will thin the inferior breast, improving access. Typically, the patient will raise her ipsilateral arm above her head, which can further thin the tissue. Cushions or foam wedges will help stabilize the patient and keep her comfortable in the position you choose— just make sure that they don't end up getting in your way.

Planning the Approach
This most difficult part of ultrasound-guided biopsy occurs before the first sample is taken. Where we place the transducer is determined by the location of the lesion, but its orientation is up to us.

Find the lesion and optimize the technical settings by adjusting the depth, focal zone, and gain. Sometimes a lesion is more clearly seen using compound or harmonic imaging. Once you identify the lesion, think about where you want to make your skin nick. Entering along the curve of the lateral breast is easiest. The tissue is thinner in the upper inner quadrant and there is less of a curve, so a more inferior approach often works well for lesions in this area. Sometimes you realize that the lesion is only well seen in one plane, and in these cases you'll need to approach the lesion with the transducer oriented in that plane in order to visualize the lesion well during sampling. Positioning the transducer so the lesion appears on the far side of the US screen from the entry site allows you to visualize a longer segment of the needle as it approaches the lesion (Fig. 20.3).

Now that you've decided on where to place your transducer, let's make it easy to get back there by marking the skin. You can mark the skin next to both sides of the

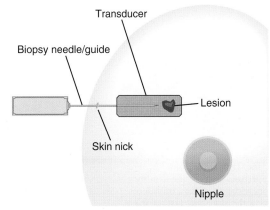

FIGURE 20-3 **Keeping Everything Aligned.** Overhead view showing alignment of the lesion, long axis of the transducer, skin nick, and coaxial guide/biopsy needle in one plane. The biopsy device is in the pre-fire position.

transducer. Another option is to mark a "T" with the top of the letter at the entry side of the transducer and the stem in the plane of the long axis of the transducer. Your skin nick will be along this path, so this also helps the technologist know where to clean the skin. The patient is next prepped and draped. Don't wash off the skin marks!

Getting Everything Lined Up
Four things need to be aligned in one plane: the lesion, transducer, skin nick, and the biopsy needle/coaxial guide (see Fig. 20-3). Place your transducer into position using your marks and be prepared to stay there for the duration of the biopsy. Be the rock! This can be tricky; when the transducer and gel are placed on the curved surface of the breast, the transducer can easily slide away from the lesion. And the harder you push, the more you seem to slide. To help keep the transducer still throughout the procedure, create a stable platform holding the transducer near the skin and rest the flat of your hand and the fourth and fifth fingers on the breast. Now you can stay on that lesion all day long.

If you are in the habit of turning to grab stuff from the tray behind you, you will find it difficult to stay on the lesion. Develop a habit of having things handed to you or have the tray immediately next to you. If you do slide away from the lesion, go back to those skin marks that you made earlier. It's also helpful to record an image of the lesion before starting the procedure, with the transducer in the position to be used for biopsy. This image can be recalled during the procedure, and landmarks adjacent to the lesion can help re-identify the lesion if it becomes indistinct during biopsy.

Making the Nick
By judging the depth of your lesion, you will determine your needle path and the location of your skin nick. For superficial lesions, the nick can be made close to the transducer (Fig. 20-4). For most deep lesions, we can use the curvature of the breast to advantage to keep our approach parallel to the chest wall. For these lesions, we make our nick farther away from the edge of the

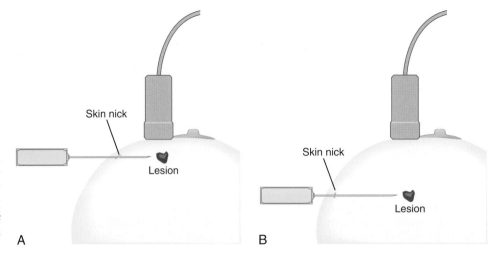

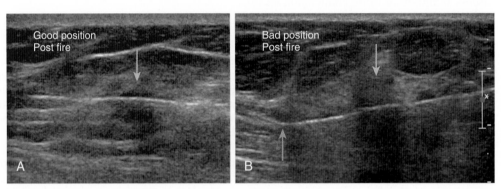

FIGURE 20-4 **Adjusting the Approach for Deeper Lesions. A,** For more superficial lesions, the skin nick is made close to the transducer. **B,** Making the skin nick farther from the transducer uses the curvature of the breast to approach deeper lesions parallel to the chest wall.

FIGURE 20-5 **Good and Bad Needle Angles.** The needle traverses the mass (*yellow arrows*) in both cases. In the first case, which is well positioned, the needle is seen in its entirety and is parallel to the chest wall. In the second case, the needle is not parallel to the chest wall and the tip abuts the pectoral muscle (*purple arrow*). Ouch!

transducer, resulting in a needle insertion close to the depth of the lesion (see Fig. 20-4).

Now that we have a plan, let's go ahead and anesthetize the skin, the path to the lesion, and the tissues surrounding the lesion along the long axis of the transducer. Watch as you inject under real-time guidance so that you can modify your approach if you discover that it is too shallow or deep. Then make the skin nick.

Needle Angle
The needle and the anterior edge of the pectoralis muscle are two lines that should never intersect! Keeping the needle parallel (or at least close to parallel) to the muscle (Fig. 20-5) is mainly a safety issue, but it also improves needle visualization by keeping the needle perpendicular to the ultrasound beam. A parallel approach is a good habit even for more superficial lesions—that way you won't ever have to worry about hitting the pectoral muscle (which hurts a LOT).

Inserting the Coaxial Guide/Biopsy Needle
Keeping the long axis of the transducer aligned with the skin nick and lesion, go ahead and insert the coaxial guide or needle through the nick. Gradually advance it toward the lesion while monitoring the process by US to be sure it is advancing at the desired depth and angle.

If you are using a coaxial guide, remove the inner cannula and slide in the biopsy needle. Maintaining real-time visualization of the needle and the lesion, advance the needle to the edge of the lesion. The biopsy needle

should remain parallel or almost parallel to the chest wall. This will allow for safe sampling with good visualization of the needle.

Help! I Can't Find My Needle!
If at any point you lose visualization of the needle or guide, it should be close to the plane of the ultrasound beam because of the steps you have taken in planning your approach. You need only to use a small waving motion of the needle from side to side to bring the needle into view. If this does not work, the alignment needs to be checked. Get good visualization of the lesion on the US screen. Then look down at the alignment of the skin nick, biopsy device, and transducer. If they are aligned, try doing the gentle wave with the needle again. If they are not in alignment, you have two choices (Fig. 20-6). You can rotate the transducer to realign it with the skin nick (keeping the lesion on the screen), or you can move the needle/skin nick (a short distance) to be in alignment with the transducer.

Getting the Sample
You now have all of the geometry working in your favor. The tip of the biopsy needle is within a few millimeters of the edge of the lesion, the angle of approach is safe, and you have good visualization of the lesion and the entire shaft of the biopsy needle. You are now ready for your first pass! Watch as you take the sample. Nice job. But wait! Before you remove the needle, scan through the lesion to ensure that the needle went through it. Take at

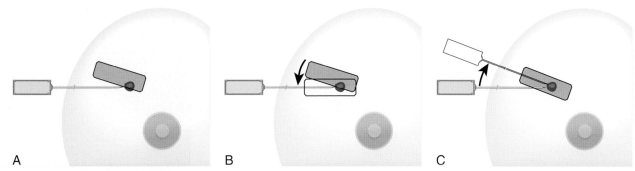

FIGURE 20-6 **Off-Angle Correction.** If you are only seeing part of the needle on the US screen, then your needle is not aligned with the transducer (**A**). To correct this problem, look down at the patient to check the alignment. You have two choices. While keeping the lesion on the US screen, you can rotate the transducer to again align with the needle and skin nick (**B**). Alternatively, you can move the needle/nick position to align with the transducer (**C**). This maneuver is usually used only for small corrections.

least a couple of pre- and post-fire images. We typically take five samples, place a marker, and then hold pressure for 5 to 10 minutes. A mammogram with light compression afterward will confirm the location of the marker.

Biopsy Etiquette

Patients are understandably very focused on everything that is said during the procedure. When taking the samples, we say things like, "You are going to hear a click," or "You may feel a little pressure now." If you ask the technologist, "Do you think that's the mass?" or say, "I'm going to fire the gun," your patient may ask you for a last meal and a cigarette.

Challenging Ultrasound–Guided Biopsies

The Deep Lesion in a Large Breast

In some cases—if the breast is very large or the lesion is very deep—using the curvature of the breast alone may not give you an acceptable approach. The lesion may be too far from the edge of the breast to access it easily. Fortunately, we can still biopsy these lesions by modifying our usual approach. Basically, we will start with a steeper approach and then depress the needle to have a safe angle as we approach the lesion.

Using a coaxial guide with this modified approach is really helpful, even if you don't typically use one. Insert the guide at least several centimeters away from the edge of the transducer and advance it under real-time visualization so its tip is near the depth of the lesion (Fig. 20-7). The angle of the coaxial guide will be steeper than usual and does not need to be parallel to the chest wall at this point. Now we'll insert the biopsy needle gradually into the coaxial guide until it just emerges from the other end of the guide.

At this point, the needle is directed toward the pectoral muscle at too steep an angle to move directly toward the lesion. So how can we keep good visualization of the needle and convert our steep approach to one that is parallel to the pec? There are two great tricks that can really help. The first is to rock the transducer *away* from the skin nick along its long axis. This directs the ultrasound beam so that it is more perpendicular to the needle, improving its visibility (see Fig. 20-7). The second trick

is to depress the coaxial guide, needle, and skin nick together (see Fig. 20-7). This is possible because of the pliability of the breast tissue (NOT recommended during biopsy of internal organs!). The result is a deeper approach that is more parallel to the chest wall. The lever effect of this action may also elevate the lesion slightly away from the pectoral muscle. Now you can advance the needle relatively parallel to the chest wall, and you're ready to take the first sample in a very safe position (see Fig. 20-7).

Using this technique, it is usually possible to obtain an excellent approach for lesions at any depth. Sometimes the needle is actually angled slightly away from the pec when you're using this technique, so you know your position is safe. If you've performed these actions and the needle is still angled slightly toward the pectoral muscle, try rocking the transducer away from you a little more. The resulting change in compression of the breast tissue by the transducer will often improve your angle of approach even more.

The Disappearing Lesion

After one or more samples are taken, some lesions become indistinct or even invisible by US. This loss of visualization can be caused by hemorrhage, air in the needle tracks, removal of portions of the mass, or rupture of a fluid-filled component. As a result, it may become difficult to obtain additional samples or accurately place a marker. Loss of visualization is most likely to occur during biopsy of a small solid mass, a mass that may be either cystic or solid by US, or a complex mass that has a small solid component. Here are a few tips for biopsy of these lesions.

The Small Mass

Injecting too much anesthetic can obscure some lesions—especially those in the several millimeters range. One trick is to inject anesthetic up to but not in the lesion and to use a separate injection to anesthetize the far side of the lesion (Fig. 20-8). If too much anesthetic is injected, simply wait a few minutes and rescan. Some of the anesthetic will have absorbed or dissipated, and the lesion will often become easier to see. Be careful to not inject air while anesthetic is being given; it may take hours or longer to absorb. If this occurs and the lesion cannot be identified with confidence, the procedure will need to be rescheduled.

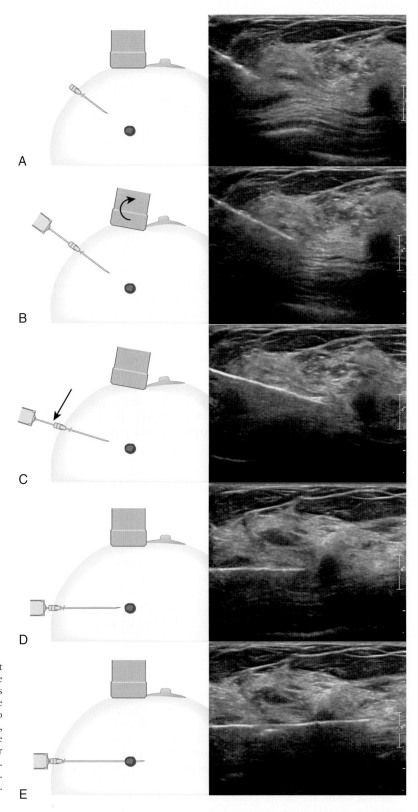

FIGURE 20-7 **Deep Lesion in a Large Breast. A,** Insert the coaxial guide several centimeters from the edge of the transducer to the approximate depth of the lesion. **B,** As you insert the biopsy needle through the guide, rock the transducer away from the entry site along its long axis to better visualize the needle. **C,** Depress the coaxial guide, needle, and skin nick together (*arrow*) to make the needle nearly parallel to the chest wall. Keep the transducer parallel to the needle to maintain good visualization. **D,** The biopsy needle is now in the pre-fire position. **E,** The post-fire image confirms successful sampling. Diagnosis: IDC.

Make the first pass count! Over 90% of malignant masses can be diagnosed by tissue obtained on the first two cores. You will never see a lesion better than before the first samples are taken, so it's important to carefully target and obtain these cores from the most suspicious portion of the lesion. This will maximize your ability to obtain diagnostic material.

Targeting the deeper part of a small lesion first is another helpful technique (Fig. 20-9). The more superficial portion will remain visible longer and will be more easily targeted on subsequent passes and during clip placement. If the more superficial portion is targeted first, air in the biopsy track has a greater chance of obscuring the remainder of the lesion.

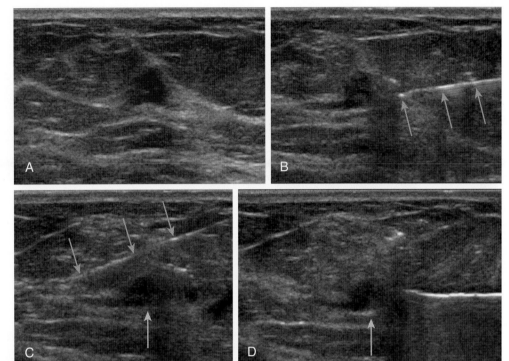

FIGURE 20-8 **Anesthetizing a Small Mass. A,** The scout image shows a small hypoechoic mass. **B,** While visualizing in real time, enter the side of the breast along the anticipated path of the coaxial guide/needle. Advance the anesthetic needle (*purple arrows*) so that the tip is close to but not through the lesion. Inject as you pull the needle back, being careful not to leave large pools of anesthetic. **C,** Next, anesthetize the breast tissue just beyond the lesion by entering near the transducer edge using a steep needle angle (*purple arrows*). **D,** The mass is still easily seen on the pre-fire image. Diagnosis: high-grade invasive mammary carcinoma.

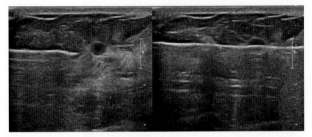

FIGURE 20-9 **Biopsy the Deeper Part First.** Pre- and post-fire images taken during biopsy of a papilloma. With small masses, sampling the deeper portion first can improve visualization of the remainder of the lesion during subsequent passes.

BOX 20-1 When Do I Need to Send Cyst Fluid to the Lab?

- Cyst fluid that is bloody has a small chance of showing atypical or malignant cells and is typically sent for cytologic analysis.
- Nonbloody (green, yellow, black) cyst fluid is benign and can be discarded.

Some small masses have pronounced shadowing that is even more conspicuous than the mass itself. When we biopsy this type of lesion, we don't want to aim *too* deep, as this may cause us to miss the lesion entirely (Fig. 20-10).

Bleeding can also obscure a small mass during biopsy. If bleeding occurs and you are losing visibility of the mass, get a couple more quick samples if you can, place a clip, and end the procedure. Remember: the first one or two well-targeted cores will likely be diagnostic. If they are not (i.e., the pathologic findings are discordant with imaging), a repeat biopsy can be performed after the hematoma has resolved (usually in a few weeks).

Vacuum-assisted biopsy can also work very well for small masses (Fig. 20-11). The vacuum needle chamber is placed posterior to the lesion. Samples are obtained anterior to the biopsy needle while the needle remains in place.

It's a good idea to have a clip ready to use throughout the procedure. That way, if you lose visualization of a mass, the clip can be placed immediately while you can still visualize the biopsy site. You can even place a clip before finishing the biopsy if the lesion is very small or disappearing during sampling. Putting the clip just deep to the lesion will help keep it from being removed if additional cores are obtained (Fig. 20-12).

Cyst versus Solid Mass

If you suspect that a hypoechoic mass may represent a cyst containing debris rather than a solid mass, aspiration can be performed first (Fig. 20-13). If the aspirate is nonbloody and the lesion completely resolves, you are done. Core biopsy is not needed, and the aspirate can be discarded. If the aspirate is bloody and the lesion disappears, send the aspirate for cytologic testing and place a clip (Box 20-1). Purulent aspirate is sent for microbiology culture and sensitivity testing. If the lesion does not resolve with aspiration, we proceed directly to core biopsy of the residual solid mass (see Fig. 20-13).

The Complex Mass

Complex masses contain cystic and solid components. These are suspicious findings with a positive predictive

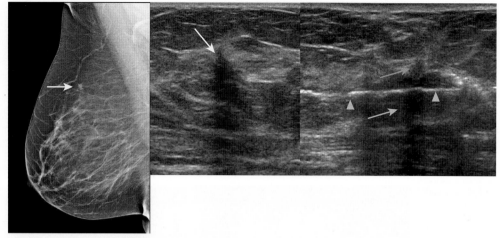

FIGURE 20-10 **Biopsy the Lesion, Not the Shadow.** A mass with spiculated margins was detected on mammography (*arrow*). US reveals a corresponding shadowing lesion. Post-fire image from the ultrasound-guided core biopsy shows that the needle (*arrowheads*) is traversing the shadow (*yellow arrow*) behind the mass rather than the mass itself (*purple arrow*). The pathologic examination showed proliferative fibrocystic changes, a finding that is discordant. Repeat ultrasound-guided biopsy showed IDC.

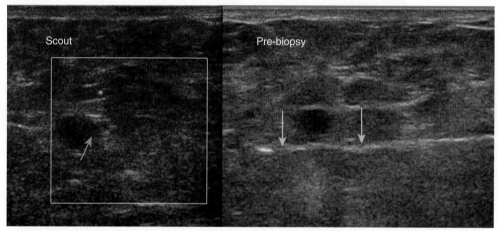

FIGURE 20-11 **Vacuum-Assisted US Biopsy.** Scout image shows a hypoechoic mass with Doppler flow at the margin suggesting an intracystic mass (*arrow*). A vacuum-assisted biopsy needle was placed directly posterior to the mass with the bevel (*yellow arrows*) directed toward the lesion. The lesion disappeared during sampling. Diagnosis: Fibrocystic change with apocrine metaplasia, which is concordant.

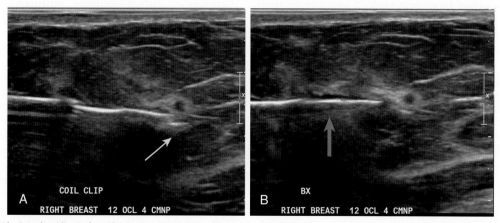

FIGURE 20-12 **Placing the Clip Before the Lesion Disappears.** Hypoechoic mass with an echogenic halo in a 51-year-old woman with a history of contralateral breast cancer. **A,** Because of the small size of the mass, the marker clip (*arrow*) was placed before core biopsy, slightly deep to the lesion. **B** shows the needle (*arrow*) in the pre-fire position. Diagnosis: fat necrosis.

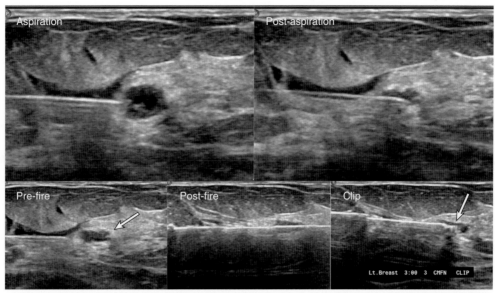

FIGURE 20-13 **Aspiration and Core Biopsy of a Complex Mass.** Biopsy was recommended for this new 5-mm screening-detected mass that had a complex appearance on US. The lesion was first aspirated, yielding bloody material. The lesion became much smaller but did not resolve after aspiration. Core biopsy of the residual lesion (*arrow*) was performed. A clip (*arrow*) was placed in the residual lesion. Diagnosis: invasive papillary carcinoma.

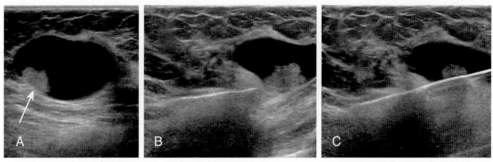

FIGURE 20-14 **Core Biopsy of a Complex Mass. A,** US of a palpable mass in a 48-year-old woman shows a solid intracystic lesion (*arrow*). **B** and **C,** During core biopsy of this mass, the solid portion is targeted for biopsy (pre- and post-fire images). Diagnosis: papilloma.

value of 20% to 30%. Most of these lesions are amenable to ultrasound-guided core or vacuum-assisted biopsy. The key to diagnosis lies in sampling of the solid component, and that should be your target (Fig. 20-14). For a small complex mass, a vacuum-assisted biopsy needle can be performed, just as for a small solid mass. For a larger complex mass that is mostly cystic, a vacuum-assisted needle can also be used, but make sure that you target the solid component (Fig. 20-15).

Although we would like to believe that we can safely and adequately sample any lesion, sometimes the patient might be better served by proceeding directly to surgical excision. This plan should be recommended if you believe that you would have difficulty obtaining representative sampling from the lesion—for example, if the solid component is so small that rupture of the fluid-filled component might preclude accurate targeting (Fig. 20-16).

Biopsy of Women with Implants

One sure sign that your biopsy skills are improving is that biopsies of women with implants are increasingly scheduled on your day. The possibility of implant rupture

occurring during biopsy is often raised by patients and should be discussed when you are obtaining consent. Patients can be reassured that this complication is very uncommon and that you will take every precaution to avoid it. However, they should also understand that the potential for rupture cannot be entirely eliminated.

Implants often lie only a few millimeters beneath the skin surface, even when in a subpectoral location. When injecting the local anesthetic and making the skin nick, keep the needle and scalpel blade as superficial as possible. Raising the skin between your fingers can make it safer to insert the needle for anesthesia and make the nick. The needle should be monitored continuously by US as anesthetic is injected.

Let's think about a dome—the U.S. Capital building or St. Paul's Cathedral, for instance. The breast tissue is like a dome overlying the implant. We need to plan our approach so that the needle will stay within the exterior portion of the dome and away from the interior living space. We can do this by keeping the needle parallel to the implant and as superficial as possible. Rather than our typical entry from the side of the breast with the

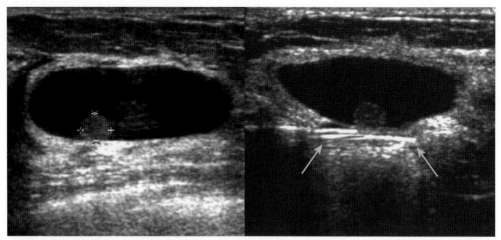

FIGURE 20-15 **Vacuum-Assisted Biopsy of a Complex Mass.** Intracystic mass demonstrated by US (*calipers*). The sampling notch of the biopsy probe (*arrows*) is positioned deep to the mass. Pathologic examination revealed papilloma.

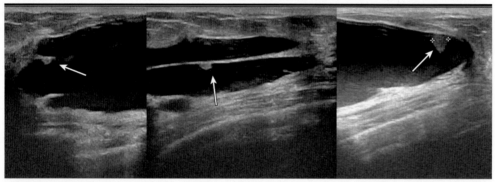

FIGURE 20-16 **Multiple Papillomas Best Left to the Surgeon.** US of a 58-year-old woman with a palpable right breast mass shows a septated cyst with multiple solid masses. Because the solid component is so small, excision was recommended and revealed multiple papillomas.

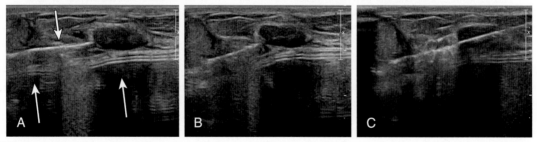

FIGURE 20-17 **Biopsy Adjacent to an Implant. A,** Pre-fire position. Note that the biopsy needle (*short arrow*) is parallel to the implant (*long arrows*). **B,** With the handle of the biopsy device gently lowered, a biopsy angle directed away from the implant is obtained. **C,** Post-fire image showing successful sampling of the lesion. Diagnosis: fibroadenoma.

needle directed toward the central breast, our path may be more sideways through the breast tissue overlying the implant. A great trick for superficial lesions in these women is to *gently* depress the handle of the biopsy device toward the chest wall. As a result of this movement, the needle is aimed away from the implant, up toward the superficial tissues (Fig. 20-17).

Occasionally, a lesion is so close to the implant—even indenting it or located within a fold in the shell—that an approach with ultrasound guidance will risk rupture. Don't panic! You have another option. Consider stereotactic guidance in these cases if the lesion is seen on

mammography (Fig. 20-18). Positioning for stereotactic biopsy is similar to that for implant-displaced views taken routinely for mammography, where the implant is moved safely out of the way. If the lesion is seen only on US and not mammography, you can still displace the implant back against the chest wall using the open compression paddle that you use for wire localization (Fig. 20-19). Ultrasound can then be used to localize the lesion by scanning through the opening. Ultrasound-guide aspiration or biopsy can be performed by either entering adjacent to the ultrasound transducer or from the side of the breast (see Fig. 20-19).

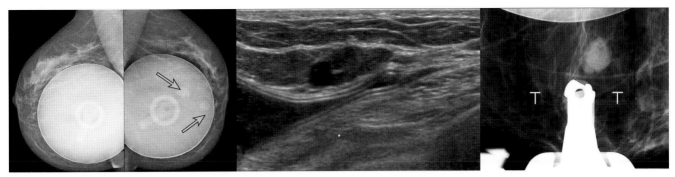

FIGURE 20-18 **Stereotactic Biopsy Using Implant-Displaced Views.** This patient with two masses (*arrows*) on her baseline mammogram required tissue diagnosis of at least one for her to be eligible for a kidney transplant. The implant was quite soft, and the masses balloted into the implant without a good path for US biopsy. The patient was therefore positioned for stereotactic biopsy, and a pre-fire image shows successful displacement of one of these masses away from implant. Diagnosis: fibroadenoma.

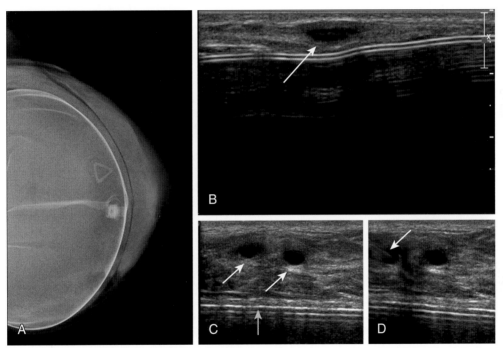

FIGURE 20-19 **Ultrasound-Guided Aspiration with Breast in Mammographic Compression. A** and **B,** Aspiration was recommended for a hypoechoic palpable mass (*arrow*) that is adjacent to her saline implant and not visible on the mammogram. Although aspiration was attempted, the mass could not be punctured by the needle due to mobility. **C,** The patient was placed in mammographic compression with the implant displaced toward the chest wall using a needle localization paddle. US performed through the paddle aperture showed two masses (*arrows*). The bright inferior band (*yellow arrow*) represents the digital receptor, not the implant. **D,** A spinal needle entering adjacent to the transducer punctured the cyst (*arrow*). Both lesions resolved with aspiration, which obtained nonbloody fluid consistent with complicated cysts.

Biopsy of Multiple Lesions

When planning ultrasound-guided biopsy of two lesions that are close together in the same breast, we generally biopsy the more subtle one first. Otherwise, this lesion could become more difficult to visualize because of anesthetic or hemorrhage from the first biopsy. In this situation, the lesions can be approached through separate nicks or through the same skin nick (Fig. 20-20).

Biopsy of Axillary Masses

Axillary biopsy has the potential for more significant complications than routine breast biopsy. The axilla is like a valley with the pectoralis muscle on the medial side and the latissimus dorsi muscle on the lateral side (Fig.

20-21). These muscles limit our approach so that a steep approach is usually needed, resulting in the needle being directed toward the bottom of the valley. The challenge is then to avoid the axillary artery and vein and the brachial plexus that lie in the bottom of the valley. Color Doppler may be used to identify the axillary vessels when you are planning your approach. You do not want to hit those—especially with a core needle—or your day could become much longer. The use of a device with a manual throw (e.g., Achieve needle, Cardinal Health, Dublin, OH) gives us more control over the procedure and is probably safer than an automated throw device.

The lymph nodes most commonly undergoing biopsy lie in the low axilla, as this is where breast cancers

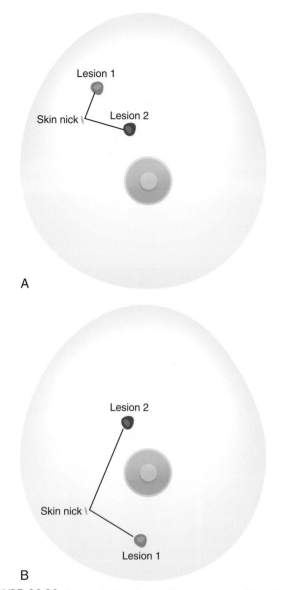

A

B

FIGURE 20-20 **Approach for Biopsy of Two Lesions.** Although two different skin nicks are perfectly acceptable, a single skin nick may suffice to access both lesions. **A,** If the lesions are near each other, a single skin nick can be made in a location that provides easy access to both lesions. Generally, the more subtle lesion is biopsied first. **B,** If the lesions are more widely spaced, (6 o'clock and 11 o'clock positions of the right breast in this example), they can be approached and biopsied through separate skin nicks or one skin nick that is made between them (at the 8 o'clock position in this example).

typically metastasize first. The approach for axillary biopsy is usually from the lateral or inferior aspect. The patient should raise the ipsilateral arm over her head. This provides wide access to the axilla and also flattens the axillary pyramid, making it shallower and easier to navigate.

Fine-Needle Aspiration versus Core Biopsy

For axillary adenopathy of unclear etiology and for axillary masses that may not represent adenopathy, core biopsy is preferred because it is more likely to provide diagnostic material. We typically obtain two or three core

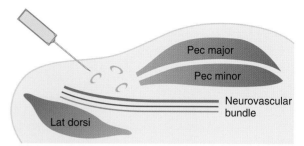

FIGURE 20-21 **Cross Section of the Right Axilla.** The latissimus and pectoralis muscles limit the approach to biopsy of the axilla. A steep needle approach is usually needed. An automated throw needle in this approach may result in damage to the axillary artery, vein, or nerves (*red*, *blue*, and *brown* lines) that lie in the base of the axilla. Use of a manual throw needle provides us with greater control.

samples in these cases. For suspected axillary nodal metastasis from known primary breast cancer, either fine-needle aspiration or core biopsy can be performed (Fig. 20-22). Fine-needle aspiration has been shown to have high sensitivity and specificity in this setting. Typically, one to three passes are made, targeting the thickened lymph node cortex.

Stereotactic Biopsy

With stereotactic core needle biopsy (SCNB), the geometric calculations needed to align the needle with the lesion are performed by computer, and the needle is kept parallel to the chest wall by patient positioning and fixation of the biopsy device. As a result, SCNB can often be learned more quickly than ultrasound-guided interventions. Prone table and "add-on" upright units are available, and each has its own advantages and limitations.

Problems that can arise during stereotactic biopsy include inability to access very posterior lesions, difficulty visualizing subtle lesions, and compressibility of the breast tissue to less than 2 to 3 cm, so that sampling cannot be performed without risking penetrating the other side of the breast (negative stroke margin). Accurate sampling can also be difficult when there is movement of the lesion after targeting. Although some of these limitations cannot be overcome, we will give you some tips for managing those that can.

Prone Table versus Add-on

Prone tables are popular. Lesions can be accessed from any angle and vasovagal reactions are very uncommon. Unfortunately, posterior lesions can be difficult to reach. Also, a room with a prone table is probably used for only a small fraction of a business day. The digital receptors used on many prone tables are not state of the art; they often use older charge coupled device (CCD) technology that can limit our ability to locate and target lesions for biopsy.

Add-on units are attached to a clinical mammography unit. Room usage is therefore high, and the detector is of

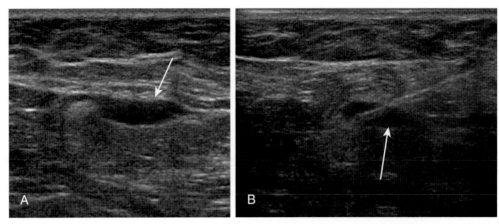

FIGURE 20-22 **Axillary Lymph Node Metastasis. A,** Focal cortical thickening (*arrow*) in a woman with ipsilateral invasive breast cancer. **B,** Core biopsy using a manual throw device shows the needle traversing the thickened cortex (*arrow*). Histologic diagnosis: metastatic carcinoma.

clinical quality. Visualization of low-density lesions is less problematic, and there is improved access to posterior lesions. Complaints about neck and shoulder pain are also less frequent with the add-on unit. Vasovagal reactions can occur when the patient is sitting, although most biopsies can be performed with the patient lying on her side.

Posterior Lesions

Positioning patients to allow targeting of very posterior lesions can be difficult on the prone table because of the thickness of the table. Posterior location is much less of an issue when using an add-on biopsy unit so long as the lesion does not overlie the muscle.

To maximize the posterior tissue that can be included in the field of view, remove the pad from the table or use a thinner one. Use gravity as much as possible by centering the breast in the aperture and making sure it can move freely away from the chest wall. Ask the patient to relax (as much as possible) into the aperture. Try different angles—such as an oblique approach—to include more of the posterior tissues. Bringing the arm through the aperture can be used to access more posterior lesions in some cases. It may seem that only former gymnasts would be able to maintain this awkward position, but in our experience, most patients are able to tolerate this approach quite well.

Thin Breast

If the breast tissue compresses to less than 2 to 3 cm, there may not be enough thickness for the device to be placed to the designated depth and fired without reaching the other side of the breast and the image receptor (negative stroke margin).

First, keep in mind that the depth calculated by the computer places the lesion at the center of the sampling notch. Lesions can often still be sampled if the probe is withdrawn by several millimeters, using the deep end

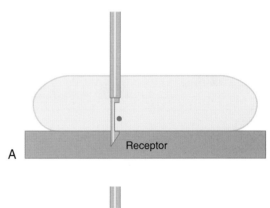

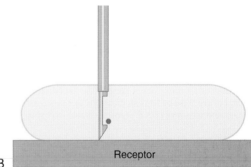

FIGURE 20-23 **Adjusting the Needle Position for a Deep Lesion.** **A,** The system centers the lesion in the notch, which may result in a negative stroke margin (i.e., the needle will hit the digital receptor). **B,** This can be avoided by adjusting the z coordinate so that the stroke margin is zero. The lesion will then be located at the far end of the notch, but adequate samples can be obtained so long as the lesion is at least 5 mm from the deep skin surface (this is the biopsy needle dead zone).

of the notch rather than the center (Fig. 20-23). Many manufacturers offer a biopsy probe with a smaller sampling aperture. Although the sample size is smaller, this alternative can allow for biopsy of some lesions that have a negative stroke margin when targeted using the standard probe. Finally, a lateral side-arm biopsy attachment can often, but not always, be used to sample a lesion in a thin breast (Fig. 20-24). When this approach is used, the needle may be quite close to the skin and sampling toward the skin is therefore best avoided (Box 20-2).

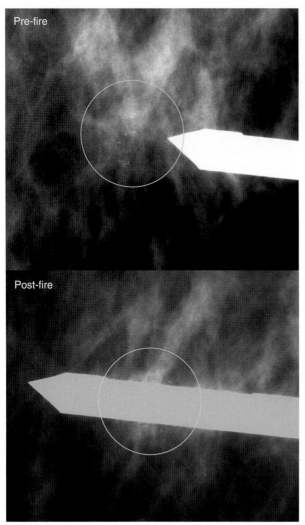

FIGURE 20-24 **Stereotactic Biopsy Using a Lateral Side-Arm.** Biopsy of amorphous calcifications in a 56-year-old woman with compressed breast thickness of 26 mm using a lateral side-arm attachment. Pre-and post-fire images are shown. The calcifications were successfully sampled. Pathologic examination revealed atypical ductal hyperplasia.

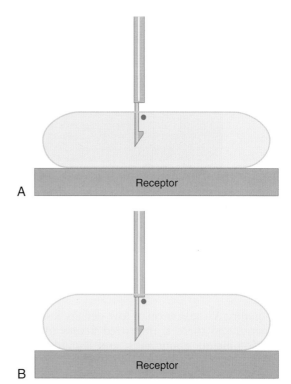

FIGURE 20-25 **Adjustment for Superficial Location. A,** The calculated target places the lesion at the center of the notch. This may result in the bevel opening above the skin, which may tear. **B,** Advance the needle so that the bevel is just below the skin. The lesion will not be at the center of the notch, but will be adequately sampled nevertheless.

BOX 20-2   Thin Breast with Negative Stroke Margin: Options for Biopsy

- Try a different approach (e.g., change from craniocaudal [CC] to lateral medial [LM]).
- Insert to the allowable depth only and sample with distal part of notch.
- Use a probe with a smaller biopsy aperture.
- Use a lateral side-arm if available.
- Build up depth with additional anesthetic.
- See if the lesion is visible by US.
- Recommend wire-localized surgical biopsy.

Superficial Lesions

Lesions that are superficial seem to make radiologists nervous. They are really pretty easy. If the sampling notch is not completely covered due to a superficial location, simply advance the needle so that the notch is just beneath the skin and go ahead with the procedure (Fig. 20-25). The lesion will be sampled at the top of the notch rather than the center. Manufacturers may provide needles with a smaller sampling notch or plastic inserts that cover the proximal portion of the notch. These options can be considered if the breast is thin and the needle cannot be advanced enough to cover the notch without reaching the receptor.

Subtle Lesions

Small soft tissue density targets (masses, asymmetries, or architectural distortion) and faint calcifications are the most difficult to visualize. This is less of an issue for add-on units. Firm compression of the breast tissue often improves visibility of the target lesion. The surface of the breast in the window of the compression paddle should be taut and smooth. "Pillowing" of the tissue should be avoided.

If you are having difficulty finding your target, try using adjacent landmarks such as a fat necrosis calcification to try to locate the finding. Another trick is putting a BB over the area using a needle localization grid attached to your clinical mammography unit, then placing that area in the target window. This approach will at least get you in the right neighborhood. Once you find the correct location, inject only a little anesthetic—just enough to get the biopsy needle in without discomfort—so as not to obscure the lesion on your pre-fire images. Additional anesthetic can easily be administered after placement of the probe.

The lateral side-arm attachment available on some units allows the biopsy needle to be inserted from the side while the breast is compressed by a full compression paddle. The more uniform compression by this type of paddle can also improve visualization of subtle lesions.

Lesion Moves from Its Original Position

Movement can occur at any point during the biopsy procedure. Patients may move, anesthetic or hemorrhage may displace a lesion, or the lesion may be displaced during insertion or firing of the biopsy device. For these reasons, images are obtained after placement of the device, prior to sampling, to confirm that a lesion has not shifted in position.

If a firm lesion is directly targeted and the needle is manually advanced, there is a chance it will be pushed deep by the probe ("snowplow" effect) rather than penetrating the tissue. In our experience, firing of the device in the breast reduces the chance of this occurring. There is little reason to not fire in the breast, so this is our routine practice.

If there is movement of a lesion in the x or y plane, remember that you may be able to use the directional capability of the device to successfully sample the lesion, even if it is a few millimeters from the notch (Fig. 20-26). If there is displacement by more than a few millimeters, retargeting is usually needed. You will need to back the needle out most of the way before repositioning it. Otherwise, moving the needle will move the lesion and surrounding tissues with it, rather than bringing the needle closer to the lesion.

Sometimes, despite all of our efforts, a lesion cannot be targeted for stereotactic biopsy. In these cases, consider using US—even for calcifications. Lesions presenting as suspicious calcifications on mammography are seen by US in 23% of cases, with larger clusters containing more calcifications most likely to be visible. US-visible calcifications are more likely to be malignant and to represent invasive carcinoma than clusters that are not visible by US. When performing ultrasound-guided biopsy of lesions that present as calcifications, we prefer vacuum-assisted biopsy to reduce the chance of undersampling (Fig. 20-27).

MRI-Guided Biopsy

If you can perform a stereotactic biopsy, then you are ready to learn MRI-guided biopsy as well. The principles are very similar. We'll just review a few problem situations.

Nonenhancing Lesion

This situation does occur, but unfortunately a nonenhancing lesion does not mean that the finding is benign. About 14% of lesions that do not enhance on the day of the biopsy are malignant. As a preemptive action, know what the enhancement pattern of the lesion was on the diagnostic MRI before you start. If it had slow initial and persistent enhancement, have the technologist take a couple extra sequences while you are looking at the first one. If the lesion is still not seen on those later ones, loosen the compression slightly and wait another minute or 2 before you do another sequence. If the lesion is still not seen, we typically reschedule the biopsy in 1 to 2 months. If the lesion is not seen, then short-term follow-up MRI in 6 months is usually recommended.

Posterior Lesions

Just as with stereotactic biopsy using a prone table, there is padding on the breast MRI coil that can be removed to bring more breast tissue into the coil. Bringing the patient's arms down by her side can relax the pectoral muscles and allow more of the breast to drop into the coil. If the lesion is lateral, try closing the aperture on the contralateral side and rolling her slightly to the ipsilateral side. This technique is also helpful when the lesion is adjacent to the pectoral muscle, because more lateral tissue will drop into the coil, often yielding an improved biopsy approach. Many devices are available with a blunt tip that can be used for lesions close to the pectoralis muscle.

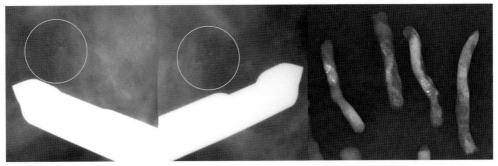

FIGURE 20-26 **Using the Directional Capability of Vacuum-Assisted Biopsy.** Amorphous calcifications (*circles*) that moved during placement of the biopsy needle. The calcifications could still be biopsied by obtaining samples from 10 o'clock to 11o'clock. Successful sampling was confirmed on specimen radiography. Diagnosis: atypical ductal hyperplasia with the same diagnosis at excision.

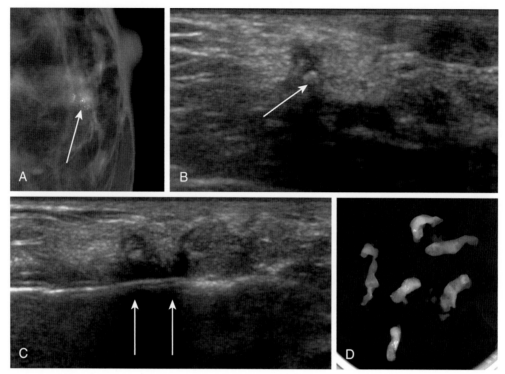

FIGURE 20-27 **Ultrasound-Guided Biopsy of Calcifications. A,** Stereotactic biopsy was attempted for these fine pleomorphic calcifications (*arrow*), but was canceled due to compressed breast thickness of 24 mm. **B,** The calcifications were identified on US (*arrow*). **C,** The vacuum-assisted biopsy needle was positioned directly posterior to the calcifications (*arrows*). **D,** Numerous calcifications were present in the specimen. Histologic diagnosis: DCIS, high grade.

Thin Breast

This approach is the same as with stereotactic biopsy. Try adjusting the depth, as in Figures 20-23 and 20-25, for deep or superficial lesions in these breasts. Switching to a probe with a smaller sampling aperture may also enable you to perform biopsy in these cases. If it is apparent that the lesion will not likely be amenable to MRI-guided core biopsy, then MRI-guided wire localization or clip placement can be performed.

Multiple Lesions

If the lesions are in the same breast, percutaneous biopsy can be performed simultaneously. Some breast coils and guidance systems also allow for biopsy of bilateral lesions, using dual localization grids. If this option is not available, you may have to schedule bilateral biopsies on different days. However, if at least one lesion can be localized using landmarks, you may be able to use your contrast for one lesion and landmarks for the second, allowing biopsy of both on the same day (Fig. 20-28).

MRI-Guided Marker Placement

If MRI-guided biopsy is not possible due to a thin compressible breast or posterior location, the patient can be scheduled for an MRI-guided wire localization for surgical biopsy. However, if you've already scanned and given

contrast, you can still place a marker through the introducer sheath (Fig. 20-29). Surgical excision can be then performed using conventional mammographic wire localization of the MRI-placed marker instead of an MRI-guided wire localization. This is also an option for women with moderate claustrophobia because the time in the scanner is reduced compared with biopsy.

Please Leave a Marker!

Few decisions are more likely to result in a call from a once-friendly surgeon than not leaving a marker after biopsy. These situations arise because the surgeon is concerned that a lesion cannot be accurately localized for excision. It may be that the lesion is no longer visible on mammography or by US following the biopsy. Even moderate-sized lesions may be obscured by a hematoma. Occasionally, lesions that were initially palpable may become impalpable after core biopsy.

Breast surgeons understand that the accurate placement of this tiny metallic marker plays a major role in the care of their patients. The marker provides an easy target for preoperative wire localization (Fig. 20-30). It allows us to confirm removal of a lesion on specimen radiography. When pathologic findings from core biopsy are benign, the marker indicates the region of biopsy that should be examined on follow-up imaging studies.

In our practices, placement of a marker is standard for every case, even after biopsy of a large highly suspicious mass. When these lesions prove malignant, neoadjuvant

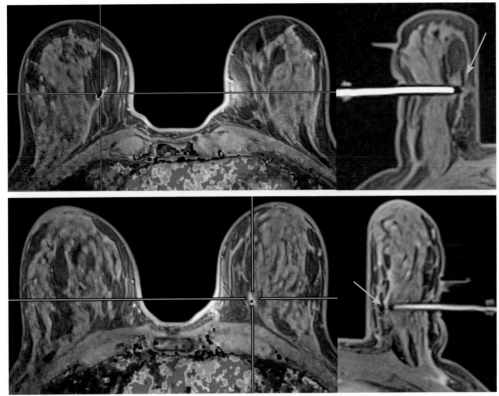

FIGURE 20-28 **Bilateral MRI-Guided Biopsy.** This high-risk screening MRI showed bilateral suspicious nonmass enhancement (*cursors*). On the right, the lesion (*arrow*) is located centrally within fat and underwent MRI biopsy using landmarks for guidance. The lesion on the left (*arrow*) is more difficult to define, and biopsy was performed with contrast. Histologic diagnosis: right—dense stromal sclerosis; left—DCIS.

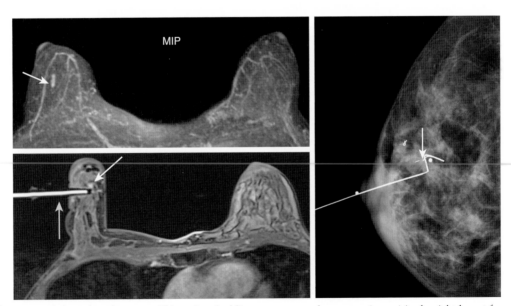

FIGURE 20-29 *MRI-Guided Marker Placement.* This patient had linear nonmass enhancement (*arrow*) in the right breast for which biopsy was recommended. However, her breast compressed to only 25 mm, and MRI-guided biopsy could not be performed. An obturator was positioned (*yellow arrow*) showing the lesion (*white arrow*) at the tip, and a marker was placed through the introducer sheath. She returned a few weeks later for a mammography-guided wire localization of the marker (*arrow*). The ribbon marker was from a previous benign ultrasound-guided core biopsy. Histologic diagnosis: stromal fibrosis.

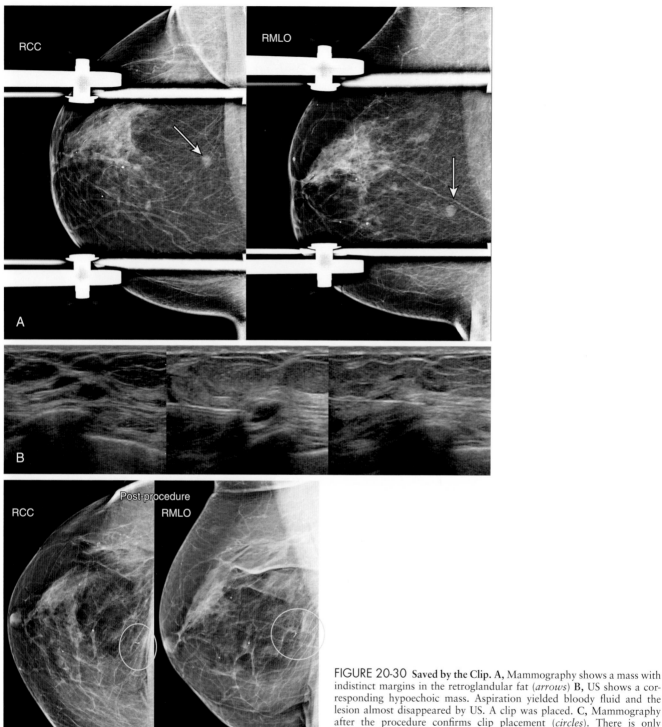

FIGURE 20-30 **Saved by the Clip. A,** Mammography shows a mass with indistinct margins in the retroglandular fat (*arrows*) **B,** US shows a corresponding hypoechoic mass. Aspiration yielded bloody fluid and the lesion almost disappeared by US. A clip was placed. **C,** Mammography after the procedure confirms clip placement (*circles*). There is only minimal residual density in the region of the mass. The aspirate yielded malignant cytologic findings, and wire-localized excision of the clip area showed grade 3 invasive lobular carcinoma (ILC).

treatment may cause the lesion to regress markedly or even disappear prior to surgery. The presence of the marker allows the region of malignancy to be excised if this occurs.

When biopsy of more than one lesion is performed, use different-shaped markers for each site. This minimizes the chance of confusion if wire localization and excision are needed. We keep three types in stock and record in the report which type of clip is placed in each location.

After placement of a marker, a mammogram is performed with light compression in orthogonal projections. In cases in which a lesion is visible on mammography, clip placement after ultrasound-guided biopsy confirms that the US and mammographic findings correspond to a single lesion, rather than representing two different lesions (see Fig. 20-1).

Please note that we use the terms "marker" and "clip" interchangeably. Most markers placed after biopsy don't actually clip onto anything, and they can occasionally migrate. If this occurs, we can help avoid confusion by clearly stating so in our report. If the patient later presents for wire localization, then it will be clear that the site of the lesion rather than the marker should be localized for excision.

Pathology-Imaging Concordance

Once the pathologic findings return from biopsy, the images should be reviewed and the pathologic diagnosis should explain the imaging finding. This is probably best performed by the person who performed the biopsy, though help may be needed from the person who did the diagnostic evaluation or read the MRI. Discussing the finding with the pathologist is also helpful, especially when concordance is unclear. The sensitivity of percutaneous breast biopsy is about 98%, but is not 100% even in the best of hands. We will all fail to adequately sample a lesion from time to time, and it is important to catch these sooner rather than later. A recommendation for excision following a benign biopsy result should not necessarily be considered a personal error.

If the pathologic findings are benign and concordant, review the screening and diagnostic images, report, and postbiopsy clip images. This is your last check to ensure that the correct lesion was adequately sampled. Imaging in 6 months to ensure stability is commonly recommended after a benign concordant biopsy. However, imaging in 1 year may be adequate if the diagnosis is very specific and benign (e.g., an oval mass that is a fibroadenoma).

Regarding high-risk lesions, atypical ductal hyperplasia on core biopsy should routinely be excised, as 20% to 50% of these women will have at least DCIS at surgery. The management of other high-risk lesions (atypical lobular hyperplasia, lobular carcinoma in situ [LCIS], radial scar, papilloma) is more controversial; however, these lesions are often excised as well. We recommend establishing a process for reviewing imaging and pathologic findings after biopsy and establishing standards in your practice for managing different types of lesions.

KEY POINTS

- Choose your guidance carefully. A lesion seen on US is not necessarily best biopsied using ultrasound guidance. If the US correlate to a mammographic or MRI finding is not convincing, reconsider the guidance method.
- Optimize your geometry. Alignment of the lesion, transducer, skin nick, and coaxial guide/biopsy needle is key to efficient, accurate ultrasound-guided biopsy. The biopsy needle should generally be parallel or at least close to parallel to the chest wall for safety and visualization of the needle.
- To sample deeper lesions, take advantage of the curvature of the breast and insert the needle farther from the transducer. If necessary, the device and skin nick can be depressed to obtain a more favorable angle. The transducer can be rocked along its long axis to optimize visualization of the needle.
- Small lesions and complex masses with small solid components may become indistinct during sampling. Numbing in front of and behind but not through the lesion will keep the mass clearly seen before biopsy. Starting with the deepest aspect will keep the lesion visible longer. A vacuum-assisted device can also make short work of these lesions with confidence.
- Axillary lesions can be safely biopsied with ultrasound guidance using a manual throw device. Color Doppler can be used to identify the axillary vessels prior to biopsy.

- Lesions in patients with implants can usually be biopsied with a free-hand technique. Alternatively, techniques that use compression to displace the lesion away from the implant may result in a less stressful day.
- Posterior lesions can be problematic for both stereotactic and MRI-guided biopsy. Removing the table pad and being flexible with positioning can often bring these lesions into biopsy range.
- A thin, compressed breast is also problematic for both stereotactic and MRI-guided biopsy. Adjustments to needle depth can allow for an adequate biopsy even though the lesion may not be centered in the notch. A probe with a smaller sampling aperture may also be used.
- If a biopsy is not possible with MRI and the patient is already there, consider placing a marker under MRI guidance. It will allow for wire localization for excision using mammography rather than MRI.
- PLEASE place a marker after every biopsy. Women with large cancers may undergo neoadjuvant chemotherapy. Although you may be able to find the lesion again, she may come to see us (or your neighboring facility) and we may have to guess which lesion you sampled. It takes only an additional minute or 2, and you will not regret it.

References

Abe H, Schmidt RA, Sennett CA, et al. US-guided core needle biopsy of axillary lymph nodes in patients with breast cancer: Why and how to do it. Radiographics 2007;27:S91-S99.

Berg WA, Campassi CI, Ioffe OB. Cystic lesions of the breast: Sonographic-pathologic correlation. Radiology 2003;227:183-191.

Doshi DJ, March DE, Crisi GM, Coughlin BF. Complex cystic breast masses: Diagnostic approach and imaging-pathologic correlation. Radiographics 2007;27:S53-S64.

Eby PR, Lehman C. MRI-guided breast interventions. Semin Ultrasound CT MR 2006;27:339-350.

Fishman JE, Milikowski C, Ramsinghani R, et al. US-guided core needle biopsy of the breast: How many specimens are necessary? Radiology 2003;226:779-782.

Harvey JA, Moran RE. US-guided core needle biopsy of the breast: Technique and pitfalls. Radiographics 1998;18:867-877.

Harvey JA, Moran RE, DeAngelis GA. Technique and pitfalls of ultrasound-guided core-needle biopsy of the breast. Semin Ultrasound CT MR 2000;21:362-374.

Krishnamurthy S, Sneige N, Bedi DG, et al. Role of ultrasound-guided fine-needle aspiration of indeterminate and suspicious axillary lymph nodes in the initial staging of breast carcinoma. Cancer 2002;95:982-988.

March DE, Hu R, Goulart RA, et al. Ultrasound-guided breast core biopsy: Analysis of factors affecting patient tolerance. J Womens Imaging 2000;2:156-160.

Parker SH, Jobe WE. Percutaneous Breast Biopsy. New York, Raven Press, 1993, Chap. 13, pp 147-163.

Parker SH, Klaus AJ. Performing a breast biopsy with a directional, vacuum-assisted biopsy instrument. Radiographics 1997;17:1233-1252.

Shulman SG, March DE. Ultrasound-guided breast interventions: Biopsy techniques and applications in patient management. Semin Ultrasound CT MR 2006;27:298-307.

Smith DN, Kaelin CM, Korbin CD, et al. Impalpable breast cysts: Utility of cytologic examination of fluid obtained with radiologically guided aspiration. Radiology 1997;204(1):149-151.

Soo MS, Baker JA, Rosen EL. Sonographic detection and sonographically guided biopsy of breast microcalcifications. Am J Roentgenol 2003;189:941-948.

Youk FH, Kim EK, Kim MF, et al. Missed breast cancers at US-guided core needle biopsy: How to reduce them. Radiographics 2007;27:79-94.

CASE QUESTIONS

CASE 20-1. Your colleague has recommended biopsy of a new mass in this 51-year-old woman recalled from screening (*arrow*). How would you proceed?

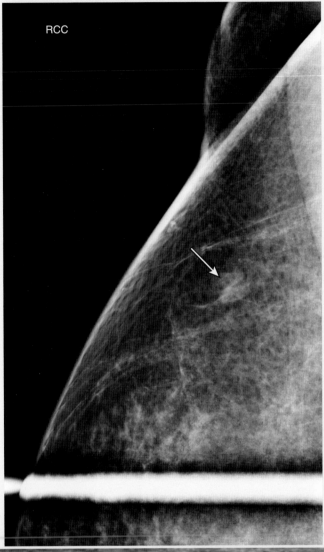

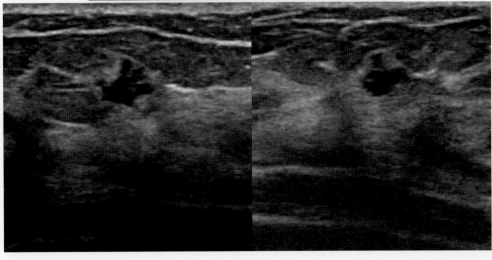

CASE 20-2. What potential challenges can you anticipate in sampling this lesion using ultrasound-guided core biopsy, and how can you avoid them?

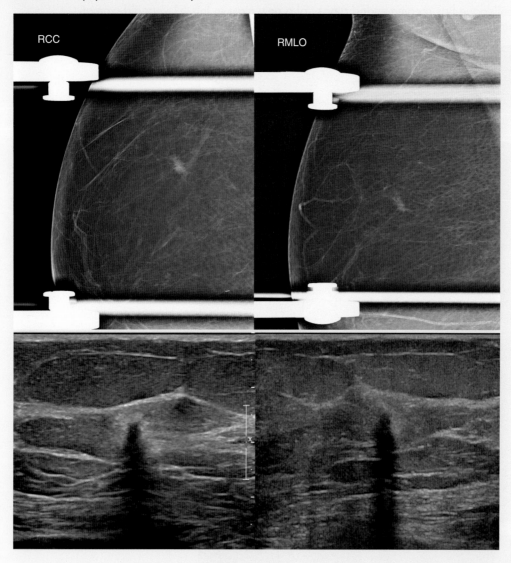

CASE 20-3. A 79-year-old woman had a mass detected on screening mammography (*circles*). A corresponding US image and representative pre- and post-fire images obtained during ultrasound-guided biopsy are shown here. Pathologic examination revealed fibrous and fatty tissue with no evidence of malignancy. Are these results concordant? If not, what is a possible explanation for sampling error? How would you manage this patient?

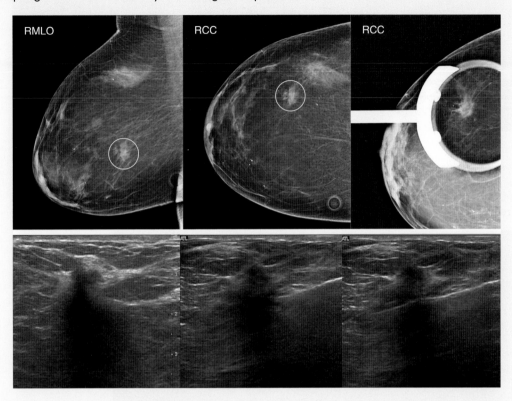

CASE 20-4. You are supervising a recently trained radiologist performing one of his first ultrasound-guided procedures. **A,** The lesion to be biopsied is shown here. **B,** The pre-fire image shows the biopsy needle (*arrows*). Is the approach acceptable? What do you recommend?

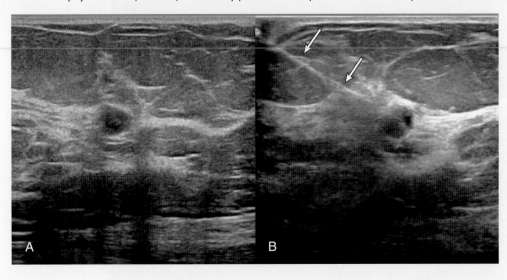

CASE 20-5. You are performing ultrasound-guided biopsy of a deep mass, as shown in the sequence of images here. What is the next step you should take?

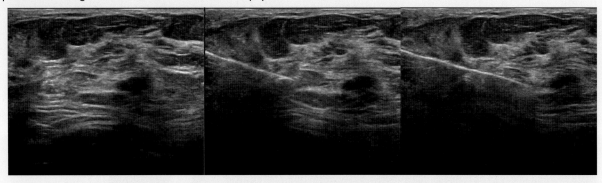

CASE 20-6. A 56-year-old woman has a new mass in her upper left breast. Mammography and US are shown here. During ultrasound-guided biopsy (shown on the next page) you see this appearance of the biopsy needle (*arrow*) and lesion in real time. What is the cause of this appearance, and what correction is needed before sampling?

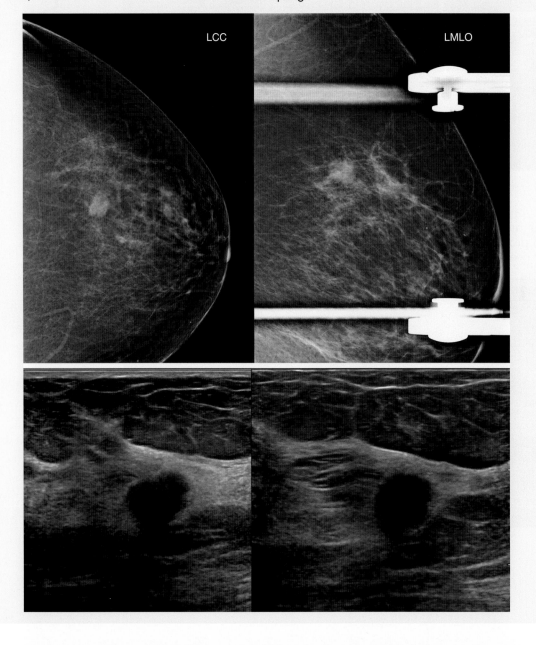

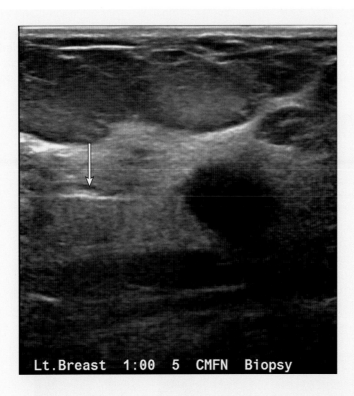

Lt.Breast 1:00 5 CMFN Biopsy

CASE 20-7. An adjustment is made during biopsy of the lesion seen in Case 20-6, leading to the appearance shown here. What further correction is needed?

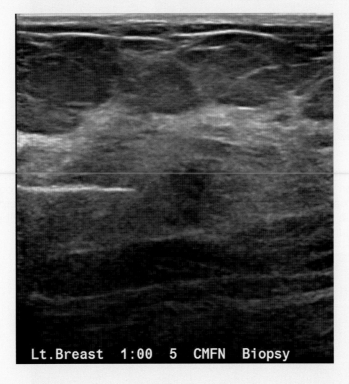

Lt.Breast 1:00 5 CMFN Biopsy

CASE 20-8. An 82-year-old woman had a new mass detected in her medial left breast (*circles*). On US, a 4-mm hypoechoic mass is seen in the 9 o'clock position (*arrow*). Ultrasound-guided core biopsy was performed, and a clip was placed. Pathologic examination revealed microcysts. Postprocedure mammography is shown here. Are the pathologic findings concordant? What do you recommend?

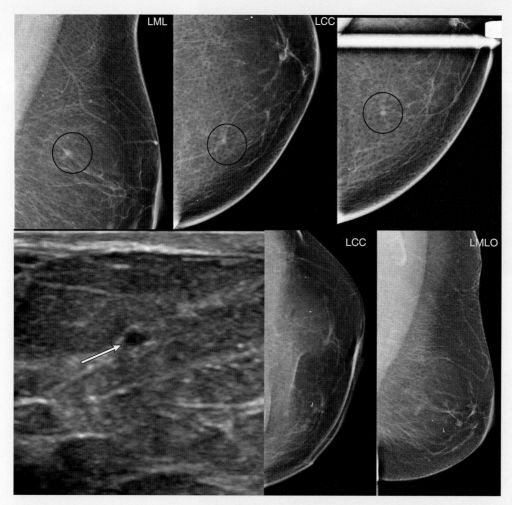

CASE 20-9. A 33-year-old woman presents with a palpable mass in her right breast. Mammography showed a circumscribed mass. US is shown here. The lesion was aspirated with US guidance, and the resulting findings are shown. The aspirate was bloody. How would you describe the lesion? If you were performing the procedure, what would you do next?

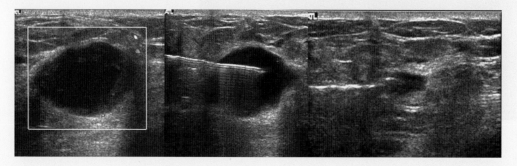

CASE 20-10. This 67-year-old woman was recalled from screening for a focal asymmetry in the right breast (*arrows*). US was negative, so stereotactic biopsy was performed. The scout and stereo pair images and postbiopsy mammogram are provided. Histologic examination shows normal breast tissue with no pathologic abnormality. How would you manage this patient?

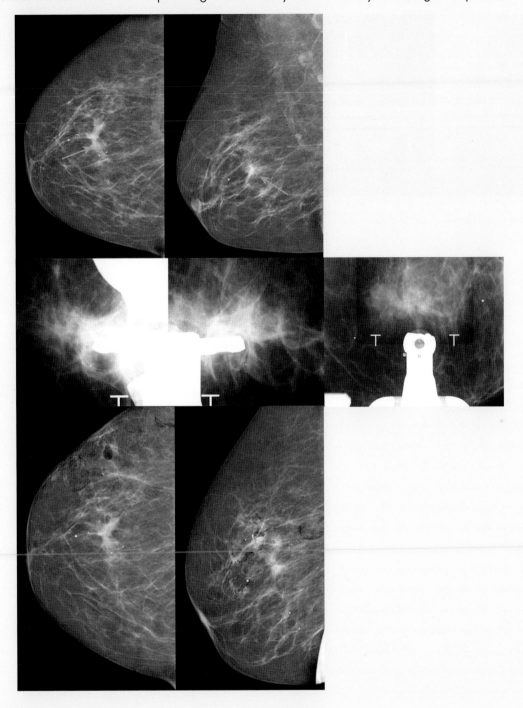

CASE 20-11. A 48-year-old woman has a mammographically detected enlarging mass in her right breast. Your partner recommended ultrasound-guided biopsy of the finding shown here. On the day of biopsy, you are not certain you can reproduce the lesion by US. What are your options?

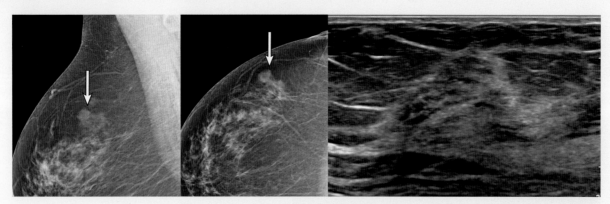

CASE 20-1. There is an irregular, markedly hypoechoic mass without posterior acoustic features. These features are suspicious. BI-RADS 4. Because the appearance on US suggests that the lesion may be partially cystic, aspiration followed by core biopsy if the lesion persists is a good plan.

The lesion was aspirated, and only minimal fluid could be obtained (images here). Core biopsy was then performed (pre- and post-fire images here) followed by clip placement. Diagnosis: IDC and DCIS.

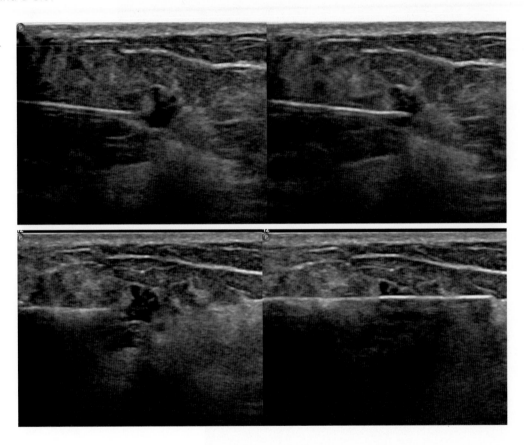

CASE 20-2. The lesion is small and irregular with pronounced shadowing. Inject enough anesthesia around the lesion to numb but not obscure it. If the most superficial portion of the lesion is sampled first, shadowing from air in the biopsy track could make it more difficult to visualize the remaining lesion for subsequent samples. However, if you sample too deep—in the region of shadowing—you may miss the lesion. Clip placement is important. Without it, the lesion could become difficult or impossible to localize after the biopsy. Diagnosis: IDC.

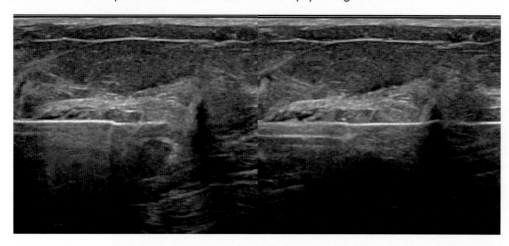

CASE 20-3. The imaging findings are highly suspicious, so the pathologic findings are discordant. Repeat biopsy is needed. Review of the US images suggests that sampling may have been deep to the lesion, in the region of shadowing. Repeat biopsy with more superficial targeting revealed ILC.

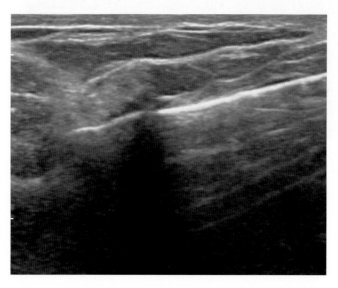

CASE 20-4. Yikes! The angle of approach is too steep! If the device were fired, it could reach the pectoral muscle. If you are watching someone else performing this procedure, now would be a good time to take control of the equipment! The device should be repositioned and the lesion approached at an angle that is more parallel to the chest wall. Diagnosis: infiltrating carcinoma with ductal and lobular features.

CASE 20-5. The angle of approach should be more parallel to the chest wall, so don't fire yet! Depress the coaxial guide, biopsy device, and skin nick together toward the chest wall to improve the angle, as shown on the images here. Diagnosis: fibroadenoma.

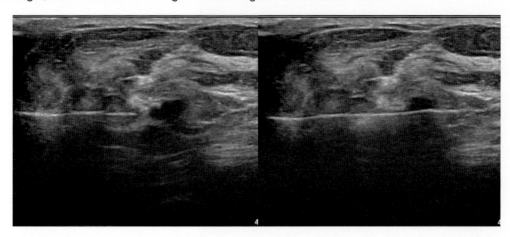

CASE 20-6. The lesion is well seen, but the shaft of the needle is incompletely seen. This means that the needle is not aligned with the long axis of the transducer. If this situation occurs, look down at the transducer and needle to see what adjustment is needed. Either the transducer can be rotated to align with the needle, or the nick/needle can be moved to align with the transducer. The biopsy needle should then be well seen along its length.

CASE 20-7. Although the needle has been brought into the plane of the ultrasound beam, the transducer has moved off the center of the mass. We are now seeing only the periphery of the lesion. The transducer needs to be repositioned over the mass, and then the biopsy needle brought into the plane of the ultrasound beam.

Now we are ready! The needle, transducer, and lesion are aligned in the pre-fire position. Go ahead and take the first pass. Diagnosis: IDC.

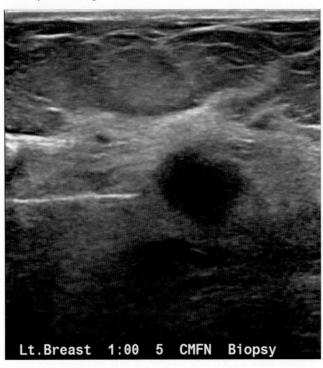

CASE 20-8. Clustered microcysts may be concordant; however, on the mammogram taken after biopsy (**A** and **B**), the clip is anterior to the mammographic finding (*arrows*). This most likely indicates the presence of two lesions—one visible by mammography and the second visible by US. Clip migration is uncommon with US biopsy. Stereotactic biopsy was performed, and the postbiopsy mammogram (**C** and **D**) shows the biopsy cavity in the region of the mass that was seen on mammography (*arrows*). Histologic diagnosis: ILC and LCIS.

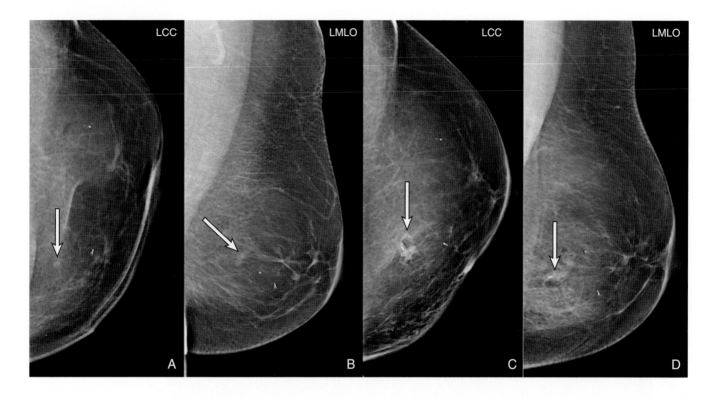

CASE 20-9. The finding is a complex mass with a thick wall. The bloody aspirate may or may not provide a diagnostic cytologic specimen. The lesion became much smaller after aspiration but did not resolve, so core biopsy of the residual lesion was performed and a clip was placed. Diagnosis: necrotic grade 3 IDC.

CASE 20-10. Although the scout and stereo pair images look like the lesion was well targeted, the postbiopsy mammogram shows that the biopsy cavity and marker (*arrows*) are at least 4 cm lateral to the lesion. Pathologic examination showed only normal breast tissue, which would not likely explain this finding. The marker location and biopsy result both suggest that the biopsy is discordant. Either repeat stereotactic biopsy, or surgical excision should be performed. In this case, wire-localized biopsy was performed, showing IDC.

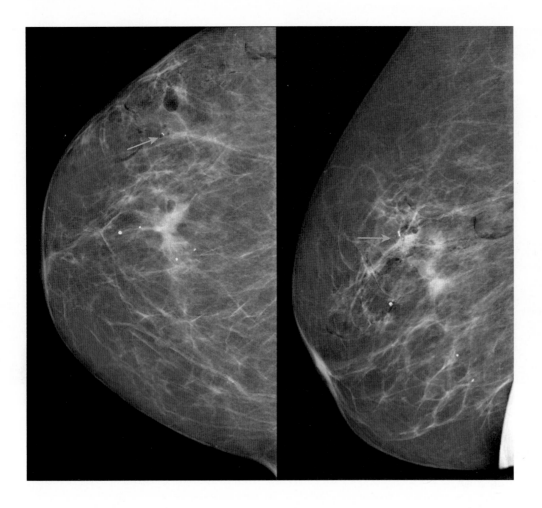

CASE 20-11. Yes, you could spend the next 45 minutes taking BB shots, but let's rethink our approach. This lesion is well seen on mammography, and the US correlate is uncertain. Let's consider changing the approach to stereotactic biopsy. In this case, stereotactic biopsy revealed pseudoangiomatous stromal hyperplasia, which is concordant.

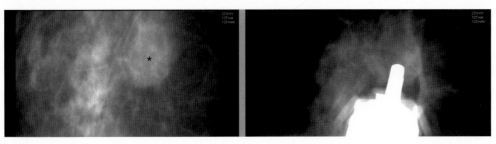

Index

Page numbers followed by "f" Indicate figures, "t" indicate tables, and "b" indicate boxes.